STEM CELL TRANSPLANTATION

A Textbook of Stem Cell
Xenotransplantation

STEM CELL TRANSPLANTATION

A Textbook of Stem Cell Xenotransplantation

E. Michael Molnar, MD

To Dr. Novak in appreciation of his interest in stem cell transplantation.

October 21, 2012   E. M. Molnar

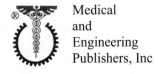

Medical and Engineering Publishers, Inc

© Medical and Engineering Publishers Inc

First published in the United States of America by
Medical and Engineering Publishers, Inc
PO Box 74
Sunshine, MD 20833-0074
USA
(http://www.mepublishers.com)

All rights reserved. No part of this book may be reproduced, stored in any retrieval system without the written permission of the publisher. This includes copying or production by any means, mechanical, photographic, electronic, or any other means, as well as translation into other languages.

Library of Congress Cataloging-in-Publication Data

Stem Cell Transplantation
E. Michael Molnar. First Edition
Includes bibliographical references and index
2006

Library of Congress Control Number: 2005936720
ISBN 978-1-930636-05-7

Copyright 2006
Medical and Engineering Publishers, Inc

Printed in Korea.

Printed on acid-free paper.

TO MY WIFE GABRIELA
and
OUR DAUGHTER MICHELE

ACKNOWLEDGEMENTS

After I made a pledge in 1976 to my prematurely deceased father that I will devote my life to search for therapies that could have saved him, it took about two years before I recognized that cell transplantation would have done it, and it is the therapy of the future. Due to my 'double life', oscillating between 70 hours a week in my private surgical practice, and whatever time and energy remained for my research, I did not come to this conclusion overnight.

Just as I recognized that I am 'running against the wall' in my country of US, I was introduced by '*New Hope Parents Association*', that educated their US members that there is a treatment for their handicapped children, to Dr. Franz Schmid, Professor of Pediatrics, Heidelberg Medical School, Germany, the biggest living expert of cell therapy. For 15 years, until his death in 1997, he was my teacher in stem cell transplantation. With the exception of a few days that we spent together when he accepted my invitation to participate in seminars in Zagreb, Croatia, and Carlsbad, Czech Republic, and then during his 3 – 4 days' long four visits in Moscow, we never worked together. But he was always there for me: whenever I had a question, I could always get him on the phone, and get advice. He never asked for any monetary compensation. When we had a pediatric patient with no diagnosis after spending weeks in the world's top medical institutions, I would send him a medical summary and close-up photos of a patient, and during the next phone call I would get the diagnosis and advice about stem cell transplantation treatment, and what else to do. He was a great physician, 'tough as a nail', a real Man!

I worked with a large number of physicians, veterinarians, biologists, in many countries, during those 27 years that I devoted my time to stem cell transplantation, and I am grateful to all of them. Most of them became my friends. There are a few that have exceptionally added to my knowledge. Prof. Dr. Sergey V. Savel'ev, a genius comparative embryologist, knows the central nervous system like no one I have ever met, and I was going to be a neurologist. Daniel Elias, DVM, PhD, DSc, a master of tissue culture, without whom our method of manufacturing would not have been born, has amazed me continuously during our 8 years of collaboration by his deep knowledge of everything to be discussed, or a flat statement that he does not have sufficient knowledge to talk about the subject.

Prof. Dr. Sreco Simic, Chief of the Hospital for Obstetrics, Gynecology and Neonatology, University of Sarajevo Medical School, was in charge of our project in Yugoslavia until he was seen on CNN to beg the warring parties to stop shooting at their hospital, killing newborn babies and pregnant women. The civil war in Yugoslavia forced us to move the project elsewhere, i.e. to USSR.

Jaroslav J. Marik, MD, my close friend of 35 years, has been the sole US physician that gave me full support in all my stem cell transplantation activities, including visiting with us in Moscow and directly participating in our cooperation with US FDA.

There were my close personal friends/non-physicians who made important contributions to our stem cell transplantation project: Mr. Vincenzo Labella of Italy, Emmy Award winning producer of 'Marco Polo' and of various famous Italian films, for his attempt to launch the project on my behalf in Peoples' Republic of China in 1987-1988, Mr. Branko Lustig of Croatia, a double Oscar-winning producer of 'Schindler's List' fame, without whom the project would not have started in Yugoslavia in 1988, Mr. Reiner Oppenheimer, our manager in Munich, Germany, who brought me to Germany in 1985, and established our project there, and Mr. Brian Keadle of USA, our 'street smart' US manager, the only one that could deal with US FDA, who unfortunately died very prematurely in 1999 of a genetic disorder of lipoprotein metabolism.

Stanislav Gavrilovich Yazvinski, one of my best friends, the former deputy director of Soviet Cosmic Program, and Director of Rocket Armies of the USSR Joint Chiefs of Staff, who made my life safer in Moscow when the 'goings became very rough' in that country due to the power struggle after 1994 that eventually forced the termination of our project in Russia.

Many thanks to Dr. Jafar Vossoughi, Technical Consulting Editor for Medical and Engineering Publishers, Inc., who encouraged and assisted me in getting the Book project go through in a timely manner. The editorial assistance of Mrs. Sharon Whitt from the Publisher's office is greatly acknowledged.

Naturally, there are many who have tried to kill this project, and continue to do so, but I will not mention them here.

E. Michael Molnar, MD

DISCLAIMER

The opinions presented in this book are the opinions of the author, and are based on his research and personal and professional experience. The book should not be used to diagnose or treat an illness. Individuals should consult physicians/healthcare professionals.

Every effort has been made to ensure the accuracy of the information presented in this book. However, due to the constant and rapid development in medical technology, neither the author, nor the publisher can accept any legal or other responsibilities for the errors, accuracy and omissions that may have occurred at the time of publication.

Contents

Acknowledgements vii

Contents ix

Preface xiii

Part I--- INTRODUCTION

1. Definitions and Basics 3
2. Stem Cell Xenotransplantation vs. Stem Cell Allotransplantation 9
3. Atlas of Comparative Histology of Various Stem Cell Transplants 15
4. History 23
5. Legislative Situation
    a. European Community 33
    b. USA 64
    c. Other Countries 115
6. Safety Issues 117

Part II--- SCIENTIFIC BASIS OF CLINICAL USE OF STEM CELL TRANSPLANTATION

7. Essential Facts 127
8. Cytology 131
9. Cell Biology 135
10. Physiology 141
11. Biochemistry 149
12. Medical Genetics 157
13. Comparative Embryology 161
14. Growth and Developments 165
15. Aging Process 177
16. Immunology 181
17. Transmission of Infection 195

18. Cancerogenesis 199
19. Pre-clinical vs. Clinical Studies 205
20. Artificial Organs and Bio-Prostheses for Reconstructive Surgery 209

Part III — MANUFACTURING OF STEM CELL XENO-TRANSPLANTS

21. Preparation and Manufacturing of Stem Cell Xenotransplants 219
22. Animal Sources for Stem Cell Xenotransplants 225
23. Closed Colony of Source Animals 231
24. Screening for Infectious Agents/Individual Qualification of Animal Sources 237
25. Procurement of Stem Cell Xenotransplants 241
26. Archiving of Medical Records and Specimens from Animal Sources 245
27. Quality control 247
28. Release and Labeling of Stem Cell Xenotransplants 249

Part IV — USE OF STEM CELL XENOTRANSPLANTS IN HUMAN MEDICINE

29. Therapeutic Goal of Stem Cell Xenotransplantation 255
30. General Principles of Therapeutic Application 267
31. Concurrent Treatment by Stem Cell Xenotransplantation and Pharmaceutical Drugs of Chemical Nature 273
32. Concurrent Treatment by Stem Cell Xenotransplantation and Medications prepared by Biotechnological Methods 275
33. Treatment of Iatrogenic Diseases by Stem Cell Xenotransplantation 281
34. Mono- vs. Poly-Therapy by Stem Cell Xenotransplantation 283
35. Description of various Stem Cell Xenotransplants 301
36. Indications/Contra-Indications 305
37. Patient's Preparation for Stem Cell Xenotransplantation 311
38. Treatment Procedure 313
39. Post-Stem Cell Xenotransplantation Precautions and Patient Monitoring 319
40. Patient's Pre- and Post-Treatment Instructions 321
41. Surveillance for Possible Transmission of Xeno-Zoonoses 325

42. Surveillance for Possible Immunological Reactions after
    Stem Cell Transplantation   329
43. Mechanism of Action   331
44. Complications   335

Part V--- CLINICAL TREATMENT BY STEM CELL XENOTRANSPLANTATION

45. Genetic Diseases   339
46. Chromosomal Disease   363
47. Neonatal and Perinatal Diseases   377
48. Aging Disease   387
49. Endocrine Diseases   401
50. Immune System Diseases   463
51. Autoimmune Diseases   481
52. Cancer Treatment   487
53. Haematological Diseases   497
54. Treatment of Radiation Injuries   507
55. Disease of Central Nervous System   509
56. Diseases of Locomotor Apparatus   535
57. Digestive System Diseases   545
58. Liver Diseases   551
59. Metabolic Diseases   559
60. Kidney Diseases   567
61. Cardiovascular Diseases   573
62. Lung Disease   585
63. Skin Diseases   589

Part VI--- BIBLIOGRAPHY   593

List of Abbreviations   615

Index

> 'An invasion of armies can be resisted,
> but not an idea whose time has come'.
> *Victor Hugo, 1802-1885, Histoire d'un Crime, [1852]*

PREFACE

Stem cell transplantation has finally been recognized during the past four years by the public, media, and a small segment of physicians as very valuable, particularly for those diseases with no known therapy, or those where the 'state-of-the-art' treatment stopped being effective. It took a century since the first patient was so treated in Western Europe, or 75 years since its official declaration in Switzerland as a new chapter in the therapeutic armamentarium of medical profession.

Medical publications by newcomers to this field in the last few years fail to mention an ample research, enormous clinical experience gained by cell transplantation treatment of over 5 million patients, multiple published papers of the past 70+ years. Medical progress has always been based on the past discoveries, as the structure and function of human body have not changed since the early medical writings of 5,000 years ago. Contrary to this principle, all that has been learned about cell transplantation over the past 100 years is ignored today, like in the Middle Ages when by the same attitude the progress of medicine was set back for centuries.

Embryonic stem cell transplantation is spoken about incessantly, even though there is no 'Mother-of-all-Cells', or 'Universal Cell', from which are made any & all of ~ 200 types of cells making up the body of any member of animal kingdom, including 'Homo Sapiens'. Human or animal bodies are created by union of sperm and ovum, but not by a cell line of one – or several - embryonic stem cell propagated in the laboratory dish. Only cancerous growth is created that way.

Umbilical cord blood of human newborn contains hematopoietic and mesenchymal stem cells only, but not 'Universal Cells'.

You may get confused when terms 'stem cell transplantation' and 'cell transplantation' are used side by side in this book. The term 'stem cell transplantation' has been favored by a group of newcomers to this field versed in laboratory techniques but not in clinical practice of cell transplantation. Experienced practitioners of cell transplantation recognized decades ago that cell transplants of various organs or tissues contain all generations of the family of a certain cell type, including those of the precursor stem cells, i.e. they treated their patients by stem cell transplantation for many years even though a term 'stem cell transplantation' was not coined yet.

Method of stem cell transplantation described in this book is not a 'magic bullet', a treatment of all known diseases. It has limited usefulness as a treatment of many diseases, e.g. chronic inflammatory diseases.

At the same time, all patients with diseases with no known treatment, e.g. genetic or chromosomal diseases, or various perinatal diseases, often with brain damage, should be treated immediately after the diagnosis was made.

There must be no competition between the standard treatment of a certain disease and stem cell transplantation. Type 1 diabetics must be treated by insulin alone until they develop complications: at that time stem cell transplantation should be added, as insulin alone cannot control the progression of retinopathy, nephropathy, peripheral arterial disease, etc., toward blindness, kidney failure, gangrene, impotence, etc.

Sometimes the cost has to be considered. Gaucher's disease is an enzymopathy, where the missing enzyme was identified, purified, and is commercially available, but at an astronomical cost that is hardly affordable by patients. Stem cell transplantation can offer the same therapeutic benefit for the fraction of the cost of the enzyme.

In the clinical part, the author has focused on diseases where there is a substantial clinical experience with stem cell transplantation, as well as a success. Such clinical knowledge can be extrapolated onto other diseases with a similar pathogenesis. If a certain single gene disorder has been successfully treated by stem cell transplantation it means that all other genetic diseases due to a single gene disorder can be treated by stem cell transplantation as well, as long as it is known in which type of cell is the gene defect located, and the diagnosis can be made early after the birth, so that the stem cell transplantation treatment program can start early, and be repeated every 3 – 4 months up until the age of 4 years.

As the diagnosis is frequently just a label used for insurance billing nowadays, the patient selection has to be based on the patophysiology of the illness(es).

The purpose of this book is to present the field of cell transplantation as it has evolved during the past 100 years, and as it is practiced today by physicians, that acquired the knowledge learned by the preceding generations of their colleagues.

You may notice that there is much less information in this textbook about the treatment of kidney, lung or skin diseases, systems exposed to the external environment of the body, by stem cell transplantation. The same applies to gastrointestinal system, with the exception of liver and pancreas.

Cell transplantation was developed primarily by brilliant clinicians responding to a challenge presented by patients advised by their physicians that therapeutically the standard medicine has nothing to offer for their untreatable or incurable disease(s). That apparently did not apply to the patients with diseases of the above four systems, perhaps due to a progress of hemodialysis, respiratory therapy, and surgery of digestive tube that historically was well ahead of urological or chest surgery, or because stem cell transplants prepared without a primary tissue culture were not as effective for treatment of autoimmune diseases of urinary, respiratory systems, digestive tube and skin.

How to use this textbook?

If you are new to the stem cell transplantation, you should read the book from cover to cover. It contains all that you have to know for a clinical practice of this new field of medicine. The author has done it all during the past 27 years: research, development of the method of manufacturing of precursor stem cell transplants, from human as well as animal fetuses, clinical practice of both fetal allo- and xeno-transplantation, and all this knowledge and experience is expressed in this book.

For those physicians that have treated their patients by stem cell transplantation already, this book can serve as a guide to show the types of diseases that can be successfully handled by this treatment modality, and at what stage of different diseases to use it.

Finally, this book explains why stem cell xenotransplantation is much more versatile than stem cell allo-transplantation, including bone marrow transplantation or umbilical cord blood stem cell transplantation, and superior in its safety. Autologous human adult stem cell transplantation cannot compete in its clinical effectiveness with stem cell xeno-transplantation. Statistical evaluation of clinical results of stem cell transplantation, similar to any surgical treatment, including organ transplantation, is not too reliable, but it proves inferior results of autologous human adult stem cell transplantation.

PART I

INTRODUCTION AND BASICS

Chapter 1

When you know a thing, to hold that you know it, and when you do not know a thing, to allow that you do not know it – this is knowledge.
Confucius, 551 – 497 BC

DEFINITIONS AND BASICS

Stem cell transplantation (SCT) is a surgical procedure in which an implantation of stem cells containing live tissue fragments of different organs and tissues, of human (allo-) or animal (xeno-) origin, from fetal, neonatal, juvenile, or adult stage, is carried out as the therapy of diseases of humans and animals.

Stem cell transplantation is the only known treatment to accomplish a repair or healing of any mal- (or non-) functioning cell type, of any tissue(s) and organ(s) damaged by disease, injury, or abnormal growth and development. The treatment is accomplished by direct stimulation of regeneration of the patient's own mal- (or non-) functioning cells of any such damaged tissue(s) or organ(s), or by transplantation of new stem cells to replace the function of those damaged or destroyed in the patient's body.

It is believed that 70% of the benefit from stem cell transplantation is due to the direct stimulation of regeneration and 30% due to the transplantation of new stem cells.

Stem cell transplantation is carried out by:

A: Implantation by an injectional route (or via minor surgery):

- intra-hepatic
- intra-venous, usually intraportal, via portal vein
- subaponeurotic (under aponeurosis of m. rectus abdominis)

- deep subcutaneous (epifascial)
- intra-muscular
- intra-omental (via laparoscopy)
- intra-peritoneal
- intra-arterial (via needle or catheter)
- intra-splenic
- intra-thymic
- intra-cerebral, or intra-ventricular via stereotactic neurosurgery
- intra-thecal via lumbar puncture
- intra-articular
- intra-osseous

B: Implantation by a major surgery:

- orthopedic
- neuro-transplantation
- reconstructive

C: Surface application of stem cells transplants for:

- treatment of deep burns requiring skin grafting
- treatment of aging surface tissues of the body

Stem cell transplantation is *a surgical procedure* that has been used successfully for over 70 years (albeit under various names depending upon the country where the progress took place, or a pioneering physician worked) for treatment of many diseases *for which modern medicine has had no therapy*, or in which *'state-of-the-art' therapies stopped being effective*. It is not a 'wonder drug', or a transplantation of some 'Mother-of-all-Cells', or 'universal stem cell', that cures everything.

Physicians have utilized cell transplantation as treatment of many ailments when they recognized that their patients need *an outright transplantation of fetal stem cells* to replace the dead or non-functioning cells, or a *direct stimulation of regeneration, i.e. repair* of the damaged (diseased) cells or tissues of various organs.

The proof of effectiveness is in an enormous number of medical references about stem cell transplantation of the past approximately 15 years that can be easily found by opening the MEDLINE of US National Library of Medicine, where thousands of summaries about stem cell transplantation could be found by searching for the following *key words*:

- stem cell transplantation
- embryonic cell transplantation
- cell transplantation
- tissue transplantation
- xenotransplantation
- xenograft
- fetal tissue transplantation
- brain tissue transplantation
- hematopoietic cell transplantation
- islets of pancreas transplantation.

It is apparent that the use of stem cell transplantation in clinical practice has not been a rarity. The most important older (but also current) medical research and clinical reports, nearly all in German and Russian, are not included in MEDLINE, and can only be found with great difficulties.

This is unfortunate because they contain groundbreaking data on which the entire field of stem cell transplantation has been based and which have been ignored in the recent Anglophone literature. Many such publications are cited and discussed in this book.

The value of these publications becomes obvious when one considers that over 5 million patients have been treated in Germany and Switzerland by various types of cell transplantation, and of those an estimated 800,000 have been treated with 'stem cells containing fresh cell transplants'. Additionally, an estimated 20 million patients received live human placental tissue implantation containing various trophoblastic cells, developed in USSR by VP Filatow.

Without trophoblasts an embryo could never become a newborn. At the beginning of conception the trophoblasts are indistinguishable from 'embryonic stem cells'. Only at the stage of 58-cell human blastocyst can the outer cells, destined to produce trophoblast of placenta, be recognized as different from the inner cells that will form embryo proper. In 107-cell human blastocyst, 8 embryo-producing cells are surrounded by 99 trophoblastic cells, a 12:1 numerical discrepancy [215]. *Genotypically trophoblastic cells are the same cells as 'embryonic stem cells'.*

Germany and USSR have been the leaders in stem cell transplantation. The author has been involved for over 27 years in the research and clinical application of the stem cell transplantation in thousands of patients in many countries.

Current medicine knows of only one treatment to help the replacement of dead cells: transplantation of organs that has been with us for a few decades. These are life saving major surgical procedures in which an entire organ, without which the recipient cannot live, is replaced by one from a living or just deceased donor. Organ transplantation has been used only as a treatment of last resort since it is a major surgery, and because the body of the receiving patient always rejects an organ allo-transplant, such patients must take immuno-suppressants for the rest of their lives, with all their side effects, some life-threatening.

Stem cell transplantation is a newer approach, one that will dominate medicine of the 21st century. Cell transplantation is a *minor procedure for the patient and* for that reason can be, and should be, *used in the earlier stages of those diseases that current medicine cannot cure or successfully treat.* There is no logical reason to wait until the end-stage, as is the case with organ transplantation, and has been the case with (stem) cell transplantation until now.

Implanted stem cell transplants are not dependent on blood circulation of the recipient, and thereby undergo no structural changes through degeneration, or outright necrosis, due to inadequate blood circulation and lack of oxygen as in organ transplantation.

In order to avoid enormous difficulties with obtaining human fetuses, haematopoietic stem cell transplantation became highly popular in the US, where the source of cells has been umbilical cord blood collected during normal deliveries.

The latest approach that avoids some of the problems with procurement of human fetuses has been the transplantation of embryonic cells obtained from early stages of division of fertilized eggs unused during *in vitro* fertilization. The advantage of the use of early embryonic cells is that there are pluripotential, i.e. they can develop into any cell of any organ of the body. The disadvantage is that besides two common problems of cell transplantation, i.e. transmission of infection, and immune reactions, there is an added problem of oncogenicity. The pluripotential embryonic cells can develop into any normal cell of any organ of the body, but also into cancerous cells. There is no such danger when precursor stem cell transplants are utilized.

Despite a daily flood of data on stem cell transplantation, physicians and medical audience continue to be confused about the subject since the reports have forgotten to mention these facts:

- it has been known for several decades that *embryonic stem cells are unusable for an actual patient treatment due to their oncogenicity.*
- *an implantation of precursor (or progenitor) stem cells, several generations older than embryonic stem cells, have been used as a treatment for over 70 years.*
- precursor stem cells from animal fetus are equally effective, and safe, for the stem cell transplantation treatment, so that all troubles with human embryonic stem cells can be avoided, i.e. moral ethical, religious, etc.
- therapeutic use of stem cell transplants originating from animal fetus in approximately one million patients over more than 70 years has accumulated sufficient data to assure that this treatment, i.e. stem cell xenotransplantation, is not dangerous to an individual patient or to a mankind.

The above number of nearly one million patients represents 99% of all patients that have received stem cell transplantation to-date, i.e. the use of stem cell allo-transplants, stem cell of human origin, have been minimal so far.

There are many published medical reports on hundreds of patients showing that changes of laboratory parameters of the immune system function before and after stem cell transplantation are minimal and statistically insignificant.

This confirms the absence of any noticeable clinical immune reactions after stem cell transplantation provided stem cell transplants have been prepared properly, such as by the method described in this book. Of estimated 5 to 25 million patients treated by cell transplantation worldwide, 99.99% underwent xeno- or allo-transplantation without immunosuppression.

Until we learn what life is, and many philosophers believe that it will never happen, and can explain many aspects of the function of the living body, we have to be satisfied with the fact that implantation of stem cell transplants prepared by the 'state-of-the-art' method does not cause clinically apparent immune reactions.

The use of immunosuppression has been one of the main reasons why the success rate of cell transplantation has been so low in those countries where the use of immunosuppression has been mandatory. Long-term immunosuppression is not only dangerous to the patients; it is detrimental to the stem cell transplants, because these very young cells are enormously sensitive to any toxins, such as immunosuppressants.

Definitions of various types of stem cells

STEM CELL is a cell from the embryo, fetus, or adult that has the ability to reproduce itself for long periods. It can give rise to specialized cells that make up the tissues and organs of the body.

EMBRYONIC STEM CELL is derived from the blastocyst of an embryo, or from fetal tissue destined to become a part of the gonads. In the laboratory, and only under special conditions, this type of stem cell can proliferate indefinitely. It is pluripotent, which means that it has an ability to give rise to all types of cells, which develop from any of the three germ layers, ectoderm, entoderm, and mesoderm, from which all the cells of the body arise. It remains in such uncommitted state until it receives a signal to develop into one of approximately 200 known specialized cell types. When maintained as a cell line, embryonic stem cells have a normal number and shape of chromosomes.

FETAL STEM CELL is an undifferentiated cell that occurs within a differentiated tissue of the fetus, renews itself for the lifetime of the organism, and differentiates into all of the specialized cell types of the tissue from which it originated. But it does not replicate indefinitely in tissue culture. Up until now it has been difficult to identify, isolate and purify. It 'homes' into its tissue of origin.

PRECURSOR (PROGENITOR) STEM CELL occurs in fetal tissues, rarely in adult tissues, and is partially differentiated. It divides and gives rise to a specialized cell of the tissue to which it belongs. It replaces damaged or dead cells, and thus maintains the integrity and function of the tissue of origin. It 'homes' to the tissue it comes from.

Chapter 2

Leave no stone unturned.
Euripides, 485-406 BC in Heraclidae

Prove all things. Hold fast that which is good.
The first Epistle of Paul the Apostle to the Thessalonians 5:21

STEM CELL XENOTRANSPLANTATION VS. STEM CELL ALLO-TRANSPLANTATION

Up until now, xenotransplantation has been used in over 99.7% of approximately 5 million patients treated by stem cell transplantation, over a period of seven decades, while the remaining 0.3% of patients have had allotransplantation. Due to the error of small numbers, it is hard to statistically evaluate the benefit of the newest forms of stem cell transplantation, i.e. umbilical cord blood stem cell transplantation and human embryonic stem cell transplantation, in actual clinical practice.

Xenotransplantation is transplantation of cells, tissues or organs between species, i.e. from animal to man, from man to animal, or from one animal species to another, such as from dog to cat, from cat to rabbit, from monkey to goat, from goat to sheep, etc.

Allotransplantation is transplantation within the same species, from one man to another, from one dog to another, from one monkey to another, etc.

Auto-transplantation is a transplantation from one part of the body to another of the same member of animal kingdom, i.e. to take a piece of skin from the abdomen of the patient and transplant it to the finger tip lost in an accident, or to take an adrenal medulla of a patient and transplant it to the striatum of his brain to treat his Parkinson's disease, etc.

There is not much difference between cell xenotransplantation and allotransplantation in clinical effects. This fact was recognized already by P. Niehans in 30's of the last century and by all major figures of German cell therapy in 50's and thereafter. For that reason the west European cell therapists were not concerned about their inability to use human embryonic and fetal stem cells in their work because of prevailing ethical, moral, and religious attitudes in European countries.

The author was brought up by the European school of *'zellentherapie'*, that in English means 'cell xenotransplantation'. As cell xenotransplantation was considered in the US 'quackery', 'Frankenstein treatment', anything but a serious scientific effort, the author switched after 1987 to allotransplantation, i.e. human fetal cell transplantation, against the opinion of top German experts. F. Schmid, the best cell therapist in the world for two decades after the death of the father of cell therapy, P. Niehans, advised that there is only one difference between Homo sapiens and the rest of mammals: the frontal lobe of the brain, that animals do not have, but the rest of the body is the same on cytological level, so why to go through all of the problems of working with human fetal cells and tissues? And trouble it has been, is, and will be. The author is one of the few scientists with extensive experience with both human fetal cell transplantation and fetal cell xenotransplantation, and that applies to the preparation/manufacture of stem cell transplants as well as their clinical application.

Human cell transplantation, i.e. allotransplantation, is not, and will not be better or superior, to cell xenotransplantation as the therapeutic tool in human medicine, until human beings will be kept in closed colonies, and euthanasia will be permitted in the preparation of human fetal cell transplants, which is (hopefully) unthinkable. The use of frozen superfluous, redundant, or not needed, human embryos from infertility clinics is another form of euthanasia. At this moment there is only one incurable illness, where human fetal brain cell transplants may be necessary for cell transplantation, i.e. Alzheimer's disease, in all other instances stem cell xenotransplantation will give the same clinical results.

Without oxygen, the human heart survives 3 ½ to 5 minutes, but after 20 - 30 seconds all oxygen reserves of the body are depleted and damage to the heart is inevitable. Initial disturbance of cardiac action must be expected after 8 – 10 systoles, i.e. in 10 seconds, and in one minute the cardiac output is reduced to one third.

Human brain post-asphyxia function is limited to 2 – 3 mimutes due to a great energy demand and very small reserves. Electrocorticogram record stops in 12 – 15 minutes, and evoked transsynaptic potentials in 2 – 4 minutes. Cell membranes depolarize in 6 – 8 minutes.

Kidneys survive for 15 – 30 minutes after asphyxia, with a chance of recovery up to 40 – 60 minutes, but none after 60 minutes.

Impairment of pulmonary function after asphyxia alone takes place in minutes to hours, but if there is an additional lung pathology present, then only a few seconds to minutes [286].

The data from the last 3 paragraphs explain why the quality of stem cell allotransplants can seldom match that of stem cell xenotransplants.

Experienced scientists and clinical specialists in the field of stem cell transplantation doubt that embryonic stem cell transplantation, that currently by erroneous definition means 'human' embryonic stem cell transplantation, could be of any value in the actual treatment of human diseases. But even if it would be, there would be serious questions about what is really helping the patient: human embryonic stem cells or the feeder mouse cells without which the human embryonic stem cells cannot survive in a laboratory dish. Is it just a feeding or is it in reality a co-culture of human embryonic stem cells and mouse feeder cells? And what is the outcome of such co-culturing? This is an important question that needs to be answered.

Our team studied the poor results in human embryonic/fetal cell transplantation (or neurotransplantation) for Parkinson's disease. With permission of the Ethics Committee of the Russian Ministry of Health, the transplantation of brain cells of various genetic mutants of Drosophila to moribund patients after severe gunshot injuries of the brain was carried out, followed by a detailed autopsy. There was no clinical effect from such neurotransplantation but also no histologic evidence of any harm. The next step was a neurotransplantation of a mixture of brain cells of various genetic mutants of Drosophila with human fetal brain cells from basal ganglia and other parts of the brain. The positive clinical results led to the treatment of posttraumatic aphasia patients, and eventually patients with Parkinson's disease using the combination of human fetal brain cells with brain cells of a genetic mutant of Drosophila. The excellent results of such neurotransplantation in Parkinson's disease have never been surpassed [220]. One of the patients described in this report died of myocardial infarction 8 months later and a permission to carry out a full autopsy of his brain was obtained. The published microphotographs show excellent synaptic connections of the host brain neurons with the implanted neurons of human fetal origin and neurons from the genetic mutant of Drosophila. There was no histologic evidence of any scar tissue between the host brain and transplant. Transplanted tissue of Drosophila consisted of large multipolar neurons 2 – 5 times larger than thalamic neurons of the host. Human neurons and Drosophila brain cells formed connections via collateral axons. Multiple bundles of 50 to 200 neuronal fibers connected host brain and transplanted tissue. Capillaries and arterioles penetrated between transplanted and host tissue running parallel with neuronal fibers.

The background of this research was the fact that human fetal brain cells are too slow in their differentiation, as the full growth and development of dendrites, axons and synapses, is not attained until 4th year of life, so that they do not make connections with neurons of the host fast enough, while in Drosophila, with a life span of only 3 months, the nerve fibers and synapses develop quickly. The enormous clinical success in transplantation of the mixture of brain cells of the genetic mutant of Drosophila and that of human fetus was explained by a hypothesis that the quickly growing and differentiating brain cells of Drosophila enabled the transplanted human fetal brain cells to establish synapses with the host neurons much faster. Obviously the excellent clinical effect was the result of the synaptic connection between neurons of the host and transplanted human fetal neurons, proven by histologic findings, but the clinical success was possible only due to mediating effect of the brain cells of genetic mutants of Drosophila [220, 221].

This example is presented to trigger a debate about the feeder cells and their use in a Petri dish in laboratory conditions or *the use of feeder cells in situ*, when a 'co-culture' takes place in the recipient organ of the host.

In Chapter 1 we alluded to a classical microphotograph of the human product of conception at the stage of blastula with 107 cells, of which only 8 cells become the embryonic stem cells, while the remaining 99 cells differentiate into trophoblastic cells of placenta. At that point of development all these cells are the same and those that will become trophoblastic cells have the same potential for growth and development as embryonic stem cells. If scientists believe in superiority of human embryonic stem cells over precursor stem cells they have to turn the attention to the trophoblastic cells where they encounter much less moral, ethical, and religious outrage, and follow the path so well lit for them by over 20 million patients that received trophoblastic cell implantation.

In the meantime, our research focus is on animal trophoblastic cells, specifically of rabbits. Most of knowledge in the field of human embryonic stem cell transplantation has been obtained from mouse embryonic stem cells. Besides karyotyping, there are no dramatic differences between human and mouse embryonic stem cells, and 99% of human genom can be found in the nucleus of mouse cells. The case is the same with rabbits.

In the field of stem cell transplantation it makes very little difference whether one is dealing with xenotransplantation or allotransplantation when it comes to science. But there is an enormous difference in medical practice, since with stem cell xenotransplantation we can treat hundreds of thousands of patients already today while with stem cell allotransplantation only a few hundred, or perhaps thousand. Stem cell xenotransplants can be manufactured in nearly limitless quantities, and ultimately at low cost.

It has been, and will be, hard to develop stem cell transplantation as a therapeutic method if there is enough therapeutic material for treatment of a few patients only: this situation has been slowing the progress for many years.

Well established scientific facts have explained the reasons why stem cell xenotransplants can be used instead of stem cell allotransplants with a 'state-of-the-art' safety:

1. It has been known since 19th century, and the entire modern cell biology is based on the fact that, *all eukaryotic cells in Nature are built and function according to the same laws.* In clinical practice of stem cell transplantation we have been dealing with eukaryotic cells (of mammals) only.

2. Main cells of the same organ or tissue are the same in Nature, (or nearly the same), regardless of the species of origin, i.e. corresponding cells of the identical organ of different animal species (including man) are biologically similar. We could make a similar statement about any of the approximately 200 types of cells of human or animal body. This scientific *'principle of organo-specificity'*, described in German and Soviet/Russian literature decades ago, is still an unknown term in Anglophone medical journals. The explanation can be found in various parts of this book.

   There are no antigenic differences between the corresponding cells of the identical organ of different animal species, including man. This is another proof of 'organospecificity'.

3. All biological systems in nature are composed of the same types of molecules. Great majority of proteins from different organisms, including man, are similar over the entire amino acid sequence, i.e. they are homologous of each other and in general carry out similar functions. The homologous proteins evolved over billions of years from a common ancestor, and logically established a *'principle of homology'*.

4. The basic law of molecular biology, *whereby DNA directs the synthesis of RNA, that in turn controls the assembly of proteins*, applies to all living beings.

   Genetic encoding is the same in most known organisms. 'Families' of similar genes encode proteins with similar functions. All that implies that life on earth evolved only once.

The described scientific data explain why it has been possible to implant live stem cell transplants prepared from sheep, cattle, pigs, horses, rabbits, and probably other mammals, in 5 million patients over the past 70 years, without any serious consequences for individual patients or mankind.

Clinical xenotransplantation of cultured pancreatic islet cells originating from pig fetuses, the first in the world, was performed at RITAOMH in 1981. Besides pig fetuses, also adult pigs, cow fetuses, and later, fetal and newborn rabbits have been used by RITAOMH.

Chapter 3

> One picture is worth more than ten thousand words.
> *Chinese proverb*

ATLAS OF COMPARATIVE HISTOLOGY OF VARIOUS STEM CELL TRANSPLANTS

For the more visually oriented readers, we are adding a few examples from the future atlas of comparative human/rabbit histology applied to stem cell transplantation, under preparation by the author and D Elias, DVM, PhD. The purpose of the atlas is to show the structural similarity between human and rabbit organs and tissues, both adult and fetal, but also the similarity between all above and the histological preparations of tissue culture of the same organs and tissues, as well as the native microphotograph of the same tissue culture taken just minutes before the collection of tissue fragments from tissue cultures whereupon they become a stem cell transplant of that particular organ or tissue. Stained histological preparations of a stem cell transplant give the patient and the transplantologist a better idea about what the patient is getting in the process of stem cell transplantation.

On each of the five plates (Figures 3.1 – 3.5), six microphotographs are presented. In the top row you see side-by-side histology of human adult and rabbit adult organs, in the middle row side-by-side histology of the same human fetal and rabbit fetal organs, and in the bottom row microphotographs of the stem cell transplant of the same organ, both as stained histological preparation and in native state under inverted microscope.

The histological preparation of the stem cell transplant is prepared by running two parallel tissue cultures, one in the regular tissue culture flasks that becomes a stem cell transplant, and the second in Layton flask, that permits processing of tissue culture as histological preparation, including the use of common staining methods. Viewing the tissue culture in native state under inverted microscope requires trained eyes of experienced tissue culture expert, and even more so when only microphotograph is available. For that reason the stained histological preparation of the tissue culture was added as more 'user-friendly'.

On five color plates, the described combination of microphotographs of Langerhans islets of pancreas, liver, adrenal cortex, ovary and cerebellum, are shown.

If you focus on one of the plates, islets of pancreas, for example, compare the microscopic structure of islets of pancreas of human adult and rabbit adult, then of human fetus and rabbit fetus, and finally compare the structure of human adult to human fetus, and rabbit adult to rabbit fetus, or in any other combination, undoubtedly you will find the similarity of structure of human and animal islets of pancreas, both at fetal stage or in adulthood, striking. Then compare the microscopic structure of organs, adult and fetal, with the histological preparation of the stem cell transplants. Although many cells and other non-cellular structures were eliminated in the process of 11-day long primary tissue culture, the basic structure of the islets is retained, and you can see the same on the native microphotograph of stem cell xenotransplants of islets of pancreas. You are at a disadvantage when you have only microphotographs to look at rather than a 3-dimentional image through the microscope.

This exercise is usually convincing to prove a visual similarity of structure of the same organ or tissue in animal kingdom, so that when you read about organospecificity in this book, you will believe that there is no real difference between islet cell xeno- and allotransplantation in clinical practice.

Cerebellum

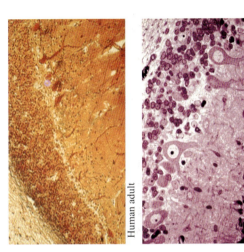

Animal adult | Human adult

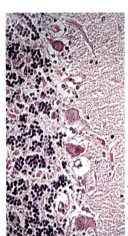

Animal embryo | Human embryo

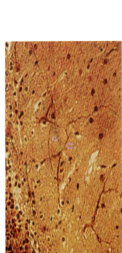
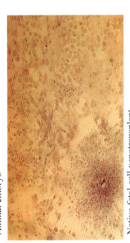

Native fetal cell xenotransplant | Stained fetal cell xenotransplant

Figure 3.1 Comparative microphotographs of stem cell transplants (Cerebellum) from rabbit and human

Insulae Langerhans

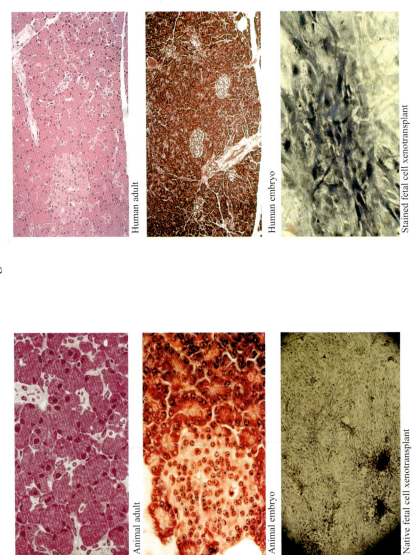

Figure 3.2 Comparative microphotographs of stem cell transplants (Insulae Langerhans) from rabbit and human

Hepar

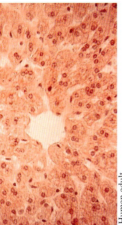
Animal adult

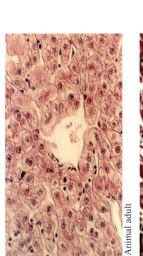
Human adult

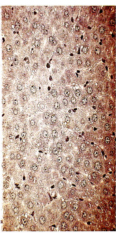
Animal embryo

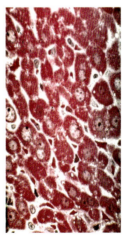
Human embryo

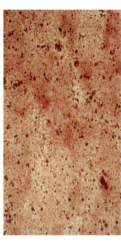
Native fetal cell xenotransplant

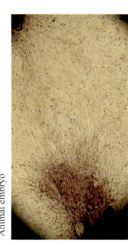
Stained fetal cell xenotransplant

Figure 3.3 Comparative microphotographs of stem cell transplants (Hepar) from rabbit and human

Ovarium

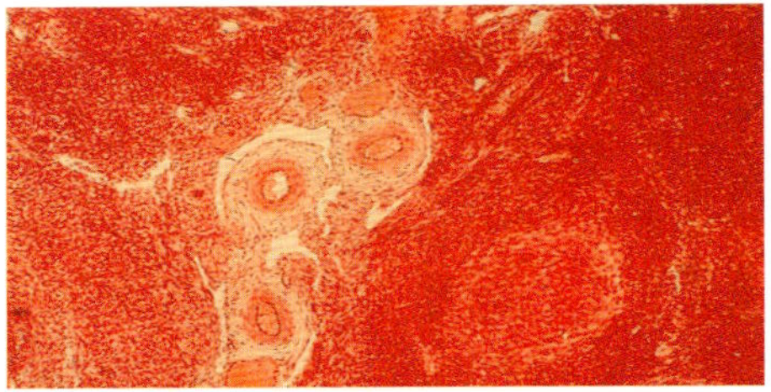

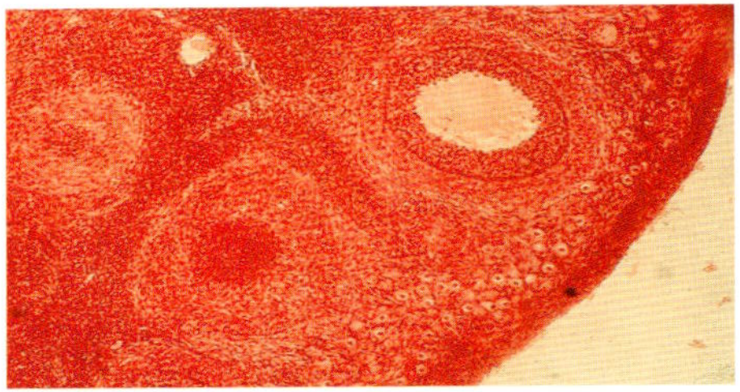

Human adult

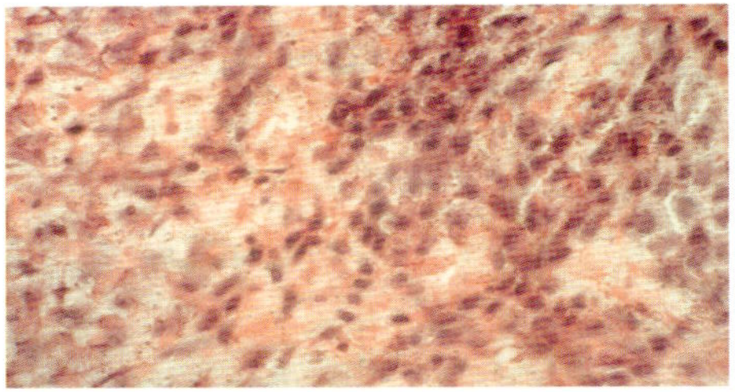

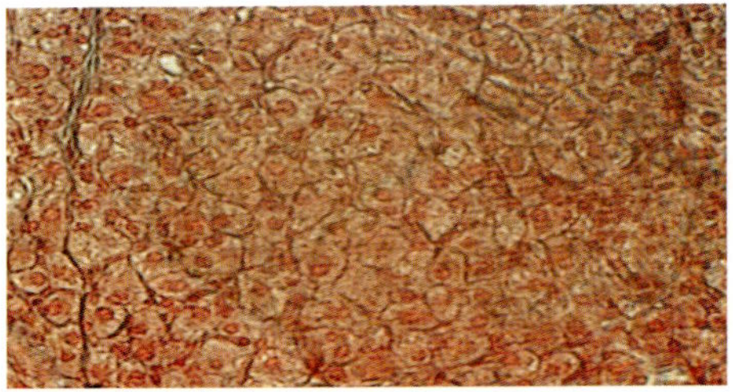

Human embryo

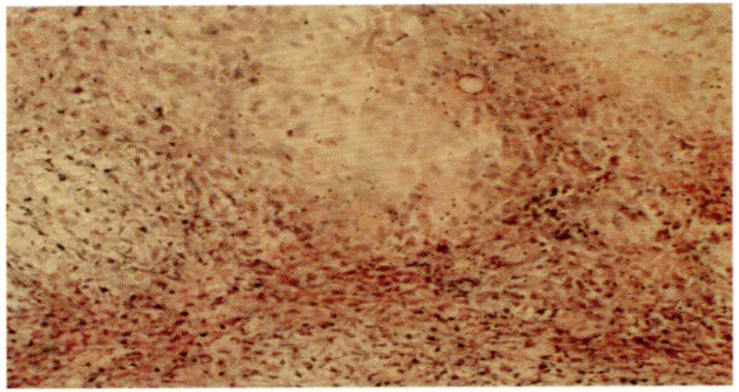

Stained fetal cell xenotransplant

Animal adult

Animal embryo

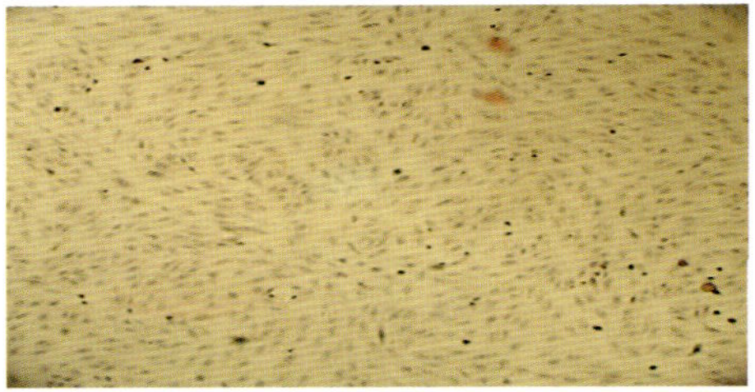

Native fetal cell xenotransplant

Figure 3.4 Comparative microphotographs of stem cell transplants (Ovarium) from rabbit and human

Supraren

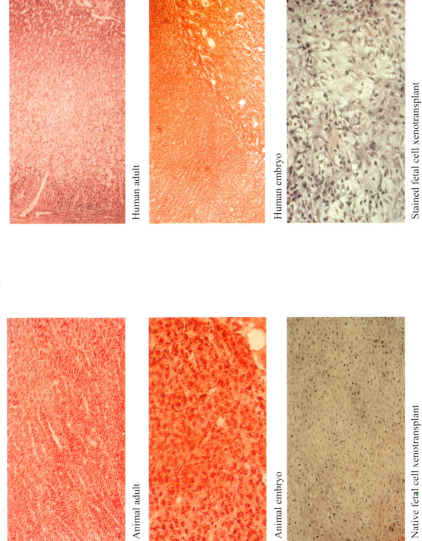

Animal adult · Human adult
Animal embryo · Human embryo
Native fetal cell xenotransplant · Stained fetal cell xenotransplant

Figure 3.5 Comparative microphotographs of stem cell transplants (Supraren) from rabbit and human

Chapter 4

A journey of thousand miles must begin with a single step.
Lao – Tzu, c. 604 – c. 531 BC

Rome was not built in one day.
John Heywood, c. 1497 – c. 1580, Proverbs

HISTORY

The history of stem cell transplantation is really a history of stem cell xenotransplantation. It was not until the late 70s of the last century when human fetal tissue transplantation (allotransplantation) began in the USSR, and from there spread into some other communist countries, i.e. Yugoslavia, Hungary, German Democratic Republic, and Peoples' Republic of China.

In the late 80s Hana Biologicals, a public corporation based in Alameda, California, began procurement of human fetal tissue transplants in cooperation with a human fetus collection company in Philadelphia, Pennsylvania. After US FDA approved clinical trial of treatment of type 1 diabetes mellitus by transplantation of cells produced by Hana Biologicals failed, all cell transplantation activity ceased in the US until 2001.

The idea was born a long time ago. The following list presents important chronological events in the development of cell transplantation:

Papyrus of Eber - 3,000 BC - described preparation of medications from animal organs.

Susruta – 1,400 BC (Mesopotamia, today Iraq) – prescribed ingestion of sex glands of young tigers as treatment of impotence.

Hippocrates – 470 – 410 BC – carried out transplantation of frog skin to treat man.

Aristoteles – 384 – 322 BC, and **Plinius the Elder** – 23 – 79 AD, described preparation and use of animal and human organ extracts for human treatment.

Paracelsus (Theofrastus Bombastus of Hohenheim) – 1493 – 1541 – wrote in his book: "**Heart heals heart, kidneys heal kidneys**" and "**Like heals like**", i.e. he discovered organospecificity, one of the scientific principles of modern stem cell transplantation.

Hooke – 1663 – used the word "cell" for the first time.

Schleiden – 1838 – discovered that cells are the structural basis of all plants.

Schwann – 1839 – discovered that cells are the structural basis of all animals.

Hunter – 1771 - and **Berthold** – 1849 – proved the substitution effect of implanted sex glands on a castrated cock.

Brown-Sequard – 1889 – presented to the fellow members of French Academy of Sciences a report on self-treatment by implantation of canine sex glands for revitalization (as an elderly widower he re-married a much younger woman that caused problems which he, the most famous physiologist of his era, resolved). This was the first documented case of cell xenotransplantation in the history of medicine. Immunosuppression was unknown then.

Virchow – 1821 –1902, father of modern pathology, stated that "all life stems from cells", and that "there is no life without cells". Or, in other words, 'cells are bearers of all life'.

Carell – 1873 – 1944, father of cell biology, (first US Nobel prize winner, in 1912, for discovering technique of surgical suture of blood vessels), succeeded in keeping a tissue culture of chick embryo cardiomyoblasts alive indefinitely, as long as the tissue culture medium was replenished at regular intervals by another containing a small amount of the same embryonic cells. Actually his tissue culture was allowed to expire after 34 years.

Cushing – 1869 – 1939, one of the fathers of neurosurgery, was also the most important endocrinologist of all times due to his pioneering research on pituitary hormones and their relations to hormones of hypothalamus, adrenals, and other peripheral endocrine organs. Niehans credited Cushing with some of his ideas that were included in the concept of cell therapy / cell transplantation.

Landsteiner – 1900 – discovered blood groups, thus making blood transfusion safe, without immunosuppression. Blood transfusion was the first widely used method of cell transplantation in clinical practice.

Kuttner – 1912 - succesfully transplanted human adult thyroid tissue to another patient after total thyroidectomy. Immunosuppression was unknown at that time.

Voronoff – 1910 – began to widely use xenotransplantation in clinical practice. His research on transplantation of animal (monkey) testes to aging men caught attention of media and brought him notoriety. Unfortunately monkeys are carriers of syphilis (which is harmless to them) and thus his patients acquired a dangerous disease, for which there was no treatment at that time. Today by following US FDA and WHO rules on manufacturing xenotransplants this kind of disaster would be absolutely impossible. No immunosuppression was used then.

Niehans – 1982 – 1971 – doctor of Lutheran theology and doctor of medicine, decorated hero of WW1 and WW2, a member of Papal Academy of Sciences, an illegitimate child of the last German Kaiser, developed between 1920 and 1931 'cell therapy'[*] that was defined by him as a transplantation of freshly obtained animal fetal tissue fragments of various, in principle all, organs for treatment of man. In 1927 he successfully used implantation of fresh calf pituitary tissue fragments for treatment of pituitary dwarfs. In 1929 he treated patients with chronic polyarthritis by a similar method with good results.

In 1931 he was asked to save the life of a woman dying of tetany due to accidental removal of all parathyroid glands during total thyroidectomy by a famous surgeon. As there was no time even for the usual minor implantation surgery, Niehans took surgical scissors and chopped down the animal parathyroid glands obtained from the slaughterhouse so that it would pass through an injection needle, and implanted the tissue fragments

---

[*]Anglophone medical literature uses the term 'cell transplantation', while German literature has used the term 'cell therapy' (zellentherapie) for implantation of tissue fragments of animal origin. German law does not recognize the term 'cell transplantation' and US FDA banned 'cell therapy' in 1956.

obtained with syringe and large-bore needle. The patient survived and lived for another 21 years. Thereby 'cell therapy' was born, created in a life or death situation, without any research or scientific discussions. This genius clinician treated more VIPs of our world than any other physician alive or dead. He did not use any immunosuppression.

In 1954, during 'Therapy Week' in Karlsruhe, Germany, around 5,000 physicians packed the auditorium, standing in vestibule and halls, in order to listen to his lectures. As a result of his teachings and that of his most glorious followers: Schmid, Stein, Schmidt, Kment, Neumann, Hoepke, Langendorff, Bernhard, Lettre, Landsberger, Andres, Wolf, Gianoli, Camerer, and others, as many as 5 million patients were treated by cell therapy (more than 4 million of that in Germany), of which around one million was treated by live cell transplants. Afterward the definition of cell therapy was enlarged to include the use of preserved cells for treatment.**

In the 1950's, Niehans received one night visitors from an insulin-maker Eli Lilly Co. with a $1,000,000 check to induce him to stop his attempts to find a treatment of diabetes mellitus by cell therapy (to find a treatment for diabetes mellitus and cancer by cell therapy was his lifelong obsession). After he refused, the pharmaceutical industry began to systematically attack cell therapy. After 1956 all publications about cell therapy/cell transplantation stopped in the US, and from that time, no US medical school library kept any German medical journals or books known to publish articles about cell therapy/cell transplantation.

In 1987, the German government banned the sale of preserved cell therapeutics in pharmacies, but when it attempted to ban cell therapy altogether in 1997, i.e. fresh cell therapy/cell transplantation, it failed.

** Here starts the discrepancy between terms 'cell therapy' and 'cell transplantation' when it comes to an implantation of tissue fragments of animal origin. 'Cell transplantation' includes only 'fresh cell therapy' as in the original definition of Niehans, but not the use of preserved cells (preservation by lyophilization causes cells to lose cell membrane and thereby they are no longer live, preservation by freezing - as it used to be done in those days – leads to death of 85 – 95% of cells, mostly during thawing process). Today in German, 'cell therapy' (zellentherapie) means use of animal preserved cells or cellular material for treatment, while 'fresh cell therapy' (frischzellentherapie) means the use of freshly obtained animal fetal tissue fragments for therapeutic implantation.

German Supreme Court ruled on February 16, 2000, that fresh cell therapy/cell transplantation is safe, and overturned the attempted ban. This decision means that cell transplantation has continued to be permitted in Germany and thereby in the entire European Union.

Filatow – 1875 – 1956 – father of transplantation of cornea, while developing his method in 1933 came across an idea to use implantation of fragments of human placenta to improve results of corneal transplantation. Implantation of human placental fragments became the most popular biological therapeutic method to-date, worldwide, known under numerous names, usually that of the clinic owner. No immunosuppression has ever been used.

Kasakow – in 1925, based on the method of Tuchnow, developed treatment by cell hydrolysates, which became well known in USSR. Subsequent to the death of the deputy chief of NKVD (predecessor of KGB), allegedly as a result of such therapy, Kasakow was sentenced to death, his governmental institute eliminated and all writings locked up for generations by KGB in a library of banned literature, until partially discovered by Bio-Cellular Research Organization (BCRO) in 1993.

Shumakow – 1979 – published in a peer reviewed journal about the success of cell transplants prepared by tissue culture in the treatment of a female with severe complications of insulin dependent diabetes mellitus, without immunosuppression; the patient was well for 21 years without any additional cell transplantation.

Bio-Cellular Research Organization (BCRO) – subsequent to US FDA issuing regulations about preparation of cell, tissue and organ xenotransplantations in September 1996, BCRO completed the development of its method of manufacturing of cell transplants of animal fetal origin, and after filing US Patent application in 1998, began manufacturing of stem cell transplants in July 1998.

BCRO has not discovered a procedure of (stem) cell transplantation, it found a method to prepare (stem) cell xenotransplants of any of around 200 kinds of cells that mammals are made of, for clinical use, that can be implanted with 'state-of-the-art' safety, and without immunosuppression. (The author has been the managing director of BCRO since its inception in 1989).

Stem cell transplantation was introduced into clinical practice in 1931 and has historically preceded organ transplantation by several decades. It shall dominate the medicine of the 21st century.

BRIEF SUMMARY OF AUTHOR'S PREVIOUS EXPERIENCE WITH STEM CELL ALLO- AND XENOTRANSPLANTATION

It all began 27 years ago, at first by the study of German and Soviet information bases of cell transplantation, and then by close cooperation with the leaders in this field in Germany between 1982 – 1997. Finally, a major clinical research work of International Institute of Biological Medicine (IIBM), a Russian corporation, created in 1991 by Bio-Cellular Research Organization (BCRO), as 51% shareholder, together with a division of the Ministry of Health Care and Health Care Industry of Russian Federation, in the field of human fetal/embryonic cell transplantation was carried out between 1990 and 1997. In 1993, the work of BCRO/IIBM in the treatment of patients with complications of diabetes mellitus attracted the attention of Sansum Medical Research Foundation, Santa Barbara, California. Sansum organized in that year the first US clinical trial in the use of the combined fetal allo-/xeno- cell transplantation for a treatment of complications of IDDM as a cooperation between BCRO and Sansum. (Dr. Sansum was the first US physician to use insulin in his medical practice).

On August 1, 1993, a total of 24 US patients with complications of IDDM, predominanly of retinopathy and nephropathy, were treated by BCRO system in the clinical facility of Sansum in Santa Barbara, California. A manuscript describing the positive clinical results of this trial was submitted for publication to 'Transplantation' by medical teams of Sansum and BCRO. It reported on the treatment of 24 patients with Type 1 diabetes mellitus with retinopathy, nephropathy or both, with duration of diabetes of 21 ± 7 years. During the 12 months follow-up, the insulin requirement was significantly reduced by 21 ± 8% (p=0.0260), systolic blood pressure significantly reduced from 120 ± 17 to 111 ± 13 (p=0.012), and diastolic blood pressure from 78 ± 8 to 72 ± 8 (p=0.005). Total body weight was reduced from 153 ± 30 to 150 ± 28 (p=0.189), and HbA1c from 7.1 ± 1.4 to 6.8 ± 1.2 (p=0.222). Plasma levels of C-peptide increased from 0.06 ng/ml before treatment to 0.186 ng/ml within one year (p=0.01). There was no further progression of retinopathy and nephropathy in any of the 24 patients during the one year follow-up. One female patient became pregnant during this time [115].

The US company, created by personnel of Sansum, organized a continuation of these clinical trials in 1995 at Los Gatos Community Hospital, Los Gatos, California [113]. On three different occasions in 1995, altogether 32 US patients with complications of IDDM (n=27) and NIDDM (n=5) were treated by BCRO system in the clinic facilities of Los Gatos Community Hospital, again by combined fetal allo-/xeno- cell transplanttation, as at Sansum in 1993. During the 12 months follow-up insulin requirement was significantly reduced by 41 ± 8% (p=0.001), blood glucose levels stabilized from 229 ± 44 mg/dl to 104 ± 21 mg/dl, and plasma levels of C-peptide increased significantly from 0.09 ng/ml to 0.49 ng/ml (p=0.001). Diabetic complications of every patient remained stable, the creatinine clearance of one patient with diabetic nephropathy improved from 39 ml/min to 58 ml/min [112]. The islet cell transplants used in the treatment of all 56 US patients were prepared from fetal/newborn rabbits.

Stem cell transplants prepared by BCRO method have been used for the patients treatment in the Emirates, Qatar, Germany, Italy, Czech Republic, Slovakia, Mexico, Switzerland, Thailand, and South Africa.

Past History

Cell transplantation/cell therapy has been around for over 70 years in several different countries: Germany, Switzerland, France, Italy, Spain, Austria, USSR, etc. Political, philosophical, professional, language, and other barriers, have caused the absence of professional and scientific communication in this new field of medicine between two pioneering countries: Germany and USSR. The principals of BCRO have succeeded in overcoming of these barriers and establishing the communication channels.

Germany has been the only country in the West where various methods of cell transplantation have been widely used since 1950's. The form of this treatment known as 'fresh cell therapy' (frischzellentherapie), has been used to this date. In February, 2000, the Bundesverfassungsgericht (German Supreme Court) in Karlsruhe, case number: 1 BvR 420/97, ruled in favor of a continuous approval of this therapeutic method. Since over 800,000 patients have been treated by fresh cell therapy in Germany during the past 70 years, this was quite an impressive statement. Additionally, more than 4 million patients have been treated during this time by frozen and lyophilized 'cell-therapeutics', registered in West Germany until 1987.

In 1984, the Ministry of Health of USSR issued 'Recommendations on the Method' (the same type of document as 'US FDA regulations') dealing with cell transplantation that amounted to the official approval of this treatment [76]. It confirmed a completion of a major pre-clinical and clinical research in this field in the USSR [78], which led to the successful treatment of a patient with complications of IDDM (by fetal allo-transplantation), already in 1979, and thereafter, hundreds of other diabetics and patients suffering of other untreatable diseases.

Since the Ministry of Health of USSR put its Research Institute of Transplantology and Artificial Organs of the Ministry of Health of USSR (RITAOMH) in charge of this work, and the transplantologists, 'big surgeons', were much more interested in organ transplantation than in 'just simple injections of cells', the method did not attract much attention within the Soviet health care system. Only after IIBM entered the field in the new Russian Federation in 1991, the cell transplantation became known as a therapeutic method, and was included in the list of approved therapies by the Ministry of Health Care of Russian Federation, and received a governmental code.

By the decree of the Minister of Health of Russian Federation on November 1994, it is now a duty of a diabetologist in Russia to refer a diabetic patient for cell transplantation, if indicated [77].

By the time of its first international symposium in December 1995, in Moscow, IIBM treated by stem cell allo- and xenotransplantation around 3,000 private patients with a variety of diseases, besides those treated under various clinical research projects. Thus in the span of 3 years (1993 - 1995) IIBM treated the same number of patients as 12 top Soviet research institutes since 1979.

The major contribution of BCRO/IIBM was its unpublished study, carried out together with the staff of RITAOMH, in which *the clinical results of cell transplantation by fetal allo- and xenotransplants were compared.* This study proved the overall superiority of cell xenotransplantation. The main reason was a much better quality of the animal (rabbit) source of cell transplants. While the animal (rabbit) material could always be obtained fresh, i.e. cells were 100% live when planted onto the tissue culture medium, the same could hardly ever be stated about human fetal material, where for obvious reasons there was always a delay between the time of death and the dissection of human fetal cadaver, often quite substantial, so that the viability of cells at the time of their planting onto the tissue culture medium varied substantially.

There were 12 major medical research institutes in 5 different republics of USSR involved in cell transplantation. It should be noted that medical science was organized in USSR under a 'pyramidal principle', i.e. in each field of science there was a central USSR institute in charge for the whole country, for example RITAOMH in transplantology, and there were central institutes in each field of medical science in charge in each of the 15 republics of USSR

Although RITAOMH was in overall control in the transplantology, the main institutes of each Republic had a lot of latitude in their actions. Some of them were carrying out only cell allo-transplantation while others only cell xenotransplantation, with bovine or porcine fetuses as sources of transplants, and some of these institutes carried out both cell allo- and xeno-transplantation.

Ultimately, cell allo-transplantation was abandoned by all of them in favor of xenotransplantation. Among the 12 research institutes involved in cell transplantation, only RITAOMH switched from bovine and porcine fetuses to the fetal (but eventually also to newborn) rabbits as a source of cell xeno-transplants, and that began in 1987. The change of the source of cell xenotransplants coincided with the fall of communism and of the USSR, which caused a major breakdown of Russian medical science, medical industry, and health care, with a subsequent decrease of medical publication activity as well.

As a result, there is much less published material about the cell xeno-transplantation with fetal and newborn rabbits as a source of transplants, as compared with bovine and porcine fetuses. In 'Bibliography' are included also dissertations for the degree of 'Candidate of Medical Sciences' (PhD), and for the degree 'Doctor of Medical Sciences', mandatory for all future professors, carried out under the roof of RITAOMH, summaries of lectures from the various 'All-USSR' congresses on cell, tissue and organ transplantation: Tenth All-USSR Symposium on Organ Transplantation, 1985, in Kiev (now Ukraine), Fourth Congress of Ukrainian Endocrinologists, 1987, in Kiev, Symposium on Transplantologic Methods of Treatment of Diabetes Mellitus, 1988, in Riga (now Latvia), Third All-USSR Congress of Endocrinology, 1989, in Tashkent (now Uzbekistan), Eleventh All-USSR Symposium on Organ Transplantation, 1990, in Lvov, (now Ukraine), and from the symposiums at RITAOMH in Moscow, as well as from the yearly International Symposia 'Transplantation of Endocrine Pancreas', organized by the Institute for Endocrinology, Diabetes and Metabolic Diseases, University Clinical Center, Belgrade, Yugoslavia.

Prior to being invited to USSR by the last Soviet Minister of Health, Prof. Dr. Chazov, Nobel Peace Prize winner, in June 1990, the author and BCRO began its work in the field of cell transplantation in Eastern Europe in September 1988 in Yugoslavia. For practical reasons, the Yugoslav colleagues decided to base the project in the Medical School in Sarajevo, today Bosnia/Hercegovina, and that decision proved ominous: in early 1990, the project was stopped by civil war, and was moved to the USSR.

Chapter 5

Where no law is, there is no transgressions.
The Epistle of Paul the Apostle to the Romans 4:15

LEGISLATIVE SITUATION

EUROPEAN COMMUNITY

On February 16, 2000, by its favorable ruling in the case 1 BvR 420/97, the German Supreme Court (Bundesverfassungsgericht) re-affirmed that 'frischzellentherapie' (fresh cell xenotransplantation with precursor stem cells) approved by the Government, and in common use by medical practitioners in Germany since early 1950's, had continued to be permitted. Thereby Germany had re-established its leadership in this field. This decision of German Supreme Court, with a power of law, applies to all Member States of the European Union.

Here are salient points of the decision of the German Supreme Court,

From a regulatory viewpoint:

1. '*Frischzellentherapeutica*' (i.e. cell xenotransplants) are outside of regulatory controls of the State because they are neither drugs nor 'therapeutica', ('*arzneimittel*' in German), but are another form of medication, individually prepared by a physician, for his specific patient, by agreement with his patient, confirmed by the signed informed consent prescribed by law.
2. They are prepared for one time use only.
3. They have no 'shelf-life'.
4. They are not distributed through the usual channels, i.e. through pharmacies.

5. They have to be implanted on a date set prior to the start of their preparation.
6. Their implantation has to be carried out by the same physician who wrote a prescription for the stem cell xenotransplants for the named patient.

The European Community Council's Directives are in harmony with this German legal concept.

Here is the ruling of the German Supreme Court in the original version. The key items are italicized in the English translation that is located right after the German official version.

BUNDESVERFASSUNGSGERICHT
Der Bund ist nach Art. 74 Abs. 1 Nr. 19 GG nicht befugt, die Herstellung solcher Arzneimittel zu regeln, die der Arzt zur Anwendung bei eigenen Patienten herstellt.

Das Herstellungsverbot in § 1 Abs. 1 der Frischzellen-Verordnung ist nichtig.

BVerfG, Urteil vom 16. 2. 2000 - 1 BvR 420/ 97 (Lexetius.com/2000, 3868 [2001/6/68])

1. In dem Verfahren über die Verfassungsbeschwerde des Herrn Dr. A ..., der Frau Dr. B ..., des Herrn Dr. J ..., des Herrn Dr. M ... - Bevollmächtigte: Rechtsanwälte Felix Busse und Partner, Oxfordstraße 21, Bonn - gegen § 1 Abs. 1 und § 2 Abs. 2 der Verordnung über das Verbot der Verwendung bestimmter Stoffe zur Herstellung von Arzneimitteln (Frischzellen-Verordnung) vom 4. März 1997 (BGBl I S. 432) hat das Bundesverfassungsgericht - Erster Senat - unter Mitwirkung des Vizepräsidenten Papier, der Richter Grimm, Kühling, der Richterinnen Jaeger, Haas, der Richter Hömig, Steiner und der Richterin Hohmann-Dennhardt aufgrund der mündlichen Verhandlung vom 9. November 1999 durch Urteil für Recht erkannt:
2. § 1 Absatz 1 und § 2 Absatz 2 der Verordnung über das Verbot der Verwendung bestimmter Stoffe zur Herstellung von Arzneimitteln (Frischzellen-Verordnung) vom 4. März 1997 (Bundesgesetzblatt I Seite 432) verletzen die Beschwerdeführer in ihrem Grundrecht aus Artikel 12 Absatz 1 des Grundgesetzes. Sie sind nichtig.

3. Die Bundesrepublik Deutschland hat den Beschwerdeführern die notwendigen Auslagen zu erstatten.
4. Gründe: A. Die Beschwerdeführer sind Ärzte. Ihre Verfassung-sbeschwerde richtet sich unmittelbar gegen § 1 Abs. 1 und § 2 Abs. 2 der Verordnung über das Verbot der Verwendung bestimmter Stoffe zur Herstellung von Arzneimitteln (Frischzellen-Verordnung) vom 4. März 1997 (BGBl I S. 432), wonach es unter Strafandrohung verboten ist, bei der Herstellung von Arzneimitteln, die zur Injektion oder Infusion bestimmt sind, Frischzellen zu verwenden. Die Verordnung ist vom Bundesministerium für Gesundheit aufgrund von § 6 des Gesetzes über den Verkehr mit Arzneimitteln (Arzneimittel-gesetz) in der Fassung der Bekanntmachung vom 19. Oktober 1994 (BGBl I S. 3018; im Folgenden: AMG) erlassen worden. § 6 Abs. 1 AMG lautet.
5. Das Bundesministerium für Gesundheit (Bundesministerium) wird ermächtigt, durch Rechtsverordnung mit Zustimmung des Bundesrates die Verwendung bestimmter Stoffe, Zubereitungen aus Stoffen oder Gegenstände bei der Herstellung von Arzneimitteln vorzuschreiben, zu beschränken oder zu verbieten und das Inverkehrbringen von Arzneimitteln, die nicht nach diesen Vorschriften hergestellt sind, zu untersagen, soweit es geboten ist, um eine unmittelbare oder mittelbare Gefährdung der Gesundheit von Mensch oder Tier durch Arzneimittel zu verhüten.
6. Die einschlägigen Vorschriften der Frischzellen-Verordnung lauten.
7. § 1. Verbot der Verwendung von Frischzellen. (1) Es ist verboten, bei der Herstellung von Arzneimitteln, die zur Injektion oder Infusion bestimmt sind, Frischzellen zu verwenden. (2) bis (5) ...
8. § 2. Straf- und Bußgeldvorschriften. (1) ... (2) Nach § 96 Nr. 1 des Arzneimittelgesetzes wird bestraft, wer entgegen § 1 Abs. 1 Frischzellen verwendet. (3) ...
9. Streitig ist, ob es auf der Grundlage des Arzneimittelgesetzes Ärzten verboten werden kann, Frischzellen zur unmittelbaren Anwendung am Patienten herzustellen.
10. I. 1. Die Frischzellen-Therapie besteht im Wesentlichen darin, lebende tierische Zellen dem Patienten zu injizieren mit der Absicht, eine revitalisierende Wirkung zu erzielen. Die Zellen werden in der Regel aus Schafsfeten gewonnen. Die Spendertiere stammen aus - in der weiblichen Linie - geschlossenen Herden; damit soll das Risiko der Übertragung bestimmter Krankheiten vermieden werden.
11. Die Frischzellen-Therapie gehört zu den so genannten alternativen Heilmethoden. Die Therapeuten gehen unter anderem davon aus, dass die eingespritzten Zellen in den korrespondierenden Organen körpereigene "Repair-Mechanismen" auslösen und dadurch

wirksam werden. Gegen die Frischzellen-Therapie wird von der Schulmedizin vor allem eingewandt, dass einem fehlenden therapeutischen Nutzen ein hohes denkbares Risiko, insbesondere Überempfindlichkeitsreak-tionen, autoimmunologische Reaktionen und die Übertragbarkeit von Infektionen, gegenüberstehen.

12. 2. Die Frischzellen-Verordnung erging aufgrund der Erkenntnisse, die das Bundesgesundheitsamt 1992 und 1994 in Gutachten niedergelegt hat, sowie unter Berücksichtigung früherer Stellungnahmen des Wissenschaftlichen Beirats der Bundesärztekammer. Das Verbot wird mit der Gefährlichkeit der Frischzellen-Therapie begründet (BRDrucks 38/ 97, S. 4 bis 7). 1987 hatte das Bundesgesundheitsamt bereits das Ruhen der Zulassung aller Arzneimittel zur Zellular-therapie angeordnet, die als Fertigarzneimittel nach der Übergang-sregelung des Arzneimittelgesetzes noch als zugelassen galten (vgl. Pharmazeutische Zeitung 1987, S. 1999).
13. II. Die Beschwerdeführer haben zur ihrer tatsächlichen Situation folgende Angaben gemacht:
14. Sie sind ausschließlich privatärztlich tätig und auf Frischzellenbehandlungen spezialisiert. Seit Jahren halten sie geschlossene Schafherden allein zur Gewinnung von Frischzellen.
15. 1. Der Beschwerdeführer zu 1) ist Arzt für Allgemeinmedizin. 1991 übernahm er eine Privatklinik, in der schon seit 1977 schwerpunktmäßig Frischzellenbehandlungen durchgeführt werden. In der Klinik mit 60 Betten werden 53 Angestellte beschäftigt. Der Umsatz beruht zu mehr als der Hälfte auf der Frischzellenbehandlung; die Anzahl der Patienten ist rückläufig.
16. 2. Die Beschwerdeführerin zu 2) übernahm von ihrem Vater ein Sanatorium mit 45 Betten, das seit 1951 Frischzellenbehandlungen anbietet. Sie beschäftigt 41 Angestellte und erwirtschaftet ihren Gewinn fast ausschließlich durch Frischzellenbehandlungen. Die meisten Patienten nehmen sie zum wiederholten Male in Anspruch.
17. 3. Der Beschwerdeführer zu 3) wendet die Frischzellen-Therapie seit 1968 an. Er beschäftigt als niedergelassener Arzt vier Personen und arbeitet mit einem Kurhotel zusammen. Die Anzahl der Patienten und die Gewinne sind rückläufig.
18. 4. Der Beschwerdeführer zu 4) ist Facharzt für Urologie. Er leitet seit 1980 eine Klinik mit 42 Betten und 29 Angestellten, die auf Frischzellen-Therapie spezialisiert ist und hiermit mehr als drei Viertel ihres Umsatzes erzielt.
19. III. Mit ihrer unmittelbar gegen § 1 Abs. 1 und § 2 Abs. 2 der Frischzellen-Verordnung gerichteten Verfassungsbeschwerde

rügen die Beschwerdeführer eine Verletzung von Art. 12 Abs. 1 und Art. 14 Abs. 1 GG.
20. Die Verfassungsbeschwerde sei zulässig. Die Beschwerdeführer würden durch das strafbewehrte Verbot in § 1 Abs. 1 der Frischzellen-Verordnung selbst und unmittelbar betroffen. Die Verfassungsbeschwerde sei auch begründet. Das Arzneimittel-gesetz ermächtige den Verordnungsgeber nicht, in die ärztliche Therapiefreiheit einzugreifen. Art. 74 Abs. 1 Nr. 19 GG begründe eine konkurrierende Gesetzgebungskompetenz des Bundes nur für den Verkehr mit Arzneimitteln, nicht für das Arzneimittelrecht schlechthin. Allein für den Arzneimittelverkehr dürfe der Bundes-gesetzgeber selbst Regelungen treffen und den Verordnungsgeber hierzu ermächtigen. Zwar betreffe der Verkehr den gesamten Umgang mit Arzneimitteln von der Herstellung bis zum Handel und Verbrauch. Die Herstellung dürfe vom Bund jedoch nur bei solchen Arzneimitteln geregelt werden, die für den Verkehr bestimmt seien. Frischzellen seien keine Arzneimittel dieser Art, da sie bestimmungsgemäß nicht in den Verkehr gebracht würden. Sie würden vom Arzt hergestellt und von ihm selbst angewendet. Damit lägen lokal abgeschlossene Einzelvorgänge vor, die im Wege der Gesundheitsaufsicht von den Ländern zu überwachen seien. Die Herstellung selbst sei überdies ungefährlich und werde nur verboten, um Ärzten, wie den Beschwerdeführern, die Therapie unmöglich zu machen.
21. Im Übrigen sei das Verbot der Frischzellenherstellung und der Frischzellen-Therapie auch unverhältnismäßig. Die tatsächlichen Bewertungen des Bundesgesundheitsamtes über die Nutzlosigkeit einerseits und die Gesundheitsgefährdung andererseits seien unzutreffend und entbehrten einer statistisch relevanten Datenbasis. Es werde auch nicht berücksichtigt, dass die Patienten umfassend aufgeklärt würden und ausdrücklich ihre Einwilligung erklärten. Für spezialisierte Kliniken hätte überdies eine Übergangsregelung gefunden werden müssen.
22. IV. Zu der Verfassungsbeschwerde haben das Bundesministerium für Gesundheit namens der Bundesregierung, das Bundesinstitut für Arzneimittel und Medizinprodukte, die Bundesärztekammer sowie der Bundesverband Deutscher Ärzte für Frischzellen-Therapie Stellung genommen.
23. 1. Das Bundesministerium für Gesundheit hält die Verfassungsbeschwerde für unbegründet. Die Frischzellen-Verordnung sei kompetenzgemäß erlassen und materiell verfassungsmäßig. Art. 74 Abs. 1 Nr. 19 GG erfasse den gesamten Umgang mit Arzneimitteln von der Herstellung bis zum Verbrauch im Interesse eines

umfassenden gesundheitlichen Schutzes der Patienten. Zur effektiven Gefahrenverhütung sei es erforderlich, in einem möglichst frühen Stadium, also bereits bei der Herstellung eines Arzneimittels, anzusetzen. Dabei sei unerheblich, ob bereits vom Herstellungsvor-gang Gefahren ausgingen. Eine Beschränkung der Gesetzgebung-skompetenz könne sich insbesondere nicht aus den Definitionen im Arzneimittelgesetz ergeben. Dieses enthalte im Übrigen auch für den Tierarzt und im Zusammenhang mit Betäubungsmitteln ebenso weitgehende Vorschriften über die Herstellung wie die angegriffene Verordnung.

24. Die Regelung entspreche dem Verhältnismäßigkeitsprinzip. Sie sei erforderlich, um Patienten vor gravierenden Gefahren für Leben und Gesundheit zu schützen. Auch bei unmittelbarer Anwendung selbst hergestellter Arzneimittel müsse das Grundprinzip ärztlichen Selbstverständnisses und Standesrechts gelten, möglichen Schaden vom Patienten abzuwenden und ihn nach bestem Wissen und Gewissen zu behandeln. Bei der Frischzellen-Therapie würden nicht einmal die einfachsten Grundregeln der Arzneimittelher-stellung beachtet. Die im Gutachten des Bundesgesundheitsamtes von 1994 beschriebenen denkbaren Schäden (allergische Sofortreaktionen, Unverträglichkeitsreaktionen, autoimmunolo-gische Reaktionen und Ansteckung mit Scrapie, BSE, Tollwut und Prokolose) rechtfertigten auch ein sofortiges Einschreiten.

25. 2. Das Bundesinstitut für Arzneimittel und Medizinprodukte vertritt die Auffassung, dass ein Fehlen der Frischzellenzu-bereitungen keinerlei Behandlungslücke hinterlasse. Auch die von den Besch-werdeführern vorgelegten Unterlagen gäben keine Veranlassung, von der bisher vorgenommenen Risikodarstellung und Risikobewertung abzuweichen.

26. 3. Die Bundesärztekammer hält nach Beratung durch ihren Wissenschaftlichen Beirat sowie durch die Arzneimittelkomm-ission der Deutschen Ärzteschaft (Fachausschuss der Bundesä-rztekammer) die Verfassungsbeschwerde für unbegründet. Der Inhalt der Frischzellen-Verordnung sei zu begrüßen. Bisher habe kein Wirksamkeitsnachweis für Frischzellen geführt werden können. Bei den einzelnen Krankengeschichten handele es sich um medizinisch nicht fundierte Einzelfallbeobachtungen. Der Nutzen sei nicht nachgewiesen; dem stehe ein mehrfaches, teils lebensgefährliches Risiko durch Virusübertragungen und Überempfindlichkeitsreak-tionen gegenüber.

27. 4. Der Bundesverband Deutscher Ärzte für Frischzellen-Therapie hält die Verfassungsbeschwerde für zulässig und begründet. Es

habe seit 1983 keine bemerkenswerten Fälle gravierender Nebenwirkungen gegeben. Nach jahrzehntelangen praktischen Erfahrungen könne man davon ausgehen, dass ein erheblicher therapeutischer Nutzen bestehe, der nur mit einem geringen Restrisiko verbunden sei. Behandelt würden überwiegend ältere Menschen, die wegen der Nebenwirkun-gen sonstiger Arzneimittel und Therapien eine alternative Behandlung suchten.

28. V. Seit März 1997 hat das Bundesverfassungsgericht die Anwendung von § 1 Abs. 1 der Frischzellen-Verordnung bis zur Entscheidung in der Hauptsache einstweilen ausgesetzt, soweit die Herstellung der dort genannten Arzneimittel zur Injektion oder Infusion für eigene Patienten der herstellenden Ärzte erfolgt.

29. VI. In der mündlichen Verhandlung haben die Beschwerdeführer und das Bundesministerium für Gesundheit ihren Vortrag erläutert und vertieft.

30. B. Die Verfassungsbeschwerde ist zulässig.

31. Die Beschwerdeführer werden durch das strafbewehrte Verbot gegenwärtig und unmittelbar betroffen. Bis zum Erlass der Verordnung waren sie befugt, die für die Behandlung ihrer Patienten erforderlichen Zelltherapeutika herzustellen. Sie benötigten weder eine Herstellungserlaubnis nach dem Arzneimitt-elgesetz noch waren die Präparate selbst zulassungspflichtig nach diesem Gesetz. Den Beschwerdeführern ist dieser für sie ganz wesentliche Teil der beruflichen Betätigung genommen worden, ohne dass es eines Vollzugsaktes bedarf.

32. Gegen die geltend gemachte Grundrechtsverletzung können die Beschwerdeführer auch nicht anderweit Rechtsschutz vor den Fachgerichten erhalten. Unter dem Gesichtspunkt der Subsidiarität der Verfassungsbeschwerde kommt eine Verweisung auf einen solchen Rechtsschutz zwar in Betracht, wenn er in tatsächlicher und rechtlicher Hinsicht geeignet ist, die unmittelbaren Normwirkungen einer gerichtlichen Prüfung zu unterziehen, die den Anforderungen des Art. 19 Abs. 4 Satz 1 GG genügt (vgl. BVerfGE 71, 305 [337]).

33. Ein derartiger Rechtsschutz wurde von den Verwaltungsgerichten hier aber nicht gewährt. Ein Normenkontrollverfahren nach § 47 Abs. 1 Nr. 2 VwGO findet gegen Verordnungen des Bundes nicht statt. Feststellungsklagen, die die Wirksamkeit der Frischzellen-Verordnung betrafen, wurden von den Verwaltungsgerichten als unzulässig angesehen, weil sie ohne das zu fordernde hinreichend konkrete Rechtsverhältnis gegenüber den landesrechtlichen Arzneimittelbehörden der Sache nach eine Normenkontrolle zum Gegenstand hätten (vgl. dazu zuletzt Urteil des Bundesverwaltung-

sgerichts vom 30. September 1999 - 3 C 39. 98 -). Die Versuche der Beschwerdeführer, vor den Verwaltungsgerichten im Wege der einstweiligen Anordnung wirkungsvollen Rechtsschutz zu erlangen, waren demgemäß erfolglos.

34. C. Die Verfassungsbeschwerde ist begründet. Das angegriffene Verbot, mit dem in die durch Art. 12 Abs. 1 GG geschützte Berufsfreiheit der Beschwerdeführer eingegriffen wird, ist nicht kompetenzgemäß erlassen. § 1 Abs. 1 und § 2 Abs. 2 der Frischzellen-Verordnung sind verfassungswidrig und nichtig.

35. I. Die Verordnung überschreitet allerdings den durch den Wortlaut der Ermächtigungsnorm in § 6 Abs. 1 AMG und durch die Systematik des Gesetzes gezogenen Rahmen nicht (1.). Diese Norm ist aber unter Berücksichtigung der Kompetenzzuweisung in Art. 74 Abs. 1 Nr. 19 GG einschränkend auszulegen; der Bund ist nur befugt, die Herstellung solcher Arzneien gesetzlich oder im Verordnungswege zu regeln, die dazu bestimmt sind, in den Verkehr gebracht zu werden. Dazu gehören nicht Arzneimittel, die der Arzt selbst herstellt und beim Patienten anwendet (2.).

36. 1. Nach seinem Wortlaut ermächtigt § 6 AMG das Bundesministerium für Gesundheit auch zum Erlass von Verordnungen, die wie die angegriffene Regelung allein die Herstellung von Arzneimitteln betreffen.

37. a) Das Gesetz über den Verkehr mit Arzneimitteln soll im Interesse einer ordnungsgemäßen Arzneimittelversorgung von Mensch und Tier die Sicherheit im Verkehr mit Arzneimitteln, insbesondere die Qualität, Wirksamkeit und Unbedenklichkeit der Arzneimittel gewährleisten (vgl. § 1). In Ergänzung der gesetzlichen Ge- und Verbote enthält § 6 Abs. 1 AMG eine Verordnungsermächtigung für das Bundesministerium der Gesundheit, nach der die Verwendung bestimmter Stoffe, Zubereitungen aus Stoffen oder Gegenstände bei der Herstellung von Arzneimitteln vorgesch-rieben, beschränkt oder verboten werden dürfen, um eine unmittelbare oder mittelbare Gefährdung der Gesundheit von Mensch oder Tier durch Arzneimittel zu verhüten. Dieser Wortlaut erlaubt daher dem Verordnungsgeber, die Arzneimittelherstellung als solche zu regeln.

38. Daneben enthält § 6 Abs. 1 AMG auch eine Ermächtigung zu solchen Regelungen, die das Inverkehrbringen von Arzneimitteln betreffen. Die Ermächtigungsnorm unterscheidet demgemäß - ebenso wie das Arzneimittelgesetz im Übrigen - zwischen der Herstellung und dem Inverkehrbringen von Arzneimitteln. Die Herstellung wird in § 4 Abs. 14 AMG definiert als das Gewinnen, das Anfertigen, das Zubereiten, das Be- oder Verarbeiten, das Umfüllen einschließlich Abfüllen, das

Abpacken und das Kennzeichnen von Arzneimitteln. Hingegen definiert § 4 Abs. 17 AMG das Inverkehrbringen als das Vorrätighalten zum Verkauf oder zu sonstiger Abgabe, das Feilhalten, das Feilbieten und die Abgabe an andere.

39. b) Die Unterscheidung zwischen der Herstellung und der Abgabe als einer der Formen des Inverkehrbringens hat für zahlreiche arzneimittelrechtliche Regelungen Bedeutung. Was unter Abgabe in Zusammenhang mit der Herstellungserlaubnis nach § 13 AMG zu verstehen ist, wird in dessen Absatz 1 Satz 3 festgelegt: Eine Abgabe an andere liegt vor, wenn die Person, die das Arzneimittel herstellt, eine andere ist als die, die es anwendet.

40. Für das Arzneimittelrecht besteht daher in Rechtsprechung und Literatur Einigkeit darüber, dass bei der Herstellung durch einen Arzt, der das von ihm hergestellte Arzneimittel selbst am Patienten anwendet oder in seinen unmittelbaren Einwirkungsbereich durch weisungsgebundene Hilfskräfte oder durch den Patienten selbst anwenden lässt, keine Abgabe in diesem Sinne vorliegt (vgl. BVerwGE 94, 341; OVG NRW, NJW 1998, S. 847 in ausdrücklicher Abkehr von NJW 1989, S. 792; Deutsch, Medizinrecht, 3. Aufl., 1997, S. 534 f.; Hoppe, MedR 1996, S. 72 [73]; Kloesel/ Cyran, Arzneimittelrecht, Kommentar, § 13 Anm. 11 [Stand: Januar 1998]; Pabel, NJW 1989, S. 759 f.; Räpple, Das Verbot bedenklicher Arzneimittel, 1991, S. 36 ff.; Wolz, Bedenkliche Arzneimittel als Rechtsbegriff, 1988, S. 40 ff.). Ärzte brauchen deshalb keine Herstellungserlaubnis, solange sie die von ihnen hergestellten Arzneimittel nicht aus der Hand geben. Wenn das Arzneimittel an die Patienten oder andere Ärzte weitergegeben wird und damit die Verfügungsgewalt über das Arzneimittel wechselt, ist hingegen unter den Voraussetzungen des § 13 AMG eine Herstellungserlaubnis erforderlich.

41. Diese Auffassung steht in Übereinstimmung mit der Begründung des 1958 vorgelegten Entwurfs eines Gesetzes über den Verkehr mit Arzneimitteln (vgl. BTDrucks 3/ 654, S. 20). Damals wurde eine einheitliche gesetzliche Regelung des gesamten Arzneimittelverkehrs, der zuvor teilweise von der Gewerbeordnung oder einzelnen Verordnungen erfasst war, für erforderlich gehalten, weil die Bevölkerung inzwischen gegenüber früheren Zeiten erleichterten Zugang zu industriell gefertigten Arzneimitteln erhalten habe (vgl. BTDrucks a. a. O., S. 15 linke Spalte). Die landesrechtlichen Vorschriften zur Überwachung von Apothekern, Ärzten und Krankenhäusern wurden aber als selbstverständlich vorausgesetzt (BTDrucks a. a. O., S. 20 linke Spalte). Insbesondere

sollte die Verordnungsfreiheit von Ärzten nicht eingeschränkt werden (BTDrucks a. a. O., S. 16 linke Spalte, S. 18 rechte Spalte und S. 20 linke Spalte). Die Anwendung (Verabreichung, Injektion) eines Arzneimittels am Patienten in der Sprechstunde sollte ausdrücklich vom Abgabebegriff ausgenommen sein (BTDrucks a. a. O., S. 20 linke Spalte).

42. Die gesetzlichen Definitionen des Arzneimittelgesetzes bewirken danach eine Abgrenzung zwischen verschiedenen Formen ärztlicher Tätigkeit. Ärzte, die ihre eigenen Arzneimittel in Verkehr bringen, werden den allgemeinen Regeln des Arzneimittelrechts unterworfen; zugleich lässt aber das Arzneimittelgesetz die Therapiefreiheit des Arztes insoweit unangetastet, als die Anwendung von Arzneimitteln bei den eigenen Patienten nicht als Abgabe im Sinne des Arzneimittelrechts verstanden wird.

43. c) Die angegriffene Verordnung enthält in § 1 Abs. 1 keine Regelung, die im Sinne des Arzneimittelgesetzes den Verkehr mit Arzneimitteln oder ihre Abgabe an andere betrifft. Sie beschränkt sich vielmehr auf ein allgemeines Herstellungsverbot. Da aber solche ausschließlich auf die Herstellung bezogenen Regelungen dem Arzneimittelgesetz nicht durchgehend fremd sind (vgl. § 4 Abs. 14, § 8 Abs. 1 1. Alternative, § 54 Abs. 1 Satz 1), lassen sich allein aus der Systematik des Gesetzes keine Bedenken gegen die vom Bundesministerium für Gesundheit in Anspruch genommene Kompetenz herleiten.

44. 2. Dem Bundesgesetzgeber ist in Art. 74 Abs. 1 Nr. 19 GG indes nur die Kompetenz zur Regelung des Verkehrs mit Arzneimitteln eingeräumt. Diese umfasst deshalb nicht die unbeschränkte Zuständigkeit zur Regelung aller Fragen des Arzneimittelrechts. Die Verfassung zieht in Art. 74 Abs. 1 Nr. 19 GG die Grenze dort, wo es um den Verkehr mit Arzneimitteln im weitesten Sinne geht. Will der Bundesgesetzgeber zur Optimierung des Gesundheitsschutzes der Bevölkerung schon bei der Herstellung verkehrsfähiger Arzneimittel ansetzen, hält er sich so lange im Rahmen dieser Zuständigkeit, wie seine Regelung Arzneimittel betrifft, die zum Zwecke des Inverkehrbringens hergestellt werden.

45. a) Präventiver Gesundheitsschutz rechtfertigt frühzeitige Kontrolle, wenn mit der zunehmenden Länge des Vertriebsweges die Wirksamkeit staatlicher Überwachung mehr und mehr abgeschwächt wird. Besteht bei der Herstellung des Arzneimittels die Absicht, dieses über Apotheken oder sonstige Verkaufsstellen in den allgemeinen Verkehr zu bringen, ist mindestens eine bundesweite Verbreitung des Arzneimittels regelmäßig

angestrebt. Deshalb gibt es gute Gründe dafür, dass der Bund insoweit eine Befugnis zur konkurrierenden Gesetzgebung hat.

46. Das gilt jedoch nicht für solche vom Arzt hergestellten Arzneimittel, die nicht zur Abgabe bestimmt sind und die der Arzt auch tatsächlich nicht an Dritte abgibt. Solche Arzneien sind herkömmlich Teil ärztlicher Therapie, die in ihren Auswirkungen lokal auf den jeweils behandelten Kreis von Patienten begrenzt ist. Heilbehandlungen finden regelmäßig nur in einem begrenzten Wirkungskreis statt. Sie sind wesentlicher Bestandteil der ärztlichen Berufsausübungsfreiheit sowie Gegenstand der ärztlichen Sorgfaltspflicht und Verantwortung, für deren Überwachung die Länder zuständig sind.

47. b) Diese Abgrenzung zwischen der ärztlichen Behandlungsfreiheit und dem Arzneimittelrecht ist bisher - soweit ersichtlich - in Rechtsprechung und Literatur zu Art. 74 Abs. 1 Nr. 19 GG nicht ausdrücklich behandelt worden.

48. Der Umfang der dem Bund zugewiesenen Kompetenz war in der bisherigen Rechtsprechung des Bundesverfassungsgerichts nicht zweifelhaft. Soweit Arzneimittelrecht Gegenstand von Verfahren war, ging es stets um Kauf oder Verkauf und damit um den Verkehr mit Arzneimitteln (vgl. BVerfGE 9, 73; 17, 269; 20, 283; 75, 166). In der Literatur wird herkömmlich der Begriff des Verkehrs weit gefasst (vgl. Maunz, in: Maunz/ Dürig, Grundgesetz, Bd. IV, Art. 74 Rn. 219 [Stand: 1984]; Kunig, in: v. Münch/ Kunig, Grundgesetz-Kommentar, Bd. 3, 3. Aufl., 1996, Art. 74 Rn. 95; Pestalozza, in: v. Mangoldt/ Klein, Das Bonner Grundgesetz, Bd. 8, 3. Aufl., 1996, Art. 74 Rn. 1342 und 1436). Andererseits ist allgemein anerkannt, dass Art. 74 Abs. 1 Nr. 19 GG keine Globalermächtigung des Bundes für den Bereich des Gesundheitswesens darstellt, sondern dass enumerativ und spezifisch einige Felder aufgeführt sind, bei denen der Bund normierungsbefugt ist (vgl. Stettner, in: Dreier, Grundgesetz, 1998, Art. 74 Rn. 89; Degenhart, in: Sachs, Grundgesetz, 2. Aufl., 1999, Art. 74 Rn. 70). Auch wenn unter "Verkehr mit Arzneimitteln" der gesamte Umgang mit diesen Mitteln von der Herstellung über den Handel bis zum Verbrauch verstanden wird, so wird doch andererseits nicht bezweifelt, dass die Bundeskompetenz im Arztrecht auf Zulassungsfragen beschränkt ist (vgl. Maunz, a. a. O., Rn. 215 und 219) und sich nicht auf die ärztliche Berufsausübung insgesamt erstreckt.

49. c) Auch die historische Entwicklung des Kompetenztitels aus Art. 74 Abs. 1 Nr. 19 GG spricht gegen seine Inanspruchnahme für eine Befugnis des Gesetzgebers, die Herstellung von Arzneimitteln

unabhängig vom Verwendungszweck des Inverkehrbringens zu regeln und Bestimmungen über die Anwendung von selbst hergestellten Arzneien durch den Arzt zu treffen.

50. Ein Verkehr mit Arzneimitteln hat sich entwickelt, seitdem Apotheker nicht mehr als Hilfskräfte des Arztes auf Einzelanweisung Arzneimittel herstellen, und statt dessen Fertigarzneimittel den Markt bestimmen (vgl. zu dieser Entwicklung BVerfGE 9, 73 [80 f.]; 94, 372 [374 f.]; Giesbert, Die Abgabe von Arzneimitteln in rechtlicher Sicht, 1970, S. 2 ff.). Bei Schaffung des Grundgesetzes fand der Verfassungsgeber eine herkömmliche Teilung zwischen gewerberechtlichen Regelungen über Herstellung und Vertrieb von Arzneimitteln einerseits und dem Arztrecht andererseits vor. Hauptausschuss und Zuständigkeitsausschuss des Parlamentarischen Rates bekräftigten ausdrücklich, dass außer dem Recht der Zulassung zu den ärztlichen Berufen das Arztrecht Ländersache bleiben sollte (vgl. JöR, N. F., Bd. 1, 1951, S. 540 bis 543).

51. Der Verkehr mit Arzneimitteln wurde weder begrifflich noch inhaltlich problematisiert. Insoweit gab es eine mehr als siebzigjährige Tradition reichsrechtlicher Regelungen, die den Begriff des Verkehrs mit Arzneimitteln bei Erlass des Grundgesetzes in einem eindeutigen Sinn belegten (vgl. die Verordnung, betreffend den Verkehr mit Apothekerwaaren, vom 25. März 1872 [RGBl S. 85]; die Verordnung, betreffend den Verkehr mit Arzneimitteln, vom 4. Januar 1875 [RGBl S. 5]; die Verordnung, betreffend den Verkehr mit Arzneimitteln, vom 27. Januar 1890 [RGBl S. 9] sowie die Folgeverordnungen vom 31. Dezember 1894 [RGBl 1895, S. 1], vom 25. November 1895 [RGBl S. 455], vom 19. August 1897 [RGBl S. 707], vom 22. Oktober 1901 [RGBl S. 380] und vom 31. März 1911 [RGBl S. 181]; vgl. auch die Verordnung über den Verkehr mit Arzneimitteln vom 4. Oktober 1933 [RGBl I S. 721] und die Verordnung über die Herstellung von Arzneifertigwaren vom 11. Februar 1943 [RGBl I S. 99]). Es stand danach bei Erlass des Grundgesetzes außer Zweifel, dass der Begriff des Verkehrs mit Arzneimitteln das Feilhalten und den Verkauf von Arzneien an den Endverbraucher betraf. Nur in diesem Zusammenhang waren auch ergänzend Regelungen über die Herstellung von Fertigarznei-mitteln erlassen worden. Die Herstellung von Arzneien und ihre unmittelbare Anwendung durch Ärzte waren niemals Gegenstand reichsgesetzlicher Vorschriften über den Verkehr mit Arzneimit-teln gewesen. Die Kompetenzregel des Art. 74 Abs. 1 Nr. 19 GG wurde daher im Parlamentarischen Rat - Ausschuss für

Zuständigkeitsabgrenzung - nach langen Debatten darüber, wie die Zuständigkeitsabgrenzung zwischen Bund und Ländern beim Arztrecht erfolgen solle, bezüglich des Arzneimittelverkehrs ohne jede Diskussion angenommen (vgl. Parlamentarischer Rat, Ausschuss für Zuständigkeitsabgrenzung [Wortprotokolle], Teil 1, Bd. 6 b; Protokoll der 3. Sitzung vom 23. September 1948, S. 162).

52. d) Dem entspricht das umgangssprachliche Verständnis, das den Verkehr mit Gegenständen, seien es Arzneimittel oder Lebensmittel, kaufmännisch als den "Umsatz oder den Vertrieb von Waren" versteht (vgl. Duden, Das große Wörterbuch der deutschen Sprache, Bd. 8, 2. Aufl., 1995, S. 3672 f.; Grimm, Deutsches Wörterbuch, Bd. 25, 1956, Spalte 625). Der Verkehr steht insoweit synonym für den Handel mit den entsprechenden Gegenständen, meint jedoch nicht jedes Erzeugen und Gebrauchmachen.

53. e) Der Kompetenztitel des Art. 74 Abs. 1 Nr. 19 GG zielt danach auf die Kontrolle von Arzneifertigwaren (Spezialitäten) oder sonst industriell hergestellten Arzneimitteln ab. Die traditionell in Länderkompetenz liegenden Systeme der Kontrolle über die Tätigkeit von Apothekern und Ärzten sollten hierdurch nicht berührt werden. Der Begriff des Arzneimittelverkehrs umfasst daher nicht die von Ärzten praktizierte Behandlungsmethode, bei ihren Patienten selbst hergestellte Arzneimittel unmittelbar anzuwenden. In die ärztliche Behandlung kann durch Rechtsvorschriften des Arzneimittelverkehrs mittelbar vor allem eingegriffen werden, soweit Regelungen für Fertigarzneimittel von den Ärzten bei ihrer Verschreibung zu beachten sind.

54. Unter Beachtung dieser verfassungsrechtlichen Vorgaben ist § 6 Abs. 1 AMG dahin auszulegen, dass die Verwendung bestimmter Stoffe bei der Herstellung von Arzneimitteln nur dann durch Rechtsverordnung des Bundes verboten werden darf, wenn die Arzneimittel zum Zwecke der Abgabe an andere hergestellt werden. Eine weitergehende Rechtsetzungsdelegation verletzte die dem Bundesgesetzgeber durch Art. 74 Abs. 1 Nr. 19 GG gezogenen Grenzen.

55. 3. Das generelle Herstellungsverbot nach § 1 Abs. 1 der Frischzellen-Verordnung und die Strafbewehrung in § 2 Abs. 2 der Frischzellen-Verordnung sind demnach nicht durch die Ermächtigung des § 6 Abs. 1 AMG gedeckt. Eine verfassungskonforme Auslegung der angegriffenen Vorschriften ist nicht möglich, weil § 1 Abs. 2 der Frischzellen-Verordnung für die Arzneimittel, die in den Verkehr gebracht werden, eine

selbständige Regelung enthält. Als Anwendungsbereich des Absatzes 1 bleiben daher nur Frischzellen, die von Ärzten hergestellt und unmittelbar angewendet werden. Nur dieser Teil der Verordnung ist mangels Regelungskompetenz des Bundes nichtig; die Verordnung im Übrigen, die mit der Verfassungsbeschwerde nicht angegriffen worden ist, bleibt unberührt.

56. Ob ein Verbot der Herstellung von Frischzellen zur unmittelbaren Anwendung beim Patienten durch den Arzt aus Gründen des Gesundheitsschutzes gerechtfertigt ist, war hier nicht zu entscheiden.

57. II. Art. 14 Abs. 1 GG kommt als Prüfungsmaßstab nicht in Betracht. Er wird hier von Art. 12 Abs. 1 GG als dem sachnäheren Grundrecht verdrängt. Art. 14 Abs. 1 GG schützt das Erworbene, die Ergebnisse geleisteter Arbeit, Art. 12 Abs. 1 GG dagegen den Erwerb, die Betätigung selbst (vgl. BVerfGE 84, 133 [157]). Hier greift die Verordnung in die Freiheit der individuellen Erwerbs- und Berufsmöglichkeiten ein, weshalb der Schutzbereich des Art. 12 Abs. 1 GG berührt ist. Die Begrenzung der Innehabung und Verwendung vorhandener Vermögensgüter, für die der Schutz des Art. 14 GG grundsätzlich in Betracht kommt, ist hier nur mittelbare Folge der angegriffenen Handlungsbeschränkung.

58. III. Die Entscheidung über die Kosten beruht auf § 34 a Abs. 2 BVerfGG.

Here is the English translation of the ruling of the German Supreme Court.

IN THE NAME OF THE PEOPLE
In the prosecution of the complaints made by the Constitutional Plaintiffs

Dr. A ....' Dr. B ....' Dr. J ....' Dr. M ....

Counsel appearing on behalf of the Plaintiffs: Felix Busse and Partners, 21 Oxford Street, Bonn -
Complaining against § sub-sections 1 and 2 of the Fresh Cell Regulations (Federal Gazette I page 432) promulgated on March 4, 1997, prohibiting the application of certain substances in the preparation of medical treatment,

Appearing before the Constitutional Court - First Chamber - with participation of the

Vice Judge President Papier,
Honourable Justices Grimm,
Kühling,
Jaeger
Haas'
Hömig'
Steiner
and Hohmann – Dennhardt,

recording reasons in writing for the judgment delivered verbatim on November 9, 1999, judgment is as follows

JUDGMENT

i. § 1 and 2 of the Fresh Cell Regulations (Federal Gazette I page 432) promulgated on March 4, 1997, which prohibits the application of certain substances in the preparation of medical treatment, are found to be inconsistent with the provisions of § 12 (1) of the Constitution., and are thus null and void.

ii. The Federal Republic of Germany furnished the Plaintiffs with the necessary documentation.

REASONS

All of the Plaintiffs are physicians. The Plaintiffs vigorously appeal against the constitutionality of § sub-sections 1 and 2 of the Fresh Cell Regulations (Federal Gazette I page 432) promulgated on March 4, 1997, prohibiting the application of certain substances in the preparation of medical treatment, under which statute, it is a criminal offense to produce the medicine for treatment, to be administered by way of injection or infusion. This Regulation was promulgated by the Federal Department of Health on October 19, 1994, in accordance with § 6 of the Drug Act regulating any dealing with medicine:

> "The Federal Department of Health (Federal Department) is granted the right by the Federal Council of States (Senate) to limit, prescribe, and prohibit the application of certain identified substances in the preparation and production of medicine, destined for treatment and to limit, prescribe, and prohibit the distribution of such medicine or treatment, which are not prepared or produced in accordance with the provisions of the statute, and to prohibit the endangerment of man and animal through administering such medical treatment".

The provisions complained about in the Fresh Cell Regulations are as follows:

§1 Prohibition of the use of Fresh Cells

(1) The use of Fresh Cells in the preparation of medical treatment to be administered by way of injection or infusion is prohibited.
(2) to (5) ...

§ 2 Criminal Offences and Fines

(1) ...

(2) Subject to § 96 number 1 of the Drug Act, it shall be a criminal offense to use fresh cells contrary to the meaning of § 1 sub-section 1.

(3) ...

It is questionable whether it was the purpose of the Drug Act to prevent the preparation of fresh cells for the purpose of administering it to patients by physicians.

A.

I.

1. In principle, fresh cell therapy entails the injection of living animal cells into patients with the anticipation of achieving a revitalising effect. In general these cells are harvested from sheep's fetus. The donor animals are of the female sex and originate from closed herds; and thereby the transmission of certain illnesses is avoided.

   Fresh cell therapy is classified as a so called alternative treatment method. Fresh cell therapists are of the opinion that the injected cells *relate to the corresponding organs' unique 'repair mechanisms' by stimulating them, and is thus helpful in the re-creation of new and healthy cells or tissues.* Orthodox medical community maintains its critical posture that improperly practiced fresh cell therapy holds the potential of high risk, especially of allergic reactions, auto-immune reactions and transmission of infections.

2. The Fresh Cells Regulation is based on the regulations issued by the Federal Department of Health in 1992 and 1994, and supported by the earlier reports of the Science Committee of the Federal Medical Council. The prohibition is founded upon the perceived danger of fresh cell therapy (Federal Republic Publishers 38/97, pages 4 to 7). *During 1987 the Federal Department of Health relaxed its position by allowing all fresh stem cell therapy*, in accordance with the interim provisions of the Drug Act, which regulations are still in force (compare the article appearing in the Pharmaceutical Newspaper 1987, page 1999).

II.

The Constitutional Plaintiffs brought the following factual arguments before the court:

They are all exclusively in private practice of medicine and specialize in fresh cell therapy. The Appellants have kept herds of sheep for several years for the specific purpose of harvesting fresh cells.

1. The First Appellant is a medical doctor, a general practicioner. In 1991 he became the proprietor of a private clinic, which has been offering intensive fresh cell therapy since its inception of 1977. The 60 bed clinic employs 53 staff members. Fresh cell therapy accounts for over half of the clinic's annual turnover, and many patients are coming back for repeat treatments.

2. The Second Appellant took a 45 bed sanatorium over from her father, who had been practicing fresh cell therapy since 1951. She employs 41 people and generates her income singularly from the provision of fresh cell therapy. Most patients visit the clinic for repetitive therapy.

3. The Third Appellant has been specialising in fresh cell therapy since 1968. He practices as a licensed medical practitioner, provides employment to 4 persons, and works in conjunction with a health spa. The number of patients and turnover is remaining the same.

4. The Fourth Appellant is a medical practitioner specializing in Urology. He has been managing a 42 bed clinic with 29 employees since 1980, concentrating on cell therapy, which represents more than three quarters of his turnover.

III.

The Constitutional Plaintiffs come before this Court after being convicted in terms of the provisions of § 1 sub-section 1 and § 2 sub-section 2 of the Fresh Cells Regulation, and complain against an infringement of their fundamental rights afforded under Article 12, sub-section 1, and Article 14, sub-section 1 of the Constitution.

This court upholds the complaint. An immediate criminal judgment under § 1 sub-section 1 of the Fresh Cells Regulation was entered against the Appellants. The complaint before this court is allowed. *The Drug Act does not grant the Regulatory Authority the right to intervene in the therapeutic freedom of medical practitioners.* Article 74 sub-sections 1, number 19 of the Constitution, allows for a concurrent legislative competence *only in as far as the distribution of drugs is concerned.* The Federal legislature is allowed to regulate only the distribution of drugs, and to delegate such legislative regulatory authority. Distribution in its ordinary meaning does not include a comprehensive dealing with drugs starting with the manufacture, the distribution, and its consumption. *The Federal legislative authority is limited to an imposition of regulations regarding the distribution of drugs. Fresh Cells are not included in this category of drugs, as they are not brought directly into distribution channels.* It is prepared by the practitioner himself and used in his own practice. This practice is governed by the local State authorities of that particular State. *The manufacture or preparation of fresh cells does not pose any significant danger and seems to be forbidden only to discourage the physicians from using fresh cell therapy.*

There is a difference between the prohibition of the manufacture of fresh cells and the fresh cell therapy itself. The factual assertion by the Federal Department of Health states that fresh cell therapy is useless on one side, without effect, and without any reliable statistics. *All patients are explained the therapeutic procedure and treatment is carried out only upon the patient's consent.* Institutions specializing in this therapy have found it necessary to introduce an interim regulation regarding this.

IV.

Appearing on behalf of the Plaintiff, the Federal Department of Health on behalf of the Federal Government, Federal Institute of Drugs and Medicinal Products, Federal Medical Council as well as the German Association of Fresh Cell Therapists, argued as follows:

1. The Federal Department of Health holds the complaints of the Constitutional Plaintiffs as unsubstantiated. The Fresh Cell Regulation was competently promulgated and is constitutional to be applied. Article 74, sub-section 1, number 19 of the Constitution, contains the dealing with drugs from manufacture to consumption, in consideration of encompassing comprehen-sive protection to patients. In consideration of extending an effective avoidance of danger, it demands to conduct research into the manufacturing process of drugs. In that way it could be determined with certainty whether the manufacturing poses any risk. It is further not possible to discern a limitation on the legislative competence in the definition section of the Drug Act. This subject further impinges on the subject of Veterinary Surgery and has relations to anaesthetic substance, as well as far reaching prescriptions regarding the manufacture, like the prohibitive clause under consideration.

   The Regulation refers to the principle of reasonability. It is desirable to protect patients from potential life threatening danger and to protect general health. Even in the instance of medical practitioners administering self manufactured drugs, the general principle of professionalism and law must prevail, to prevent harm from coming to patients and to treat patients to his best knowledge and ability. Fresh cell therapy does not observe these general principles in the manufacture of drugs. The 1994 publication of the Federal Department of Health issued a warning against perceived dangers (immediate allergic reactions, rejection reactions, auto-immunological reactions and the transmission of Scrapie, mad cow disease, rabies and Procolosis), which justifies an immediate limitation.

2. The Federal Institute of Drugs and Medicinal Products maintains the position that an error in the preparation of fresh cells is risky because there is no margin of safety in this treatment. *The documentation presented by the Constitutional Plaintiffs provides no valid reason for existence of such risk and thereby any need for an avoidance of risk.*

3. The Federal Medical Council supported by the German Medical Practitioners' Drugs Commission (special committee to the Medical Council) negates the validity of the Constitutional Plaintiffs defense. The provisions of the Fresh Cell Regulations are welcomed. To date no working document regarding fresh cells is available. Little mention of fresh cells is found in medical history, and it is normally limited to preliminary observations only. The use of fresh cell

therapy has no conclusive proofs, and triggers multiple life threatening risks through virus transmission and allergic reactions.

4. *The German Medical Association of Fresh Cell Therapists supports the case brought forward by the Constitutional Plaintiffs. Since 1983 no significant cases of side effects were recorded. Years of practical experience has taught that a medical therapeutic use does exist, with only a slight risk.* The majority of patients are elderly people for whom, through the side effects of other drugs, no alternative treatment is available.

V.

Since March 1997 the Constitutional Court avoided to decide upon the precise interpretation of § 1 sub-section 1 of the Fresh Cell Regulation, insofar the production of medications mentioned within the provisions of the statute for the purposes of injection or infusion to patients by medical doctors who prepare their own cells.

VI.

The oral presentations made by the Plaintiffs and the Federal Department of Health accentuated the case.

B.

The Constitutional Complaints are allowed. The Constitutional Plaintiffs had the immediate judgment of the prohibition entered against them. *Until the enactment of the Regulation they were allowed to practice the treatment of their patients by self prepared fresh cells. They were not required to hold specific permit under the Drug Act for the production of medications nor was the prepared substance the subject of licensing under the Act. The Constitutional Plaintiffs were not party to any unlawful activity* for a great part of their professional careers.

The Constitutional Plaintiffs are not allowed to approach another specialist Court in the light of the complaints of infringement of fundamental rights. The viewpoint that the constitutional complaint makes no direct reference to lawful protection of a fundamental right, for which it is entitled to, and that the immediate judicial hearing is needed, is in accordance with the mentioned Article 19 sub-section 4 sentence 1 of the Constitution.

Such legal protection is not guaranteed by the judiciary. A norm control check in accordance with § 47 sub-section 1 number 2 VwGO did not take place according to the Federal guidelines. The complaints regarding the Fresh Cell Regulation were not allowed by the judiciary, as it did not hold any relation to the local State Drug Agencies (compare the judgement of the Federal Administrative Court of September 30, 1999 - 3 C 39.98 -). The attempts by the Constitutional Plaintiffs to secure legal protection were unsuccessful.

C.

The constitutional complaint is allowed. The complained about prohibition limiting the entrenched freedom of profession in accordance with Article 12 sub-section 1 of the Constitution, was not competently promulgated. *§ 1 sub-section 1 and § 2 sub-section 2 of the Fresh Cell Regulation is not consistent with the constitution and is null and void.*

I.

The Regulation is inconsistent with the wording of the rights granting § 6 sub-section 1 of the Drug Act. In retrospect, the norm inferred by the competency clause contained in Article 74 sub-section 1 number 19 of the Constitution must be construed with limitation, that the Federal authority is competent to prescribe the manufacture of drugs destined for public distribution only. *Drugs manufactured by the physician himself to be administered to his patients do not form part of this category.*

1. The Federal Department of Health is permitted subject to the wording of § 6 of the Drugs Act to issue regulations like that of the complained about regulations, regarding the manufacturing of drugs.

    a) The Act must, regarding the distribution of drugs, achieve quality, effectiveness, and harmlessness in the interest of legal certainty for the provision of safety of drugs for use by humans and animals. To complement the statutory provisions and prohibitions, the Federal Department of Health is granted rights by a regulatory authority to regulate the application of certain substances, preparations made from a substance or restrictions on the manufacturing of drugs, to limit, or to prohibit, direct or indirect risk or danger to the health of human or animal through drugs.

§ 6 of the Drug Act further contains the authority to regulate the distribution of drugs. The norm of authority, as found within the confines of the Drug Act, differentiates between the manufacturing and the distribution of drugs. Manufacturing is defined in § 4 sub-section 14 of the Drug Act, to include profit, manufacture, preparation, processing, pouring, decanting, packaging and labeling and identification of drugs. In contrast, § 4 sub-section 17 of the Drug Act defines distribution as the keeping of stock for the purpose of sale, or other handling , the offer for sale, and the handling thereof, and other.

b) The difference between the manufacturing and the handling as one of the forms of distribution has application to many Drug Regulations. Meaning is lent to the term handling in conjunction with the authority to manufacture by § 13 subsection 1 sentence 3 of the Drug Act: a *handling occurs when the person manufacturing the drug is a different person from who administers it.*

Legal literature and legal precedents agree that the *person manufacturing drugs for treatment of his patients or direct administration by patients themselves does not constitute handling. Medical doctors, therefore, do not require any permission to manufacture, as long as the manufactured drugs do not leave their hands.* The moment the drug is distributed or supplied to other physicians or patients, this action falls within the scope of § 13 of the Drug Act, and requires the issuance of specific permission.

This supposition is in accordance with the provisions of a 1958 Bill dealing with the distribution of drugs. This Bill had as its purpose the consolidation of statutory regulation of the distribution of drugs, which was previously regulated by a singular statute, in an era where people had more easy access to manufactured medication. The consolidation of State regulation of pharmacies, doctors' surgeries and hospitals, was a purpose. *It was not the purpose of the statute to limit the medical profession. The administering of medicine to patients during consultation was specifically not included as having the meaning of handling* and if indeed it did contain the meaning it would have been removed.

The statutory definition included in the Drug Act aims to curb the disparity between different forms of activities performed by medical doctors. Medical doctors who manufacture and distribute their products are the subject of the Act. On the other hand *the Act sanctifies the freedom of treatment of doctors who provide medicine they themselves have prepared for treatment of their own patients*, and the Act does not construe these activities as being handling.

c) The complained about § 1 sub-section 1 does not contain any provision pertaining to the distribution or handling of drugs. They limit themselves much more by pleading a general prohibition on manufacturing. The regulations governing manufacturing is of single importance and is not alien to this type of proceedings, although the structure of the Drug Act does not leave any doubt about the origin of the Federal Department of Health's legislative competence.

2. The Federal Legislature in Article 74 subsection 1 number 19 of the Constitution *grants only the authority to regulate the distribution of drugs. This does not mean that the legislature have an unlimited competence to regulate every aspect of the law relating to medicine.* The Constitution therefore imposes a limit to the distribution thereof.

   a) Preventive health regulation justifies additional control, when in the light of increasing business the control by the State diminishes. If the purpose of manufacture is the distribution to pharmacies or other such sale points, the extension of regulation is needed nationwide. It is, therefore, desirable for the legislature to posses such statutory powers. The latter *does not apply to medical doctors who manufacture for the exclusive purpose of not distributing it to third parties. This type of prepared medicine or medication is classified as medical therapy, given to the patient dedicated as the treatment on the spot. The freedom to use a certain therapy must form a significant part of the medical doctor's freedom to exercise his profession, whilst not neglecting his primary responsibility to the wellbeing of the patient.* The regulation of such practice should be the responsibility of the local State Government.

   b) The proper delimitation of the freedom of exercising a profession and the law of medicine has not been dealt with exhaustively by literature and legal precedent.

   The previous legal precedents have left no doubt as to the extend of the awarded legislative competence to the Constitutional Court. In its simplest form the matter of regulating the legal position of medicine is still that of supply and demand on the open market, i.e. distribution. Researching the meaning of distribution, the majority of legal literature teaches us that distribution lends itself to a wide interpretation. On the other hand it could be argued that Article 74 sub-section 1 number 19 of the Constitution does not recognize an unqualified authority by the government to regulate the medical profession, but rather suggests a selective or specific regulation. In the instance where the weighing up of distribution of medicine or drugs and manufacturing to the end user is under consideration, it is still only concerned about the distribution and consumption of drugs by the consumer and does not touch the freedom of therapy and profession awarded to every physician.

c) Historically, Article 74 subsection 1 number 19 of the Constitution, *makes a distinction between the legislative authority of the government regarding the manufacture of drugs, manufactured for the purpose of general public distribution and preparation of medicine destined only for the purposes determined by the doctor.*

Dealings with medicine underwent significant development during the last years. Traditionally the chemist was the physician's first port of call in the assistance with the preparation of medication. Since then, mass produced drugs are readily available to the patient and the doctor. When the Constitution was drafted, the Constitutional Assembly found themselves confronted with the rights of the government to regulate the manufacturing and the distribution of medicine to the market on the one hand and the legal rights of the medical doctor on the other. The scale was finally balanced, when the Constitutional Assembly acknowledged the government's rights to set standards for the medical profession, and further recommended that the regulation of the medical profession is a matter for local State regulation.

The water did not remain clear for long. The concept of dealing with medicine was severely complicated by a plethora of legislation promulgated during the last and its preceding centuries, (compare the provisions of the Dealing in Pharmaceutical Products Regulation of march 25, 1872, Dealing in Drugs Regulation of January 4, 1875, Dealing in Drugs Regulation of January 27, 1890, Consequences Regulation of December 31, 1894, RGBI 1895 page 1, RGBI of November 25, 1895 page 455, of August 19, 1897 page 707, October 22, 1901 page 380, of March 31, 1911 page 181,

October 4, 1933 page 721, The Manufacturing of Ready Made Drugs Regulation of February 11, 1943 page 99). The legal uncertainty surrounding the dealing, manufacturing, distribution and sale of drugs, was to be expected. However, *the imperial legislation does not impinge upon the rights of the doctor to prepare drugs for immediate dispatch to his patients.* The legislative authority of the Federal Government invited long sessions of debate by the members of the Constitutional Assembly. A virtual stand-off resulted therein when some members sought to protect the rights of the local state to regulate the medical profession in its jurisdiction. In the end, the Federal Government's authority to regulate dealing in drugs was upheld (Minutes of the Constitutional Assembly of September 23, 1948, page 162).

d) Ordinary language lends an inclusive meaning to the word 'dealing' as having the meaning of 'turnover or the sale of goods' (Duden, The Great Dictionary of the German Language Volume 8 page 3672 and Grimm, German Dictionary page 626). Dealing is brought in direct context with trade as its synonym, although in this context it does not bare such a meaning by every manufacturer and user.

e) It appears that Article 74 subsection 1 number 19 of the Constitution, has as its principal purpose the regulation of ready-made drugs manufactured *en masse* by industry. The rights of the local State to regulate the activities of pharmacists and doctors within its jurisdiction is left unaffected. *The term dealing or distribution of drugs does not include the preparation of drugs by doctors for the treatment of their own patients.* However, the dealing in ready-made drugs remains a regulated activity under the authority of the Federal Government.

Considering this, *it is apparent that the provisions of § 6 subsection 1 of the Drug Act only bring on sanctions contained in the Act in the event of a person manufacturing drugs for distribution to other people. The statutory authority of the legislature overstepped the boundaries of the limitations clause contained in Article 74 subsection 1 number 19 of the Constitution.*

3. The general prohibitory clauses contained in § 1 subsection 1 and § 2 subsection 2 of the Fresh Cells Regulation, is not covered under the provisions of § 6 subsection 1 of the Drug Act. It is not possible for

this Court to strike the complained legislation down as it is not applicable to this situation but rather to the situation where drugs are manufactured and distributed to others. *Only subsection 1 of the Fresh Cells Regulations is held to be null and void,* the rest of the statute remains in force.

The Court finds that it is not needed to decide whether doctors manufacturing drugs for the treatment of their own patients is in the best interest of the protection of health.

II.

Article 14, sub-section 1, of the Constitution did not play any role in discharging the burden of proof in this instance. The provisions of Article 12, subsection 1, of the Constitution replaced the application of Article 14 in this instance. Article 14 protects the rights of the acquisition, the result of the action, whereas Article 12 protects the acquired, action itself. This matter was decided on the individual freedom of the employee, or freedom of profession, i.e. Article 12.

III.

The award of costs in the matter shall be determined in accordance with § 34 a subsection 2 BverfGG.

The above decision of the German Supreme Court is legally related to certain parts of the 2001/83/EC European Community Council Directive, which in turn had become incorporated in national laws of all Member States of European Union, as mandated by Maastricht Treaty. Since the entire 2001/83/EC Directive, created as a replacement of all regulations related to medical therapeutics issued by the European Parliament and Council since 1965, is too long to include in this book, the pertinent parts are extracted here. Parts related to the stem cell xenotransplantation are italicized.

The following paragraphs are taken verbatim from 2001/83/EC.

**Directive 2001/83/EC
of The European Parliament and of The Council
of November 2001
On the Community Code Relating to Medicinal Products
for Human Use**

THE EUROPEAN PARLIAMENT AND THE COUNCIL OF THE EUROPEAN UNION

Having regard to the Treaty establishing the European Community, and in particular Article 95 thereof; having regard to the proposal from the Commission; having regard to the opinion of the Economic and Social Committee; and acting in accordance with the procedure laid down in Article 251 of the Treaty, whereas:

(1) Council Directive 65/65/EEC of January 26, 1965 on the approximation of provisions laid down by law, regulation or administrative action relating to medicinal products, Council Directive 75/318/EEC of May 20, 1975 on the approximation of the laws of Member States relating to analytical, pharmaco-toxicological and clinical standards and protocols in respect of the testing of proprietary medicinal products, Council Directive 75/ 319/EEC of May 20, 1975 on the approximation of provisions laid down by law, regulation or administrative action relating to proprietary medicinal products, Council Directive 89/342/EEC of May 3, 1989 extending the scope of Directives 65/65/EEC and 75/319/EEC and laying down additional provisions for immuno-logical medicinal products consisting of vaccines, toxins or serums and allergens, Council Directive 89/343/EEC of May 3, 1989 extending the scope of Directives 65/65/EEC and 75/319/EEC and laying down additional provisions for radiopharmaceuticals, Council Directive 89/381/EEC of June 14, 1989 extending the scope of Directives 65/65/EEC and 75/319/EEC on the approximation of provisions laid down by law, regulation or administrative action relating to medicinal products and laying down special provisions for proprietary medicinal products derived from human blood or human plasma, Council Directive 92/25/EEC of March 31, 1992 on the wholesale distribution of medicinal products for human use, Council Directive 92/26/EEC of March 31, 1992 concerning the classification for the supply of medicinal products for human use, Council Directive 92/27/EEC of March 31, 1992, on the labelling of medicinal products for human use and on package leaflets, Council Directive 92/28/EEC of March 31, 1992, on the advertising of medicinal products for human use, Council Directive 92/73/EEC of September 22, 1992, widening the scope of Directives 65/65/EEC and 75/319/EEC on the approximation of provisions laid down by law, regulation or administrative action relating to medicinal products and laying down additional provisions on homeopathic medicinal products, have been frequently and substantially amended. In the interests of clarity and rationality, the said Directives should therefore be codified by assembling them in a single text.

(2) The essential aim of any rules governing the production, distribution and use of medicinal products must be to safeguard public health.

(3) However, this objective must be attained by means which will not hinder the development of the pharmaceutical industry or trade in medicinal products within the Community.

(4) *Trade in medicinal products within the Community is hindered by disparities between certain national provisions, in particular between provisions relating to medicinal products* (excluding substances or combinations of substances which are foods, animal feeding-stuffs or toilet preparations), *and such disparities directly affect the functioning of the internal market.*

(5) *Such hindrances must accordingly be removed; whereas this entails approximation of the relevant provisions.*

(6) *In order to reduce the disparities which remain, rules should be laid down on the control of medicinal products and the duties incumbent upon the Member States' competent authorities should be specified with a view to ensuring compliance with legal requirements.*

(12) With the exception of those medicinal products which are subject to the centralized Community authorization procedure established by Council Regulation (EEC) No 2309/93 of July 22, 1993 laying down Community procedures for the authorization and supervision of medicinal products for human and veterinary use and establishing a European Agency for the Evaluation of Medicinal Products *a marketing authorization for a medicinal product granted by a competent authority in one Member State ought to be recognized by the competent authorities of the other Member States* unless there are serious grounds for supposing that the authorization of the medicinal product concerned may present a risk to public health. In the event of a disagreement between Member States about the quality, the safety or the efficacy of a medicinal product, a scientific evaluation of the matter should be undertaken according to a Community standard, leading to a single decision on the area of disagreement binding on the Member States concerned. Whereas this decision should be adopted by a rapid procedure ensuring close cooperation between the Commission and the Member States.

(30) In this connection persons moving around within the Community have the right to carry a reasonable quantity of medicinal products lawfully obtained for their personal use. *It must also be possible for a person established in one Member State to receive from another Member State a reasonable quantity of medicinal products intended for his personal use.*

TITLE II
Article 5

A Member State may, in accordance with legislation in force, and to fulfil special needs, exclude from the provisions of this Directive medicinal products supplied in response to a bona fide unsolicited order, formulated in accordance with the specifications of an authorized health care professional, and for use by his individual patients on his direct personal responsibility.

TITLE III
Article 10

1. In derogation of Article 8(3)(i), and without prejudice to the law relating to the protection of industrial and commercial property:

    (a) The applicant shall not be required to provide the results of toxicological and pharmacological tests or the results of clinical trials, if he can demonstrate:
    (i) either that the medicinal product is essentially similar to a medicinal product authorized in the Member State concerned by the application, and that the holder of the marketing authorization for the original medicinal product has consented to the toxicological, pharmacological and/or clinical references contained in the file on the original medicinal product being used for the purpose of examining the application in question;
    (ii) that the constituent or constituents of the medicinal product have a well established medicinal use, with recognized efficacy and an acceptable level of safety, by means of a detailed scientific bibliography;
    (iii) *that the medicinal product is essentially similar to a medicinal product which has been authorized within the Community, in accordance with Community provisions in force, for not less than six years* and is marketed in the Member State for which the application is made. This period shall be extended to 10 years in the case of high-technology medicinal products

having been authorised according to the procedure laid down in Article 2(5) of Council Directive 87/22/EEC. Furthermore, a Member State may also extend this period to 10 years by a single Decision covering all the medicinal products marketed on its territory where it considers this necessary in the interest of public health. Member States are at liberty not to apply the six-year period beyond the date of expiry of a patent protecting the original medicinal product. However, where the medicinal product is intended for a different therapeutic use from that of the other medicinal products marketed, or is to be administered by different routes, or in different doses, the results of appropriate toxicological and pharmacological tests and/or of appropriate clinical trials must be provided.

   (b) In the case of new medicinal products containing known constituents not hitherto used in combination for therapeutic purposes, the results of toxicological and pharmacological tests, and of clinical trials relating to that combination must be provided, but it shall not be necessary to provide references relating to each individual constituent.

2. Annex I shall apply by analogy where, pursuant to point (ii) of paragraph 1, (a), bibliographic references to published data are submitted.

TITLE VI
Article 71

1. Medicinal products shall be subject to medical prescription where they:

   - are likely to present a danger, either directly or indirectly, even when used correctly, if utilized without medical supervision,
   - are frequently and to a very wide extent used incorrectly, and as a result are likely to present a direct or indirect danger to human health,
   - contain substances, or preparations thereof, the activity and/or adverse reactions of which require further investigation,
   - are normally prescribed by a doctor to be administered parenterally.

2. Where Member States provide for the sub-category of medicinal products subject to special medical prescription, they shall take account of the following factors:

   - the medicinal product contains, in a non-exempt quantity, a substance classified as a narcotic or a psychotropic substance

within the meaning of the international conventions in force, such as the United Nations Conventions of 1961 and 1971,
- the medicinal product is likely, if incorrectly used, to present a substantial risk of medicinal abuse, to lead to addiction or be misused for illegal purposes,
- the medicinal product contains a substance which, by reason of its novelty or properties, could be considered as belonging to the group envisaged in the second indent as a precautionary measure.

3. Where Member States provide for the sub-category of medicinal products subject to restricted prescription, they shall take account of the following factors:

- the medicinal product, because of its pharmaceutical characteristics, or novelty, or in the interests of public health, is reserved for treatments which can only be followed in a hospital environment,
- the medicinal product is used in the treatment of conditions which must be diagnosed in a hospital environment, or in institutions with adequate diagnostic facilities, although administration, and follow-up, may be carried out elsewhere, or
- the medicinal product is intended for outpatients, but its use may produce very serious adverse reactions requiring a prescription drawn up as required by a specialist, and special supervision throughout the treatment.

4. A competent authority may waive application of paragraphs 1, 2 and 3 having regard to:

- the maximum single dose, the maximum daily dose, the strength, the pharmaceutical form, certain types of packaging; and/or
- other circumstances of use which it has specified.

5. If a competent authority does not designate medicinal products into sub-categories referred to in Article 70, it shall nevertheless take into account the criteria referred to in paragraphs 2 and 3 of this Article in determining whether any medicinal product shall be classified as a prescription-only medicine.

Article 72

Medicinal products not subject to prescription shall be those which do not meet the criteria listed in Article 71.

USA

Since US medical authorities frowned upon cell xenotransplantation for decades, and US FDA actually banned cell therapy in 1956, it was a great surprise when US FDA issued the 'Draft of PHS Guidelines on Infectious Disease Issues in Xenotransplantation' on September 23, 1996, (Federal Register FR 49920), that then on January 19, 2001, became...

PHS Guideline on Infectious Disease Issues in Xenotransplantation

Preamble

Background
Several developments have fueled the renewed interest in xenotransplantation- the use of live animal cells, tissues and organs in the treatment or mitigation of human disease. The world-wide, critical shortage of human organs available for transplantation and advances in genetic engineering and in the immunology and biology of organ/tissue rejection have renewed scientists' interest in investigating xenotransplantation as a potentially promising means to treat a wide range of human disorders. This situation is highlighted by the fact that in the United States alone, 13 patients die each day waiting to receive a life-saving transplant to replace a diseased vital organ.

While animal organs are proposed as an investigational alternative to human organ transplantation, xenotransplantation is also being used in the effort to treat diseases for which human organ allotransplants are not traditional therapies (e.g. epilepsy, chronic intractable pain syndromes, insulin dependent diabetes mellitus, and degenerative neurologic diseases such as Parkinson's disease and Huntington's disease). At present, the majority of clinical xenotransplantation procedures utilize avascular cells or tissues rather than solid organs in large part due to the immunologic barriers that the human host presents to vascularized xenotransplantation products. However, with recent scientific advances, xenotransplantation is viewed by many researchers as having the potential for treating not only end-organ failure but also chronic debilitating diseases that affect major segments of the world population.

Although the potential benefits may be considerable, the use of xeno-transplantation also presents a number of significant challenges. These include (1) the potential risk of transmission of infectious agents from source animals to patients, their close contacts, and the general public; (2) the complexities of informed consent; and (3) animal welfare issues.

On September 23, 1996, the US Department of Health and Human Services (DHHS) published for public comment the *Draft PHS Guideline on Infectious Disease Issues in Xenotransplantation* to address the infectious disease concerns raised by xenotransplantation (61 Federal Register 49919). The Draft Guideline was jointly developed by five components within DHHS-the Centers for Disease Control and Prevention (CDC), Food and Drug Administration (FDA), Health Resources and Services Administration (HRSA), National Institutes of Health (NIH), all parts of the US Public Health Service (PHS), plus the DHHS Office of the Assistant Secretary for Planning and Evaluation. This Draft Guideline discusses general principles for the prevention and control of infectious diseases that may be associated with xenotrans-plantation. Intended to minimize potential risks to public health, these general principles provide guidance on the development, design, and implementation of clinical protocols to sponsors of xenotransplantation clinical trials and local review bodies evaluating proposed xenotrans-plantation clinical protocols. The Draft Guideline emphasizes the need for appropriate clinical and scientific expertise on the xenotransplan-tation research team, adequate protocol review, thorough health surveillance plans, and comprehensive informed consent and education processes.

In response to the Draft Guideline, the DHHS received over 140 written comments reflecting a broad spectrum of public opinion (Federal Register docket No. 96M-0311). Comments were received from a variety of stakeholders, including representatives of academia, industry, patient, consumer, and animal welfare advocacy organizations; professional, scientific and medical societies, ethicists, researchers, other government agencies and private citizens.

In revising the Draft Guideline, careful consideration was given to recent scientific findings, each of the written comments, as well as to public comments received at several national, international, and DHHS-sponsored workshops. These meetings constituted critically important public forums for discussing the scientific, public health, and social issues attendant to xenotransplantation.

The DHHS sponsored two public workshops on xenotransplantation during 1997 and 1998. The first meeting, held in July 1997, focused on virology and documented evidence of cross species infections. Titled "Cross-Species Infectivity and Pathogenesis", the meeting addressed current knowledge about the mechanisms and consequences of infectious agent transmission across species barriers. Discussions also focused on the possibility that an infectious agent might cross from an animal donor organ or tissue to human xenotransplantation product recipients. The conference also highlighted gaps in knowledge about the emergence of new infections in humans, especially as a result of xenotransplantation. The basic consensus of the meeting was that while there were examples of animal infectious agents crossing species barriers to infect, and even cause diseases in humans, the actual likelihood of this in xenotransplantation product recipients cannot be ascertained at this time. Small adequate and well-controlled clinical trials designed to test the safety and efficacy of xenotransplantation were considered to be appropriate. One anticipated outcome of such trials would be to both minimize and better understand the risks of transmission of infectious agents.

In January 1998, a second DHHS workshop titled "Developing US Public Health Service Policy in Xenotransplantation", focused on the current and evolving US public health policy in xenotransplantation. Among other issues, the regulatory framework, a national xenotransplantation database, and a national advisory committee were discussed.

During this workshop, several themes were raised repeatedly and echoed many of the written public comments on the Draft Guideline. First, there was a broad consensus that the Draft Guideline was important and should be implemented, albeit with some modifications. For example, it was expressed that there could be more public awareness and participation in the development of public health policies in the field of xenotransplantation. Second, there was strong support for the DHHS proposal to establish a national xenotransplantation advisory committee, not only to facilitate analysis and discussion of the scientific, medical, ethical, legal, and social issues raised by xenotransplantation, but also to review and make recommendations about proposed clinical trial protocols. There was broad support for proceeding cautiously with xenotransplantation trials; however, some participants held that a national moratorium on clinical trials in xenotransplantation might be advantageous until the national xenotransplantation advisory committee is established and operational. While there is no definitive scientific evidence that xenotransplantation would promote cross-species infectious agent transmission *leading to disease*, there are data providing a reasonable basis for caution [see revised guideline, section 6., references D.1.a; e.; f.; i.; l; o.; q.; r.& s.]. Some members of the scientific and medical community and concerned citizens expressed the opinion that there is a perceived greater risk from the use of xenotransplantation products procured from nonhuman primates (as opposed to other species) because of potential public health risks and animal welfare concerns.

The January 1998 workshop also included presentations by representatives of the World Health Organization (WHO), the Organization for Economic Cooperation and Development (OECD), and several nations engaged in developing policies on xenotransplantation. These presentations placed the US policy in global context and enhanced international dialogue on important public health safeguards. Because of the potential for the secondary transmission of infectious agents, the public health risks posed by xenotransplantation transcend national boundaries. International communication and cooperation in the development of public health policies are critical elements in successfully addressing the global safety and ethical challenges inherent in xenotransplantation. To this end, several countries, including Canada, France, Germany, the Netherlands, Spain, Sweden, the United Kingdom, and the United States and several international organizations such as the WHO, OECD, and the Council of Europe are actively engaged in international workshops and consultations on xenotransplantation. [see revised guideline, section 6.C.7. for a partial bibliography of guidance documents and websites from national and international bodies].

Major Revisions and Clarifications to the Guideline

Major revisions and clarifications to the Draft Guideline are briefly summarized and discussed below. These revisions were prompted by public comments submitted to the Draft Guideline docket, concerns expressed at public workshops, evolving science, and developing international policies. PHS intends to address related issues that go beyond the scope of this Guideline in future guidance documents. In the future the Guideline may be amended as needed to appropriately reflect the accrual of new knowledge about cross-species infectivity and pathogenesis, new insights into the potential risks associated with xenotransplantation, policies currently under development (e.g. the Secretary's Advisory Committee on Xenotransplantation and the National Xenotransplantation Database), and other evolving public health policies in this arena.

Definition of Xenotransplantation and Xenotransplantation Product
The definition of "xenotransplantation" has been revised from that used in the Draft Guideline. For the purposes of this document and US PHS policy, xenotransplantation is now defined to include any procedure that involves the

transplantation, implantation, or infusion into a human recipient of either (a) live cells, tissues, or organs from a nonhuman animal source or (b) human body fluids, cells, tissues or organs that have had *ex vivo* contact with live nonhuman animal cells, tissues, or organs. Furthermore, xenotransplantation products have been defined to include live cells, tissues or organs used in xenotransplantation. The term xenograft, used in previous PHS documents, will no longer be used to refer to all xenotransplantation products.

Clinical Protocol Review and Oversight

A variety of opinions were expressed regarding the appropriate level of protocol review and oversight of clinical trials in the US For example, the American Society of Transplant Surgeons stated that the Draft Guideline represented an unnecessary intrusion of government regulation into the performance of transplant surgery. In contrast, some organiza-tions with commercial interests in the development of xenotransplantation contended that an inappropriate share of the burden for oversight of clinical trials had been assigned to local review committees and that the responsibility for this oversight should reside at the national level with the FDA. Several academic veterinarians, a group of 44 virologists, and other concerned citizens asserted that strict regulations should accompany the Guideline and that the major responsibility for determining the suitability of any animals as sources of nonhuman animal live cells, tissues or organs used in xenotransplantation must reside with the FDA.

The revised Guideline makes clear that, in addition to review by appropriate local review bodies (Institutional Review Boards, Institutional Animal Care and Use Committees, and the Institutional Biosafety Committees), the FDA has regulatory oversight for xenotransplantation clinical trials conducted in the US. Xenotransplantation products (i.e. live cells, tissues, or organs from a nonhuman animal source or human body fluids, cells, tissues, or organs that have had *ex vivo* contact with live cells, tissues, or organs from nonhuman animal sources and are used for xenotransplantation) are considered to be biological products, or combination products that contain a biological component, subject to regulation by FDA, under section 351 of the Public Health Service Act (42 USC 262), and under the Federal Food, Drug, and Cosmetic Act (21 USC 321 et seq.). In accordance with the applicable statutory provisions, xenotransplantation products are subject to the FDA regulations governing clinical investigations and product approvals (e.g. the Investigational New Drug [IND] regulations in 21 CFR Part 312, and the regulations governing licensing of biological products in 21 CFR Part 601). Investigators should submit an application for FDA review before proceeding with xenotransplantation clinical trials. Sponsors are strongly encouraged to meet with FDA staff in the pre-submission phase. In addition to the guidances referred to below, the FDA is considering further regulations and/or guidances regarding, for example, the development of xenotransplantation protocols and the technical and clinical development of xeno-transplantation products.

Xenotransplantation clinical protocols may also be reviewed by the Secretary's Advisory Committee on Xenotransplantation. The scope and process for this review will be described in future publications [see revised guideline, sections 2.3, 5.3].

Responsibility for Design and Conduct of Clinical Protocols
The Draft Guideline originally proposed that clinical centers, source animal facilities, and individual investigators share the responsibilities for various aspects of the clinical trial protocol, including pre-xenotransplantation screening programs, patient informed consent procedures, record keeping, and post-xenotransplantation surveillance activities. The revised Guideline clarifies that primary responsibility for designing and monitoring the conduct of xenotransplantation clinical trials rests with the sponsor (as provided under, e.g. 21 CFR 312.23(a)(6)(d) and 312.50).

Informed Consent and Patient Education
Virologists, infectious disease specialists, health care workers, and patient advocates emphasized the need for the sponsor to offer assistance to xenotransplantation product recipients in educating their close contacts about potential infectious disease risks and methods for reducing those risks. The Guideline has been revised to state that the sponsor should ensure that counseling regarding behavior modification and other issues associated with risk of infection is provided to the patient and made available to the patient's family and other close contacts prior to and at the time of consent, and that such counseling should continue to be available thereafter. The revised Guideline clarifies and strengthens the informed consent process for xenotransplantation product recipients and the education and counseling process for recipients and their close contacts, including associated health care professionals. It also emphasizes the need for xenotransplantation product recipients to comply with long-term or life-long surveillance regardless of the outcome of the clinical trial or the status of the graft or other xeno-transplantation product [see revised guideline, sections 2.5.3, 2.5.4, 2.5.7.].

Deferral of Allograft and Blood Donors
The 1996 Draft Guideline recommended that xenotransplantation product recipients refrain from donating body fluids and/or parts for use

in humans. Some infectious disease specialists and an infectious disease control practitioner organization suggested that this be strengthened to active deferral of xenotransplantation product recipients, and that consideration also be given to the deferral of close contacts of xenotransplantation product recipients. This issue was addressed by the FDA Xenotransplantation Subcommittee of the Biological Response Modifiers Advisory Committee (December, 1997).

The committee recommended that xenotransplantation product recipients and their close contacts be counseled and actively deferred from donation of body fluids and other parts. A proposed FDA policy was then later presented to FDA's Blood Products Advisory Committee for further discussion (March, 1998). At the time of both of these advisory committee meetings the operative definition of xenotransplantation did not include, as it does now, the use of certain products involving limited *ex vivo* exposure to xenogeneic cell lines or tissues. FDA has published a draft guidance document (Guidance for Industry: Precautionary Measures to Reduce the Possible Risk of Transmission of Zoonoses by Blood and Blood Products from Xenotransplantation Product Recipients and Their Contacts) for public comment, which was again discussed by the FDA Xenotransplantation Subcommittee of the Biological Response Modifiers Advisory Committee on January 13, 2000. FDA will further consult with its advisors to identify the range of xenotransplantation products for which recipients and/or their contacts should be recommended for deferral from blood donation. Additionally, the range of contacts that should be deferred from blood donation will be clarified after further public discussion. The Guideline has been revised to reflect comments made at the FDA advisory committee meetings [see revised guideline, sections 2.5.11].

Xenotransplantation Product Sources
Strong opposition to the use of nonhuman primates as xenotransplantation product sources was voiced by many individuals and groups, including 44 virologists, scientific and medical organizations such as the American Society of Transplant Physicians, the American College of Cardiology, private citizens, and commercial sponsors of xenotransplantation clinical trials. The concerns focused on the ethics of using animals so closely related to humans, as well as the risk of transmission of infectious diseases from nonhuman primates to humans. Many recommended that the Guideline state that clinical xenotransplantation trials using xenotransplantation products for which nonhuman primates served as source animals should not occur until a closer examination of infectious disease risks can be adequately carried out.

Scientific findings, since the publication of the Draft Guideline, have also resulted in revisions. For example, the ability of simian foamy virus (SFV) to persistently infect human hosts has been further characterized [see revised guideline, section 6., references D.2.m. & D.4.d.], the persistence of microchimerism with anatomically dispersed baboon cells containing SFV, baboon cytomegalovirus (CMV), and baboon endogenous retrovirus (BaEV), in human recipients of baboon liver xenotransplantation products has been documented [see revised guideline, section 6., references D.3.a. & D.4.h.], and new viruses capable of infecting humans have been identified in pigs [see revised guideline, section 6., references D.2.a., b., f., g., h., i., v., w., x., bb., cc., ee., & gg.]. The active expression of infectious porcine endogenous retrovirus from multiple porcine cell types, and the ability of porcine endogenous retrovirus variants A and B to infect human cell lines *in vitro* has been demonstrated [see revised guideline, section 6., references D.1.q., s.; D.2.jj.; D.3.i.; D.4.a., e., f., m., s. & t.], giving scientific plausibility to concerns that this retrovirus from porcine xenotrans-plantation products may be able to infect recipients *in vivo*.

Diagnostic tests for porcine endogenous retrovirus, BaEV, and other relevant infectious agents have been developed [see revised guideline, section 6., references D.4.a., b., d., g., h., l., n., p., q., t. & u.] and studies are currently underway to assess the presence or absence of infectious endogenous retroviruses and other relevant infectious agents in both porcine and baboon xenotransplantation products and in the recipients of these xenotransplantation products [see revised guideline, section 6., references D.3.a.; D.4.c., h., j., l. & n.]. The risk of endogenous retrovirus infection, however, is multi-factorial and it is not known whether results from these studies will be predictive of the potential infectious risks associated with future xenotransplantation products. One factor that impacts porcine endogenous retrovirus infectivity is its sensitivity to inactivation and lysis by human sera, yet the virus becomes resistant to inactivation after a single passage through human cells [see revised guideline, section 6., references D.2.jj. & D.4.m.]. It is hypothesized that pre-xenotransplantation removal of naturally occurring xenoreactive antibodies from the recipient and other modifications intended to facilitate xenotransplantation product survival, such as the procurement of xenotransplantation products or nonhuman animal live cells, tissues or organs used in the manufacture of xenotransplantation products from certain transgenic pigs, may also modulate the infectivity of endogenous retroviruses for xenotransplantation product recipients [see revised guideline, section 6., references D.1.d., o., q., s.; D.2.k., jj.; D.3.i.; D.4.e., k., m. & r.].

As the science regarding porcine endogenous retroviruses summarized above began to emerge, the FDA placed all clinical trials using porcine xenotransplantation products on hold (October 16, 1997) pending development by sponsors of sensitive and specific assays for (1) preclinical detection of infectious porcine endogenous retrovirus in porcine xenotransplantation products, (2) post-xenotransplantation screening for porcine endogenous retrovirus and clinical follow-up of porcine xenotransplantation product recipients, and (3) the development of informed consent documents that indicate the potential clinical implications of the capacity of porcine endogenous retrovirus to infect human cells *in vitro*. These issues were discussed publicly by the FDA Xenotransplantation Subcommittee of the Biological Response Modifiers Advisory Committee (December, 1997).

In response to concerns articulated by scientists and other members of the public regarding the use of nonhuman primate xenotransplantation products, the FDA, after consultation with other DHHS agencies, has issued a "Guidance for Industry: Public Health Issues Posed by the Use of Nonhuman Primate Xenografts in Humans" containing the following conclusions:

1. "... an appropriate federal xenotransplantation advisory committee, such as a Secretary's Advisory Committee on Xenotransplantation (SACX) currently under development within the DHHS, should address novel protocols and issues raised by the use of nonhuman primate xenografts, conduct discussions, including public discussions as appropriate, and make recommendations on the questions of whether and under what conditions the use of nonhuman primate xenografts would be appropriate in the United States.
2. clinical protocols proposing the use of nonhuman primate xenografts should not be submitted to the FDA until sufficient scientific information exists addressing the risks posed by nonhuman primate xenotransplants. Consistent with FDA Investigational New Drug (IND) regulations [21 CFR 312.42(b)(1)(iv)], any protocol submission that does not adequately address these risks is subject to clinical hold (i.e. the clinical trial may not proceed) due to insufficient information to assess the risks and/or due to unreasonable risk.

3. at the current time, FDA believes there is not sufficient information to assess the risks posed by nonhuman primate xenotransplantation. FDA believes that it will be necessary to have a public discussion before these issues can be adequately addressed..."

While the document "Guidance for Industry: Public Health Issues Posed by the Use of Nonhuman Primate Xenografts in Humans" specifically addresses the issue of nonhuman primates as sources for xenotransplantation products, the DHHS recognizes that other animal species have been used and/or are proposed as sources of xenotransplantation products and that all species pose infectious disease risks. Accordingly, the principles for source animal screening and health surveillance described in the revised Guideline apply to all candidate source animals regardless of species. These principles will need to be reassessed as new data become available.

Source Animal Screening and Qualification

Many groups and individuals expressed concern that the Draft Guideline did not set forth sufficiently stringent principles and criteria for source animal husbandry and screening, source animal facilities, and procurement and screening of xenotransplantation products. This view was expressed by virologists, veterinarians, infectious disease specialists, concerned citizens, commercial producers of laboratory animals, industrial sponsors of xenotransplantation trials, and a number of professional, scientific, medical, and advocacy organizations, such as the American Society of Transplant Surgeons, Doctors and Lawyers for Responsible Medicine, the American College of Cardiology, Biotechnology Industry Organization (BIO - representing 670 biotech companies), and the Association for Professionals in Infection Control and Epidemiology. Others expressed concern that the stringency of the Draft Guideline imposed high economic burdens on producers of xenotransplantation product source animals and/or on sponsors of xenotransplantation clinical trials. However, in order to reduce the potential public health risks posed by xenotransplantation, strict control of animal husbandry and health surveillance practices are needed during the course of development of this technology.

The Guideline has been revised to clarify the animal husbandry and pre-xenotransplantation infectious disease screening that should be performed before an animal can become a qualified source of xenotransplantation products. The revised Guideline now emphasizes that risk minimization precautions appropriate to each xenotransplantation product protocol should be employed during all steps of production and that screening, quarantine, and surveillance protocols should be tailored to the specific clinical protocol, xenotransplantation product, source animal and husbandry history. Breeding programs using cesarean derivation of animals should be used whenever possible. Source animals should be procured from closed herds or colonies raised in facilities that have appropriate barriers to effectively preclude the introduction or spread of infectious agents. These facilities should actively monitor the herds for infectious agents. The revised Guideline clarifies and strengthens the infectious disease screening and surveillance practices that should be in place before a clinical trial can begin.

Specimen Archives and Medical Records
A number of infectious disease specialists, veterinarians, epidemiologists, industry sponsors of xenotransplantation trials, biotechnology companies, professional organizations such as the American Society of Transplant Physicians, and consumer advocates requested clarification regarding the collection and usage of, and access to biological specimens obtained from both source animals and xenotransplantation product recipients.

The revised Guideline clarifies the recommended types, volumes, and collection schedule for biological specimens from both source animals and xenotransplantation product recipients. It also clearly distinguishes between biological specimens archived for public health investigations [see revised guideline, sections 4.1.2. and 3.7.] and specimens archived for use by the sponsor in conducting surveillance of source animals and post-xenotransplantation laboratory surveillance of xenotransplantation product recipients. The revised Guideline also states that health records and biologic specimens should be maintained for 50 years, based on the latency periods of known human pathogenic persistent viruses and the precedents established by the US Occupational Safety and Health Administration with respect to record-keeping requirements.

National Xenotransplantation Database
A number of infectious disease specialists, epidemiologists, transplant physicians, and a state health official emphasized the need for accurate and timely information on infectious disease surveillance and xenotransplantation protocols and their outcomes. They further supported the concept of a national xenotransplantation database as described in the Draft Guideline.

The revised Guideline describes the development of a pilot national xenotransplantation database to identify and implement routine data collection methods, system design, data reporting, and general start-up and to assess routine operational issues associated with a fully functional national database. The revisions also discuss plans to expand this pilot into a national xenotransplantation database intended to compile data from all clinical centers conducting trials in xenotransplantation and all animal facilities providing source animals for xenotransplantation.

Secretary's Advisory Committee on Xenotransplantation
Xenotransplantation research brings to the fore certain challenges in assessing the potential impact of science on society as a whole, including the role of the public in those assessments. The broad spectrum of public opinions expressed since the publication of the Draft Guideline indicates that there is neither uniform public endorsement nor rejection of xenotransplantation. The fields of research involved are rapidly moving ones, at the leading edge of medical science. Furthermore, in many instances the clinical trials are privately funded and the public may not even be aware of them. However, public awareness and understanding of xenotransplant-ation is vital because the potential infectious disease risks posed by xenotransplantation extend beyond the individual patient to the public at large. In addition to these safety issues, a variety of individuals and groups have identified and/or raised concerns about issues such as animal welfare, human rights, community interest and consent, social equity in access to novel biotechnologies, and allocation of human allografts versus xenotransplantation products. For all of these reasons, public discourse on xenotransplantation research is critical and necessary.

The revised Guideline acknowledges the complexity, importance, and relevance of these issues, but emphasizes that the scope of the Guideline is limited to infectious disease issues. The revised Guideline discusses the development of the Secretary's Advisory Committee on Xenotransplantation (SACX) as a mechanism for ensuring ongoing discussions of the scientific, medical, social, and ethical issues and the public health concerns raised by xenotransplantation, including ongoing and proposed protocols. The SACX will make recommendations to the Secretary on policy and procedures and, as needed, on changes to the Guideline.

PHS GUIDELINE ON INFECTIOUS DISEASE ISSUES IN XENOTRANSPLANTATION

TABLE OF CONTENTS

1. Introduction

    1.1. Applicability
    1.2. Definitions
    1.3. Background
    1.4. Scope of theDocument
    1.5. Objectives

2. **Xenotransplantation Protocol Issues**

   2.1. Xenotransplantation Team
   2.2. Clinical Xenotransplantation Site
   2.3. Clinical Protocol Review
   2.4. Health Screening and Surveillance Plans
   2.5. Informed Consent and Patient Education Processes

3. **Animal Sources for Xenotransplantation**

   3.1. Animal Procurement Sources
   3.2. Source Animal Facilities
   3.3. Pre-xenotransplantation Screening for Known Infectious Agents
   3.4. Herd/Colony Health Maintenance and Surveillance
   3.5. Individual Source Animal Screening and Qualification
   3.6. Procurement and Screening of Nonhuman Animal Live Cells, Tissues or Organs Used for Xenotransplantation
   3.7. Archives of Source Animal Medical Records and Specimens
   3.8. Disposal of Animals and Animal By-products

4. **Clinical Issues**

   4.1. Xenotransplantation Product Recipient
   4.2. Infection Control
   4.3. Health Care Records

5. **Public Health Needs**

   5.1. National Xenotransplantation Database
   5.2. Biologic Specimen Archives
   5.3. Secretary's Advisory Committee on Xenotransplantation (SACX)

6. **Bibliography**

1. **Introduction**

1.1. Applicability

This guideline was developed by the US Public Health Service (PHS) to identify general principles of prevention and control of infectious diseases associated with xenotransplantation that may pose a hazard to public health. It is intended to provide general guidance to local review bodies evaluating proposed xenotransplantation clinical protocols and to sponsors in the development of xenotransplantation clinical protocols, in preparing submissions to FDA or the Secretary's Advisory Committee on Xenotransplantation (SACX, section 5.3.), and in the conduct of xenotransplantation clinical trials. Such clinical trials conducted within the United States are subject to regulation by the FDA under the Public Health Service Act (42 U.S.C. 262, 264), and the Federal Food, Drug, and Cosmetic Act (21 U.S.C. 321 et seq.). This guidance document represents PHS's current thinking on certain infectious disease issues in xenotransplantation. It does not create or confer any rights for or on any person and does not operate to bind PHS or the public. This guidance is not intended to set forth an approach that addresses all of the potential health hazards related to infectious disease issues in xenotransplantation nor to establish the only way in which the public health hazards that are identified in this document may be addressed. The PHS acknowledges that not all of the recommendations set forth within this document may be fully relevant to all xenotransplantation products or xenotransplan-tation procedures. Sponsors of clinical xenotransplantation trials are advised to confer with relevant authorities (the FDA, other reviewing authorities, funding sources, etc) in assessing the relevance and appropriate adaptation of the general guidance offered here to specific clinical applications.

1.2. Definitions

This section defines terms as used in this guideline document.

1. **Allograft** - a graft consisting of live cells, tissues, and/or organs between individuals of the same species.
2. **Closed herd or colony** - herd or colony governed by Standard Operating Procedures that specify criteria restricting admission of new animals to assure that all introduced animals are at the same or a higher health standard compared to the residents of the herd or colony.
3. **Commensal** - an organism living on or within another, but not causing injury to the host.
4. **Good Clinical Practices** - A standard for the design, conduct, performance, monitoring, auditing, recording, analyses, and reporting of clinical trials that provides assurance that the data and reported results are credible and accurate, and that the rights, integrity, and confidentiality of trial subjects are protected.
5. **Infection Control Program** - a systematic activity within a hospital or health care center charged with responsibility for the control and prevention of infections within the hospital or center.
6. **Infectious agents** - viruses, bacteria (including the rickettsiae), fungi, parasites, or agents responsible for Transmissible Spongiform Encephalopathies (currently thought to be prions)

capable of invading and multiplying within the body.
7. **Institutional Animal Care and Use Committee (IACUC)** - a local institutional committee established to oversee the institution's animal program, facilities, and procedures. IACUC carry out semiannual program reviews and facility inspections and review all animal use protocols and any animal welfare concerns. (See PHS Policy on Humane Care and Use of Laboratory Animals, September 1986; reprinted March 1996).
8. **Institutional Biosafety Committee (IBC)** - A local institutional committee established to review and oversee basic and clinical research conducted at that institution. The IBC assesses the safety of the research and identifies any potential risk to public health or the environment. (See Section IV-B-2 of the NIH Guidelines for Research Involving Recombinant DNA Molecules).
9. **Institutional Review Board (IRB)** - A local institutional committee established to review biomedical and behavioral research involving human subjects in order to protect the rights of human subjects (See 45 CFR Part 46, Protection of Human Subjects, and 21 CFR Part 56, Institutional Review Boards).
10. **Investigator** - an individual who actually conducts a clinical investigation (i.e. under whose immediate direction the drug [or investigational product] is administered or dispensed to a subject). In the event an investigation is conducted by a team of individuals, the investigator is the responsible leader of the team (see 21 CFR 312.3(b)).
11. **Nosocomial infection** - an infection acquired in a hospital.
12. **Occupational Health Service** - an office within a hospital or health care center charged with responsibility for the protection of workers from health hazards to which they may be exposed in the course of their job duties.
13. **Procurement** - the process of obtaining or acquiring animals or biological specimens (such as cells, tissues, or organs) from an animal or human for medicinal, research, or archival purposes.
14. **Recipient** - a person who receives or who undergoes *ex vivo* exposure to a xenotransplantation product (as defined in xenotransplantation).
15. **Secretary's Advisory Committee on Xenotransplantation (SACX)** - the advisory committee appointed by the Secretary of Health and Human Services to consider the full range of issues raised by xenotransplantation (including ongoing and proposed protocols) and make recommendations to the Secretary on policy and procedures.

16. **Source animal** - an animal from which cells, tissues, and/or organs for xenotransplantation are obtained.
17. **Source animal facility** - facility that provides source animals for use in xenotransplantation.
18. **Sponsor** - a person who takes responsibility for and initiates a clinical investigation. The sponsor may be an individual or a pharmaceutical company, government agency, academic institution, private organization or other organization. The sponsor does not actually conduct the investigation unless the sponsor is a sponsor-investigator (see, e.g. 21 CFR 312.3(b)).
19. **Transmissible spongiform encephalopathies (TSEs)** - fatal, subacute, degenerative diseases of humans and animals with characteristic neuropathology (spongiform change and deposition of an abnormal form of a prion protein present in all mammalian brains). TSEs are experimentally transmissible by inoculation or ingestion of diseased tissue, especially central nervous system tissue. The prion protein (intimately associated with transmission and pathological progression) is hypothesized to be the agent of transmission. Alternatively, other unidentified co-factors or an as-yet unidentified viral agent may be necessary for transmission. Creutzfeldt-Jakob disease (CJD) is the most common human TSE.
20. **Xenogeneic infectious agents** - infectious agents that become capable of infecting humans due to the unique facilitating circumstances of xenotransplantation; includes zoonotic infectious agents.
21. **Xenotransplantation** - for the purposes of this document, any procedure that involves the transplantation, implantation, or infusion into a human recipient of either (A.) live cells, tissues, or organs from a nonhuman animal source or (B.) human body fluids, cells, tissues or organs that have had *ex vivo* contact with live nonhuman animal cells, tissues, or organs.
22. **Xenotransplantation Product(s)** - live cells, tissues or organs used in xenotransplantation (defined above). Previous PHS documents have used the term "xenograft" to refer to all xenotransplantation products.
23. **Xenotransplantation Product Recipient** - a person who receives or undergoes *ex vivo* exposure to a xenotransplantation product.
24. **Zoonosis** - A disease of animals that may be transmitted to humans under natural conditions (e.g. brucellosis, rabies).

1.3. Background

The demand for human cells, tissues and organs for clinical transplantation continues to exceed the supply. The limited availability of human allografts, coupled with recent scientific and biotechnical advances, has prompted the renewed development of investigational therapeutic approaches that use xenotransplantation products in human recipients.

The experience with human allografts, however, has shown that infectious agents can be transmitted through transplantation. HIV/AIDS, Creutzfeldt-Jakob Disease, rabies, and hepatitis B and C, for example, have been transmitted between humans via allotransplantation. The use of live nonhuman cells, tissues and organs for xenotransplantation raises serious public health concerns about potential infection of xenotransplantation product recipients with both known and emerging infectious agents.

Zoonoses are infectious diseases of animals transmitted to humans via exposure to or consumption of the source animal. It is well documented that contact between humans and nonhuman animals -- such as that which occurs during husbandry, food production, or interactions with pets -- can lead to zoonotic infections. Many infectious agents responsible for zoonoses (e.g. Toxoplasma species, Salmonella species, or Cercopithecine herpesvirus 1 (B virus) of monkeys) are well characterized and can be identified through available diagnostic tests. Infectious disease public health concerns about xenotransplantation focus not only on the transmission of these known zoonoses, but also on the transmission of infectious agents as yet unrecognized. The disruption of natural anatomical barriers and immuno-suppression of the recipient increase the likelihood of interspecies transmission of xenogeneic infectious agents. An additional concern is that these xenogeneic infectious agents could be subsequently transmitted from the xenotransplantation product recipient to close contacts and then to other human beings. An infectious agent may pose risk to the patients and/or public if it can infect, cause disease in, and transmit among humans, or if its ability to infect, cause disease in, or transmit among humans remains inadequately defined.

Emerging infectious agents may not be readily identifiable with current techniques. This was the case with the several year delay in identifying HIV-1 as the etiologic agent for AIDS. Retroviruses and other persistent infections may be associated with acute disease with varying incubation periods, followed by periods of clinical latency prior to the onset of clinically evident malignancies or other diseases. As the HIV/AIDS pandemic demonstrates, persistent latent infections may result in person-to-person transmission for many years before clinical disease develops in the index case, thereby allowing an emerging infectious agent to become established in the susceptible population before it is recognized.

1.4. Scope of the Document

This guideline addresses the public health issues related to xenotransplantation and recommends procedures for diminishing the risk of transmission of infectious agents to the recipient, health care workers, and the general public. While it is beyond the scope of this document to address the array of complex and important ethical issues raised by xenotransplantation, this guideline describes a mechanism for ensuring ongoing broad public discussion of ethical issues related to xenotransplantation (section 5.3). Other publications and reports of public discussions (section 6., references C.7.a., c., d., h., I.; D.1.b. & I.) have addressed issues such as animal welfare, human rights, and community interest.

This guideline reflects the status of the field of xenotransplantation and knowledge of the risk of xenogeneic infections at the time of publication. The general guidance in this document will be augmented by public discussion, new advances in scientific knowledge and clinical experience, and specific FDA guidance documents intended to facilitate the implementation of the principles set forth herein. HHS may ask the Secretary's Advisory Committee on Xenotransplantation (SACX) to review the Guideline on a periodic basis and recommend appropriate revisions to the Secretary (section 5.3).

1.5. Objectives

The objective of this PHS guideline is to present measures that can be used to minimize the risk of human disease due to xenogeneic infectious agents including both recognized zoonoses and non-zoonotic infectious agents that become capable of infecting humans due to the unique facilitating circumstances of xenotransplantation. In order to achieve this goal, this document:

- Outlines the composition and function of the xenotransplantation team to ensure that appropriate technical expertise can be applied (section 2.1).
- Addresses aspects of the clinical protocol, clinical center, and the informed consent and patient education processes with respect to public health concerns raised by the potential for infections associated with xenotransplantation (sections 2.2-2.5).
- Provides a framework for pre-transplantation animal source screening to minimize the potential for transmission of xenogeneic infectious agents from the xenotransplantation product to the

human recipient (section 3, particularly sections 3.3-3.6).
- Provides a framework for post-xenotransplantation surveillance to monitor transmission of infectious agents, including newly identified xenogeneic agents, to the recipient as well as health care workers and other individuals in close contact with the recipient (section 4, particularly sections 4.1.1. and 4.2.3.).
- Provides a framework for hospital infection control practices to reduce the risk of nosocomial transmission of zoonotic and xenogeneic infectious agents (section 4.2.).
- Provides a framework for maintaining appropriate records, including human and veterinary health care records (section 4.3. and 3.7), standard operating procedures of facilities and centers (sections 3.2, 3.4), and occupational health service program records (section 4.3).
- Provides a framework for archiving biologic samples from the source animal and the xenotransplantation product recipient. These records and samples will be essential in the event that public health investigations are necessitated by infectious diseases and other adverse events arising from xenotransplantation that could affect the public health (sections 3.7, 4.1.2., and 5.2).
- Discusses the creation of a national database that will enable population based public health surveillance and investigation(s). (section 5.1).
- Discusses the creation of a Secretary's Advisory Committee on Xenotransplantation (SACX) that will consider the full range of complex and interrelated issues raised by xenotransplantation, including ongoing and proposed protocols (sections 2.3. and 5.3.).

2. Xenotransplantation Protocol Issues
2.1. *Xenotransplantation team*

The development and implementation of xenotransplantation clinical research protocols require expertise in the infectious diseases of both human recipients and source animals. Consequently, in addition to health care professionals who have clinical experience with transplantation, the xenotransplantation team should include as active participants: (1) infectious disease physician(s) with expertise in zoonoses, transplanttation, and epidemiology; (2) veterinarian(s) with expertise in the animal husbandry issues and infectious diseases relevant to the source animal; (3) specialist(s) in hospital epidemiology and infection control; and (4) experts in research and diagnostic microbiology laboratory methodologies. The sponsor should ensure that the appropriate expertise is available in the development and implementation of the clinical protocol, including the onsite follow up of the xenotransplantation product recipient.

2.2. Clinical Xenotransplantation Site

Any sites performing xenotransplantation clinical procedures should have experience and expertise with and facilities for any comparable allotransplantation procedures.

All xenotransplantation clinical centers should utilize CLIA'88 (Clinical Laboratory Improvements Act, amended in 1988) accredited virology and microbiology laboratories.

2.2.1. The safe conduct of xenotransplantation clinical trials should include the active participation of laboratories with the ability to isolate and identify unusual and/or newly recognized pathogens of both human and animal origin. Each protocol will present unique diagnostic, surveillance, and research needs that require expertise and experience in the microbiology and infectious diseases of both animals and humans. The sponsor should ensure that persons and centers with appropriate experience and expertise are involved in the study development, clinical application, and follow up of each protocol, either on-site or through formal and documented off-site collaborations.

2.3. Clinical Protocol Review

All clinical trials involving xenotransplantation are subject to regulation by the FDA under the Public Health Service Act (42 U.S.C. 262, 264) and the Federal Food, Drug, and Cosmetic Act (21 U.S.C. 321 et seq.).

Sponsors are responsible for ensuring reviews by local review bodies as appropriate, (Institutional Review Boards (IRBs), Institutional Animal Care and Use Committees (IACUCs), Institutional Biosafety Committees (IBCs)), the FDA, and the SACX (upon implementation by the Secretary, HHS). The scope and process for SACX review will be described in subsequent publications.

Institutional review of xenotransplantation clinical trial protocols should address: (1) the potential risks of infection for the recipient and contact populations (including health care providers, family members, friends, and the community at large); (2) the conditions of source animal husbandry (e.g. screening program, animal quarantine); and (3) issues related to human and veterinary infectious diseases (including virology, laboratory diagnostics, epidemiology, and risk assessment).

2.4. Health Screening and Surveillance Plans

Clearly defined methodologies for pre-xenotransplantation screening for known infectious agents and post-xenotransplantation surveillance are essential parts of clinical xenotransplantation trials and should be clearly developed in all protocols. Pre-xenotransplantation screening includes screening of the source herd (sections 3.2. - 3.4.), the source animal(s) (section 3.5.), and the nonhuman animal live cells, tissues or organs used in the manufacture of the xenotransplantation product or the product itself (section 3.6.). Post-xenotransplantation surveillance includes surveillance of the recipient(s) (section 4.1.), selected health care workers or other contacts (section 4.2.), and the surviving source animal(s) (section 3.6.). The screening methods used and the specific agents sought will differ depending on the procedure, cells, tissue, or organ used, the source animal, and the clinical indication for xenotransplantation. Details of these screening and surveillance plans, including a summary of the relevant aspects of the health maintenance and surveillance program of the herd and the medical history of the source animal(s) (section 3) and written protocols for hospital infection control practices regarding both xenotransplantation product recipients and health care workers (section 4.2.) should be described in the materials submitted for review by the SACX, the FDA, and the local review bodies.

2.5. Informed Consent and Patient Education Processes

In the process of obtaining and documenting informed consent, the sponsor and investigators should comply with all applicable regulatory requirement(s) (e.g. Title 45 Code of Federal Regulations Part 46; Title 21 Code of Federal Regulations Parts 50 and 56), and should adhere to Good Clinical Practices and to the ethical principles derived from the Belmont Report of the National Commission for the Protection of Human Subjects of Biomedical and Behavioral Research and to recommendations from the National Bioethics Advisory Board (NBAB). The local IRB may consider having the consent process observed by a patient advocate (See e.g. 45 CFR 46.109(e)). In addition, the sponsor should ensure that counseling regarding behavior modification and other issues associated with risk of infection is provided to the patient and made available to the patient's family and contacts prior to and at the time of consent. Such counseling should remain available on an ongoing basis thereafter.

The informed consent discussion, the informed consent document, and the written information provided to potential xenotransplantation product recipients should address, at a minimum, the following points relating to the potential risk associated with xenotransplantation:

2.5.1. The potential for infection with zoonotic agents known to be associated with the nonhuman source animal species.
2.5.2. The potential for transmission to the recipient of unknown xenogeneic infectious agents. The patient should be informed of the uncertainty regarding the risk of infection, whether such infections might result in disease, the nature of disease that might result, and the possibility that infections with these agents may not be recognized for an extended period of time.
2.5.3. The potential risk for transmission of xenogeneic infectious agents (and possible subsequent manifestation of disease) to the recipient's family or close contacts, especially sexual contacts. The recipient should be informed that immunocompromised persons may be at increased risk of xenogeneic infections. The recipient should be counseled regarding behavioral modifications that diminish the likelihood of transmitting infectious agents and relevant infection control practices. (sections 4.2.1.1., 4.2.1.2., 4.2.1.5., and 4.2.3.1.).
2.5.4. The informed consent process should include a documented procedure to inform the recipient of the responsibility to educate his/her close contacts regarding the possibility of xenogeneic infections from the source animal species and to offer the recipient assistance with this education process, if desired. Education of close contacts should address the uncertainty regarding the risks of xenogeneic infections, information about behaviors known to transmit infectious agents from human to human (e.g. unprotected sex, breast-feeding, intravenous drug use with shared needles, and other activities that involve potential exchange of blood or other body fluids) and methods to minimize the risk of transmission. Recipients should educate their close contacts about the importance of reporting any significant unexplained illness through their health care provider to the research coordinator at the institutions where the xenotransplantation was performed.
2.5.5. The potential need for isolation procedures during any hospitalization (including to the extent possible the estimated duration of such confinement and the specific symptoms/situation that would prompt such isolation), and any specialized precautions needed to minimize acquisition or transmission of infections following hospital discharge.
2.5.6. The potential need for specific precautions following hospital discharge to minimize the risk that livestock of the source animal species and the recipient of the xenotransplantation product will represent biohazards to each other. For example, if a recipient comes into contact with the animal species from which the xenotransplantation product was procured, the xenotransplantation product (and therefore the recipient) may have an increased risk from exposures to

agents infectious for the xenotransplantation product source species. Conversely, the recipient may represent a biohazard to healthy livestock if the presence of the xenotransplantation product enables the recipient to serve as a vector for outbreaks of disease in source species livestock.

2.5.7. The importance of complying with long-term or life-long surveillance necessitating routine physical evaluations and the archiving of tissue and/or body fluid specimens for public health purposes even if the experiment fails and the xenotransplantation product is rejected or removed. The schedule for clinical and laboratory monitoring should be provided to the extent possible. The patient should be informed that any serious or unexplained illness in themselves or their contacts should be reported immediately to the clinical investigator or his/her designee.

2.5.8. The responsibility of the xenotransplantation product recipient to inform the investigator or his/her designee of any change in address or telephone number for the purpose of enabling long-term health surveillance.

2.5.9. The importance of a complete autopsy upon the death of the xenotransplantation product recipient, even if the xenotransplantation product was previously rejected or removed. Advance discussion with the recipient and his/her family concerning the need to conduct an autopsy is also encouraged in order to ensure that the recipient's intent is known to all relevant parties.

2.5.10. The long term need for access by the appropriate public health agencies to the recipient's medical records. To the extent permitted by applicable laws and/or regulations, the confidentiality of medical records should be maintained. The informed consent document should include a statement describing the extent, if any, to which confidentiality of records identifying the subject will be maintained (45 CFR 46.116 or 21 CFR 50.25(A)(5)).

2.5.11. As an interim precautionary measure, xenotransplantation product recipients and of their contacts should be deferred indefinitely from donation of Whole Blood, blood components, including Source Plasma and Source Leukocytes, tissues, breast milk, ova, sperm, or any other body parts for use in humans. Pending further clarification, contacts to be deferred from donations should include persons who have engaged repeatedly in activities that could result in intimate exchange of body fluids with a xenotransplantation product recipient. For example, such contacts may include sexual partners, household members who share razors or toothbrushes, and health care workers or laboratory personnel with repeated percuta-neous, mucosal, or other direct exposures. These recommendations may be revised based on ongoing surveillance of xenotransplantation product recipients and their contacts to clarify the actual risk of acquiring xenogeneic infections, and the outcome of deliberations between FDA and its advisors.

FDA has published a draft guidance document (Guidance for Industry: Precautionary Measures to Reduce the Possible Risk of Transmission of Zoonoses by Blood and Blood Products from Xenotransplantation Product Recipients and Their Contacts) for public comment and will consult with its advisors to identify the range of xenotransplantation products for which recipients and/or certain of their contacts should be recommended for deferral from blood donation. Additionally, the range of contacts who should be deferred from blood donation will be clarified after further public discussion.

2.5.12. Xenotransplantation product recipients who may wish to consider reproduction in the future should be aware that a potential risk of transmission of xenogeneic infectious agents not only to their partner but also to their offspring during conception, embryonic/fetal development and/or breast-feeding cannot be excluded.

2.5.13. All centers where xenotransplantation procedures are performed should develop appropriate xenotransplantation procedure- specific educational materials to be used in educating and counseling both potential xenotransplantation product recipients and their contacts. These materials should describe the xenotransplantation procedure(s), and the known and potential risks of xenogeneic infections posed by the procedure (s) in appropriate language. Those activities that are considered to be associated with the greatest risk of transmission of infection to contacts should be described. Education programs should detail the circumstances under which the use of personal protective equipment (e.g. gloves, gowns, masks) or special infection control practices are recommended, and emphasize the importance of hand washing. The potential for transmission of these agents to the general public should be discussed.

3. Animal Sources for Xenotransplantation

Recognized zoonotic infectious agents and other organisms present in animals, such as normal flora or commensals, may cause disease in humans when introduced by xenotransplantation, especially in immunocompromised patients. The risk of transmitting xenogeneic infectious agents is reduced by procuring source animals from herds or colonies that are screened and qualified as free of specific pathogenic infectious agents and that are maintained in an environment that reduces exposure to vectors of infectious agents. Precautions intended to reduce risk should be employed in all steps of production (e.g. during animal husbandry, procurement and processing of nonhuman animal live cells, tissues or organs used in the manufacture of xenotransplantation products) and should be appropriate to each xenotransplantation protocol. Before an animal species is used as a source of xenotransplantation product(s), sponsors should adequately address the public health issues raised. These issues are delineated in more detail below.

Procedures should be developed to identify incidents that negatively affect the health of the herd. This information is relevant to the safety review of every xenotransplantation product application. Such information, as well as the procedures to collect the information, should be reported to FDA.

Some experts consider that nonhuman primates pose a greater risk of transmitting infections to humans. The PHS recognized the substantial concerns about this issue that has been raised within the scientific community and the general public. In its April 6, 1999 guidance on nonhuman primate xenotransplantation products "Guidance for Industry: Public Health Issues Posed by the Use of Nonhuman Primate Xenografts in Humans". FDA concluded, after consulting with other PHS agencies, that at the current time there is not sufficient information to assess the risks posed by nonhuman primate xenotransplantation. The FDA has determined that:

1. "...an appropriate federal advisory committee, such as the Secretary's Advisory Committee on Xenotransplantation (SACX) currently under development within the DHHS, should address novel protocols and issues raised by the use of nonhuman primate xenografts, conduct discussions, including public discussions as appropriate, and make recommendations on the questions of whether and under what conditions the use of nonhuman primate xenografts would be appropriate in the United States.
2. clinical protocols proposing the use of nonhuman primate xenografts should not be submitted to FDA until sufficient scientific information exists addressing the risks posed by nonhuman primate xenotransplantation. Consistent with FDA Investigational New Drug (IND) regulations [21 CFR 312.42(b) (1)(iv)], any protocol submission that does not adequately address these risks is subject to clinical hold (i.e. the clinical trial may not proceed) due to insufficient information to assess the risks and/or due to unreasonable risk..."

3.1. Animal Procurement Sources
All xenotransplantation products pose a risk of infection and disease to humans. Regardless of the species of the source animal, precautions appropriate to each xenotransplantation product protocol should be

employed in all steps of production (animal husbandry, procurement and processing of nonhuman animal live cells, tissues or organs) to minimize this risk. Source animal procurement and processing procedures should include, at minimum, the following precautions:

3.1.1. Cells, tissues, and organs intended for use in xenotransplantation should be procured only from animals that have been bred and reared in captivity and that have a documented, well characterized health history and lineage.

3.1.2. Source animals should be raised in facilities with adequate barriers, i.e. biosecurity, to prevent the introduction or spread of infectious agents. Animals should also be obtained from herds or colonies with restricted admission of new animals. Such closed herds or colonies should be free of infectious agents that are relevant to the animal species and that may pose risk to the patient and/or the public. An infectious agent may pose risk to the patients and/or public if it can infect, cause disease in, and transmit among humans, or if its ability to infect, cause disease in, or transmit among humans remains inadequately defined. In this regard, persistent viral infections are of particular concern. Source animals should specifically be free of infection with any identifiable exogenous persistent virus. Breeding programs utilizing caesarean derivation of animals reduce the risk of maternal-fetal transmission of infectious agents and should be used whenever possible. The prevalence of exposure to these agents should be documented through periodic surveillance of the herd or colony using serologic and other appropriate diagnostic methodologies.

3.1.3. Animals from minimally controlled environments such as closed corrals (captive free-ranging animals) should not be used as source animals for xenotransplantation. Such animals have a higher likelihood of harboring adventitious infectious agents from uncontrolled contact with arthropods and/or other animal vectors.

3.1.4. Wild-caught animals should not be used as source animals for xenotransplantation.

3.1.5. Animals or live animal cells, tissues, or organs obtained from abattoirs should not be used for xenotransplantation. Such animals are obtained from geographically divergent farms or markets and are more likely to carry infectious agents due to increased exposure to other animals and increased activation and shedding of infectious agents during the stress of slaughter. In addition, health histories of slaughterhouse animals are usually not available.

3.1.6. Imported animals or the first generation of offspring of imported animals should not be used as source animals for xenotransplantation unless the animals belong to a species or strain (including transgenic animals) not available for use in the United States and their use is scientifically warranted. In this case, the imported animals should be documented to have been bred and continuously maintained in a manner consistent with the principles in this document. The source animal facility, production process and records are subject to inspection by the FDA (Federal Food, Drug and Cosmetic Act, [21 USC 374]). The US Department of Agriculture (USDA), Animal and Plant Health Inspection Service (APHIS), Veterinary Services (VS) regulates the importation of all animals and animal-origin materials that could represent a disease risk to US livestock and poultry (9 CFR Part 122). Importation or interstate transport of any animal and/or animal-origin material that may represent such a disease risk requires a USDA permit. In addition, plans for testing and quarantine of the imported animals as well as health maintenance and surveillance of the herd or colony into which imported animals are introduced should be conducted by a veterinarian who is either specifically trained in or who otherwise has a solid background in foreign animal diseases.

3.1.7. Source animals from species in which transmissible spongiform encephalopathies have been reported should be obtained from closed herds with documented absence of dementing illnesses and controlled food sources for at least 2 generations prior to the source animal (section 3.2.6.3). Xenotransplantation products should not be obtained from source animals imported from any country or geographic region where transmissible spongiform encephalopathies are known to be present in the source species or from which the USDA prohibits or restricts importation of ruminants or ruminant products due to concern about transmissible spongiform encephalopathies.

3.1.8. The CDC, Division of Quarantine, regulates the importation of certain animals, including nonhuman primates (NHP), because of their potential to cause serious outbreaks of communicable disease in humans (42 CFR Part 71). Importers must register with CDC, certify imported NHP will be used only for scientific, educational, and exhibition purposes, implement disease control measures, maintain records regarding each shipment, and report suspected zoonotic illness in animals or workers. Further, the importation and/or transfer of known or potential etiological agents, hosts, or vectors of human disease (including biological materials) may require a permit issued by CDC's Office of Health and Safety.

3.2. Source Animal Facilities

Potential source animals should be housed in facilities built and operated taking into account the factors outlined in this section.

3.2.1. Source Animal Facilities (facilities providing source animals for xenotransplantation) should be designed and maintained with adequate barriers to prevent the introduction and spread of infectious agents. Entry and exit of animals and humans should be controlled to minimize environmental exposures/inadvertent exposure to transmissible infectious agents. Source Animal Facilities should not be located in geographic proximity to manufacturing or agricultural activities that could compromise the biosecurity of these facilities.

3.2.2. Source Animal Facilities should have veterinarians on staff who possess expertise in the infectious diseases prevalent in the animal species and the emergency clinical care of the species. Facilities should also have persons with expertise in research virology and microbiology either on staff or as established consultants. These facilities should also maintain active and documented collaboration with accredited microbiology laboratories.

3.2.3. Procedures should be in place to assure the humane care of all animals (see e.g. the Animal Welfare Regulations as amended in 1985 (9 CFR Parts 1, 2, and 3) and the PHS Policy on the Humane Care and Use of Laboratory Animals).

3.2.4. Source Animal Facilities should incorporate procedures consistent with those set forth for accreditation by the Association for Assessment and Accreditation of Laboratory, Animal Care International (AAALAC International) and should be consistent with the National Research Council's Guide for the Care and Use of Laboratory Animals (1996).

3.2.5. Source Animal Facilities should have a documented health surveillance system.

3.2.6. The Source Animal Facility standard operating procedures should thoroughly describe the following: (1) criteria for animal admission, including sourcing and entry procedures, (2) description of the disease monitoring program, (3) criteria for the isolation or elimination of diseased animals, including a diagnostic algorithm for ill and dead animals, (4) facility cleaning and disinfecting arrange-ments, (5) the source and delivery of feed, water and supplies, (6) measures to exclude arthropods and other animals, (7) animal transportation, (8) dead animal disposition, (9) criteria for the health screening and surveillance of humans entering the facility, and (10) permanent individual animal identification.

>**3.2.6.1.** Animal movement through the secured facility should be described in the standard operating procedures of the facility. All animals introduced into the source colony other than by birth should go through a well defined quarantine and testing period (section 3.5). With regard to the reproduction and raising of

suitable replacement animals, the use of methods such as artificial insemination (AI), embryo transfer, medicated early weaning, cloning, or hysterotomy/hysterectomy and fostering may minimize further colonization with infectious agents.

3.2.6.2. During final screening and qualification of individual source animals and procurement of live cells, tissues or organs for use in xenotransplantation, the potential for transmission of an infectious agent should be minimized by established standard operating procedures. One method to accomplish this is a step-wise "batch" or "all-in/all-out" method of source animal movement through the facility rather than continuous replacement movement. With the "all-in/all-out" or "batch" method, a cohort of qualified animals is quarantined from the closed herd or colony while undergoing final screening qualification and xenogeneic biomaterial procurement. After the entire cohort of source animals is removed, the quarantine and xenogeneic biomaterial processing areas of the animal facility are then cleaned and disinfected prior to the introduction of the next cohort of source animals.

3.2.6.3. The feed components, including any antibiotics or other medicinals or additives, should be documented for a minimum of two generations prior to the source animal. Pasteurized milk products may be included in feeds. The absence of other mammalian materials, including recycled or rendered materials, should be specifically documented. The absence of such materials is important for the prevention of transmissible spongiform encephalopathies and other infectious agents. Potentially extended periods of clinical latency, severity of consequent disease, and the difficulty in current detection methods highlight the importance of eliminating risk factors associated with transmissible spongiform encephalopathies.

3.2.7. The sponsor should establish records linking each xenotransplantation product recipient with the relevant health history of the source animal, herd or colony, and the specific organ, tissue, or cell type included in the xenotransplantation product or used in the manufacture of the xenotransplantation product. The relevant records include information on the standard operating procedures of the animal procurement facility, the herd health surveillance, and the lifelong health history of the source animal (s) for the xenotransplantation product (sections 3.2. - 3.7.).

3.2.7.1. The sponsor should maintain these record systems and an animal numbering or their system that allows easy, accurate, and rapid linkage between the information contained in these different record systems and the xenotransplantation product recipient for 50 years beyond the date of xenotransplantation. If record systems are maintained in a computer database, electronic back ups should be kept in a secure office facility and back up on hard copy should be routinely performed.

3.2.7.2. In the event that the Source Animal Facility ceases to operate, the facility should either transfer all animal health records and specimens to the respective sponsors or notify the sponsors of the new archive site. If the sponsor ceases to exist, decisions on the disposition of the archived records and specimens should be made in consultation with the FDA.

3.2.8. All animal facilities should be subject to inspection by designated representatives of the clinical protocol sponsor and public health agencies. The sponsor is responsible for implementing and maintaining a routine facilities inspection program for quality control and quality assurance.

3.3. Pre-xenotransplantation Screening for Known Infectious Agents

The following points discuss measures for appropriate screening of known infectious agents in the herd, individual source animal and the nonhuman animal live cells, tissues or organs used in xenotransplan-tation. The selection of assays for pre-transplant screening should be determined by the source of the nonhuman animal live cells, tissues or organs and the intended clinical application of the xenotransplantation product. General guidance on adventitious agent testing may be found in "Points to Consider for the Characterization of Cell Lines Used to Produce Biologicals" (FDA, CBER, 1993), and a guidance document from the International Conference on Harmonization: "Q5D Quality of Biotechnological/Biological Products: Derivation and Characterization of Cell Subsets Used for Production of Biotechnological/Biological Products".

3.3.1. The design of preclinical studies intended to identify infectious agents in the xenotransplantation product and/or the nonhuman animal live cells, tissues or organs intended for use in the manufacture of xenotransplantation products should take into consideration the source animal species and the specific manner in which the xenotransplantation product will be used clinically. These studies should identify infectious agents and characterize their potential pathogenicity and tropism for human cells by appropriate *in vivo* and *in vitro* assays. Characterization of persistent viral infections and endogenous retroviruses present in source animals cells, tissues or organs is particularly important. The information from these studies is necessary for the identification and development of appropriate assays for xenotransplantation product screening programs.

3.3.2. Programs for screening and detection of known infectious agents in the herd or colony, the individual source animal, and the xenotransplantation product itself or the nonhuman animal live cells, tissues or organs used in the manufacture of xenotransplantation products should take into account the infectious agents associated with the source animals used, the stringency of the husbandry techniques employed, and the manner in which the xenotransplan-tation product will be used clinically. These programs should be updated periodically to reflect advances in the knowledge of infectious diseases. The sponsor should develop an adequate screening program in consultation with appropriate experts including oversight and regulatory bodies.

3.3.3. Assays used for screening and detection of infectious agents should have well defined and documented sensitivity, specificity, and reproducibility in the setting in which they are employed. In addition to assays for specific infectious agents, the use of assays capable of detecting broad ranges of infectious agents is strongly encouraged. *In vivo* assays involving animal models may require different standards for evaluation. Assays under development may complement the screening process.

3.3.4. Samples from the xenotransplantation product itself or of the nonhuman animal live cells, tissues or organs used in the manufacture of the xenotransplantation product, whenever possible, or from an appropriate biologic proxy should be tested preclinically with co-cultivation assays. These assays should include a panel of appropriate indicator cells, which may include human peripheral blood mononuclear cells (PBMC), to facilitate amplification and detection of endogenous retroviruses and other xenogeneic viruses capable of producing infection in humans. Agents that may be latent are of particular concern and their detection may be facilitated by using chemical and irradiation methods.

3.3.5. All xenotransplantation products should be screened by direct culture for bacteria, fungi, and mycoplasma (see, e.g. 21 CFR Part 600-680). In addition, universal PCR probes for the presence of micro-organisms are available and should be considered to complement the screening of xenotransplantation products.

3.4. Herd/Colony Health Maintenance and Surveillance

The principal elements recommended to qualify a herd or colony as a source of animals for use in xenotransplantation include: (1) closed herd or colony of stock (optimally caesarian derived) raised in barrier facilities; and (2) adequate surveillance programs for infectious agents.

The standard operating procedures of the animal facility with regard to the herd or colony health maintenance and surveillance programs relevant to the specific xenotransplantation product usage should be documented and available to appropriate review bodies. Medical records for the herd or colony and the specific individual source animals should be maintained by the animal facility or the sponsor, as appropriate, for 50 years beyond the date of the xenotransplantation.

3.4.1. Herd or colony health measures that constitute standard veterinary care for the species (e.g. anti-parasitic measures) should be implemented and recorded at the animal facility. For example, aseptic techniques and sterile equipment should be used in all parenteral interventions including vaccinations, phlebotomy, and biopsies. All incidents that may affect herd or colony health should be recorded (e.g. breaks in the environmental barriers of the secured facility, disease outbreaks, or sudden animal deaths). Vaccination and screening schedules should be described in detail and taken into account when interpreting serologic screening tests. Prevention of disease by protection from exposure is generally preferable to vaccination, since this preserves the ability of serologic screening to define herd exposures. In particular, the use of live vaccines is discouraged, but may be justified when dead or acellular vaccines are not available and barriers to exposure are inadequate to prevent the introduction of infectious agents into the herd or colony.

3.4.2. In addition to standard medical care, the herd/colony should be monitored for the introduction of infectious agents which may not be apparent clinically. The sponsor should describe the monitoring program, including the types and schedules of physical examinations and laboratory tests used in the detection of all infectious agents, and document the results.

3.4.3. Routine testing of closed herds or colonies in the United States should concentrate on zoonoses known to exist in captive animals of the relevant species in North America. Since many important pathogens are not endemic to the United States or have been found only in wild-caught animals, testing of breeding stock and maintenance of a closed herd or colony reduces the need for extensive testing of individual source animals. Herd or colony geographic locations are relevant to consideration of presence and likelihood of pathogens in a given herd or colony. The geographic origin of the founding stock of the colony, including quarantine and screening procedures utilized when the closed colony was established, should be taken into consideration. Veterinarians familiar with the prevalence of different infectious agents in the geographic area of source animal origin and the location where the source animals are to be maintained should be consulted.

3.4.3.1. As part of the surveillance program, routine serum samples should be obtained from randomly selected animals representative of the herd or colony population. These samples should be tested for indicators of infectious agents relevant to the species and epidemiologic exposures. Additional directed serologic analysis, active culturing, or other diagnostic laboratory testing of individual animals should be performed in response to clinical indications. Infection in one animal in the herd justifies a larger clinical and epidemiologic evaluation of the rest of the herd or colony. Aliquots of serum samples collected during routine surveillance and specific disease investigations should be maintained for 50 years beyond the date of sample collection. The Source Animal Facility or the sponsor should maintain these specimens (either on- or off-site) for investigations of unexpec-ted diseases that occur in the herd, colony, individual source animals, or animal facility staff. These herd health surveillance samples, which are not archived for PHS investigation purposes, should nonetheless be made available to the PHS if needed (section 3.7.).

3.4.3.2. Any animal deaths, including stillbirths or abortions, where the cause is either unknown or ambiguous should lead to full necropsy and evaluation for infectious etiologies (including transmissible spongiform encephalopathies) by a trained veteri-nary pathologist. Results of these investigations should be documented.

3.4.4. Standard operating procedures that include maintenance of a subset of sentinel animals are encouraged. Monitoring of these animals will increase the probability of detection of subclinical, latent, or late-onset diseases such as transmissible spongiform encephalopathies.

3.5. Individual Source Animal Screening and Qualification

The qualification of individual source animals should include documentation of breed and lineage, general health, and vaccination history, particularly the use of live and/or live attenuated vaccines (section 3.4.1). The presence of pathogens that result in acute infections should be documented and controlled by clinical examination and treatment of individual source animals, by use of individual quarantine periods that extend beyond the incubation period of pathogens of concern, and by herd surveillance indicating the presence or absence of infection in the herd from which the individual source animal is selected. The use of any drugs or biologic agents for treatment should be documented. During quarantine and/or prior to procurement of live cells, tissues or organs for use in xenotransplantation, individual source animals should be screened for infectious agents relevant to the particular intended clinical use of the planned xenotransplantation product. The screening program should be guided by the surveillance and health history of the herd or colony.

3.5.1. In general, individual source animals should be quarantined for 3 weeks prior to procurement of live cells, tissues or organs for use in xenotransplantation. During the quarantine, acute illnesses due to infectious agents to which the animal may have been exposed shortly before removal from the herd or colony would be expected to become clinically apparent. It may be appropriate to modify the need for and duration of individual quarantine periods depending on the characterization and surveillance of the source animal herd or colony, the design of the facility in which the herd is bred and maintained, and the clinical urgency. When the quarantine period is shortened or eliminated, justification should be documented and any potentially increased infectious risk should be addressed in the informed consent document.

3.5.1.1. During the quarantine period, candidate source animals should be examined by a veterinarian and screened for the presence of infectious agents (bacteria including rickettsiae when appropriate, parasites, fungi, and viruses) by appropriate serologies and cultures, serum clinical chemistries (including those specific to the function of the organ or tissue to be procured), complete blood count and peripheral blood smear, and fecal exam for parasites. Evaluation for viruses which may not be recognized zoonotic agents but which have been documented to infect either human or nonhuman primate cells *in vivo* or *in vitro* should be considered. Particular attention should be given to viruses with demonstrated capacity for recombination, complementation, or pseudotyping. Surveillance of a closed herd or colony (as described in section 3.4.3.) will minimize the additional screening necessary to qualify individual member animals. The nature, timing, and results of surveillance of the herd or colony from which the individual animal is procured should be considered in designing appropriate additional screening of individual animals. These tests should be performed as closely as possible to the date of xenotransplantation while ensuring availability of results prior to clinical use.

3.5.1.2. Screening of a candidate source animal should be repeated prior to procurement of live cells, tissues or organs for use in xenotransplantation if a period greater than three months has elapsed since the initial screening and qualification were performed or if the animal has been in contact with other non-quarantined animals between the quarantine period and the time of cells, tissue or organ procurement.

3.5.1.3. Transportation of source animals may compromise the microbiologic protection ensured by the closed colony. Careful attention to conditions of transport can minimize disease exposures during shipping. Microbiological isolation of the source animal during transit is critically important. Source animals should be transported using a system that reliably ensures microbiological isolation. Transported source animals should be quarantined for a minimum period of three weeks after transportation, during which time appropriate screening should be performed. The sponsor may propose a shorter quarantine period if appropriate justification (that reflects the level of containment and the duration of the transportation) is provided. When source animals are transported intact, the sponsor should consult the FDA about further details of appropriate transport, quarantine, and screening. If the animals are transported across state or federal boundaries the USDA should be consulted.

3.5.1.4. For the reasons cited above, it is preferable, whenever feasible, to procure live cells, tissues or organs for use in xenotransplantation at the animal facility. Precautions employed during transport to ensure microbiological isolation of the procured xenotransplantation product or live cells, tissues or organs should be documented.

3.5.2. All procured cells, tissues and organs intended for use in xenotransplantation should be as free of infectious agents as possible. The use of source animals in which infectious agents, including latent viruses, have been identified should be avoided. However, the presence of an infectious agent in certain anatomic sites, for example the alimentary tract, should not preclude use of the source animal if the agent is documented to be absent in the xenotransplantation product.

3.5.3. When feasible a biopsy of the nonhuman animal live cells, tissues or organs intended for use in xenotransplantation, the xenotransplantation product itself, or other relevant tissue should be evaluated for the presence of infectious agents by appropriate assays and histopathology prior to xenotransplantation, and then archived (section 3.7).

3.5.4. The sponsor should ensure that the linked records described in section 3.2.7. are available for review when appropriate by the local review bodies, the SACX, and the FDA. These records should include information on the results of the quarantine and screening of individual xenotransplantation source animals. In addition to records being kept at the Source Animal Facility, a summary of the individual source animal record should accompany the xenotransplantation product and be archived as part of the medical record of the xenotransplantation product recipient.

3.5.5. The Source Animal Facility should notify the sponsor in the event that an infectious agent is identified in the source animal or herd subsequent to procurement of live cells, tissues or organs for use in xenotransplantation (e.g. identification of delayed onset transmissible spongiform encephalo-pathies in a sentinel animal).

3.5.6. The sponsor should ensure that the quarantine, screening, and qualification program is appropriately tailored to the specific source animal species, the animal husbandry history, the process for procuring the xenogeneic biomaterial and preparing the xenotransplantation product, and the clinical application. The sponsor should also ensure that the results of these procedures are reviewed and approved by persons with the appropriate expertise prior to the clinical application.

3.6. Procurement and Screening of Nonhuman Animal Live Cells, Tissues or Organs used for Xenotransplantation

3.6.1. Procurement and processing of cells, tissues and organs should be performed using documented aseptic conditions designed to minimize contamination. These procedures should be conducted in designated facilities which may be subject to inspection by appropriate oversight and regulatory authorities.

3.6.2. Cells, tissues or organs intended for xenotransplantation that are maintained in culture prior to xenotransplantation should be periodically screened for maintenance of sterility, including screening for viruses and mycoplasma. The FDA publications entitled "Guidance for Industry: Guidance for Human Somatic Cell Therapy and Gene Therapy (1998)"; "Points to Consider in the Characterization of Cell Lines used to Produce Biologicals (1993)"; and "Points to Consider in the Manufacture and Testing of Therapeutic Products for Human Use Derived from Transgenic Animals (1995)" should be consulted for guidance. The sponsor should develop, implement, and stringently enforce the standard operating procedures for the procurement and screening processes. Procedures that may inactivate or remove pathogens without compromising the integrity and function of the xenotransplantation product should be employed.

3.6.3. All steps involved in the procuring, processing, and screening of live cells, tissues, organs, or xenotransplantation products, to the point of xenotransplantation, should be rehearsed preclinically to ensure repro-ducible quality control.

3.6.4. If nonhuman animal live cells, tissues, or organs, for use in xenotransplantation, are procured without euthanatizing the source animal, the designated PHS specimens should be archived (PHS specimens are discussed in section 3.7.1.) and the animal's health should be monitored for his entire life. When source animals die or are euthanatized, a complete necropsy with gross, histopathologic and microbiological evaluation by a trained veterinary pathologist should follow, regardless of the time elapsed between xenogeneic biomaterial procurement and death. This should include evaluation for transmissible spongiform encephalopathies. The sponsor should maintain documenttation of all necropsy results for 50 years beyond the date of necropsy as part of the animal health record (sections 3.2.7. and 3.4.). In the event that the necropsy reveals findings pertinent to the health of the xenotransplantation product recipient(s) (e.g. evidence of transmissible spongiform encephalopathies) the finding should be communicated to the FDA without delay (see e.g. 21 CFR 312.32).

3.7. Archives of Source Animal Medical Records and Specimens

Systematically archived source animal biologic samples and record keeping that allows rapid and accurate linking of xenotransplantation product recipients to the individual source animal records and archived biologic specimens are essential for public health investigation and containment of emergent xenogeneic infections.

3.7.1. Source animal biologic specimens designated for PHS use (as outlined below) should be banked at the time of xenogeneic biomaterial procurement. These specimens should remain in archival storage for 50 years beyond the date of the xenotransplantation to permit retrospective analyses if a public health need arises. Such archived specimens should be readily accessible to the PHS and remain linked to both source animal and recipient health records.

At the time of procurement of nonhuman animal live cells, tissues or organs for use in xenotransplantation, plasma should be collected from the source animal and stored in sufficient quantity for subsequent serology and viral testing. In addition, the sponsor should recover and bank sufficient aliquots of cryopreserved leukocytes for subsequent isolation of nucleic acids and proteins as well as aliquots for thawing viable cells for viral co-culture assays or other tissue culture assays. Ideally at least ten 0.5 cc aliquots of citrated or EDTA-anticoagulated plasma should be banked. At least five aliquots of viable (1×10^7) leukocytes should be cryopreserved. It may also be appropriate to collect paraffin-embedded, formalin fixed, and cryopreserved tissue samples from source animal organs relevant to the specific protocol at the time of xenogeneic biomaterial procurement. Additionally, cryopreserved tissue samples representative of major organ systems (e.g. spleen, liver, bone marrow, central nervous system, lung,) should be collected from source animals at necropsy. The material submitted for review by FDA and, when appropriate, the Secretary's Advisory Committee on Xenotransplantation (under development, see section 5.3) should justify the types of tissues, cells, and plasma taken for storage and any smaller quantities of plasma and leukocytes collected.

3.7.2. The sponsor should maintain archives of designated PHS specimens (section 3.7.1.) and serum collected for herd surveillance for 50 years beyond the date of collection (section 3.4.3.1.), and animal health records for 50 years beyond the date of the animal's death (sections 3.2.7.).

3.8. Disposal of Animals and Animal By-products

The need for advanced planning for the ultimate disposition of source and sentinel animals bred for xenotransplantation, especially animals of species ordinarily used to produce food, should be anticipated. Generally source and sentinel animals should not be used as pets, breeding animals, sources of human food via milk or meat, or as ingredients of feed for other animals because of their potential to enter the human or animal food chain.

3.8.1. There may be species specific situations where animals from xenotransplant facilities can be considered to be safe for human food use or as feed ingredients when disposed of through rendering. FDA's Center for Veterinary Medicine (CVM) regulates animal feed ingredients and also establishes conditions for the release of animals to the USDA Food Safety Inspection Service for inspection as food for humans. Persons wishing to offer animals into the human food or animal feed supply, or who have food safety questions, should consult with CVM. Food safety issues will be referred to CVM.

3.8.2. Animals from biomedical facilities that have not been authorized for release by CVM into the human food or animal feed supply may be adulterated under the Federal Food, Drug and Cosmetic Act (21 USC 321 et seq.), unfit for food or feed, and potentially infectious. They should be disposed of in a manner consistent with infectious medical waste in compliance with federal, state and local requirements.

4. Clinical Issues

4.1. Xenotransplantation Product Recipient

4.1.1. Surveillance of the xenotransplantation product recipient

Post-xenotransplantation clinical and laboratory surveillance of xenotransplantation product recipients is critical, as it provides the means of monitoring for any introduction and propagation of xenogeneic infectious agents in the xenotransplantation product recipient. The sponsor should carry out, and ensure documentation of, the surveillance program. Life-long post-xenotransplantation surveillance of xenotransplantation product recipients is appropriate.

4.1.1.1. Recipients should be evaluated throughout their lifetime for adverse clinical events potentially associated with xenogeneic infections.

4.1.1.2. Laboratory surveillance of the xenotransplantation product recipient should be instituted when xenogeneic infectious agents are known or suspected to be present in the xenotransplantation product. Minimally, laboratory surveillance should be conducted for evidence of recipient infection with all identified xenotropic endogenous retroviruses known to be present in the source animal. The intent of active screening in this setting is detection of sentinel human infections prior to dissemination in the general population. Serum, PBMCs, tissue or other body fluids should be assayed at intervals post-xenotransplantation for xenogeneic agents known or suspected to be present in the xenotransplantation product. Laboratory surveillance should include frequent screening in the immediate post-xenotransplantation period (e.g. at 2, 4, and 6 weeks after xenotransplantation) that decreases in frequency if evidence of infection remains absent.

It is critical that adequate diagnostic assays and methodologies for surveillance of known infectious agents from the source animal are available prior to initiating the clinical trial. The sensitivity, specificity, and reproducibility of these testing methods should be documented under conditions that simulate those employed at the time of and following the xenotransplantation procedure. As with pre-xenotransplantation screening, assays under development may complement the surveillance process (see section 3.3.3.).

The laboratory surveillance should include methods to detect infectious agents known to establish persistent latent infections in the absence of clinical symptoms (e.g. herpesviruses, retroviruses, papillomaviruses) and that are known or suspected to have been present in the xenotransplantation product. When the xenogeneic viruses of concern have similar human counter-parts (e.g. simian cytomegalovirus), assays to distinguish between the two should be used in the post-xenotransplantation laboratory surveillance. Depending upon the degree of immuno-suppression in the recipient, serological assays may be or may not be useful. Methods for analysis may include co-cultivation of cells coupled with appropriate detection assays.

4.1.2. Xenotransplantation Product Recipients' Biologic Specimens Archived for Public Health Investigations (PHS Specimens).
Biological specimens obtained from the xenotransplantation product recipients and designated for public health investigations (as distinct from specimens collected for clinical evaluation or laboratory surveillance) should be archived for 50 years beyond the date of the xenotransplantation to allow retrospective investigation of xenogeneic infections. The type and quantity of specimens archived may vary with the clinical procedure and the age of the xenotransplantation product recipient. In the application for FDA review, which may also be reviewed by the SACX, the sponsor should justify the amount and types of specimens to be designated for PHS use, including any differences from the recommendations described below.

At selected time points, at least three to five 0.5 cc aliquots of citrated or EDTA-anticoagulated plasma should be recovered and archived. At least two aliquots of viable (1×10^7) leukocytes should be cryopreserved. Specimens from any xenotransplantation product that is removed (e.g. post-rejection or at the time of death) should be archived.

The following schedule for archiving biological specimens is recommended: (1) Prior to the xenotransplantation procedure, 2 sets of samples should be collected and archived one month apart. If this is not feasible then two sets should be collected and archived at times that are separated as much as possible. One set should be collected immediately prior to the xenotransplantation. (2) Additional sets should be archived in the immediate post-xenotransplantation period and at approximately one month and six months after xenotransplan-tation. (3) Collection should then be obtained annually for the first two years after xenotransplantation. (4) After that, specimens should be archived every five years for the remainder of the recipient's life. More frequent archiving may be indicated by the specific protocol or the recipient's medical course.

4.1.2.1. In the event of recipient's death, snap-frozen samples stored at -70° C, paraffin embedded tissue, and tissue suitable for electron microscopy should be collected at autopsy from the xenotransplantation product and all major organs relevant to either the xenotransplantation or the clinical syndrome that resulted in the patient's death. These designated PHS specimens should be archived for 50 years beyond the date of collection.

4.1.2.2. The sponsor should maintain an accurate archive of the PHS specimens. In the absence of a central facility (section 5.2), these specimens should be archived with the safeguards necessary to ensure long-term storage (e.g. a monitored storage freezer alarm system and specimen archiving in split portions in separate freezers) and an efficient system for the prompt retrieval and linkage of data to medical records of recipients and source animals.

The sponsor should maintain these archives and a record system that allows easy, accurate, and rapid linkage of information among the different record systems (i.e. the specimen archive, the recipient's medical records and the records of the source animal) for 50 years beyond the date of xenotransplantation. If record systems are maintained in a computer database, electronic back ups should be kept in a secure office facility and back up on hard copy should be routinely performed.

4.1.2.3. A clinical episode potentially representing a xenogeneic infection should prompt notification of the FDA, which will notify other federal and state health authorities as appropriate. Under these circumstances, the PHS may decide that an investigation involving the use of these archived biologic specimens is warranted to assess the public health significance of the infection.

4.2. Infection Control
4.2.1. Infection control practices

4.2.1.1. Strict adherence to recommended infection control measures will reduce the risk of transmission of xenogeneic infections and other blood borne and nosocomial pathogens. Standard precautions should be used for the care of all patients. Standard precautions includes hand washing before and after each patient contact, appropriate use of barriers, and care in the use and disposal of needles and other sharp instruments.

4.2.1.2. Additional infection control or isolation precautions (e.g. Airborne, Droplet, Contact) should be employed as indicated in the judgment of the hospital epidemiologist and the xenotransplantation team infectious disease specialist. For example, appropriate isolation precautions for each hospitalized xenotransplantation product recipient will depend upon the type of xenotransplantation, the extent of immunosuppression, and patient symptoms. Isolation precautions should be continued until a diagnosis has been established or the patient symptoms have resolved. The appropriateness of isolation precautions and other infection control measures should be reassessed when the diagnosis is established, the patient's symptoms change, and at the time of readmission and discharge. Discharge instructions should include specific education on appropriate infection control practices following discharge, including any special precautions recommended for disposal of biologic products. The most restrictive level of isolation should be used when patients exhibit respiratory symptoms, because airborne transmission of infectious agents is most concerning.

4.2.1.3. Health care personnel, including xenotransplantation team members, should adhere to recommended procedures for handling and disinfection/sterilization of medical instruments and disposal of infectious waste.

4.2.1.4. Biosafety level 2 (BSL-2) standard and special practices, containment equipment and facilities should be used for activities involving clinical specimens from xenotransplantation product recipients. Particular attention should be given to sharps management and bioaerosol containment. BSL-3 standard and special practices and containment equipment should be employed in a BSL-2 facility when propagating an unidentified infectious agent isolated from a xenotransplantation product recipient.

4.2.2. Acute Infectious Episodes

Most acute viral infectious episodes among the general population are never etiologically identified. Xenotransplantation product recipients are at risk for these infections and other infections common among immunosuppressed allograft recipients. When the source of an illness in a recipient remains unidentified, despite standard diagnostic procedures, it may be appropriate to perform additional testing of body fluid and tissue samples. The infectious disease specialist, in consultation with the hospital epidemiologist, the veterinarian, the clinical microbiologist, and other members of the xenotransplantation team should assess each clinical episode and make a considered judgment regarding the significance of the illness, the need and type of diagnostic testing, and specific infection control precautions. Other experts on infectious diseases and public health may also need to be consulted.

4.2.2.1. In immunosuppressed xenotransplantation product recipients, assays of antibody response may not detect infections reliably. In such patients, culture systems, genomic detection methodologies and other techniques may detect infections for which serologic testing is inadequate. Consequently, clinical centers where xenotransplantation is performed should have the capability to culture and to identify viral agents using *in vitro* and *in vivo* methodologies either on site or through active and documented collaborations. Specimens should be handled to ensure viability and to maximize the probability of isolation and identification of fastidious agents. Algorithms for evaluation of unknown xenogeneic pathogens should be developed in consultation with appropriate experts, including persons with expertise in both medical and veterinary infectious diseases, laboratory identification of unknown infectious agents and the management of biosafety issues associated with such investigations.

4.2.2.2. Acute and convalescent sera obtained in association with acute unexplained illnesses should be archived when judged appropriate by the infectious disease physician and/or the hospital epidemiologist. This would permit retrospective study and perhaps the identification of an etiologic agent.

4.2.3. Health Care Workers

The risk to health care workers who provide post-xenotransplantation care to xenotransplantation product recipients is undefined. However, health care workers, including laboratory personnel, who handle the animal tissues/organs prior to xenotransplantation will have a definable risk of infection not exceeding that of animal care, veterinary, or abattoir workers routinely exposed to the source animal species provided equivalent biosafety standards are employed.

The sponsor should ensure that a comprehensive Occupational Health Services program is available to educate workers regarding the risks associated with xenotransplantation and to monitor for possible infections in workers. The Occupational Health Service program should include:

4.2.3.1. Education of Health Care Workers. All centers where xenotransplantation procedures are performed should develop appropriate xenotransplantation procedure-specific educational materials for their staff. These materials should describe the xenotransplantation procedure(s), the known and potential risks of xenogeneic infections posed by the procedure(s), and research or health care activities that may pose the greatest risk of infection or nosocomial transmission of zoonotic or other infectious agents. Education programs should detail the circumstances under which the use of Standard Precautions and other isolation precautions are recommended, including the use of personal protective equipment handwashing before and after all patient contacts, even if gloves are worn. In addition, the potential for transmission of these agents to the general public should be discussed.

4.2.3.2. Health Care Worker Surveillance. The sponsor and the Occupational Health Service in each clinical center should develop protocols for monitoring health care personnel. These protocols should describe methods for storage and retrieval of personnel records and collection of serologic specimens from workers. Baseline sera (i.e. prior to exposure to xenotransplantation products or recipients) should be collected from all personnel who provide direct care to xenotransplantation product recipients, and laboratory personnel who handle, or are likely to handle, animal cells, tissues and organs or biologic specimens from xenotransplantation product recipients. Baseline sera can be compared to sera collected following occupational exposures; such baseline sera should be maintained for 50 years from the time of collection. The activities of the Occupational Health Service should be coordinated with the Infection Control Program to ensure appropriate surveillance of infections in personnel.

4.2.3.3. Post-Exposure Evaluation and Management. Written protocols should be in place for the evaluation of health care workers who experience an exposure where there is a risk of transmission of an infectious agent, e.g. an accidental needle stick. Health care workers, including laboratory personnel, should be instructed to report exposures immediately to the Occupational Health Services. The post-exposure protocol should describe the information to be recorded including the date and nature of exposure, the xenotransplantation procedure, recipient information, actions taken as a result of such exposures (e.g. counseling, post-exposure management, and follow-up) and the outcome of the event. This information should be archived in a health exposure log (section 4.3.) and maintained for at least 50 years from the time of the xenotransplantation despite any change in employment of the health care worker or discontinuation of xenotransplantation procedures at that center. Health care and laboratory workers should be counseled to report and seek medical evaluation for unexplained clinical illnesses occurring after the exposure.

4.3. Health Care Records

The sponsor should maintain a cross-referenced system that links the relevant records of the xenotransplantation product recipient, xenotransplantation product, source animal (s), animal procurement center, and significant nosocomial exposures. These records should include: (1) documentation of each xenotransplantation procedure, (2) documentation of significant nosocomial health exposures, and (3) documentation of the infectious disease screening and surveillance records on both xenotransplantation product source animals and recipients. These records should be updated regularly and cross-referenced to allow rapid and easy linkage between the clinical records of the source animal(s) and the xenotransplantation product recipient.

To the extent permitted by applicable laws and/or regulations, the confidentiality of all medical and research records pertaining to human recipients should be maintained (section 2.5.10.).

4.3.1. The documentation of each xenotransplantation procedure includes the date and type of the procedure, the principal investigator (s) (PI), the xenotransplantation product recipient, the xenotransplantation product (s), the individual source animal (s) and the procurement facilities for these animals, as well as the health care workers associated with each procedure.

4.3.2. The documentation of significant nosocomial health exposures includes the persons involved, the date and nature of each potentially significant nosocomial exposure (exposures defined in the written Infection Control/Occupational Health Service protocol), and the actions taken.

4.3.3. The documentation of infectious disease screening and surveillance includes: (a) a summary of the source animal (s) health status; (b) the results of the pre-xenotransplantation screening program for the source animal (s); (c) the results of the pre-xenotransplantation screening program for the xenotransplantation product; (d) the post-xenotransplantation surveillance studies on the xenotransplantation product recipient; and (e) a summary of significant relevant post-xenotransplantation clinical events.

5. Public Health Needs

5.1. National Xenotransplantation Database

A pilot project to demonstrate the feasibility of, and identify system requirements for a National Xenotransplantation Database is currently underway. It is anticipated that this pilot would be expanded into a fully operational Database to collect data from all clinical centers conducting trials in xenotransplantation and all animal facilities providing animals or xenogeneic organs, tissues, or cells for clinical use. Such a database would enable: (a) the recognition of rates of occurrence and clustering of adverse health events, including events that may represent outcomes of xenogeneic infections; (b) accurate linkage of these events to exposures on a national level; (c) notification of individuals and clinical centers regarding epide-miologically significant adverse events associated with xenotransplan-tation; and (d) biological and clinical research assessments. When such a Database becomes functional, the sponsor should ensure that information requested by the Database is provided in an accurate and timely manner. To the extent allowed by law, information derived from the Database would be available to the public with appropriate confidentiality protections for any proprietary or individually identifiable information.

5.2. Biologic Specimen Archives

The sponsor should ensure that the designated PHS specimens from the source animals, xenotransplantation products, and xenotrans-plantation product recipients are archived (sections 3.7.1, 3.5.3, and 4.1.2.). The biologic specimens should be collected and archived under conditions that will ensure their suitability for subsequent public health purposes, including public health investigations (sections 4.1.2.3.). The location and nature of archived specimens should be documented in the health care records and this information should be linked to the National Xenotransplantation Database when the latter becomes functional. DHHS is considering options for a central biological archive, e.g. one maintained by a private sector organization under contract to DHHS. Designated PHS specimens would be deposited in such a repository.

5.3. Secretary's Advisory Committee on Xenotransplantation (SACX)

The SACX is currently being implemented by DHHS. As currently envisioned, the SACX will consider the full range of complex issues raised by xenotransplantation, including ongoing and proposed protocols, and make recommendations to the Secretary on policy and procedures. The SACX will also provide a forum for public discussion of issues when appropriate. These activities will facilitate DHHS efforts to develop an integrated approach to addressing emerging public health issues in xenotransplantation. The structure and functions of the SACX as well as procedures for SACX review of protocols and issues will be described in subsequent publications. Inquiries about the status and function of, and access to the SACX should be directed to the Office of Science Policy, Office of the Secretary, DHHS, or the Office of Biotechnology Activities (OBA), formerly known as the Office of Recombinant DNA Activities (ORDA), Office of the Director, NIH.

6. BIBLIOGRAPHY.

A. Federal Laws
1. The Public Health Service Act (42 USC §§ 262 et seq.)
2. The Federal Food, Drug, and Cosmetic Act (21 USC §§ 321 et seq.)
3. The Social Security Act (42 USC § 1320b-8)
4. The National Organ Transplant Act (42 USC §§ 273 et seq.)
5. The Animal Welfare Act (7 USC §§ 2131 et seq.)

B. Federal Regulations
1. 21 (CFR) Parts 50, 56, 312, 314, 600 - 680
2. 45 (CFR) Part 46, 71
3. 9 (CFR) Parts 1, 2, 3, and 122

C. Guidance Documents
1. Food and Drug Administration
    a. Guidance for Industry. Guidance for Human Somatic Cell Therapy and Gene Therapy (3/30/98) (see also Quarterly List of

Guidance Documents at the Food and Drug Administration, July 6, 1998;63 FR 36413). **(www.fda.gov/cber/guidelines.htm)
b. Points to Consider in the Characterization of Cell Lines used to Produce Biologicals; (August 12, 1993; 58 FR 42974)*
c. Application of Current Statutory Authorities to Human Somatic Cell Therapy Products and Gene Therapy Products; (October 14, 1993; 58 FR 53248)*
d. Bovine Derived Materials; Agency Letters to Manufacturers of FDA Regulated Products; (August 29, 1994; 59 FR 44591)
e. Points to Consider in the Manufacture and Testing of Therapeutic Products for Human use Derived from Transgenic Animals; (August 24, 1995; 60 FR 44036)
f. Q5D Quality of Biotechnological/Biological Products: Derivation and Characterization of Cell Substrates used for Production of Biotechnological/Biological Products (September 21, 1998; 63 FR 50244)
g. Q5A Viral Safety Evaluation of Biotechnology Products Derived from Cell Lines of Human or Animal Origin; (September 24, 1998; 63 FR 51074)
h. Guidance for Industry: Public Health Issues Posed by the use of Nonhuman Primate Xenografts in Humans; (Notice of Availability: April 6, 1999; 64 FR 16743-16744)
i. Guidance for Industry: Precautionary Measures to Reduce the Possible Risk of Transmission of Zoonoses by Blood and Blood Products from Xenotransplantation Product Recipients and Their Close Contacts; (Notice of Availability: December 30, 1999; 64 FR 73562 - 73563)

[Please note that the documents identified with an asterisk "*" can be obtained from FDA/CBER/Office of Communication, Training and Manufacturers Assistance via FAX by dialing 1-800-835-4709 or via mail by calling 301-827-1800. In addition, documents marked with two asterisks "**" can be found on the internet at the indicated website].

2. **National Institutes of Health/Centers for Disease Control and Prevention**
   a) Guidelines to Prevent Simian Immunodeficiency Virus Infection in Laboratory Workers and Animal Handlers; (MMWR 1988;37:693-4, 699-700),
   (www.cdc.gov/epo/mmwr/preview/mmwrhtml/00001303.htm)
   b) Guidelines for Investigating Clusters of Health Events; (MMWR Recommendations & Reports 1990;39; RR-11),

www.cdc.gov/epo/mmwr/preview/mmwrhtml/00001797.htm
and www.cdc.gov/epo/mmwr/preview/mmwrhtml/00001798.htm
c) CDC-NIH. Biosafety in Microbiological and Biomedical Laboratories. US Department of Health and Human Services, Public Health Service, Centers for Disease Control and Prevention, and the National of Health; 3rd edition, March 1993. US Government Printing Office, Washington, DC. HHS Publication No. (CDC) 93-8395, (http://www.cdc.gov/od/ohs/biosfty/bmbl/bmbl3toc.htm)

3. National Institutes of Health

a) NIH. The NIH Guidelines for Research Involving Recombinant DNA Molecules, as amended May 1999. (64 FR 25361),
b) The Public Health Service Policy on Humane Care and Use of Laboratory Animals. Revised September 1986; Reprinted March 1996. Office for the Protection from Research Risks, 9000 Rockville Pike, Building 31, Room 4B09, Bethesda, Maryland 20892, Telephone 301- 496-7005,
(http://www.nih.gov/grants/olaw/references/phspol.htm).

4. Centers for Disease Control and Prevention

a) CDC. Update: Universal Precautions for Prevention of Transmission of HIV, Hepatitis B Virus, and other Blood borne Pathogens in Health-Care Settings. MMWR 1988;37:377-88, (www.cdc.gov/epo/mmwr/preview/mmwrhtml/00000039.htm)
b) CDC. Guidelines for Prevention of Transmission of Human Immunodeficiency Virus and Hepatitis B Virus to Health-Care Workers and Public-Safety Workers. MMWR 1989;38:No. S-6, (www.cdc.gov/epo/mmwr/preview/mmwrhtml/00001450.htm)
c) CDC. The Guideline for Hand washing and Hospital Environmental Control (published in 1985; PB85-923404)*
d) Garner JS, CDC Hospital Infection Practices Advisory Committee. Guideline for Isolation Precautions in Hospitals. Infection Control and Hospital Epidemiology 1996;17:53-80 and American Journal of Infection Control 1996; 24: 24-52,
(http://www.cdc.gov/ncidod/hip/isolat/isolat.htm)
e) NIOSH. Guidelines for Protecting the Safety and Health of Health-Care Workers. Cincinnati, Ohio: US Department of Health and Human Services, Public Health Service, CDC, 1988; DHHS publication no. (NIOSH)88-119,
(http://www.cdc.gov/niosh/hcwold0.html)
(Notice of Availability: MMWR 1990;39:417)
(www.cdc.gov/epo/mmwr/preview/mmwrhtml/00001649.htm)

[Please note that the documents identified with an asterisk "*" can be purchased from]:

The National Technical Information Service or NTIS
5285 Port Royal Road
Springfield, Virginia 22161
telephone (703) 487-4650]

US Department of Agriculture
Barbeito, et al. Recommended biocontainment features for research and diagnostic facilities where animal pathogens are used. Rev. sci. Tech. Off. Int. Epiz., 1995;14:873-887

National Research Council
NRC. Guide for the Care and Use of Laboratory Animals, Institute of Laboratory Animal Resources, Commission on Life Sciences, National Research Council, 2101 Constitution Avenue NW, Washington, DC 20418

National Academy Press, Washington DC, 1996
(http://www.nap.edu/readingroom/books/labrats/)

National and International Bodies
a) Advisory Group on the Ethics of Xenotransplantation. Animal tissue into humans.
United Kingdom Department of Health, London, UK Stationery Office, 1996.
b) Council of Europe. Recommendation on Xenotransplantation, September 1997.
c) Health. Proposed Canadian Standard for Xenotransplantation. The Expert Working Group on Xenotransplantation. July 1999. (Available on the internet: http://www.hc-sc.gc.ca/hpb-dgps/therapeut/zfiles/english/ bgtd/xeno_std_e.html).
d) Health Canada. Report of the National Forum on Xenotransplantation: Clinical, Ethical, and Regulatory Issues, November 6-8, 1997, Health Canada. (Internet: Full report: http://www.hc-sc.gc.ca/hpbdgps/therapeut/ zfiles/english/bgtd/frmrptx_e.html, Summary: http://www.hc-sc.gc.ca/hpb-gps/therapeut/zfiles/english/ bgtd/forumsummary_e.html)

e) Health Council of the Netherlands: Committee on Xenotransplantation. Rijswijk: Health Council of the Netherlands, 1998; publication no. 1998/01E.
f) Institute of Medicine. Xenotransplantation: Science, Ethics, and Public Policy. Washington, DC National Academy Press, 1996.
g) Nuffield Council on Bioethics. Animals-to-human transplants. The ethics of xenotransplantation. London, Nuffield Council on Bioethics, 1996
h) Organization for Economic Cooperation and Development. Xenotransplantation: International Policy Issues. OECD Proceedings prepared by Elettra Ronchi, OECD Secretariat. OECD Publications, Paris, France, 1999. (OECD website for xenotransplantation international policy issues: Internet: http://www.oecd.org/dsti/sti/s_t/biotech/prod/xeno.htm).
i) Subcommission of Xenotransplantation of the Permanent Commission of Transplants of the Interterritorial Council of the National Health System. Xenotransplantation: Recommendations for the Regulation of these Activities in Spain. Available in Spanish or English translation from: Organizacion Nacional de Trasplantes, C/ Sinesio Delgado, 8, 28029 Madrid, Tel: (44) 91 314 24 06; Fax: (44) 91 314 29 69; E-mail: bmiranda@msc.es
j) Swedish Committee on Xenotransplantation. From one species to another - transplantation from animals to humans. A report by the Swedish Committee on Xenotransplantation, Stockholm 1999. Swedish Government Official Report No. 1999:120. Ministry of Health and Social Affairs. The complete report in Swedish or a short version (Summary and Statutory Proposals) in English are available upon request from: Stefan Reimer, Secretary, The Swedish Committee on Xenotransplantation, P.O. Box 187,S-201 21 MALMO, Sweden. E-mail: stefan.reimer@hsb.dom.se.
k) Transplantation Society of Australia and New Zealand, Inc. Xenotransplantation: A report to the Research Committee (Public Health and Medical), the National Health and Medical Research Council, from an Ad Hoc Working Party, August 1998. Revised December 1998. (Internet: http://www.racp.edu.au/tsanz/xenomain.htm).
l) United Kingdom Department of Health.

The Government Response to Animal Tissues into Humans. The Stationary Office, London, January 1997. (Further information is available on the United Kingdom Xenotransplantation Interim Regulatory Authority (UKXIRA) website: http://www.doh.gov.uk/ukxira.htm

m) World Health Organization. Report of WHO consultation on xenotransplantation,
Geneva, Switzerland, 28-30 October, 1997
World Health Organization, 1998 (document WHO/EMC/ZOO/98.2; available from Division of Emerging and Other Communicable Diseases Surveillance and Control, World Health Organization, 1211 Geneva 27, Switzerland).
(Internet: http://www.who.int/emc-documents/zoonoses/whoemczoo982c.html)

n) World Health Organization. Xenotransplantation: Guidance on infectious disease prevention and management. World Health Organization, Geneva, Switzerland, November 1998 (document WHO/EMC/ ZOO/98.1; available from Division of Emerging and Other Communicable Diseases Surveillance and Control, World Health Organization, 1211 Geneva 27, Switzerland)
(Internet: http://www.who.int/emc-documents/zoonoses/whoemczoo981c.html)

o) Xenotransplantation: Scientific Frontiers and Public Policy. Proceedings of an OECD/NY Academy of Sciences Workshop on Xenotransplantation. Edited by J Fishman, D Sachs, and R Shaikh. Annals of the New York Academy of Science 1998; volume 862.

D. Scientific Articles and Other Reports

The above regulation, the best in the world when it comes to the prevention of the transmission of xenoses, unfortunately declared cell, tissue or organ xenotransplants 'products', and thereby made the whole regulatory situation illogical. How can a baboon heart be classified a 'product' is hard to conceive.

Likewise lumping together cell, tissue and organ xenotransplantation, and thereby giving an impression that *cell (or tissue)* xenotransplantation belongs in the same group as *organ* xenotransplantation, has been somewhat misleading. Cell (or tissue) xenotransplantation have been around officially since 1931, and used for treatment of a huge number of patients, but that has not applied to organ xenotransplantation, and will be so for many years to come. Immunological issues of cell (or tissue) xenotransplantation have been solved for all practical purposes, as you can learn from this book, but with organ xenotransplantation it has been just the opposite, and it will take a long time before organ xenotransplantation becomes a standard treatment, the way cell (or tissue) xenotransplantation is already today.

F. Schmid was invited by US FDA to their Headquarters in May 1996 to lecture on and discuss the subject of cell xenotransplantation prior to the issuance of the 'Draft...' of the xenotransplantation regulation. Unfortunately he did not convince US FDA officials to recognize that around 5 million of patients were treated by cell therapy in Europe during a period of 65 years by then, and that an enormous clinical experience was acquired there.

The largest problem is that the above US FDA regulation is the only one about cell (or tissue) xenotransplantation that the US FDA has ever issued. In all other aspects of application for a license the usual drug regulations have to be used and it is against all logic to have to refer to the regulations applicable to drugs of chemical origin when submitting the documentation dealing with live cells for stem cell transplantation.

Stem cell transplantation is, as its name states, a transplantation, a surgical procedure, and not a therapy by mass produced drugs. All surgical operations are 'individualized therapeutic procedures'. Double blind studies have never been used for the evaluation of results of surgical procedures. Stem cell xenotransplants are not, and will not become, 'mass-produced' therapeutics.

OTHER COUNTRIES

In the absence of a specific laws dealing strictly with cell xenotransplantation, such as those in European Union, Russian Federation, and to some degree in the US, any dealing with regulatory authorities about stem cell xenotransplantation is usually difficult. Although the principle of individualized therapy as a matter between a physician and his patient can be found in laws of some countries, e.g. Mexico, the central government does not respect it. In Switzerland, where cell xenotransplantation was born, the old regulations disappeared, and what is left amounts to four lines in the Codex.

The regulatory situation in other countries is even worse because there are no laws or regulations regarding stem cell transplantation, allo- or xeno-, whatsoever. Since stem cell xenotransplantation definitely does not fit under the laws on drugs and other mass produced therapeutics (!), the sole possibility of finding a solution are the laws on organ and tissue transplantation.

Chapter 6

Salus populi suprema lex (The people's safety is the highest law.)
Latin (Roman) political maxim

SAFETY ISSUES

SAFETY ISSUES RELATED TO THE POSSIBLE TRANSMISSION OF XENOSES

In 1997, the German government submitted to the German Supreme Court reports about possible transmission of zoonoses via *'frischzellentherapie'*, including infections allegedly caused by prions. The court discovery process showed that the sole case of 'possible' serious complication directly related to the fresh cell therapy was that of a patient who died of post-infectious encephalitis some time after fresh cell therapy in 1983, many years before the SBE panic, and the appearance of prions. As a result of the decision of the German Supreme Court on February 16, 2000, and since Germany is a scrapie-free country, the members of the Association of German Physicians for Fresh Cell Therapy have continued to use sheep as a source of fresh cell therapeutica.

Niehans, both a human and veterinary surgeon of high reputation earned in military during WW1, selected in the 30's sheep as an animal source for cell xenotransplantation (that he named *'cell therapy'*), because sheep had been known as the healthiest of all domestic farm animals in Europe [157]. Based on advice of a major Australian sheep producer, that there has not been a single case of cancer in 40,000 mountain black sheep in three decades [157], he set-up a farm near his clinic in Vevey, Switzerland, where he raised that breed of sheep to serve as the animal source for fresh cell therapy. To the end of his days he argued that patients treated by the implantation of black sheep cells are resistant to cancer. Despite his convictions, Niehans did not hesitate to use pigs as animal sources of certain, in particular endocrine, organs and tissues, when he started an industrial production of lyophilized cell therapeutica in 50's, and the tests showed that clinical effectiveness of some of the pig cells was superior to his favored sheep.

In the 1950's, when Niehans decided to widen the impact of cell therapy by offering preserved cells to the medical profession, his veterinarian, J. Miller, disagreed with his choice of lyophilization as the best method for cell preservation, and created a company that used quick freezing for the same purpose. Miller preferred horse fetuses for the production of cryopreserved 'cell-therapeutica'. Some smaller companies used cattle fetuses instead. Thus the 'grand-fathers' proved the point, that as long an animal source fulfills the criteria of AAALAC, many different animals could be used for the manufacture of cell xenotransplants, and when new animal comes onto the scene, it is not necessary to start the research all over again starting from the 'big bang'.

In USSR/Russia, the reason for a switch to rabbits was an economic disaster. In US it may be an ecologic disaster: a discovery of a transmissible-to-man retro-virus in pigs may force elimination of pigs from consideration. But then, the recent attempt in Australia to eliminate rabbits on a grand scale by introduction of viruses into rabbit populations may lead to another ecologic disaster that may disqualify rabbits as an animal source of cell xenotransplants, whereby guinea pigs, rats, or mice, or fowl, or fish, become animal sources of stem cell transplants in the future. But it makes no difference: in all instances the rules of cell biology, including that of organospecificity, are the same and all clinical experience collected to-date with cell transplantation using precursor stem cells containing tissue fragments originating from animal or human fetuses still apply. If cell xenotransplantation is to become a widespread method, 'practical considerations and out-right cost-effectiveness' [37] come into play.

SAFETY DATA RELATED TO IMMUNE REACTIONS

An experience with cell xenotransplantation was reviewed by the German Supreme Court over many years; in February 2000 the Court ruled that 'fresh cell therapy' is safe. Comparing with Russia, German medicine continues to be one of the best in the world, and Germans, the exemplary bureaucrats, tightly control everything, nothing ever happens 'under the table', so that German data are very reliable. Review of the court documents from Germany, as provided by Prof. Dr. Wimmer, who represented the Association of German Physicians for Fresh Cell Therapy in the lawsuit against the German government, shows that of the estimated 800,000 patients treated worldwide by fresh cell therapy over the period of more than 70 years, there was only one serious complication 'possibly' directly related to fresh cell therapy [104]. These statistics are remarkable, because the method of preparation of cell xenotransplants by the school of fresh cell therapy has not changed for the past 70 years, and is, in the author's opinion, scientifically outdated. Method of fresh cell therapy exposes a patient/recipient to unnecessarily large antigen load, and it does not permit testing of cell xenotransplants for the possible presence of zoonotic infectious agents. Let's analyze these two issues.

German government submitted to the German Supreme Court reports of German 'official' immunologists describing dangerous acute rejection reactions as a logical consequence of cell xenotransplantation. The specialists in fresh cell therapy have not seen such reactions in their clinical practices, although the immunosuppression that they have used has consisted of no more than one small oral dose of cortison/ antihistamine combination given to the patient 20 minutes before treatment [104]. This is a fact that must be explained. US immunologists are starting to publish data about 'anergy', 'tolerance', etc., and these terms express what they have recognized in their work, i.e. minimal reactions after discordant cell xenotransplantation.

If there have been no serious immune reactions after fresh cell therapy, with all the deficiencies of the old method of preparation of fresh cell implants, it is not surprising that modern methods of preparation of stem cell xenotransplants by tissue culture have eliminated them completely. This permitted the Ministry of Health of USSR to state in 1984 in the 'Regulations on Cell Transplantation' that immunosuppression is not necessary with cell transplantation, including when intraportal implantations are used, etc., if a correct method of tissue culture is used in the preparation of stem cell transplants.

From 1991 until 1997, the IIBM team under the leadership of the author never used immunosuppression with cell transplantation, even in newborns and small children, treated every 4 months, several times in a sequence, and reported during its December 1995 symposium in Moscow a complete lack of overt immune reactions in the treatment of around 3,000 private patients and many other patients included in multiplicity of clinical trials carried out at 15 top governmental medical research centers.

It was well known by the practitioners of cell therapy [184], that there was a lack of success in the treatment of certain diseases, including diabetes mellitus.

There are legends about the obsession of Niehans to solve the problem of treatment of diabetes mellitus. Despite his genius, he did not succeed. RITAOMH team proved that it could not have been done without the preparation of cell transplants by tissue culture. Despite the lack of overt immune reactions, there are apparently some other kinds of reactions, not detectable by the current laboratory tests, perhaps autoimmune, that destroy implanted cell transplants prepared by the outdated method of fresh cell therapy to such a degree that their overall clinical effect is minimal to none, as in IDDM. With the continued improvement of methods of preparation of cell xenotransplants, an area in which our team earned a major victory, the results of treatment of complications of IDDM have improved as well [146, 147].

The preparation of fresh cell therapeutica in Germany triggered a persistent criticism. By comparing BCRO Method of stem cell xenotransplantation and fresh cell therapy the reasons became obvious.

The scientific principle behind stem cell xenotransplantation (SCXT) and fresh cell therapy (FCT) is the same. In both instances live cells of any & all animal organs and tissues from animal fetuses are implanted in a patient for the treatment of those disease(s), where such therapeutic method is indicated, essentially for a direct stimulation of regeneration of diseased organ systems, organs and tissues of the recipient.

However, there is a vast difference in the safety between FCT as still practiced today, and that of SCXT when transplants are prepared by the method described in this book.

Preparation of fresh tissue fragments for FCT has not changed for the past 70 years, while stem cell xenotransplants preparation by the described method from fetal and newborn rabbits follows the European Community Council Directive 2001/83/EC, and filed for US Patent (pending) and know-how includes pertinent parts of "PHS Guidelines on Infectious Disease Issues in Xenotransplantation" of January 19, 2001 (Federal Register, Vol. 66, No. 19, pages 8120 – 8121).

The key goal of the US PHS regulations is to increase the safety of SCXT for the benefit of the recipient patient, but also to minimize, or abolish, the medico-legal exposure of the treating physician, as well as of manufacturer.

The above US PHS regulations demand that the link between female rabbit as the source of the fetal and newborn rabbits used for procurement of stem cell xenotransplants, and a patient/recipient of SCXT, is not interrupted throughout the entire preparation and treatment cycle, i.e. that it is forever known that stem cell xenotransplants implanted in a body of a named patient were obtained from a specific, well identified group of fetal and newborn rabbits, with a documented genetic lineage, bred and reared in captivity, that in turn originate from a specific, well characterized group of female rabbits, bred and reared in captivity in a well established, licensed, closed colony of rabbits.

This link is thoroughly and permanently documented, and such documentation, as well as tissue samples from each such female rabbit, and samples of each stem cell xenotransplant used for the treatment of a named patient, are stored for five years in liquid nitrogen.

These frozen samples can be, at any time, compared with various specimens obtained from the recipient patient. In this way, any doubts about a possible origin of any new illness in the patient/recipient of SCXT can be completely and quickly eliminated.

FCT has not followed such regulations, and for that reason, it has always had great difficulty defending against accusations of transmission of zoonoses while under the attack by the pharmaceutical industry media campaign. Specifically, the differences between SCXT and FCT are:

A. All BCRO stem cell xenotransplants are prepared by a primary tissue culture, whereby there is ample time for a close observation, i.e. eleven days, to ascertain that each tissue culture is free of any disease. The tissue culture is not required by EC Directive 2103/83/EC, or by US PHS regulations, it is a part of BCRO's patented procedure (US Patent Pending) and know-how.

In FCT, the dissection of the sheep (or other animal source) is carried out in a hurry. The tissue fragments are immediately loaded in syringes, and implanted within two hours from the time of hysterotomy, i.e. so there is no time whatsoever to pay attention to the quality and safety of the implanted tissue fragments.

B. The most important feature of BCRO's procedure of preparation of stem cell xenotransplants is an attainment of an almost complete immunological tolerance of stem cell xenotransplants by the recipient, as a result of which there is no need for an immunosuppression, or even a premedication, as practiced by FCT, since clinically detectable reactions of patient's immune system to SCXT are not observable or measurable.

With BCRO's method of preparation of cell xenotransplants, an elimination of 99% of cellular ballast of each cell xenotransplant takes place, whereby the patient's immunological load is decreased, and then antigenicity of cell xenotransplants is cut to a minimum as described in this book (section on manufacturing steps).

None of this happens with FCT, and that's why immune reactions to the implantation of 'frischzellen' are unavoidable. Because of that, the 'official' immunologists cannot be convinced of the safety of FCT.

C. In SCXT-preparation, described in this book, all fetal and newborn rabbits used as animal sources of stem cell xenotransplants originate from a closed colony.

A closed colony is an enclosed unit, suitably ecologically located, where rabbits with selected genetic lineages are bred and reared for generations, in order to be protected from the dangers of the surrounding world to the highest degree possible. They cannot get infected from other rabbits, other animals, or by insects or vermin, or by humans: only a minimum number of rabbit handlers and a veterinarian are permitted an entry into the closed colony, and all are subjected to regular medical examinations. They are properly attired and are excluded from entry when ill.

Feed is pasteurized and prepared by a certified manufacturer.

If a numerical expansion of the colony is necessary by intake of new rabbits, they have to come from a similar closed colony, and pass through a quarantine room, where they are observed and medically tested for 4 weeks to ascertain their good health. Once a rabbit is taken out of colony it is never allowed to return.

When a new closed colony is established, the group of rabbits with pure genetic lineages, from similar colonies, has to be bred and reared together for at least 25 generations, i.e. around 24 months, before the colony can receive a designation 'closed'. During this time of observation, any genetic abnormalities, a carrier-state of some dormant infections, and other pathological conditions, etc., become noticeable in the new rabbit colony, and the affected animals can be eliminated.

FCT has never used source animals from a closed colony.

D. The rabbits are observed daily by experienced personnel, and at least once a week by a veterinarian. The medical record of each rabbit is kept indefinitely, and is linked to *those of its predecessors for generations back. Thus the health status of the whole colony can be evaluated instantly, also historically during its entire existence.*

The blood and excreta of each female rabbit are tested every 6 months, and the blood samples are kept frozen for 5 years.

Upon death, each female rabbit undergoes a full autopsy. Samples of blood and four organs are obtained and kept frozen for 5 years.

At the first step of the manufacturing, each fetal and newborn rabbit cadaver, the source of cell xenotransplants, is dissected by an experienced veterinary pathologist, and discarded if even the slightest abnormality is observed.

None of the above has ever been done with FCT.

E. During the procurement, each tissue culture is inspected daily, macro- and micro-scopically, by a tissue culture expert.

Parallel with each tissue culture, another culture is grown in Layton flask that is processed histologically to verify that each tissue culture included in the final (released) stem cell xenotransplant originates from a correct organ or tissue, and such histological preparations are kept for 5years.

At the time of harvesting of a final cell xenotransplant, a small sample of a supernatant of each cell xenotransplant is placed in a vial and stored in liquid nitrogen for 5 years. At the same time, bacteriological testing and a test for bacterial endotoxins are carried out for each cell xenotransplant.

The manufacturing facility, equipment, supplies, personnel, and the entire manufacturing process, packaging, labeling, and release of each batch of cell xenotransplant to be used for a treatment of a named patient, etc., are supervised by the Quality Control department, and compared with standard procedures.

There is a full documentation of the preparation of each cell xenotransplant, as required by GMP (Good Manufacturing Practice) standards, which is kept indefinitely.

None of the above is carried out with FCT.

F. Clinical practice of SCXT by BCRO method.

The BCRO procedure of preparation of stem cell xenotransplants by a primary tissue culture procedure, that is the final step in obtaining a nearly complete loss of immunogenicity, permits implantation of stem cell xenotransplant directly into the blood circulation, or into various parts of any organ, including brain, and cerebrospinal fluid, without immunosuppression (!), and that markedly widens therapeutic possibilities.

One of the key reasons for the high therapeutic success rate of SCXT, carried out by BCRO clinical method, is the fact that no immunosuppression has to be used with implantation. But a better understanding of what happens in the organism of the recipient after SCXT, or of interrelationships of various simultaneously implanted stem cell xenotransplants, plays a decisive role in such success. Some 27 years ago, BCRO took the clinical experience of 'zellentherapie' as the basis for further study, and its current state-of-the-art clinical method is the result of many years of research and of diligent clinical observation.

TOXICOLOGICAL STUDIES

No toxicological studies of cell xenotransplants have ever been carried out as they would be meaningless. Incidentally, studies of acute, subacute, and chronic toxicity were carried out a few decades ago with lyophilized preparations of a variety of organs by Prof. Dr. Neuman in Germany, and even doses that were 50 times higher than therapeutic doses did not cause any harm [95].

PART II

SCIENTIFIC BASIS OF CLINICAL USE OF STEM CELL TRANSPLANTATION

Chapter 7

> Human subtlety ... will never devise an invention more beautiful, more simple or more direct than does Nature, because in her inventions nothing is lacking, and nothing is superfluous.
> Leonardo da Vinci, 1452 - 1519

ESSENTIAL FACTS

In order to *comprehend stem cell transplantation*, you ought to visualize that everything in the living body is in constant motion, i.e. electrons, protons, and other elementary particles of each atom, all atoms, all molecules, all cell organelles of every cell, as well as all fluids, which represent between 75 and 55% of body weight (depending upon age), and there is electromagnetic radiation associated with all that action. The same applies to stem cell transplants, and there is a transfer of information between stem cell transplants and the same cells of the malfunctioning organ of the recipient/patient, and the communication is on both the material and energetic levels. When the flow of electromagnetic energy in the animal body stops, the body is dead.

Next, you ought to be aware that every cell in an animal body is programmed to die, i.e. is subject to apoptosis, and that with the exception of neurons and fatty cells, all the cells are being continuously replaced: statisticians calculated that every 7 years the human body consists of a completely new set of cells, with the above two exceptions, so it seems that every 7 years a human being 'becomes a new person'. For example, our blood cells, intestinal crypt cells, cells of basal layer of epidermis, spermatocytes, are populations containing precursor stem cells that are in a steady-state equilibrium in which cell production equalizes cell loss.

Every disease means that more principal cells of a diseased organ die than are replaced by mitosis. When there are too few main cells of any organ of human body left, that organ stops its function, and if the organ cannot be replaced, the human body will stop functioning. This of course depends if it is an organ without which we cannot live, e.g. heart or brain.

Current medicine has known of only one treatment to help the replacement of dead cells: organ transplantation.

Some organs or systems cannot be transplanted, e.g. brain, immune system, so that many diseases cannot be treated in this manner.

On the other hand every diseased organ of the body can be treated by stem cell transplantation. It is a matter of finding out what type of cells to use for transplantation, and that requires knowledge and clinical sense, since our diagnostic means are still inadequate.

If stem cells are properly prepared, they can be implanted without immunosuppression, and thereby all complications caused by the use of such medications are avoided.

Besides being a replacement for the deceased cells of a diseased organ, the transplanted cells can regenerate damaged cells of the organ that actually are still alive, but not capable of functioning for some reasons, or wake up those in a 'dormant state'.

Stem cell transplantation is the only therapy known to directly stimulate regeneration of the damaged tissues of all organs, or to accomplish an outright transplantation of the new cells, which by being fetal, prepared in the proper culture media as a primary cell culture, have largely lost their immunogenicity, and thus are accepted by the body of the patient as 'self', i.e. not rejected.

One of the reasons why stem cell transplantation is such a simple procedure for a patient to go through is the principle of 'homing'. (Read more about 'Homing' in Chapter 10).

The stem cell transplants can originate from embryonic, fetal, newborn or adult stage of development of any member of the animal kingdom, from Homo sapiens to fish. Each of these possibilities has advantages and disadvantages. For example, while there has been a shortage of human organs, tissues and cells for transplantation, the same is not true for the cells, tissues, and organs of animal origin for transplantation. As a result, stem cell xenotransplantation can be used for the treatment of thousands of sick people, suffering from those diseases that cannot be cured or treated by any other therapy. Compare that to the difficulties encountered by those in need of procurement of aborted human fetuses as a source of human fetal cell transplants.

In the following chapters we will touch upon those basic science data that bear a relationship to the main scientific principles behind the established method of stem cell transplantation described in this book, i.e. organospecificity, homing, direct stimulation of regeneration, cell transplantation without immunosuppression, transfer of xenoses, implantation of precursor stem cells, transfer of information between the stem cell transplants and the recipient/patient, relationship of matter and energy, and what science cannot explain today: "transplantation of life, or vitality", from the prepared stem cell to the malfunctioning cells of the treated organ or tissue of the recipient/patient.

A repetition of what can be found in classical basic medical science textbooks is preferably avoided: the facts are presented only in the context of what is important for explanation of stem cell xenotransplantation.

Chapter 8

> I formulate the doctrine of pathological generation …in simple terms: omnis cellula a cellula. (All cells come from pre-existing cells).
> Rudolf Virchow, 1821 – 1902, Cell Pathology [1858]

CYTOLOGY

CELL

Cell is the smallest unit of live organisms. No smaller unit than a cell is capable to fulfill the basic functions of living organism: metabolism, motility, growth, reproduction, and inheritance.

Growth, reproduction and inheritance require mitosis, i.e. cell division.

Somatic cells divide into two daughter cells after duplication of the set of chromosomes, while germ cells during meiosis divide the set of chromosomes into two halves. Each cell capable of mitosis goes through the cell cycle, in which each mitosis of 30 - 120 minutes duration is separated from the next mitosis by an interphase of 6 - 36 hours.

Certain "*labile cells*" with short lifespan go continuously through the cell cycle, and thereby instantly replace all deceased cells so that the cell count of each organ and tissue is constant. Epithelial cells of different tissues i.e. epidermis, mucosa of mouth, vagina and uterine cervix, of salivary glands, gastrointestinal tract, biliary passages, of uterus and lower urinary tract, and bone marrow cells, are "labile cells". During mitosis one daughter cell remains usually undifferentiated, i.e. stem cell, and the other daughter cell gradually differentiates into no longer dividing cell, such as erythrocyte, granulocyte, or spermatogonia.

Some "*stable cells*", or "resting cells", do not proliferate. After mitosis, they enter resting state, known as phase G_0. Parenchymal cells of liver, kidneys, pancreas, and connective tissue and mesenchymal cells, i.e. fibroblasts, endothelial cells, chondrocytes, osteocytes, leiomyocytes, are "resting cells". Only a tissue loss, or a major injury of tissue, reactivates the cells in the G_o phase so that they re-enter mitosis. For example, normally only 1% of hepatocytes undergoes mitosis, but after injury as much as 10% of hepatocytes enters cell division. *Stem cell transplantation increases the rate of mitosis in stable, but also labile cells.*

Transition from G_o to G phase, as well as the stimulation of cell proliferation in general, requires binding of growth factors, or hormones, to the specific receptors, usually located on the cell surface. Receptors for growth factors are activated, with subsequent phosphorylation of various proteins of signaling chain until the cell nucleus is reached, DNA synthesis is stimulated, and cell division takes place.

Division of some resting cells is minimal without stem cell transplantation, i.e. neurons, peripheral and heart myocytes, etc.

Regulation of labile or resting cell cannot alone, i.e. by itself, reconstruct the original structure of the entire damaged tissue. For that an intact extracellular matrix is necessary, capable to direct shape, growth, migration and differentiation of cell. *Extracellular matrix* consists of fibrillar structural proteins, i.e. collagen I, II, V, elastin, and of adhesive glycoproteins of intercellular matrix, i.e. fibronectin, laminin, immersed in gel of proteoglycans and glucosaminoglycans. Integrins are cell membrane proteins that connect *extracellular matrix* with intracellular cytoskeleton and transmit signals for growth, migration and differentiation of cells.

In case of severe injury with extensive damage of extracellular matrix, the repair is by scar tissue, unless proliferation of the resting connective tissue and mesenchymal cells is triggered, that possesses the ability of secretion of extra-cellular matrix and that *can be directly stimulated only by stem cell transplantation.*

CELL ANATOMY

Cell membrane functions like a hydrophobic barrier around the cell, so that water-soluble compounds and ions do not readily pass across. A similar membrane surrounds cell organelles. Thus, there is a need for transporters to regulate flow in and out of cells and cell organelles. The most important function of a membrane is to maintain a specific microenvironment inside of a cell, or a cell organelle, by controlling the entry and exit of molecules and inorganic ions. The cell is not just a 'bag' of various components, it is a highly organized collection of interacting compartments whose separation optimizes the efficiency.

Cell nucleus contains the most important portion of genetic material, and regulates all cell function. *At gastrulation, the nucleus begins to regulate the further cell development.*

Mitochondria transform the chemical energy of metabolites in cytoplasm into energy that is easily accessible by the cell.

Protein synthetic machinery is centered on ribosomes associated with the endoplasmic reticulum.

Lysosomes are sites of intracellular digestion and turnover of cellular components.

CELL DEATH

Eukaryotic cells can disappear in two different ways: 1) necrosis as a result of damage, i.e. induced death; and 2) apoptosis, i.e. programmed cell death. Apoptosis does not lead to cell membrane damage and leak of intracellular contents that triggers an induction of inflammatory response. Apoptosis is a physiological way of maintaining homeostasis and tissue regeneration.

1. **Necrotic cell death**
   Survival of cells depends upon maintenance of normal intracellular environment. Lack of oxygen and insufficient production of ATP are two key factors that disrupt the intracellular milieu.

   Insufficient supply of oxygen causes switching of energetic metabolism to anaerobic glycolysis. Production of lactic acid, dissociating to lactate and H^+, causes intracytoplasmatic acidosis with subsequent interference with function of intracellular enzymes, whereby glycolysis slows down and so the last source of ATP dries out.

   Inadequate energy supply exposes the cell to oxidative damage because all protective mechanisms against O_2-radicals depend upon ATP. There is a threat of cell membrane destruction due to lipid peroxidation with the release of intracellular macromolecules into the extracellular space. Since immune system is normally not exposed to intracellular macromolecules, and thereby no immuno-tolerance has ever developed, the immune system is activated, inflammatory reaction takes place, and that leads to further cell damage.

2. **Apoptotic cell death**

Hundreds of billions of cells are eliminated in our body daily and replaced by new daughter cells provided by mitosis. Apoptosis is the programmed cell death regulated by physiologic mechanisms that serve the adaptation of tissues to varying demands, elimination of redundant quantity of cells, as well as the elimination of harmful cells, i.e. cancerous, virus-infected, or immunocompetent cells that turned against 'self' antigens.

Pathologically increased apoptosis, not planned by organism, causes excessive elimination of functionally necessary cells, leading to an organ insufficiency. In this way apoptosis of neurons can lead to neurodegenerative diseases, i.e. Parkinson's disease, Alzheimer's disease, ALS, transverse myelitis with paralysis, multiple sclerosis, etc., apoptosis of liver cells to liver insufficiency, β-cells of islets of pancreas to IDDM, erythropoietic cells to aplastic anemia or lymphocytes to immunodefi-ciency, AIDS, etc.

Pathologically decreased apoptosis of virus-infected cells becomes the cause of persistent infections. Cells without apoptosis become cancerous. Decreased apoptosis of immunocompetent cells that turned against 'self'-antigens become a cause of autoimmune diseases. Insuficient apoptosis leads to disturbances of embryonic development, i.e. syndaktylia.

Replacement of a cell lost by apoptosis is a function of regeneration, and regeneration can be therapeutically stimulated only by stem cell transplantation.

Chapter 9

> Man can learn nothing unless he proceeds from the known to the unknown.
> Claude Bernard, 1813 – 1878, Bulletin of New York Academy of Medicine, Vol. iv, 1928, p. 997

CELL BIOLOGY

When you place human and animal embryonic stem cells side-by-side, or human and animal precursor stem cells of the same type, you find out that they look alike and even most of the available cell-surface markers are the same.

The only way to tell the cells of one species from another is by their karyotype, the number and shape of chromosomes that are temporary structures created from the genetic material of each cell during one short phase of the mitosis.

The embryonic stem cells have a unique capability to renew themselves, i.e. proliferate, and are pluripotent, which means that they have the potential to differentiate into any and all specialized cells of the body, with a characteristic shape, and function.

They remain in an undifferentiated state, uncommitted, until they get a signal to develop into one of specialized cells of the body.

A puzzling problem is that embryonic stem cells apparently do not exist for any prolonged period of time in a living embryo, only in the laboratory dish. Up until now, their survival in laboratory conditions has been completely dependent upon the presence of a layer of 'feeder mouse cells'.

The current optimism about embryonic stem cells is based on theoretical expectation of:

- their enormous ability to proliferate that makes them suitable for a factory level manufacturing of cells for therapeutic use,
- their capability to be manipulated so that they differentiate into any desired cell type to be used for cell transplantation treatment of patients.

The unlimited potential of embryonic cells to proliferate sounds wonderful, but only until one realizes that *in cancer growth likewise one kind of cell stopped responding to the commands of the patient's body, became independent, and decided to become a 'cell factory'.*

Manipulation of embryonic skin cells into differentiation, whereby precursors/progenitors of any and all specialized cells of the body are created in a laboratory dish, is an exciting feat, but a formidable task, currently without a solution.

But since precursor stem cells cannot create in a laboratory conditions a three-dimensional body, or an organ, or even a tissue, the question arises whether these cells grown in a laboratory dish are indeed the same precursor stem cells that can be obtained from a fetus, where they have developed in a natural way, and where they created three-dimensional tissues and organs.

The kind of environment in which stem cells are growing, i.e. either in tissue culture or in live human and animal body, makes a lot of difference for the direction of cell differentiation.

Let's now focus on Precursor Stem Cells

When the precursor stem cells are taken from fetus, that have already reached the stage of organogenesis, such stem cells are no longer pluripotential but are committed to follow a predetermined path of differentiation along one lineage only, in other words, such stem cells are directed to produce cells specific for the kind of tissue where these stem cells normally reside, and to follow the body commands. At the same time they retain the ability to proliferate without pre-determined differentiation for a long time, i.e. capability of long term self-renewal. (Those precursor stem cells obtained by manipulation of embryonic stem cells in a laboratory dish remain pluripotential to some degree). This is because in fetal body the undifferentiated stem cells live in a milieu of various specialized (differentiated) cells, and there is a lot of interaction between them, which is not the case when undifferentiated stem cells grow in tissue culture.

It appears more physiological to take precursor stem cells for transplantation from their natural environment in the fetal body. That means taking them along with other cells of the same 'family', in a cell-to-cell contact with cells of the same 'family', together with cells of various generations of the same 'family', and then grow them in a primary tissue culture in order to have sufficient time for observation and safety tests, as well as to minimize their immunogenicity so that they can be implanted without immunosuppression.

Following this principle, the described *method of preparation of stem cell transplants is based on the primary tissue culture of tissue fragments, or cell clusters, and not on the primary cell culture of dispersed cells*. It has been proven beyond any doubt that cells in the tissue fragments communicate via contact, via soluble factors, and also via their electromagnetic fields. All of these factors are missing in the cell culture of dispersed cells.

Besides that the process of disintegration of an explant into individual cells requires the use of chemicals and proteolytic enzymes that damage cell membranes, sometimes even cell nuclei, so that the cell culture begins with decreased quantity of intact healthy cells. In our method of tissue culture, a much more physiological mechanical disintegration is utilized, so that the quality of cultured cells is superior.

The *use of cell lines for preparation of stem cell transplants* is another questionable area. Cell transplants prepared from cell lines have never been used for the patient treatment in the past: it has been a "res ipsa loquitur" for practicing cell transplantologists in Europe. There has been a strong opinion that *cell transplants prepared from cell lines are not clinically effective* due to the following facts.

Development of cells *in an organ or tissue culture* is influenced by a variety of interactions between cells, and due to a lack of such interactions the growth of dispersed cells in a cell culture is difficult to impossible. Culturing of dispersed embryonic stem cells growing outside their natural environment is possible only on the cell matrices, currently known as "feeder layer" of cells. The only other way is by culturing stem cells in their natural environment, inside of a living organism. Bone marrow, for example, is a perfectly structured micro-environment for 'production' of stem cells. Hematopoetic stem cells are capable of growth and development into structurally and functionally competent units only under influence of unique stimuli of all types of cells in the given micro-environment.

In cell lines of one type of cells only, as a result of prolonged living in an artificial conditions of cell culture, the cells are almost always heteroploid, and due to the influence of selection so changed, that they often cannot be recognized as derived from their tissue (or organ) of origin. In cell lines sex chromatin disappears, the mitoses run without any controls, there is a decreased production of acids released into the culture medium, cell membranes of daughter cells are incomplete, there is a lack of histotypical differentiation. Cell lines have lowered resistance against viral infections.

On the other side, the primary tissue cultures, as used in the described method of preparation of stem cell transplants, have a limited lifespan, determined by the lifespan of the tissue source of the culture, or of the donor. In primary tissue cultures the cells maintain diploid set of chromosomes, typical for the normal somatic cells of the animal source of the tissue culture. They do not differ from the cells of the original organ or tissue planted on the tissue culture neither structurally, nor biochemically. These cells grow in practically the same functional environment as when they were a part of an organism from which they were taken.

The author believes that *adult stem cells have a low therapeutic potential*, despite their apparent ability of long-term self-renewal, differentiation along a predetermined cell lineage, and ability to give rise to just one cell type for the purpose of maintenance of homeostasis. Therapeutic potency of autologous adult stem cells can be substantially increased by co-culture with precursor stem cells of the same organ or tissue of animal fetal origin.

Stem cells obtained from the fetus are much more numerous than rare adult stem cells, and they possess certain unique properties, such as:

- high level of readiness to differentiate and undergo changes in response to environmental stimuli, or in accordance with their own genetic make-up,
- easy adaptability, due to the plasticity of tissues (including growth, migration, mobility, ability to create cell-to-cell contacts), that in the course of normal fetal development gradually decreases, and finally disappears at the completion of development,
- much more frequent and faster cell division, and proliferation, as compared with adult stem cells, depending upon the type of tissue and stage of fetal development,
- production of large amounts of various biological substances, i.e. growth factors, etc., that facilitate the survival and growth of stem cells after implantation, and stimulate damaged cells, tissues and organs of the host,

- lowered immunogenicity, with a consequently much weaker immune response of the host, as compared with an implantation of adult cells or tissues,
- ability to survive on energy supplied by glycolysis alone, i.e. on lesser amount of oxygen, that is an important factor during the preparation of stem cell transplants, and during the first hours after implantation,
- lack of cell extensions easily damaged during processing of cell transplants.

HOMING

"Homing" means that the respective stem cells do not have to be implanted into a damaged organ, i.e. liver stem cells into liver, they can be implanted into more accessible superficial tissues, as for example under the aponeurosis of the rectus abdominis muscle, because they find their way into the damaged organ from there, as if 'attracted' by it.

Lymphocyte spends most of its life within solid tissues, entering the circulation only periodically to migrate from one resting place to another. At any moment only 1% of the total lymphocytes are found in blood; this part of lymphocytes is in motion, shuttling through organs, surveying body for foci of infection or foreign antigens. Lymphocytes in the blood are attracted back into solid tissues by way of specialized blood vessels known as high endothelial venules, modified form of postcapillary venules found in all lymphoid organs. Some lymphocytes passing through these venules tend to bind tightly to the specialized endothelium and then infiltrate between endothelial cells and penetrate into the tissue.

Binding occurs because proteins known as *"homing receptors"* on the lymphocyte surface have a strong affinity for determinants, called vascular *addressins*, on the high endothelial venules. *High endothelial cells in different target organs express addressins that are characteristic of that organ, and are recognized by a specific type of homing receptor.* When a circulating lymphocyte expresses a particular homing receptor, it tends to bind to and infiltrate only a tissue or organ with the corresponding addressin.

High endothelial venules are a constant feature of lymphoid organs but may also *appear transiently at any site in the body where an immune response is occurring, i.e. in a diseased organ or tissue.* They arise by differentiation of pre-existing capillaries in response to IFN-χ produced locally by activated CD4 T cells. *These cells serve as a portal for circulating lymphocytes to enter the site and join in an immune response.* By such means the lymphocytes and other reactive cells can accumulate wherever they are needed in the body [108, 165, 180].

A cascade of adhesive molecules, of which L-selectin is expressed on naive T lymphocytes, interacts with vascular addressins, with the resulting homing of naive T cells to lymphoid organs. In order for naive T cells to cross endothelial barrier into the lymphoid tissue two other types of adhesion molecules are necessary: integrins, and the immunoglobulin superfamily [165].

This homing principle has been recognized to be of key importance for a successful long-term engrafment of stem cells in bone marrow transplanttation [20]. After intravenous injection hematopoietic stem cells circulate through organs, such as the liver, lungs, kidneys, spleen, where they undergo few mitoses and form small colonies. But, they seed only bone marrow, and establish sustained hematopoiesis there. Homing represents a *cascade of adhesive interactions* between hemopoietic cells and bone marrow extracellular matrix [21, 179]. Interestingly, only 75% of labeled cells could be accounted for in these experiments [19].

Intrathymic transplantation of syngeneic islets into mice significantly reduced the severity of insulinitis, and development of diabetes mellitus, but not of sialitis, which proved that *it induced a tissue specific protection*. Subsequently there was a marked decline of thymic insulin content within 48 hours post-implantation, which indicated a rapid loss of implanted islet cells from thymus. Within a week the thymic insulin content was <1% of the initial content. Histology confirmed the rapid elimination of the islet syngrafts, and by the 7th day only an occasional granulated β-cell, as well as non-β endocrine cells, were seen, and 20 weeks post-implantation no surviving islet cells were detectable in the thymus. Thymus histology and thymic insulin content revealed a rapid loss of implanted β-cells, and *despite that there was tolerance induction by adoptive transfer of splenic leukocytes to another breed of mice* [10].

Let's compare the modern scientific facts of the last two paragraphs with the description of findings of the school of cell therapy of a few decades ago. Schmid states that the implanted cells disappear from the implantation site, with different speed, usually within 48 hours, and that the removal is effected by macrophages, and the vitally stained cells are mostly incorporated in the respective organ or tissue, following the rules of *"organospecificity"*. He also refers to the "Halsted principle" according to which implanted cells migrate to the *place of need*, i.e. damaged organ or tissue, the fact that is difficult to prove or refute by way of experiment [95].

Chapter 10

> Every experiment is like a weapon which must be used in its particular way – a spear to thrust, a club to strike. Experimenting requires a man who knows when to thrust and when to strike, each according to need and fashion.
> *Philippus Aureolus Paracelsus, 1493 – 1541, 'Surgeon's book', [1605]*

PHYSIOLOGY

Our focus here is on *organotropic effect of cell transplants*, i.e. the stimulation of healing of the same organ of the recipient by cell transplant; heart by cardiomyoblasts, kidney by epithelial cells of nephron, liver by hepatocytes, etc., as was postulated by Paracelsus at the beginning of 16th century [332].

The direct stimulation by cell transplantation is recognizable as an increase of cell count of growing organs or tissues, intensification of metabolism, or of a certain specific function, such as accentuation of anabolism. Such direct stimulation can be triggered only by implanted cell transplant of the corresponding organ, but not by transplantation of cells of other organs.

Since it is rare that an individual organ is malfunctioning, more commonly the entire organ system is diseased, it is necessary to treat all involved organs by corresponding cell transplants. The list of cell transplants necessary for treatment of each patient has to be individually designed in terms of cell composition, dosage, and date of implantation.

In 1916, Murphy and Danchakoff incubated chicken eggs for 7 days, then opened the shells, and placed a small piece of spleen, liver, bone marrow, kidney, on the chorio-allantoic membrane, then re-sealed the egg and continued the incubation. On the 17th day the shells were re-opened and spleens were found to be markedly enlarged, kidneys moderately enlarged, while liver did not enlarge at all. Subsequently an implantation of tissues of peripheral muscles, bone, cartilage and sarcoma, were done in the same way but no change of size of spleen was observed. They observed the presence of an effect that was limited to the tissue of the corresponding organs, i.e. organospecificity. This study was repeated in 1956. Implantation of spleen pulp caused a considerable progress in tissue differentiation of embryonic spleen, while application of gelatin, or a drop of milk, inhibited a differentiation, and implantation of splenic homogenate, or of splenic tissue subjected to 60 °C heat for one hour, had no effect whatsoever, thus proving that effect of an accelerated development of spleen was dependent upon an implantation of intact live splenic cells [324].

Subsequently Weiss and Taylor carried out classical experiments on the *in vivo* influence of homologous organ pulp on the growth rate of embryonic organs [325].

In 1909, Halsted succeeded in transplanting parathyroid glands from one dog into the spleen or muscle of another dog, but *only after he had previously produced a hypofunction, and therefore a 'need' in the recipient animal*, by a partial removal of the parathyroid glands before the transplantation. *The more extensive damage of an organ or tissue causes even higher proportion of the transplanted cells to 'home' into the same organ or tissue.* This has been known in cell therapy as "Halsted principle" [143], or today as *'homing principle'*, described in Chapter 9.

Demonstration of the organ-specific effect of a cell transplant required a proper experimental set-up that included an induced damage of the recipient organ. Eventually the organospecificity was proven by multiple experiments in 50's and 60's with liver (Walter, Allman, Mahler; Marshak, Walker), heart (Tumanishvili, Jandieri, Svanidze; Walter, Allman, Mahler), lacrimal glands (Teir), skin (McJunkin, Matsui), thymus (Roberts, White), Langerhans islets of pancreas (DuBois and Gonet). Kalb demonstrated organ-specific stimulating factors in the blood serum of rats 4 to 5 days after implantations of liver tissue. *All described effects were independent of the species used for an experiment, but the results were always limited to homologous organs* [95, 158, 216, 217, 219, 326].

In clinical practice it was the field of endocrinology where the *organospecificity* was recognized first. In 1771, Hunter, and then in

1849 Berthold, demonstrated the organotropic effect of implanted testis in the castrated cock. Then in 1889, Brown-Sequard reported to the French Academy of Sciences about self-treatment by extract prepared by himself from dog testes. In 1906, Morris transplanted human ovaries into a castrated woman, and menstruation re-started 4 months later. In 1912, Herrmann and Sutten transplanted the testis from a human cadaver to a castrated male. In 1925, Comolli removed one parathyroid gland during thyroidectomy and transplanted it to another patient suffering from tetany. In 1931, Dolby transplanted pancreas from still-born babies into diabetic patients.

In the 1930's, the interest in glandular transplantation waned because of rapid development of hormone therapy. Soon the drawbacks of hormonal therapy were recognized, i.e. that the effect of hormones is only temporary, and over-dosage or continuous application cause trouble because of atrophy of the gland from inactivity.

In 1927, Niehans began transplantation of anterior lobe of the pituitary from calves to the patients with nanismus, that caused the height increase up to 32 cm. In 1928 he transplanted the anterior lobe of pituitary from sheep to women with primary amenorrhea with good to very good results. In 1929 he began to transplant the posterior lobe and a stalk of pituitary into the patients with diabetes insipidus, and adrenal glands into patients with polyarthritis. And then in 1931 came the famous case when he saved the life of a female patient with a post-thyroidectomy tetany by the first *cell transplantation of minced tissue* of parathyroid with syringe and needle [18, 216, 219].

It was recognized that a hormonal effect lasted only a short time, and the real effect of cell transplantation came only some weeks later that was due to something else, not hormones. The insufficiency of an endocrine gland could be eliminated only by an implantation of tissues from the same gland: a tetany due to the removal of parathyroids responded only to the implantation of parathyroids, i.e. following the rules of organospecificity.

This was tested in experimental animals with thyroid gland insufficiency (Goos, Sturm, Kment), anterior lobe of pituitary deficiency (Maischein). But animal models of human hypo-endocrinopathies were not adequate, as they did not correspond to human illnesses. So human testing began in those endocrine diseases where the hormone production could be tested by urinary excretion of various fractions of 17-ketosteroids and corticoids: pituitary gland, sex glands, adrenal cortex. Implantation of tissue fragments of any of the three endocrine glands caused a dramatic increase in the excretion of the respective fractions of 17-keto steroids, with a maximum after 8 to 14 days, and then gradual disappearance of the effect during several months. The implantation of non-endocrine tissues caused no change in 17-keto-steroid excretion [95, 157, 158, 216, 219].

Implantation of placenta caused an increase of all 17-keto-steroid fractions to levels that exceeded even those after an implantation of anterior lobe of pituitary. Schubert showed a change of vaginal epithelium from an atrophic state to normal in post-menopausal women after an implantation of placenta that due to a lyophilization was free of any estrogen or gonadotropin [95, 327].

Niehans stressed the *implantation of hypothalamus in the treatment of diseases with disturbed neurosecretory regulations.* If transplants of anterior lobe of pituitary were implanted after the hypothalamic cells, a marked increase of excretion of all fractions of 17-keto-steroids was observed [327].

Cell transplantation is a vastly different approach to medical treatment and cannot be immediately understood by the mind accustomed to deal with (chemical) drug therapy.

The therapeutic effect of drugs of chemical origin is not as broad as those of any of the over 200 known types of cells transplanted into a diseased body with insufficient quantity or quality of a particular cell type(s).

Compare any publication about the treatment of diabetes with insulin or oral anti-diabetics with those discussing various aspects of treatment of diabetes mellitus by stem cell transplantation.

For example, the effect of different site of implantation of stem cell transplants on the course of experimental diabetes was tested in the search for a way to decrease the immune response to cell transplantation by implanting cell transplants into various "immunologically privileged" regions: intrahepatic, intrasplenic, intraportal, intrapancreatic, subcapsular (kidney), intraperitoneal, intraomental, intramuscular, intracerebral, intraspinal cord, intraocular (anterior chamber), intratesticular, intrathymic, etc. [37]. The immunoprivileged areas are unusual in two ways:

1. the communication between the privileged site and the body is *atypical in that the extracellular fluid in these sites does not pass through lymphatics*, and
2. certain humoral factors affecting immune system are produced in the privileged sites, such as TGFβ, which leave the sites along with antigens, and induces T_H1 rather than T_H2 responses. So *immunoprivileged sites do not prevent the interaction of antigens with T cells, but instead of eliciting a destructive immune reaction, such interaction induces tolerance* [165].

Another issue is that after transplantation of fetal islet cells, their function is *slow to develop, because further growth and differentiation of endocrine tissue* is necessary for the therapeutic effect to take place. About 2 - 3 months has to pass for that to happen. Compare it with the transplanted adult islets, that reverses diabetes in 1 - 2 weeks [170, 181].

Concept of critical mass of the transplanted endocrine tissue of islets necessary to accomplish insulin-independence represented an enormous step forward [130]. When a sufficient β-cell mass was transplanted, the subsequent replication of β-cells was normal, and the transplanted β-cell mass remained unchanged. If an insufficient β-cell mass was transplantted, a limitation in β-cell replication was found after transplantation, and the β-cell mass of the graft declined progressively.

When normoglycemia was restored by transplantation, the replication of transplanted β-cells was similar to that of pancreatic β-cells of normal animals. When islet transplants were sufficient to restore normoglycemia, the β-cell mass of the graft on days 10 and 30 post-transplantation was similar to the originally transplanted β-cell mass, and on day 30 the grafted β-cells had an increased size when compared to other transplanted groups.

When an insufficient islet tissue was transplanted, an initial increase in replication was found after 10 days of hyperglycemia, however, after 18 and 30 days of severe hyperglycemia, this increased replication was not maintained, which was an indication that the capacity of transplanted β-cells to grow was limited.

In chronically hyperglycemic animals, despite the increased β-cell replication by day 10, there was a continuous decline in β-cell mass of the grafts: increased β-cell destruction "over-powered" the β-cell replicative capacity. After 30 days, β-cell mass was significantly lower, and despite the persistent hyperglycemia the replication was no longer increased. A significant portion of the fall in β-cell mass was due to increased cell death.

When hyperglycemia persists after transplantation of an insufficient β-cell mass, both limited β-cell replication and accelerated cell death are found, leading to a progressive reduction in β-cell mass and failure of transplant. In contrast, when sufficient β-cell mass is transplanted, a balance among β-cell replication, β-cell hypertrophy, and β-cell death is obtained, and β-cell mass remains reasonably constant.

In normal recipients the transplanted β-cell mass dramatically diminished at days 10 and 30, despite normal replication of β-cells. This reduction was confirmed by a similar decrease in the insulin content of the graft. This was a result of downregulation in order to protect from the effect of excessive β-cell mass causing hypoglycemia [47]. This is another proof of 'Halsted Principle'.

Thus, a critical islet mass, higher than predicted, must be transplanted to achieve normoglycemia, and late failures depend on the number of initially transplanted islets. Islets exposed to sustained hyperglycemia have shown an impairment of β-cell function, limited replicative response and reduced β-cell mass.

Outcome of islet cell transplantation was improved when islets were transplanted to insulin treated diabetic mice with long-term normoglycemia and normal glucose tolerance: in such case transplanted β-cells maintained a normal insulin content. Also, *insulin treatment reduced significantly the β-cell mass needed to cure DM in transplanted mice: only 10 - 30%* of normal islet tissue was necessary to maintain normoglycemia as compared when normoglycemia had to be restored in hyperglycaemic mice not treated by insulin.

When islet cell implants were removed *14 days after transplantation, transplanted islets were already vascularized and able to sense and respond more appropriately to changes of blood glucose*. Islets transplanted to insulin-treated mice were able to increase their β-cell mass when insulin was withdrawn; this capacity of β-cell mass to adapt to changes in functional demand is essential to maintain normoglycemia. On day 60 the transplanted β-cell mass was similar to the initially transplanted mass. Even in those non-insulin-treated mice that eventually achieved normoglycaemia, there was an abnormal glucose tolerance, suggesting that *β-cell function was impaired in the islets that had been previously exposed to sustained hyperglycemia* [45].

The functioning of transplanted pancreatic islets was proved by the fact, that after removal of an organ into which islets were transplanted, the hyperglycemia, glycosuria and other symptoms of diabetes mellitus, recurred [134].

Timing of stem cell transplantation is extremely important: the sooner after the onset of disease it is carried out, the better are the results. When cultured islet cells were implanted under the kidney capsule of syngeneic mice already 3 weeks after the induction of diabetes mellitus, the capillaries of retina and kidneys maintained normal thickness of basal membrane, however, when implantation was delayed 7 months after the induction of diabetes, the basal membrane of glomerular capillaries became thicker, although the basal membrane of retinal capillaries maintained normal thickness [133].

Morphometric study of kidneys before and 4 months after cell transplantation showed decreased percentage of damaged glomeruli, widening of lumen of glomerular capillaries, and decrease of mesangial accumulation of class C immunoglobulins and complement [132]. In long-term diabetic rats with nephropathy, 6 weeks after the transplanttation of islets the phagocytosis and clearance capacity of the mesangial cells was restored and the mesangial enlargement reversed [172]. In rats with induced diabetes mellitus the transplantation of islets reduced within two weeks significantly the mesangial thickening and mesangial staining for IgG, IgM, and complement C3 [173].

Chapter 11

All intelligent thoughts have already been thought; what is necessary is only to try to think them again.
Johann Wolfgang von Goethe, 1749 – 1832, Proverbs in Prose

BIOCHEMISTRY

An important benefit of stem cell transplantation is the restoration of normal digestion and metabolism, i.e. *improved function of the entire digestive system, and harmonization of the regulation of metabolic function of all cells of the body*, as one of the key requirements for regeneration of damaged organs and tissues.

Digestion and metabolism are *enzymatic events*. Enzymes increase the biochemical reaction rates by at least a factor of one million. An enzyme is a protein that takes a molecule of a substrate and converts it into a product molecule by catalytic action. Enzymes usually work in a series, in pathways, or cycles, so that the product of one enzymatic reaction is used as a substrate by the next enzyme to produce a new product. In turn, this new compound is used by the third enzyme to yield a third product. This occurs because each enzyme catalyzes a specific reaction, and usually a string of different reactions is required to generate the desired end product.

When a product of chemical reaction is more complex than the initial substrate that entered the chain of reactions, such sequence of enzymatic reactions is called anabolic, i.e. conversion of glucose molecules into a long-branched polymer called glycogen, assembly of polypeptides and proteins from amino acids, synthesis of lipids from fatty acids and glycerol. All such reactions require energy provided by the molecule of adenosine triphosphate, ATP.

Similarly, larger molecules can be taken apart by a sequence of specific enzymatic actions to produce smaller, simple molecules. Such pathways are usually associated with the production of energy via generation of energy storing molecule of ATP. Such sequences of enzymatic actions involved in the breakdown of substrates are called catabolic, i.e. breakdown of glucose molecule into a smaller pyruvate, that is then converted into acetyl-CoA, breakdown of amino acids, or nucleotides, from disassembly of nucleic acids, or breakdown of fatty acids.

All catabolic pathways contribute to the production of acetyl-CoA, that can be used in further catabolic sequence of Krebs cycle, in which CO_2 is released, and energy is conserved with the formation of reduced co-enzymes nicotinamide-adenine dinucleotide (NADH) and nicotinamide-adenine dinucleotide phosphate (NADPH). This cycle is associated with respiratory electron transport cascade that produces water, and oxidative phosphorylation that drives the formation of ATP using the power supplied by electron transport cascade.

Metabolism is the total sum of all enzyme reactions in the body, both anabolic and catabolic.

DIGESTION

Enzymes secreted in gastrointestinal tract facilitate the breakdown of ingested food components. Proteolytic enzymes in the stomach and intestine, mostly produced in exocrine pancreas and stomach, break down peptide bonds in proteins, down to amino acids and a few di- and tri-peptides, that are taken up by the cells of intestinal mucosa.

High carbohydrates are degraded by amylase from saliva and exocrine pancreas to simple sugars, and other glycosidases break bonds between the simple sugars in the intestine to yield glucose, that is then absorbed by the intestinal mucosal cells.

Ingested fat, such as triacylglycerides, is broken down by lipases, mostly from exocrine pancreas, down to fatty acids and monoacylglycerides (one fatty acid attached by ester linkage to glycerol) and all these are absorbed by the mucosal cells of the intestine.

Simple molecules that are absorbed following digestion are used by the body to construct its own complex molecules. Glucose is used by various tissues for synthesis of glycogen, while amino acids for synthesis of proteins. Glucose is the first fuel substrate used for generation of ATP.

Fatty acids and monoacylglycerides are re-synthesized back into triacylglycerides within the same intestinal mucosal cells that absorbed them, and then released to blood as parts of lipoprotein particles to be distributed to various body tissues. At their target locations triacylglycerides are broken down in the blood into simpler molecules yet again that are then taken in by the nearby cells to be used in triacylglyceride synthesis and as fuel substrates for generation of ATP.

CELL METABOLISM

Complex molecules are broken down in various catabolic pathways. Glycogen is degraded to glucose-1-phosphate that is subsequently broken down in a pathway called glycolysis. In glycolysis, glucose is converted to pyruvate that is further metabolized to acetyl-CoA.

Acetyl-CoA enters Krebs cycle, or citric acid pathway, or circular enzyme pathway that eventually releases CO_2, to be exhaled by the lungs, and produces also the reduced co-enzymes NADH and (flavin adenine dinucleotide) $FADH_2$. These co-enzymes have energy of reduction, and the passage of their electrons down the electron transport chain releases energy. Oxygen is the final recipient of these electrons, and its reduction yields water. The respiratory chain is linked to oxidative phosphorylation that uses energy released during the passage of electrons to drive the synthesis of ATP from ADP and inorganic phosphate.

Proteins can be degraded by proteolytic enzymes that hydrolyze peptide bonds and yield amino acids. In turn, amino acids can be stripped of their amino groups, and the carbon skeletons, as pyruvate, acetyl-CoA, oxaloacetate, etc., are further broken down in Krebs cycle. So proteins can be used to provide energy as well, but because of their diverse functional roles and importance for muscles, they are used as major fuel sources only under extreme circumstances, i.e. starvation.

Quantitatively, the most important stored molecules that act as fuel substrates are fats, i.e. triacylglycerides. They are broken down to fatty acids that can be degraded through a pathway of β-oxidation. Acetyl-CoA is produced in β-oxidation that enters Krebs cycle.

All normal and usual catabolic paths converge to a small number of simple molecules, of which acetyl-CoA is central to all three: proteins, fats, and carbohydrates.

Under normal circumstances, there is a balance between catabolic and anabolic processes. While a protein molecule, for example that of albumin, is broken down within the circulation after 20 days, there is a balancing synthesis of albumin by the liver so that albumin concentration in blood remains the same.

Triacylgyceroles and glycogen build up in the body after food ingestion by synthesizing these complex storage molecules from glucose and fatty acids. Between meals, the body can draw on the reserves to provide fuel for the ongoing daily activities. If food ingestion is higher than necessary for daily activities, a fat storage ensues. During starvation the fat stores are diminishing.

METABOLIC PATHWAYS

Glycolysis is the splitting of six carbon glucose-6-phosphate into two three carbon molecules of pyruvate. Two molecules of ATP are created per one molecule of glucose entering glycolysis.

Within the mitochondria, pyruvate loses CO_2, and acetyl-CoA is formed by re-cycling of Co-enzyme A. Acetyl-CoA enters the Krebs cycle, with the production of reduced co-enzymes NADH and $FADH_2$, that serve as a source of electrons for the respiratory chain cascade that in turn provides energy for the ATP synthesis. In a complete breakdown of one molecule of glucose through glycolysis, Krebs cycle, and respiratory chain cascade altogether 36 to 38 molecules of ATP are made (38 molecules of ATP in the liver, while only 36 molecules of ATP in the brain and muscles). So eventually the molecule of glucose is broken down to CO_2 and water, and *about 40% of its energy is conserved in ATP.*

Gluconeogenesis occurs when the level of glucose is falling, and glucose is needed for the brain function. It starts by conversion of pyruvate into oxaloacetate and then steps of glycolysis are reversed.

When there is too much glucose in the blood, as after food ingestion, glycogen synthesis pathways opens up to turn excessive glucose into glycogen.

Glucose can also go through hexose monophosphate pathway, also known as pentose phosphate shunt, in which five carbon sugars are produced, which are important for the synthesis of nucleic acids.

With excessive food ingestion fatty acyl-CoA, along with a glycerol derivative, synthesizes triacylglyceride. During starvation, triacylglycerides degrade down to acyl-CoA that is further degraded by β-oxidation pathway in the mitochondrial matrix to acetyl-CoA to be used in Krebs cycle. The complete breakdown of fatty acids through β-oxidation and Krebs cycle generates considerably more ATP than that of glucose.

A complete breakdown of 16 carbon palmitic acid requires 7 repetitions of β-oxidation sequences, that generates 7 molecules of each $FADH_2$ and NADH, and those are then used in respiratory electron transport chain cascade and oxidative phosphorylation to generate 14 and 21 molecules of ATP, respectively. Then 8 acetyl-CoA molecules enter Krebs cycle, and each turn generates 12 ATP's on the basis of generation of $FADH_2$ and NADH, and their passage through electron transport chain and oxidative phosphorylation. Thus one molecule of palmitoyl-CoA yields 131 molecules of ATP via β-oxidation, Krebs cycle and electron transfer with oxidative phosphorylation.

With 131 molecules of ATP 146 molecules of water is released in mitochondria.

Acetyl-CoA can also turn into ketone bodies. When there is more acetyl-CoA from β-oxidation than Krebs cycle can handle, the excessive acetyl-CoA enters a secondary pathway that generates acetoacetate, β-hydroxybutyrate and acetone, i.e. ketone bodies. This occurs primarily in the mitochondria of hepatocytes. They are water-soluble fuel substrates, than can reverse to acetyl-CoA in any tissue, even in brain, and enter Krebs cycle.

Acetyl-CoA can also be formed during the breakdown of carbon residues of various amino acids. Carbon skeletons of amino acids can enter Krebs cycle as pyruvate, fumarate, oxaloacetate, or succinyl-CoA.

Amino groups of amino acids are converted via urea pathway in the liver into urea, eliminated in urine. Without this pathway amino acids would turn into toxic ammonia.

Anabolic and catabolic reactions make use of different pathways as the former require energy, while the later generate energy. *Anabolic and catabolic pathways are usually located in different compartments of cell: anabolic reactions take place in cytosol, while catabolic in mitochondria.* This physical separation optimizes the conditions for each type of reactions, as well as regulatory controls.

Catabolic pathways lead to the formation of ATP, NADH, and NADPH, and these molecules are then used as sources of electrons or energy in various steps of anabolic pathways. Concentration of these co-factors, and ATP, help regulate the speed of anabolic and catabolic pathways within the cell. The ADP/ATP ratio, AMP/ATP ratio, NAD^+/NADH ratio, are critical in control of glycolysis and Krebs cycle, and rising values of these ratios trigger increased rates of glycolysis and Krebs cycle.

Glycolysis is present in all cells, while Krebs cycle is absent in erythrocytes that lack mitochondria, and is not too active in leukocytes. There is no activity of β-oxidation pathway of fatty acids in the brain, except in starvation, as brain prefers glucose as fuel source. Gluconeogenesis takes place predominantly in liver and kidneys.

There is often a cooperation of various cell types of different organs in processing substrates. Lactate, the end product of glucose catabolism in erythrocytes and muscles during strenuous activity, enters blood, and is picked up by the liver and converted by gluconeogenesis to glucose.

Various catabolic pathways do not function simultaneously. Following food ingestion there is usually sufficient glucose in the body for energy needs, so that there is no need to degrade triacylglycerides. On the contrary fat stores are built-up after food ingestion. Likewise, there is no need to use protein for energy after food ingestion. In contrast, fasting leads to a breakdown of triacylglycerides, and breakdown of fatty acids provides ATP for most tissues, sparing glucose to be used as fuel for the brain. During fasting, the brain can use ketone bodies as a source of fuel.

Different organs behave differently when it comes to fuel metabolism. The brain prefers only one fuel, glucose, and the metabolic regulation assures that there is sufficient supply of glucose for the brain. *Liver is the main provider of fuel for all organs.* If blood sugar drops down, liver turns on glycogenolysis, and gluconeogenesis for glucose synthesis. Muscles likewise consume fuel, except they will take in fatty acids from triacylglycerides as well, along with glucose. *Muscles do not provide glucose for other organs and tissues, i.e. do not release glucose into blood.* Adipose tissue collects all fuel substrates and stores them as energy reserves.

Since all cells of the body require a continuous supply of fuel substrates to maintain adequate levels of ATP, and there is no continuous ingestion of food to supply these fuels, fuels derived from food have *to be stored in a* convenient form. The granules of glycogen are in abundance in the liver and muscle. But triacylglycerides are the most abundant form of stored fuel, and fat makes up the bulk of fuel reserves.

In adult male there are on average 135,000 kcal stored in fat, 900 kcal in glycogen, and 24,000 kcal in protein. One kilogram of fat can sustain a starving 70-kg male for 3 – 4 days, and his total fat reserves last for 2 months.

Carbohydrate yields 4 kcal/g, while fat 9 kcal/g.

The advantage of fat is that it is stored in anhydrous condition, whereas the strongly polar glycogen must be stored in hydrated form, which takes much more space. On the other side, simple sugars can be produced much quicker from glycogen while fatty acids are not mobilized as fast from stored fats.

The caloric requirements depend upon the level of physical activity, and environmental temperature. More calories are needed for survival in the Arctic than on Tropical Island.

Fat metabolism and carbohydrate metabolism are directly connected, and under hormonal control. Many tissues use glucose as a fuel source when food ingestion is adequate, and fat in times of fasting and starvation.

Under normal conditions there is a dynamic balance between protein breakdown and synthesis in protein metabolism. There is a constant turnover of proteins, old molecules are destroyed and new ones made to take their place.

Protein synthesis relies on availability of the 20 amino acids, derived from food ingestion or from the breakdown of existing in the body proteins. Non-essential amino acids can be made from other amino acid, or intermediates formed in glycolysis, Krebs cycle or hexose monophosphate pathway. Essential amino acids have to be supplied by food.

Breakdown of proteins in the body is carried out by proteases, which utilize water to break peptide bonds between amino acids. Inside the cells proteolysis takes place within two compartments: lysosomes, and cytosol.

Only in prolonged fasting/starvation, and in diabetes mellitus, is there a net loss of proteins, when they are used to provide fuel or carbon sources for gluconeogenesis.

Chapter 12

> Man with all his noble qualities … with his godlike intellect which has penetrated into the movements and constitution of the solar system … still bears in his bodily frame the indelible stamp of his lowly origin.
> *Charles Robert Darwin, 1809 – 1882, The Descent of Man*

MEDICAL GENETICS

Mouse and human genome separated phylogenetically only one million years ago. Mice have nearly the same genes as humans, except organized in 40 chromosomes, and their genes grouped on the same chromosomes are similar to the grouping in man, except in man such group of genes is on a different chromosome.

A similar statement could be made about the genome of primates and humans, but mice are more important for stem cell transplantation.

Genetic code is universal, i.e. the same for all organisms and non-repetitive. A partial exception is the genetic code of mitochondrial DNA, which is not universal, and is somewhat repetitive.

DNA in all eukaryotic cells is the same that means that DNA in hepatocytes, myocytes, lymphocytes, etc., of the same organism is the same. Why is then the structure and function of these cells so different? Is it due to the character of genes, their expression or their end products specific for various types of cells? The transcription of some genes is active only during some stages of development of an organism.

One molecule of human DNA is substantially larger than that of any other protein.

Mutation is a process that causes permanent changes of DNA, positive or negative. Mutations can be *major*, i.e. loss, duplicity, structural change of chromosomes, or *minimal*, i.e. *"point mutations"*, when loss, duplicity or structural change applies to only one nucleotide, or a miniscule portion of DNA.

Spontaneous mutations outnumber the induced mutations many times over. It is believed to be the result of spontaneous errors during replication and repair of DNA, or during spontaneous chemical reactions. *During human lifetime every gene is subject to 100 million to 10 billion of such mutations.* But *nearly all damage due to such mutations is repaired, or causes cell death without any consequences for other cells.* But the danger of erroneous mitosis leading to cancer is always looming.

Radiation is 2 - 3 times more effective to induce mutation when delivered as an acute dose rather than chronic. The younger the ovaries and sperms are at the time of radiation exposure the less sensitive they are to the irradiation.

Chemicals are much more dangerous mutagens than radiation.

Types of mutation caused by viruses do not differ from those caused by chemicals or radiation. Mutagenic effect of named viruses is not specific.

Absolute majority of DNA mutations is immediately repaired in the organisms. In humans there are two major repair methods that involve a complex of enzymatic steps:

1. base excision repair, an excision of damaged purine or pyrimidine base;
2. nucleotide excision repair, an excision of damaged nucleotide.

Gene mutations often take place only in some tissues. For example, a gene for Huntington chorea is expressed in many tissues, but mutations take place only in certain parts of the brain. Similarly retinoblastoma gene is expressed everywhere but genetic mutations occur only in retina.

Mutations can cause a gain of new function as often happens in cancer.

Overproduction of normal gene product can become pathologic, which is the usual mechanism for activation of protooncogens in cancer cells. The same is typical for hereditary sensory and motor neuropathy type 1A, known as Charcot-Marie-Tooth disease type 1A.

Identical phenotype can be caused by mutations of two or more different genes.

Different mutations in the same locus can sometimes cause similar phenotype, but sometimes completely different clinical signs. An example is congenital methemoglobinopathy, autosomal recessive disorder, where there are increased levels of hemoglobin with trivalent $Fe3^{+}$-methemoglobin, with much stronger bond to oxygen than normal hemoglobin, so that oxygen cannot be released in the tissues as necessary. If level of methemoglobin reaches 15% of total hemoglobin, cyanosis becomes apparent, at 40% dyspnea, at higher levels ataxia, stupor and coma, and death at 85% concentration of methemoglobin.

Gene imprinting causes a completely different phenotype due to the same chromosomal damage depending on whether the inheritance is from father or mother, i.e. deletion of long arm of chromosome 15 will cause *Prader-Willi syndrome*, if inherited from father, i.e. already in infancy observed difficulty to drink, unique cry or a lack of cry, failure to thrive, delayed speech, round face without mimicry, genital hypoplasia, or *Angelman syndrome, if* inherited from mother, with psychomotor retardation, ataxia, hypertonia of extremities with hypotonia of trunk musculature, severe speech disturbance, attacks of laugh, spasms, and typical EEG findings.

Chapter 13

> Ontogenesis, or the development of the individual, is a short and quick recapitulation of phylogenesis, or the development of the tribe to which it belongs, determined by the laws of inheritance and adaptation.
> Ernst Heinrich Haeckel, 1834 – 1919, The History of Creation [1868]

COMPARATIVE EMBRYOLOGY

This and the next chapters return again to *'organospecificity'* i.e. similarity of the same cell type in the animal kingdom. *The series of facts in italics will help you to identify the important issues.*

Organisms are divided into two major groups, their classification depending on whether their cells possess a nuclear envelope. *Prokaryotes* lack a true nucleus, such as bacteria, blue-green algae. *Eukaryotes* have a well formed nuclear envelope surrounding their chromosomes, i.e. protists, fungi, plants, animals.

Multicellular organisms that pass through embryonic stages of development are called *Metazoans*.

Birds and mammals are descendants of reptilian species. Mammalian development parallels that of reptiles and birds. Gastrulation movements of reptilian and avian embryos, which evolved around yolky eggs, are retained even in mammalian embryo despite the lack of large amount of yolk. The mammalian inner mass is sitting atop of an imaginary ball of yolk, following instructions typical for its ancestors.

Mammalian embryonic epiblast, that is believed to contain all the cells that generate the actual embryo, is similar to the avian epiblast.

While the mammalian embryonic epiblast is undergoing cell movements reminiscent of those seen in reptilian or avian gastrulation, the extraembryonic cells are making the distinctly mammalian tissue that enable the fetus to survive within the maternal uterus, i.e. *placenta*.

Although the initial trophoblastic cells of mice and man appear like regular cells, i.e. cytotrophoblast, they give rise to a population of cells wherein nuclear division occurs in the absence of cytokinesis: syncytiotrophoblast. The cytotrophoblast adheres to the endometrium through a series of adhesion molecules, and in humans contains proteolytic enzymes that enable these cells to enter uterine wall and remodel uterine blood vessels so that the maternal blood bathes fetal blood vessels. Syncytiotrophoblast furthers the penetration of the embryo into the uterine wall. This proteolytic activity ceases after 12 weeks of pregnancy.

Syncytiotrophoblast produces three hormones essential for mammalian development. Chorionic gonadotropin causes i.a. other placental cells to produce progesterone. Placental progesterone is used by the fetal adrenal gland as a substrate for corticosteroid hormones. Chorionic somatomammotropin is responsible for promoting maternal breast development, enabling milk production later.

The new extra-embryonic organ, which consists of trophoblast and blood vessel-containing mesoderm, is called *chorion*. Chorion acts to exchange gases and nutrients between mother and fetus but is also an endocrine gland. Chorion protects the fetus from the immune response of the mother as well. Human fetus expresses major histocompatibility antigens from both parents, and mother's body ought to reject it as 'nonself' because it contains also paternally-derived antigens. Chorion has evolved several mechanisms that inhibit the immune response of pregnant female against the fetus until the moment of birth.

EARLY VERTEBRATE DEVELOPMENT

There is a famous quote from the best embryologist of his time, Karl Ernst von Baer, according to which he forgot to label two small embryos preserved in alcohol, and was unable to determine the genus to which they belong, because they could be lizards, small birds, or mammals. In other words, different groups of animals share certain common features during early embryonic development, and their features become more and more characteristic of their species as development proceeds.

From his study of comparative embryology *Von Baer derived four laws*:

1. The general features of animals of a certain genus appear earlier in embryo earlier than do specialized features. All developing vertebrates appear very similar shortly after gastrulation. For example, all vertebrate embryos have gill arches, notochords, spinal cords, and pronephric kidneys.

2. Less general characteristics are developed from the more general, until finally the most specialized appear. As examples, all vertebrates have initially the same type of skin, early development of the limb is essentially the same in all vertebrates.

3. Each embryo of a given species, instead of passing through the adult stages of other animals, departs more and more from them. For example, the visceral clefts of embryonic birds and mammals resemble visceral clefts of embryonic fishes and other embryonic vertebrates rather than gill slits of adult fishes.

4. Early embryo of higher animal is never like the adult of lower animal, but is like its early embryo.

Von Baer recognized that there is a common pattern to all vertebrate development: *three germ layers give rise to different organs, and this derivation of the organs is constant whether the organism is a fish, a frog, or a chick.* Ectoderm forms skin and nerves, endoderm forms respiratory and digestive tubes, and mesoderm forms connective tissue, blood cells, heart, urogenital system, and parts of most internal organs.

In 1898, Wilson reported on his observation that in various genes (flatworms, mollusks annelids) the same organs always originated from the same group of cells, i.e. organospecificity [148].

In vertebrates a dorsal mesoderm signals ectodermal cells on the top of it to develop into the columnar neural plate cells, and as a result of this neural induction, the cells of the prospective neural plate are distinguished from the surrounding ectoderm, destined to become epidermis. *This interaction between dorsal mesoderm and its overlying ectoderm is one of the most important interactions during the development of all vertebrates, for it initiates organogenesis, the creation of specific tissues and organs.* In this interaction, the chordamesoderm directs the ectoderm to form the hollow neural tube, i.e. *neurulation*.

The mechanism of neural tube formation is similar in amphibians, reptiles, birds, and mammals.

Differentiation of the neural tube into the various regions of CNS occurs simultaneously in three different ways. Grossly anatomically, the neural tube and its lumen bulge and constrict, to form the chambers of the brain and spinal cord. On the tissue level, the cell populations within the wall of the neural tube rearrange themselves in various ways to form the different functional regions of CNS. On the cellular level, neuroepithelial cells differentiate into the numerous types of neurons and supportive (glial) cells present in the body [148].

Chapter 14

In our description of nature the purpose is not to disclose the real essence of the phenomena but only to track down, so far as it is possible, relations between the manifold aspects of our experience.
Niels Bohr, 1885 – 1962, Atomic Theory and the Description of Nature [1934]

GROWTH AND DEVELOPMENT

As stated in the previous chapter, the early development of most vertebrate CNS is similar. The early mammalian neural tube is a straight structure. The most anterior part of the tube balloons into three primary vesicles: forebrain, midbrain, and hindbrain. By the time the posterior end of the neural tube closes, optic vesicles bulge laterally from each side of the developing forebrain.

The forebrain subdivides into the anterior telencephalon, and caudal diencephalon. Mesencephalon does not divide. Rhombencephalon subdivides into anterior metencephalon and posterior myelencephalon.

Neural tube closure in mammals is initiated at several places along the AP axis. Failure to close the posterior neuropore at day 27 results in spina bifida. Failure to close anterior neural tube results in lethal anencephaly, where the forebrain remains in contact with amniotic fluid and inevitably degenerates.

The reader is advised to pay attention to the following explanation of *the reason for intraventricular implantation of stem cell transplants.*

The original neural tube is composed of a one-layer thick germinal neuroepithelium. It is a rapidly dividing cell population. DNA synthesis, i.e. S phase of mitosis, occurs while the nucleus is at the external side of the tube, and as mitosis proceeds the nucleus migrates luminally. Mitosis occurs on the luminal side of the cell layer.

During early mammalian development 100% of neural tube cells divide. Shortly thereafter, certain cells stop participating in mitosis. These post-mitotic cells, neuronal and glial, differentiate on the external side of the neural tube, while those that continue to participate in mitosis, i.e. the germinal cells, are on the luminal side of the neural tube. *The neurons that stopped participating in mitosis always migrate away from the luminal side of the neural tube.*

The time when the neuron precursor divided last time is the neuron's 'birthday'. Cells with the earliest birthdays migrate the shortest distances. Cells with later birthdays, i.e. younger, migrate through all layers to form the more superficial regions of the brain cortex. This forms an *'inside-out gradient of development'*. Subsequent differentiation of these precursor cells is dependent upon the position in terms of cell layer that these neurons occupy once outside the layer of dividing cells.

A single stem cell in the ventricular layer can produce neurons (and glial cells) that end up in any of the cortical layers. Different types of neurons and glial cells have different 'birthdays'. Determination of laminar identity, i.e. which layer a cell migrates to, is made during the final cell division.

Cells on the luminal side of the neural tube, i.e. germinal layer, later on called *'ependymal cells'*, continue to divide, while the migrating cells form a second layer, progressively thicker by a continuous addition of new cells from ependyma, *the mantle zone.*

In the mantle zone, the migrating cells differentiate into neurons and glial cells. Neurons develop dendrites to make connections between themselves, and send forth axons away from the lumen, and axons create a cell-poor marginal zone. Eventually, glial cells cover many axons with myelin sheaths, thereby giving this part of the marginal zone a whitish appearance, 'white matter of the brain'. The portion the mantle zone with neuronal bodies is referred to as 'gray matter of the brain'.

Cell migration, differential growth, and selective apoptosis, produce modifications of the three-zone pattern in the brain that is quite apparent when one compares the cortex of cerebrum and cerebellum.

Cerebrum is organized in two distinct ways:

1. *vertically* into layers that interact with each other. Certain neuroblasts from the mantle zone migrate upon glia (see below

about 'glial guidance') through the white matter to create the second zone of neurons. This newly created mantle zone is called 'neopallial cortex'. It eventually stratifies into six layers of cell bodies. *It takes up until the middle of childhood before these neurons attain adult forms.* Each layer of the cerebral cortex differs from the other in its functional properties, the types of neurons found therein, and the type of neuronal connections that develop.

2. *horizontally* into over 40 regions that regulate geographically distinct processes and functions.

Neither vertical nor horizontal organization is clonally specified. On the contrary, there is a lot of cell movement that *mixes the progenies of various precursor stem cells.*

The primary mechanism for positioning young neurons within the developing mammalian brain is "glial guidance". Neurons ride the "glial monorail" to their respective destinations. When the neuronal cell membrane first makes contact with the glial membrane, the glial cell stops proliferating and begins to differentiate and extends its glial process. *This process is controlled by glial cells and not by neurons. Neuron binds to the glial cell and begins to express calcium ion channels.* Influx of calcium ions is necessary for the motility of the neuron's leading process. The neuron wraps this long leading process around the glial fiber, and as it migrates along the glial process, it continues to signal the glial cells to retain its differentiated form. Neurons maintain its adhesion to the glial cell through a number of proteins, the most important being the adhesion protein astrotactin.

While 80% of the young neurons migrates radially, abut 12% migrates laterally from one functional region of the cortex into another. Neural descendants of a single germinal cell are dispersed across the functional regions of the cortex. *Specification of these cortical areas into specific functions occurs after neurogenesis.*

The human brain continues to develop at fetal rates even after birth. At birth, humans are prepared for independent life much less than primates, and continuous fast brain development is mandatory. For that reason, some feel that *during our first year of life we are essentially 'extrauterine fetuses'.* Much of human intelligence comes from the stimulation of the nervous system during the first year after birth.

Human cerebral cortex has no neuronal connections at 12 weeks gestation, therefore, *cannot move in response to a thought, nor experience consciousness or fear*. Measurable electrical activity characteristic of neural cells, i.e. EEG, is first seen at 7 months gestation.

Human brain consists of 100 billion neurons associated with 1 trillion of glial cells. *At birth cortical neurons have very few dendrites, but during the first year after birth each cortical neuron develops so many dendrites that it can accommodate 100,000 connections with other neurons.*

Each neuron has one axon, which may extend for several feet. It is an extension of neuronal body. To prevent dispersion of the electrical signal and to facilitate its conduction, each axon in CNS is insulated by myelination, a processes handled by oligodendrocytes. Oligodendrocyte wraps itself around the developing axon, and then produces a specialized cell membrane rich in myelin basic protein that spirals around the central axon. In the peripheral nervous system another glial cell called Schwann cell accomplishes the same.

Axon must be specialized for secreting a specific neurotransmitter across the synaptic clefts that separate axon of one neuron from the surface of its target cell.

Development of neural crest cells of most vertebrates is similar. Derived from ectoderm, neural crest cells originate at the dorsal-most region of the neural tube and migrate extensively to *generate a large number of differentiated cells types*:

1. neurons and glial cells of sensory, sympathetic, and parasympathetic nervous systems,
2. *the epinephrine-producing medulla cells of adrenal gland,*
3. *pigment containing cells of the epidermis,*
4. skeletal and connective tissue of the head.

Neural crest is divided into:

1. *cephalic* neural crest, the cells of which migrate dorso-laterally to produce the craniofacial mesenchyme; these cells also enter pharyngeal arches to give rise to *thymic cells*, odontoblasts, cartilages of inner ear and mandible,
2. *trunk* neural crest: those cells that migrate dorso-laterally become *melanocytes*, while those that migrate ventro-laterally

form either *dorsal root ganglia, or sympathetic ganglia, adrenal medulla and para-aortic bodies*,
3. *vagal and sacral* neural crest, the cells of which generate the *parasympathetic (enteric) ganglia of the gut*,
4. *cardiac* neural crest, the cells of which develop into melanocytes, neurons, mesenchyme of the 3rd, 4th, 6th pharyngeal arches, and musculo-connective tissue wall of the large arteries as they arise from the heart, and septum that separates the pulmonary circulation from aorta.

Comprehension of neural crest cells development is of great help in selecting the cell types for treatment of certain pathological conditions by stem cell transplantation.

Neural crest cells are exceptionally strongly pluripotential.

There is an interaction of oral plate ectoderm and neural tube: the root of oral ectoderm forms Rathke's pouch that becomes anterior lobe of pituitary.

Epidermis: We lose and replace 1.5 gm of dried epidermal cells a day. The replacement is coming from the population of stem cells. In adult skin, a cell born in the Malpighian layer takes approximately 8 weeks to reach stratum corneum, and remains there for about 2 weeks. In psoriasis, characterized by exfoliation of enormous numbers of epidermal cells, the time cells spend in stratum corneum is only 2 days. This is due to the over-expression of transforming growth factor TGF-α.

In male pattern baldness, the scalp follicles revert back to producing under-pigmented and very fine vellus hair of newborn. There appears to be a pluripotent epidermal stem cell the progeny of which can become epidermis, sebaceous gland or hair follicle.

MESODERM

The formation of mesodermal and endodermal organs occurs synchronously with neural tube formation.

Mesoderm is *divided into*:

1. *chorda-mesoderm*, that *forms notochord* without which the neural tube formation is not possible,

2. *somatic dorsal mesoderm*, that becomes *somites*, blocks of mesodermal cells on both sides of neural tube that produce many kinds of connective tissue of the back,
3. *intermediate* mesoderm that forms *urinary system and genital ducts*,
4. *lateral plate* mesoderm that gives rise to the *heart, blood vessels, blood cells of the circulatory system, lining of body cavities*, all mesodermal components of the limbs except the muscles, and *all extraembryonic membranes*,
5. *head mesenchyme* necessary for the development of the *face*.

The mechanism for creating mesodermal somites and body cavity linings has changed little throughout vertebrate evolution.

Somites are transient structures, any cells of which can become any of the somite derived structures.

Myogenesis cannot take place without cell-cell-recognition and cell fusion. But *species specificity is not necessary, i.e. myoblasts fuse only with other myoblasts but those myoblasts need not be of the same species.*

Osteogenesis: There are two major modes of bone formation, and both involve transformation of a pre-existing mesenchymal tissue into bone tissue:

1. *Intramembraneous ossification* is a direct conversion of mesenchymal tissue into bone: some mesenchymal cells develop into capillaries, others into osteoblasts capable to secrete bone matrix. The secreted collagen-glycosaminoglycan matrix binds calcium salts brought in by capillaries, and thereby the matrix calcifies. External layer of mesenchymal cells creates periosteum, and the cells on the inner surface of periosteum also become osteoblasts.
2. *Endochondral ossification*, where mesenchymal cells differentiate into cartilage first, and cartilage is later replaced by bone. The cartilage tissue becomes a model for the bone that is created during the next step. *This remarkable process coordinates chondrogenesis with osteogenesis.*

Cardinal difference from intramembraneous ossification is that *in the endochondral ossification "epiphyseal plates"* are created, the cartilagineous regions at the end of long bones, through which bone lengthens. *The proliferation of epiphyseal plate is controlled by hormones: growth hormone and insulin-like growth factor.* At the end of puberty, high levels of estrogen or testosterone cause the remaining epiphyseal plate cartilage to hypertrophy, leading eventually to the death of cartilage cells and their replacement by bone. *Without cartilage cells the growth of bone ceases.*

As new bone tissue is added by the periosteal osteoblasts, there is a hollowing out of the internal region of bone to form the bone marrow cavity. This destruction of bone tissue is carried out by osteoclasts, multinucleated cells that enter the bone from capillaries and dissolve both the organic and inorganic portions of matrix. *Osteoclasts are derived from the same precursor stem cells as granulocytes and macrophages.*

Blood vessels import the blood-forming cells that eventually reside in the bone marrow for the duration of life.

Kidneys: Mammalian nephron contains over 10,000 cells and 12 different cell types. Each cell type is located in a particular place in relation to the other cell types along the length of nephron.

Circulatory System is the first functioning system in the developing fetus and the heart is the first functioning organ. *The presumptive heart cells originate in the early primitive streak, just posterior to the Hensen's node, which* at the age of 20 days migrate anteriorly between ectoderm and endoderm. The direction of this migration is controlled by endoderm. The presumptive heart cells of birds and mammals form a double walled tube consisting of an inner endocardium and outer epimyocardium. Pulsations of the heart begins while the paired primordial chambers are still fusing, and the pacemaker function is assumed by the sinus venosus.

Haematopoietic System: *We lose and replace 100 billion of red blood cells each day.* The replacement is coming from the population of hematopoietic stem cells.

Red blood cells, white blood cells, i.e. granulocytes, lymphocytes, monocytes, macrophages, osteoclasts, platelets, share a common precursor: the pluripotential hematopoietic stem cell. *Hematopietic stem cells die without the growth factors of bone marrow, produced also by stromal cells*, i.e. fibroblasts and other connective tissue elements of bone marrow, and other growth factors traveling through blood. *In the spleen stem cells are committed predominantly to erythroid development, while in the bone marrow granulocyte development dominates.*

In mammals, the location of the sites of early hematopiesis has not been completely elucidated. In the fetus, the main hematopoietic organ is the liver, and it is believed that stem cells from liver migrate to the bone marrow. In the adult the major source of blood cells is bone marrow, although in mice, the spleen also participates.

ENDODERM

We lose and replace 100 billion of intestinal cells each day and the replacement is coming from the population of stem cells in intestinal mucosa.

The second pharyngeal pouch (PP) gives rise to the walls of tonsils, the third PP to thymus and one pair of parathyroid bodies, and the second pair of parathyroids comes from 4th pharyngeal pouch. Small central diverticulum is formed between two 2nd pharyngeal pouches and this pocket of endoderm and mesenchyme will migrate down and become thyroid.

Between the 4th pharyngeal pouches the laryngotracheal groove extends ventrally.

Lungs *are among the last of mammalian organs to fully differentiate.* They must be able to draw in oxygen with the first baby's breath. To accomplish this, alveolar cells secrete a surfactant into the fluid bathing the lungs. This surfactant, consisting of phospholipids such as sphingomyelin and lecithin, is secreted very late in gestation, and reaches useful level for full performance at 34th week of human gestation. It enables the alveolar cells to touch one another without sticking together [148].

DIFFERENTIATION

Differentiation **is the development of specialized cell types from the single fertilized egg.** Such change in biochemistry and function of a cell is preceded by a process involving the covert commitment of a cell to a particular fate. **After the commitment, the cell does not appear** *phenotypically different from its uncommitted state*, but somehow its developmental fate has become restricted.

The commitment takes place in various ways:

1. *autonomous specification*, where each cell becomes specified by the type of cytoplasm it acquires during mitosis, and cell fate is thereby determined *without any relationship to neighboring cells*;
2. *conditional specification*, where the cells originally have the ability to follow more than one path of differentiation, but the *interaction of these cells with other cells or tissues restricts the fates of one or both participants.* Here the future of the cell *depends upon the conditions in which it finds itself.* This is a pattern of embryogenesis called *regulative development*, that brings on *secondary inductions*.

Organs are complex structures composed of numerous types of tissues. The precise arrangement of tissues cannot be disturbed without damaging its function. *In the construction of organs, there is a coordination between groups of cells whereby one group of cells changes the behavior of an adjacent set of cells, causing them to change their shape, mitotic rate, or differentiation.* This action at close range, called "*secondary induction*", or "*proximate interaction*", enables one group of cells to respond to a second group of cells, and then via such change, to alter a third set of cells.

In "*instructive interaction*" *a signal from the inducing cell is necessary for initiating new gene expression in the responding cell.* Without the inducing cell, the responding cell is not capable of differentiating in that particular way.

In *"permissive interaction" the responding cell or tissue contains all the potentials to be expressed, but it requires an environment that allows the expression of these traits.* At the same time the *responding cell must be 'competent' to respond*, i.e. a cell must synthetize a receptor for the inducing molecule, or a cell must synthetize a specific protein that allows the receptor to function, or a cell must repress the inhibitor.

Among interactions the epithelio-mesenchymal ones are the best known, where *epithelial sheets from any germ layer interact with mesenchymal cells*, usually neural crest cells or loose mesodermal cells.

Ectodermal or endodermal epitheliums respond differently to different regionally specific mesenchymes, i.e. liver, intestine or lungs, but only as far as their genomes would permit. The *instructions sent by mesenchymal tissue can cross species barriers, and are always organospecific. They continue until an organ is formed with organ specific mesenchymal cells and organ specific epithelia* [148].

Local induction occurs via cell-cell contact, cell-matrix contact, or a diffusion of soluble signals, i.e. *paracrine factors*. Distant induction is carried out by diffusible regulators of development that travel through the blood to *cause changes in the differentiation and morphogenesis of other tissues, i.e. hormones* [148].

In 1950, a report on embryonic transplantation via vascular route concluded that injected ground early embryonic tissue survived in the blood stream of the recipient, infiltrated into the tissues, reached their 'normal' sites, and multiplied and differentiated there in a typical fashion, i.e. *description of "organospecificity", and of "homing"* [189].

In 1952, Moscona showed that "cells destined to give rise to cartilage or kidney, when initially isolated and then reassembled and grown in tissue culture, continue in their erstwhile course of histogenesis, producing cartilage and nephric tubules, respectively... ..and if provided with proper stroma, a glandular blastema may give rise to.... ...3-D morphogenesis"...[190].

Andres observed that random scrambled embryonic cell suspension incorporated in the yolk sac of chick embryo can develop into organized, very complex bodies, containing many different and well-differentiated organ parts (brain, ganglia, skeleton with joints and muscles, skin with feathers, etc.) [190].

Cells from chick embryonic kidneys, liver, and skin, were minced and then deposited on the chorio-allantoic membrane of 8-days old chick embryos. *The same organs were recreated with a typical architectural pattern*, including connective and vascular tissue, polarization, and evidence of functional activity. Since the transplanted tissue fragments *accomplished on a neutral test site a second organogenesis, strictly corresponding to the organ from which they had been isolated*, they must have achieved this by *virtue of 'information' distinctive of the kind of organ which they had formed part of* and must have been capable of translating that 'information' into a repeat performance [190].

Only about 33 animal body plans (Bauplans) are presently used on this planet. *These constitute all animal phyla in existence today.* Eukaryotic cells emerged some 1.4 billion years ago, and all known Metazoan phyla were formed in the Cambrian radiation which began 544 million years ago, and lasted some 10 million years and no new morphological pattern (Bauplan) has been added since then. A new bauplan could be created only by a modification of existing bauplan in the earliest stages of the development of an organism [148].

DEVELOPMENTAL MECHANISMS

During the evolution, 17 types of multicellular organisms emerged from the single-celled organisms. But *only three groups, those that generated fungi, plants and animals, evolved the ability to form multicellular aggregates that differentiate into particular cell types*, i.e. embryo.

Only those that retained or produced non-ciliated cells learned how to divide cells. Those that differentiated cilia never learned how to divide cells, while those that had no cilia, i.e. lacked motility, learned to migrate inside of blastocoel, and create a federation of cells. *Blastula arose as a means of joining autonomous cells into a federation, i.e. each cell gave up its autonomy in order to create a community of cells. While individual cells were totipotent, in the aggregate each cell restricted its potency, and that applied to all its neighboring cells. Once one inside population of blastocoel could interact with another, or with an outside population, induction events could occur that had given rise to new organs.*

In 1891, Metchnikoff wrote that evolution consists of *modifying embryonic organisms, not adult ones*. Organisms evolved through changes in their embryonic development. Re-arrangement of development during early embryonic stage brings about new types of organization that are the key mechanisms for establishing new phyla and classes [148].

Early developmental changes can be affected by changing the localization of cytoplasmatic determinants, changing the ratio of mitosis of one cell, or a group of cells, relative to the others, and changing the positions of the cells as they divide.

Von Baer stated that *animals of different species but of the same genus diverge very late in their development.* The more divergent are the species, the earlier can one distinguish (recognize) their embryos [148].

Vertebrates are thought to have arisen from invertebrates in several steps that involved the formation of and modification of new cell types. *The ability of mesoderm to form a notochord, and its overlying ectoderm to become a neural tube, separated chordates from the lower invertebrates.* The development of neural crest cells, and the epidermal placodes that give rise to the sensory nerves of the face, distinguish vertebrates from the protochordates. *Once a vertebrate, it is difficult to develop into anything else due to the constrains imposed upon evolution:* physical, morphogenetic construction rules, historical restrictions based on genetics of the development of an organism. In 1915, Conklin stated that we are vertebrates, because our mothers were vertebrates, and produced eggs of the vertebrate pattern [148].

In 1937, Bobshansky stated that *evolution means changes in gene frequencies in a population over time.* When the interaction between genes is changed, new cellular phenotypes can arise. *The creation of a new cell type is a rare event in nature and often can change the entire phenotype of an organism.* Mutations in regulatory genes can create large changes in morphology. Large morphological changes seen during evolutionary history could be explained by the accumulation of small genetic changes. But in 1976, Van Valen expressed an alternative opinion that *evolution can be defined as the control of the development by ecology [148].*

Chapter 15

> Old age is the most unexpected of all the things that happen to a man
> *Leon Trotsky, 1879 – 1940, Diary in Exile, [1935]*
>
> Every man desires to live long, but no man would be old.
> *Jonathan Swift, 1667 – 1745, Thoughts on Various Subjects [1711]*

AGING PROCESS

Aging is a normal unavoidable process that ends by death. While average lifespan of a newborn was around 10 years just 50,000 years ago, and in old Rome 25 years, today it is between 38 (in some Third World countries) and 80 years (in Japan). In the past, it was neonatal mortality and infectious diseases, mostly in children. Today diseases of old age are the most common cause of death: in 50% cardiovascular diseases, and in 25% cancer. Diseases prohibit reaching the maximum 'theoretic' lifespan of 120 years. The actual maximum lifespan has not changed for centuries.

CAUSES OF AGING

Only a few cell types are immortal, i.e. those with unlimited proliferation: germ cells, cancer cells, hematopoietic stem cells. All other cells die and have to be replaced, and a *disease is a lack of cell replacement*. Aging disease is one of them.

Aging and lifespan are genetically determined. In Werner's disease, known as 'progeria', the mutation of gene coding DNA-helicase brings about other somatic DNA mutations, and shortening of telomerase, that causes limitations of mitosis and subsequent premature aging. Experience with patients suffering from *genetic disease with shortened lifespan and phenotypic signs of premature aging* provide additional proofs: Down syndrome, Cockayne syndrome, ataxia telangiectasia, Seip syndrome, Klinefelter syndrome, Turner syndrome, myotonic dystrophy. There is an increased incidence of certain genetic diseases due to the higher age of father (Apert syndrome, Marfan syndrome, achondroplasia, myositis ossificans, etc.) or due to the age of a mother past 35 (all trisomies).

This idea is actually quite old, because other proofs have been collected for decades. With age there is a growing number of aneuploid cells, in particular hypodiplod cells with loss of chromosomes X and Y in lymphocytes of peripheral blood and bone marrow. Classical mutagens, i.e. X-rays, increased temperatures, UV radiation, shorten lifespan in protosoa's. There is a 1.6% growth a year in a number of mutations found in human lymphocytes.

With age, there is a significant decrease of effectiveness of human respiratory cascade, as well as progressive accumulation of deletions of mitochondrial DNA, identical to deletions in Kearns-Sayre syndrome. Another proof of "mitochondrial theory of aging" is an incidence of negativity of cytochrom C oxidase in myocardial and peripheral muscle fibers, which shows the mosaic of aging changes in human tissues.

Hypothetically, cell aging is caused by mutations of dominant or co-dominant type.

Secondarily, many genetic diseases and polygenetic risks influence lifespan. But *studies of monozygotic twins showed that 2/3 of variability of lifespan are not of genetic nature.*

In the course of aging, various body functions are reduced: maximum voluntary ventilation, oxygen consumption, cardiac index, glomerular filtration rate, etc. Weight of muscles and bones decreases for hormonal reasons. Generalized weakness is characterized by lowered muscle strength, prolongation of reflexes, limitations of motion, balance disturbances, lack of endurance that results in falls, fractures, limitations of daily physical activities, and loss of independence. Cause of muscle weakness is not only physiological processes of aging and wear and tear, but also lack of motion, all combined in a vicious circle. Memory loss of old age depends mostly on damage of long-term potentiation in cortex and hippocampus, with lowered density of glutamate receptors in gyrus dentatus.

Oxidative damage of membrane lipids, DNA, is another cause of aging, as well as accumulation of protein damage due to oxygen radicals, and diminution of activity of enzymes protecting against oxidation in the course of aging, all pointing to the environmental cause.

Let's now focus on the revitalization effect of cell transplants, especially of *placenta and gonads*, as researched extensively by Kment [256, 257]. It is less a targeted stimulation of specific organs, and more a general improvement of elementary functions of the entire organism, and thereby increased vitality. Term "revitalization" was created by Niehans, as he wanted to clarify that "rejuvenation" is not possible because biological clocks cannot be moved backward. But that does not mean that a discrepancy between the chronological age and biological age is not correctible. The premature aging shows as an excessive wear and tear and psychosomatic exhaustion.

Rietschel described the *revitalization effect of cell transplantation as an improvement of the general state of health*. Majority of patients suffering from various diseases very seldom state that their "heart condition, digestive function, or breathing, etc., is better after cell transplantation", but *speak of subjectively improved general state of health*. In other words *patients do not notice the better function of a single organ, even if that organ is malfunctioning and thus of deep concern to the patient*. They observe rather a better appetite, or change of taste for more appropriate foods, adjustment of weight, healthier skin color (from better blood circulation through skin), disappearance of wrinkles, stable emotions, more active mental and physical state, i.e. *increased vitality*. Physical and psychological factors overlap and are inseparable in patients' descriptions of their condition. There are positive changes of metabolism which are the basis of regeneration of damaged organs, and that is what is perceived by the patients as revitalization. On the basis of the 378 of own patients studied, the revitalization rate of 93.5% is reported after cell transplantation. The effect lasted on the average 6 to 12 months, occasionally 2 years or longer [255].

Studies on experimental animals are difficult to carry out, and there are always *questions whether results of such animal studies are of any value to a patient with aging disease, i.e. does it improve the therapeutic possibilities*. Multiple experimental animal studies, carried out in particular by Kment and his group in Vienna, Austria, were based on recognition of close relationship between wear and tear and aging process, and the ties of aging process to the vitality and various diseases of the older age. For studies of aging, wear and tear, involution, lowered vitality, they used controlled experiments in rats on elasticity and tear resistance of aorta and skin, collagen performance, tissue respiration in aorta, heart, liver, and kidney, mitochondrial function of myocardial fibers and hepatocytes, spontaneous activity, resorption, distribution, and elimination of V-Penicillin, in relation to age. *Cell transplantation of placenta and gonads significantly improved all measured parameters* [256, 257, 259].

Others proved that cell transplantation improves tissue oxygenation, thyroid function, reverses atrophy of vaginal epithelium, prolongs lifespan, etc., but if all such positive results are taken together it still gives no answer to the key question about vitality. One can repeat after Galileo Galilei "to measure what is measurable, and make measurable what has not been measured yet" but *vitality still cannot be directly measured*. Medicine has not been a pure science but also an art and one has to trust the wisdom of patients: the *repeated cell transplantation treatment by countless patients seeking revitalization by their own volition is a scientific fact like any other.*

Chapter 16

> Necessity knows no law except to prevail.
> *Publius Syrus, First Century BC, Maxim 553*
>
> The greater the ignorance the greater the dogmatism.
> *Sir William Osler, 1849 – 1919, Montreal Medical Journal [1902]*
>
> All great truths begin as blasphemies.
> *George Bernard Shaw, 1856 – 1950, Annajansha [1919]*

IMMUNOLOGY

H. Schmidt of Marburg, Germany, the father of immunobiology, was so puzzled by the alleged lack of immune reactions after fresh cell therapy that he decided to visit Niehans, the father of *zellentherapie*, in his clinic in Vevey, Switzerland, to see with his own eyes what happens after the transplantation of fresh cells to patients. He watched nervously the implantations to the patients, and when he did not see any anaphylactic shock, or other serious immune reactions, he admitted that his 20 years of work in immunobiology was "annihilated by just one injection". This happened in the 1950's.

No one has been able to explain this puzzle to this date [143, 95]. Niehans stated in his book that he did not know for what reason these considerable quantities of foreign albumins introduced parenterally into the organism, and repeatedly, fail to produce an anaphylactic reaction. He commented that professors with experience in the matter of anaphylaxis extended over a number of years came to his clinic and observed this astonishing fact.

He brought up the words of Halsted that in 1909 stated that the *mechanism of immunization did not work when the organism needed cell transplantation* to repair damaged organ or tissue and that an *impaired organism in need of young cells to ensure its recovery tolerates them extraordinarily well* [18]. Perhaps not a purely scientific statement, but it reflects a reality observed daily in the clinical practice of stem cell transplantation.

Modern immunology has avoided confrontation on this issue by taking an "ostrich" approach: if no immunosuppression is used then the rejection of the cell xenotransplants must take place, and if the clinician does not see it, then the clinician is incompetent.

In this chapter you will find, in *Italic*, the scientific facts which refute the common belief that cell xenotransplantation must trigger a rejection reaction.

In view of the above, it is interesting and sad to read the about Lafferty, one of the pioneers of islet transplantation in the West, on the right track when he dared to state that cell xenotransplantation can be carried out without "hypercute rejection", and then being quickly accused of a scientific fraud by a "prince" of modern immunology, P.B. Medawar. It turned out that Lafferty was correct and Medawar was wrong [170]. It is not the first case when "Princes" stopped progress in human history, and also a justification of mandatory retirement of the chiefs of departments at the universities past certain age regardless of their fame.

Let's now focus on explaining the *reasons why immunosuppression is not required after stem cell xenotransplantation.*

Some of the more recent publications indicate that immunologists are beginning to pay attention to the observed clinical data.

Immune responses to all protein antigens require initial processing and presentation of the antigen to T cells by antigen-presenting cells (APC's): dendritic cells, macrophages, and B lymphocytes are the only cell types that express also the specialized co-stimulatory molecules, which enable them to activate the naive T cells [165]. T cells recognize foreign antigens only when they are first broken down into short peptides that are then displayed, in association with major histocompatibility complex (MHC) proteins, on the cell surfaces of APC's. Thus the role of APC's is to offer antigenic peptides complexed with MHC proteins to the available repertoire of T cells. MHC molecules are obligatory components of the antigen complex recognized by T cells. The ability of T cells to recognize specific features of MHC proteins is critical for their survival in the thymus, and for the ability of the immune system to discriminate "self" from "non-self".

Human leukocyte antigens (HLA), and genes that encode them, are subdivided into classes I, II, and III. Class I and II molecules are structurally similar cell surface glycoproteins, involved in antigen presentation to T cells. HLA class I proteins are expressed on all somatic cells, while HLA class II proteins are found only on a few cell types. Class II MHC proteins are required for the presentation of the antigen to $CD4^+$ (helper) T cells, whereas $CD8^+$ (cytotoxic) T cells respond to antigens presented by class I MHC molecules.

All genes of human MHC complex are located on the short arm of chromosome 6. There are 3 genes within the class I region: HLA-A, HLA-B, and HLA-C loci, and there are 3 genes within the class II region: HLA-DP, HLA-DQ, and HLA-DR loci. Each of these genes exists in multiple, different allelic forms: 24 alleles of HLA-A and 50 alleles of HLA-B are known. Each person inherits two copies of chromosome 6, and so expresses 6 (3+3) class I and 6 (3+3) class II alleles, but because of extreme polymorphism of these loci the probability that any two individuals would express identical sets of HLA proteins is very low [108].

The peptide binding sites of both class I and II MHC proteins are similar, and have similar degenerate specificity, i.e. can bind a fairly wide range of peptides, but the peptides bound by class I MHC proteins are uniformly 8 - 10 aminoacids long, while the peptides bound by class II MHC proteins are 10 - 18 aminoacids long. Both T cell subsets use the same antigen receptors [108].

Although class I and class II MHC proteins have considerable structural homology, they function differently in antigen presentation. They present antigenic peptides to different T cell types: class I presents to $CD8^+$ cells, and class II presents to $CD4^+$ cells. The two classes of MHC proteins associate with peptides that have been created by different processing pathways within the cell. Class I MHC molecules bind peptides derived from endogenously synthetized proteins, i.e. viral protein in virus-infected cells, while class II MHC molecules bind peptides derived from exogenous proteins, i.e. those in the external medium, that have been internalized by APCs. Thus cells that harbor intracellular infectious agents are recognized and attacked by class I (cytotoxic) T cells, whereas class II (helper) T cells respond to the universe of soluble antigens, providing activating signals for antibody production by B lymphocytes [108].

It has been speculated that the evolutionary drive behind allotransplant rejection mediated by cytotoxic T lymphocytes had been the need to eliminate virus infected cells within the organism. In contrast, the defense mechanisms against infection with macroparasites, such as helminths, that are large, multicellular and because of its size cannot be eliminated by phagocytosis, and express both MHC antigens and carbohydrate epitopes, have striking similarities with the findings in the xenotransplant rejection [62].

Class I MHC proteins bind peptides during their synthesis in rough endoplasmic reticulum (RER), and this binding actually helps synthesis and promotes transport of class I molecules from RER to the cell surface. In contrast, class II molecules must be transported from RER to an endosome compartment first, where they lose an invariant chain, and can bind peptides from endocytosed, exogenous protein. *Thus class I MHC proteins and class II MHC proteins travel different routes and encounter antigens in different cellular compartments.* This difference in routing determines the source of peptide that becomes associated with each class: either endogenously synthesized and transported to the endoplasmic reticulum (endogenous pathway, class I), *or exogenous, subsequently endocytosed and degraded in an endosomal compartment (exogenous pathway, class II)* [108].

Virtually all somatic cells express class I MHC proteins, and therefore can present endogenous antigens to $CD8^+$ T cells, i.e. when infected by a virus, and killed usually by the lymphocyte as a result. *In contrast only a few cell types express class II MHC proteins, and are uniquely able to present exogenous antigens to $CD4^+$ helper T cells, so that they are important for almost all immune responses:* "*antigen-presenting cells*". The best known are *macrophages* with prodigious phagocytic activity, also producing various regulatory peptides, such as TNF, IL-1, that control lymphocyte proliferation, differentiation, and effector function; and then *B-lymphocytes*, and *dendritic* cells, derived from a common bone marrow precursor [108].

Lymphocytes become activated when specific ligands bind to receptors on their surfaces. The required ligands are different for T cells and B cells, but the response itself is similar in many respects for all types of lymphocytes. Only highly polymeric proteins, or polysaccharides, are capable to activate B-lymphocytes alone, and they are rare in nature. Usually, *the activation of B cells requires the simultaneous presence of a common antigen, binding an individual immunoglobulin on the surface of B cell, and of an activated $CD4^+$ T cell*, that interacts with non-immunoglobulin receptors on the surface of B cell to generate a second signal.

Similarly, T cell responses to most antigens require two types of simultaneous stimuli:

1. an antigen properly displayed by MHC molecule on APC, and
2. a presence of 'co-stimulator': in case of $CD4^+$ T cells a contact with a specific ligand on the surface of APC, or in case of $CD8^+$ T cells the presence of IL-2, secreted by activated $CD4^+$ T cells [165]. Thus all T cells must cooperate with APC's, while B cells depend on $CD4^+$ cells, ($CD8^+$ cells depend on $CD4^+$ cells, too), and *these interactions require either surface-to-surface contact or mediation by labile cytokines acting only over extremely short distances*, and by an array of adhesion molecules on the surface of the cells with which T lymphocyte interacts, so that *all this usually takes place in the secondary lymphoid organs, where lymphocytes, antigens, and APC's are close to each other at all times* [108, 165].

Dendritic cells, which are found in the T cell areas of lymphnodes, are the most efficient inducers of naive T lymphocytes. Their responsibility is to detect viruses that do not induce MHC class II and co-stimulatory molecules on macrophages [165].

REJECTION REACTION

According to the leading theory in "discordant" organ xenotransplantation in the un-manipulated recipient, a rapid and violent rejection reaction destroys the graft within minutes to a few hours. In "concordant" organ xenotransplantation, where a "hyperacute xenograft rejection" does not take place, or in discordant xenotransplantation where all anti-donor antibodies or complement were removed from the recipient, a delayed form of rejection: "acute vascular xenograft rejection", occurs 2 - 5 days later, which causes a failure of the transplanted xeno-organ [39].

Hyperacute rejection is due to natural immunity. It is initiated by the specific binding of xeno-reactive natural antibodies, usually IgM, to blood vessels of the donor organ. But in some species combination the hyperacute rejection depends primarily upon the activation of the specific alternative complement pathway [39].

In a given species combination the hyperacute rejection occurs nearly every time, *but not all the time*. Lack of hyperacute rejection may be due to the variable level of expression of xeno-antigens [39], or due to occasional lack of action by complement, for whatever reasons. For example, *organ xenotransplant of liver appears to be resistant to hyperacute rejection for reasons unknown* [31].

Besides liver, several tissues which require neovascularization by the recipient, such as skin grafts, pancreatic islets, etc., are resistant to hyperacute rejection, but not so bone marrow cells [31]. Isolated islets from discordant species apparently do not suffer a high rate of hyperacute rejection either [37]. Naturally occurring cytotoxic xenoreactive antibodies do not cause hyperacute rejection of the transplanted fetal porcine islet cell clusters [58]. Porcine fetal pancreatic islet cells carry determinants for human natural antibodies but are neither sensitive to the direct cytotoxic effect of antibodies nor are they sensitive to antibody-dependent cellular cytotoxicity destruction mediated by natural antibodies, and such islet cells can reconstitute streptozotocine induced DM, indicating that fetal porcine islet-cell clusters can survive *in vivo* [12]. Discordant cell xenotransplants do not have a high rate of primary non-function, in any case not any higher than cell allotransplants [35].

In neo-vascularized cell xenotransplants, such as skin or pancreatic islets, the hyperacute rejection is prevented by the absence of initial vascularization, which means a lack of endothelial cells [57, 59, 60, 150]. Rejection of these tissues appears several days after implantation and is assumed to be mediated mainly by the cellular mechanism [62].

Even if the hyperacute rejection would somehow be avoided, an "acute vascular xenotransplant rejection" takes place, for which the complement system is not necessary. Since the "acute vascular xenotransplant rejection" is unavoidable, the treatment appears futile and the best approach is prevention [39].

Sometimes when anti-donor antibodies and/or complement are depleted from the recipient for a period of time before xenotransplantation, acute vascular rejection does not occur, and the xenotransplant continues to function even after antibodies and complement have been restored. An *"accommodation"* has taken place. *If accommodation could be achieved, the continuous immunosuppression of patients could be avoided* [39, 33].

Microenvironment of liver, that includes phagocytosis of antigen by Kupffer cells, plays a unique role in the success of the induction of immune unresponsiveness to islet xenotransplants by the pre-treatment with intrahepatic transplantation of small number of islets [3], or to cardiac graft by intraportal transplantation of donor splenocytes [5]. The same applies to thymus as intrathymic implantation of splenocytes with ALS leads to indefinite cardiac allograft survival, and prolonged xenotransplant survival [44].

Adult islet allo-transplant rejection is dependent on the activity of $CD8^+$ cells, with $CD4^+$ acting as "helper" [59, 61]. But $CD4^+$ T cells alone play a pivotal role in the allo-transplant response to the purified islet tissue, xenotransplant response, and expression of the autoimmune disease process [13].

Strong T cell immunity against allo-antigens is partially due to their similarities to self-antigens, since T cells are selected in the thymus for their affinity to self-antigens. Therefore, *T cells might actually have weaker affinity for more discordant xeno-antigens.* Other molecular interactions involved in allogeneic responses, besides receptor-antigen binding, may *not operate efficiently when there are species differences* [34].

Xenotransplants are essentially always rejected faster than allo-transplants if similar types of tissues are transplanted under similar circumstances. But after the depletion of $CD4^+$ T cells, just the opposite happens: the xenogeneic reaction becomes weaker than allogeneic [31]. The rejection of pig islet xenotransplant is a $CD4^+$ dependent process, with only a minor participation of $CD8^+$ cells [11, 59, 61]. In reality, *helper and cytotoxic T cell responses to xenotransplants are generally weaker than to allo-transplants* [31, 34]. Complete rejection of islets across discordant species barrier is slower than across a closely related barrier and may be occurring by a different rejection process [1].

Reduction of immunogenicity of donor tissues prior to transplantation by elimination of donor-type hematopoietic APC's has been based on the theory that donor-derived APC's serve as major stimulators for triggering the rejection of tissue allo-transplants. Such treatment does not eliminate transplant antigen. The transplanted tissue retains its antigenic components but *the loss of APC's eliminates tissue immunogenicity, that is, the capacity to activate an immune response in the host.* One cannot assume that *antigenicity, as the capacity to be recognized by the immune system, and immunogenicity, as the capacity to activate a response in the immune system*, are regulated by the same process: antigen recognition. Antigenicity is involved in both these processes, indeed. However, immunogenicity requires the provision of a co-stimulatory signal in conjunction with antigen recognition by the specific immunocyte, and a co-stimulatory activity provided by active APC's [170].

It appears that the capacity of APC's to stimulate T cells against xenogeneic cells is generally deficient: in vitro the T cell reactivity to xenogeneic APC's tends to decrease as the phylogenetic disparity increases between the stimulating APC and responding T cell, yet *in vivo* rat islet xenotransplants are rejected more vigorously than islet allo-transplants. Thus the mechanism of islet allo-transplant and xenotrans-plant rejection differs in their dependence on donor type APC [61].

In the xenotransplant rejection, a progressive cellular infiltrate, consisting mainly of eosinophilic granulocytes and macrophages with only a small number of T lymphocytes, was detected [64]. Thus non-T cells, or T cells lacking the conventional T-cell phenotype, but expressing $CD4^+$ antigen, are the major cellular components mediating xenogeneic rejection [12]. The xenotransplant rejection is different from the allo-transplant rejection in that the major cellular components are macrophage-like $CD4^+$ cells, and not T cells [57, 62]. The absence of immunoglobulins and/or complement depositions in the early rejection phase may indicate a pure cellular cytotoxic mechanism exerted by a macrophage-like cell [12]. But, it is important to realize here, that macrophages should not be normally capable of activating T lymphocytes in the absence of microbial infection [165].

In vitro, the interactions of $CD4^+$ or $CD8^+$ T cells with their respective ligands on MHC proteins may be weak when bound antigens are from a different and discordant species. Also, some lymphokines produced by stimulating lymphocytes of one species do not function well with receptors for these lymphokines expressed on T cells of another species. A theory was proposed whereby *MHC bound xeno-antigens of the donor species may be so different in structure from the MHC bound xeno-*

antigens of the recipient species that the T cell repertoire of the recipient will not contain receptors capable of directly recognizing those MHC bound xeno-antigens of the donor. And then, apparently some animal species are likely to elicit more defective human T-cell responses than others [21]. All this is remarkable in view that the cell populations mediating xenogeneic responses, and the target antigens recognized by xeno-active T cells, are largely the same as those found in allogeneic responses [34].

TOLERANCE

The induction of "tolerant state", in which the recipient's immune system regards donor antigens as 'self' prior to cell xenotransplantation, would be essential for a full clinical success of this therapeutic method [150]. There are three known mechanisms for induction of 'tolerance': anergy, suppression, and deletion. Tolerance among T cells could be either 'central', occurring at the time of T cell development in the thymus, or "peripheral", occurring after T cell moved from the thymus to the periphery [30].

In the thymus there is a positive selection of thymocytes followed by a negative selection of self-reactive cells that leads to the death of undesirable cells by apoptosis. The same can happen in the periphery [108].

MHC is important for "determinant selection", the multistage process by which each individual's immune system selects the specific immunogens (and the specific epitopes from within complex immunogens) to which it will respond. Any given allelic form of MHC protein can bind only a finite range of peptides. Thus, an individual with a particular subset of class II genes may lack a class II MHC protein capable of binding a peptide from a particular foreign protein, so that no part of that protein can be presented to helper T cell, in which case no immune response would occur [108]. Xenogeneic class II MHC protein/antigen complex is the principal target recognized by xeno-specific helper T cells [34]. Immunoalteration occurs either via a loss of class II MHC antigen cells, or via a loss of class I MHC antigen cells, which should be expected to directly stimulate $CD8^+$ cell. There is much evidence that xenotransplant rejection occurs via indirect presentation of antigens, and therefore the direct stimulation of the $CD8^+$ cell by a class I MHC antigen would not be a major factor in xenotransplant immunogenicity [37].

A lymphocyte is considered *"anergic"* if an encounter with the antigen, that its clonally distributed surface receptor specifically recognizes as non-self, does not fully activate the cell. It can be induced in T cells when antigen is presented without an adequate co-stimulation, as T cells require additional "co-stimulatory" signal from APC's in addition to those provided by the MHC-antigenic peptide complex presented to the T cell receptor, as well as when the milieu of the regional lymphnode is lacking. The anergic T cells cannot produce IL-2, so that they cannot respond when they encounter an antigen, even if properly presented by APC. *In view of the great phylogenetic disparity between humans and rabbits, it seems that many co-stimulatory, adhesive, and cytokine mediated interactions between the two species may be defective, resulting in greater ease of tolerance induction* [30, 165].

In some systems studied, the delivery of 'minimal signals' results in 'anergy', or non-response of the T cells. Stimulation with the specific antigen, in the absence of other signals, can result in development of anergy (or non-response to that antigen on a normal antigen-presenting cell) at later times. Providing one signal to a macrophage, without other signals that are needed to activate that macrophage, results in a transcription of certain genes without their translation, that then makes those macrophages normally become non-responsive to the later delivery of the other signals [33]. Macrophages cannot generate specific immune response on their own, but have to be linked to the target cell by accessory factors, such as antibodies or complement [62].

"Suppressive" cell populations or antibodies may inhibit the responses of donor-reactive T or B cells. There are two subsets of $CD4^+$ T cell with different function [11]: T_H1 subset, T-helpers with a type 1 response, that is pro-inflammatory, indirectly involved in the rejection of allo-transplants and xenotransplants, producing IL-2, IFN-χ and TFN-β; and T_H2 subset, T-helpers with a type 2 response, that is tolerogenic, associated with allo-transplant and xeno-transplant acceptance, producing IL-4, IL-5, IL-6 and Il-10 [30].

While naive $CD8^+$ cells emerging from thymus are predestined to become cytotoxic cells, the fate of $CD4^+$ cells is decided only during their first encounter with the antigen: they become either inflammatory T_H1 cells leading to the cell-mediated immunity, or helper T_H2 cells providing humoral immunity [165].

Peripheral xenogeneic immune unresponsiveness induced by intraportal implantation of cultured rat islet cells in diabetic mice is transferrable via splenocytes to a second diabetic recipient, and T lymphocytes are the mediators. These T lymphocytes appear to be anergic, and they suppress TH1 lymphocytes either by releasing IL-4 and IL-10, which suppression is reversible by IL-2, or alternatively by competing with them for ligands on the APC membrane [7].

Clonal "deletion" of T or B cells with reactivity to donor is clinically the most promising. If there are no lymphocytes with reactivity to donor, then no specific response to donor antigens could be induced, regardless of what immunologic stimuli would be encountered. T cell tolerance can be induced across allogeneic histocompatibility barriers by transplanting pluripotent hematopoietic stem cells that induce intrathymic deletional tolerance [30], as well as across concordant xenogeneic barriers [38]. Tolerance can be induced across concordant xenogeneic barrier also by intrahepatic or intrathymic islet transplantation together with anti-lymphocyte serum [8, 44]. Pre-treatment by liver hematopoietic cells induced neonatal tolerance to cardiac organ allo-transplants [4], and the same applies to intrathymic splenocytes [43].

B cell tolerance could be achieved either by eliminating any cells that express an autoreactive antibody (clonal deletion) or by permitting such cells to survive in a functionally inactive state (clonal anergy). Clonal deletion takes place among early B lymphocytes in the bone marrow: contact of surface immunoglobulins with a self antigen at this stage transmits a signal that arrests further development of the early B cell and causes the subsequent death of the arrested cell. Several forms of clonal anergy have been observed among mature B cells in the periphery. A contact of surface immunoglobulins with a non-self antigen in the absence of appropriate $CD4^+$ T cell, or when helper cell is anergic, may be crucial in initiating various forms of B cell anergy. At other times, the affected B cells fail to express surface immunoglobulins, or if they are expressed, they fail to transmit an effective signal to the cell upon binding the non-self antigen [108].

Immunologically incompetent embryos and neonates readily accept grafts from xenogeneic donors, which proves that cells of different species are not innately incompatible. On the contrary, in the absence of immune response, *transplant and host cells of like histogenicity from widely divergent species show remarkable affinities.* The ability to reject foreign transplants depends on the maturation of the ability to respond immunologically [32, 166].

A comprehensive picture of immunological research on cell xenotransplantation, as presented here, is applicable to organ xenotransplantation, but not to the stem cell xenotransplantation when stem cell xenotransplants are prepared by described in this book method.

EXPERIMENTS ON AVOIDANCE OF IMMUNOSUPPRESSION

In 1965, insulin producing Langerhans islets were isolated in guinea pigs [123]. Later on the same was accomplished with several other vertebrates, fetal, newborn and adult, and also with human fetuses [171, 176 - 178, 188]. Lately an industrial method of isolation of islets from human adult cadavers was described.

Experiments with auto-, iso-, allo-, and xeno-transplantation of microfragments of fetal or adult pancreas, of isolated islets, either subjected to tissue culture or without culture, of cultured dispersed islet cells, have been carried out. Immunological reactions have been of major concern: they are minimal in case of auto- and iso-transplantation, but allegedly should be very serious with allo- and xeno-transplantation.

In the mid 1980's, a theory of the rejection of cell allo- and xenotransplants was presented, whereby class II MHC antigens carrying group of cells, so called 'leukocytes-passengers', were responsible for an induction of a rejection reaction. Dendritic cells, lymphocytes, macrophages and capillary endothelial cells, belong to this group [127, 170]. Several experiments proved that the survival of cell allo- and xenotransplants in the body of the recipient can be substantially prolonged if class II MHC antigens carrying cells are removed from the transplant. *This can be accomplished by sufficiently long tissue culture of pancreatic islets, during which endocrine cells survive, while class II MHC antigen carrying cells die* [122, 128].

Alteration and/or elimination of "leukocytes-passengers" is caused by tissue culture at 24 - 26° C [1, 2], together with 95% O_2 [170], or with anti-lymphocytic serum, or with anti-thymocytic globulin, or with monoclonal antibodies against dendritic cells, or with immunotoxin, or with growth-transforming factor [36, 122, 128, 169, 174, 181]. Tissue culture of pancreatic islets causes death of majority or all exocrine cells, and cessation of their enzymatic activity, while the islet cells proliferate, and differentiate, and thereby increase their hormone-producing capability [129].

Also UV light exposure, gamma irradiation, exposure to various chemicals, etc., have been used in an attempt to lower the antigenicity of cells and prolongation of the survival of the transplants. More recently diffuse capsules of semi-permeable membranes (alginate-polylysine, agar gel, etc.), permitting passing through of substances with molecular weight of less that 100,000 D, i.e. glucose or insulin, but blocking cell-destroying antibodies, have been used to encase islet cells. They protect islet cells for a few weeks or months, but ultimately lymphoid infiltration surrounds the capsules, followed by vascularized connective tissue, that becomes a complete barrier between implanted cells and the recipient [36].

New, less toxic and less dangerous to the recipient, methods of immunosuppression have been tried, such as treatment with anti-T cell monoclonal antibodies, or antilymphocytic serum [1-3, 8, 9], or pre-transplantation injection of donor-specific splenocytes. Also, pre-treatment plasmapheresis has been tested.

Let's return, yet again, to the subject of *"organospecificity"*. The theoretical basis of cell transplantation is *the absence of antigenic differences of corresponding cells of humans and animals from different taxonomic groups, i.e. organospecificity*. This is applicable to pancreatic islets, as well as all other organs and tissues [127]. It appears that US cell transplantologists came here to the same conclusion as pioneers of cell therapy 50 years earlier.

Antibodies reacting to the cell surface of viable rat islet cells are present in serum of children with IDDM. Human diabetic serums yielding positive immunofluorescence with rat islet cells were equally reactive with beta-cell suspensions from ob/ob mouse. *In vitro* physiologic characteristics of isolated islets from human pancreas seem to be similar to those of rats or mice. Thus organospecific, non-species-specific, antibodies reactive with the cell surface of viable rat islet cells are present in serum from many children with IDDM, and *the cell-surface immunoreactions caused by human diabetic serums are specific for islet cells of any species, i.e. organospecific* [116].

A typical characteristic of antibodies to the surface of islet cells is the organospecificity, and due to this phenomenon such antibodies can be identified with the help of islet cells of not only human origin, but also from other animals, specifically rats and mice. Antibodies to the surface of islet cells do not cross-react with rat hepatocytes and splenocytes. There is significant physico/chemical and immunochemical similarity between the basic protein of an auto-antigen of islet cells of man and of rat [117].

Antibody assays and immunofluorescence studies of the membrane protein antigens of isolated hepatocytes from man, rat and rabbit demonstrate a complete organospecificity of such surface antigens [118].

Rat islet cells were perfused with an immunoglobulin fraction of diabetic patients, and in every case there was an inhibition of the glucose-induced insulin release, which indicates the presence of antibodies interfering directly with rat beta-cell function. Immunoprecipitation of lysates of mouse pancreatic islets and rat insulinoma cells, and immunofluorescence of mouse and rat islet cells by sera of diabetic children support the fact that islet cell autoantibodies are "cell-specific", but "not species-specific" [119].

Chapter 17

People in general have no notion of the sort and amount of evidence often needed to prove the simplest matter of fact
Peter Mere Latham, 1789 – 1875

TRANSMISSION OF INFECTION

Xenosis (or xeno-zoonosis) is a term for an infectious disease introduced into human through procedures involving transplantation of xenogeneic cells or tissues.

The disease producing potential of an infection is a function of the relation between the host and the infecting agent. The pathogenic potential of an infection can change in an unpredictable fashion when the infecting microbe is transmitted from its natural host into a new species. The effect xenogeneic tissue may have on antigen presentation and the targeting of effective immune responses to new pathogens is not known [55].

Endogenous retroviruses, widely present in mammalian species, presumably originated as exogenous viruses that became permanently integrated into the host germ line: they are transmitted from mother to child now. In the host species they are benign. Endogenous viruses are frequently xeno-tropic: although the original host is refractory to infection, the viruses can infect other species. Endogenous retroviruses may recombine in humans after xenotransplantation. Standard diagnostic tests are not available for most of these retroviruses [55].

In xenotransplantation, the spread of zoonoses could be minimized by using gnotobiotic or SPF animals as a source of cell xenotransplants, but that would be impractical as their production is difficult and costly, and thus they would not be available in large numbers. Unrecognized endogenous viruses, passed from mother to offspring, are maintained as genomic material and are neither observed nor recovered from adult tissue. They would not be eliminated by use of gnotobiotic or SPF animals. Animals from closed colony suffice for this purpose. One has to accept the fact that infectious agents are universal, and that a clear understanding of the specificity of infectious agents is often lacking and/or is not clearly defined. An alien species infected by certain agents may change the virulence of that agent. *Many agents are host-specific and not infectious when crossing species barriers* [53].

Zoonoses are generally initiated in immunologically naive individuals, and are devastating to such population, i.e. to xenotransplant patients. Infectious agents causing zoonoses are frequently of little hazard in the host of origin: infection is usually subclinical, recognized only by a production of antibodies. Overtly sick animal would not be considered for xenotransplant donation. *It is the latent infections, which are not discernible, which may be activated as a result of transplanttation.* Endogenous agents are also unknown factors. *Immunosuppression frequently permits non-pathogenic organisms to become pathogenic. Continuing need for immunosuppression and the conceivable danger of infection is the major negative feature of transplantation in general. Clinically significant infection occurs in 75% of all allo-transplant recipients and is the leading cause of death* [53].

Cell xenotransplantation in around 5 million patients during the period of over 70 years has not cause a single fatality.

There is a potential for the co-infection of human recipient cells by porcine and human retroviruses, whereby they would form a chimeric virus with an unknown pathogenic potential. Recombination is common in cells infected by retroviruses [49]. The development of encapsulation for immunologic isolation of xenogeneic tissue and creation of transgenic animals whose organs are intended to survive immune surveillance after transplantation may increase the potential for viral recombination or reassortment [55].

There is much less controversy with xenoses as compared with immunological issues. *Despite the presence of many known potential pathogens among different donor species, there will almost certainly be less transmission of known infections by xenotransplantation than by allo-transplantation. Most investigators believe that xenotransplantation is exceedingly unlikely to lead to the generation of new pathogens.*

These are actually quotes taken from an Internet press release by one of the US companies. The above is particularly true if the animal source of cell xenotransplants is a domestic animal. *Proximity of humans to domestic animals would have caused such an event already if it were likely to happen [150]. When no immunosuppression is used the minimal chance of transmission of xenoses is further substantially diminished.* The danger of transmission of zoonoses exists, but its degree can be controlled by following regulations, such as that of US FDA, to a great degree. Main concerns are the future infections not known to us yet, such as a unique circumstance where a retrovirus of animal species would recombine with a human retrovirus.

Rabbits do not seem to present any potential problem as a source of xenoses in cell xenotransplantation today, as could be expected due to their phylogenetic and taxonomic distance from man. According to Dr. Grachev of Section on Biologics, World Health Organization, Geneva, Switzerland, an organization that supervises worldwide production of vaccines and sera, rabbit kidney cell cultures have been used extensively for vaccine production, and thus far have not shown that rabbits represent any potential danger for transmission of viral zoonoses. Thus rabbit is a good choice as a source animal for production of cell xenotransplants. Rabbits are also the only laboratory animals in which no endogenous retroviruses have been identified to-date [200, 201, 202] (See also Section on 'Manufacturing').

Review of infections transmitted by large and small laboratory animals shows that generally in rabbits the following infections can occur [54]:

- campylobacteriosis (rare),
- leptospirosis (low prevalence in hosts, or as a zoonosis),
- salmonellosis (low/moderate prevalence in hosts, unknown frequency as zoonoses), and
- dermatomycosis (low prevalence in hosts, low frequency of zoonosis)

Plague and psittacosis have a broad host range, including rabbits. Rabbits are natural hosts for a parasitic disease trichostrongylosis. Rabbits are laboratory hosts for common skin mites, and ticks Dermacentor variabilis (rickettsiosis).

Detailed didactic review of viral diseases in rabbits discusses the situation worldwide. Under the column of "public health significance" for each virus found in rabbits there is a statement such as "man is not susceptible to the myxoma virus", and the same applies for fibroma virus, rabbit pox virus (close to the vaccinia virus), papilloma virus, oral papilloma virus, rabbit kidney vacuolating virus, adenovirus, herpes virus, etc. There are known natural cases of rabies infection in rabbits potentially transmissible to man. This is of no significance in newborn or fetal rabbits, however. Arborvirus infections have been isolated in hares, but no human diseases have been reported to-date [51]. Besides that, arboviruses require a vector for transmission from one host to another and are not a transplant problem [53].

Review of potential transmission of retrovirus infections by mammals and poultry produced for food failed to demonstrate an association between human disease and these viruses. Lack of antibodies in apparently exposed groups of persons suggests an absence of infection, and/or lack of immune responsiveness of humans to infection with these viruses. Rabbits, per se, are not even mentioned in this report [50].

In recent years the number of donations and clinical allo-transplants of cornea, bone, skin, heart valve, and other tissues have exceeded that of xeno-organs, and there have been infection transmissions reported. A high rate of bacterial contamination was found with human fetal tissue donations, and two actual cases of infection from cryopreserved islet cell infusions were found [52].

Chapter 18

> Cure the disease and kill the patient.
> Francis Bacon, 1561 – 1626

> There are some remedies worse than the disease.
> Publius Syrus, First century BC, Maxim 301

CANCEROGENESIS

As many as *350 billion mitoses occur in each person every day*. **With each cell division there is a possibility that both resulting cells will be malignant.** Yet, very few cancers actually develop in any individual. Cells capable of forming cancers develop at certain frequency but a majority is never able to form observable tumors. The reason is that a solid tumor, like any other rapidly dividing tissue, needs O_2 and nutrients to survive. *Without a blood supply, potential tumors either die or remain dormant.* When dormant, such "microtumors" remain a stable cell population wherein dying cells are replaced by new cells.

Most victims of cancer do not die from the original cancer but from *metastases*. To enter a blood vessel, a tumor cell has to lyse the collagenous matrix surrounding the new capillaries, and that is done by secretion of plasminogen activator, a proteolytic enzyme, very similar to that assuring the implantation of blastocyst into the uterine wall.

Mitosis is precisely adapted to the actual needs of cells by a local release of growth factors. Besides mechanisms that increase proliferation there are factors that decrease growth via interruption of excessive mitosis. Mutations of relevant proliferation genes can lead to the development of oncogenes, the products of which called *oncoproteins* are active even without physiologic stimulators, and can trigger mitoses independently of physiologic growth factors.

Mutations can be caused by viruses, chemicals, radiation, etc., and malfunctions of DNA repair mechanism support their continuation. *Cells are prone to mutations particularly during mitosis, i.e. proliferating tissue is subject of mutations more often than differentiated tissue.* This happens particularly with tissue inflammation and tissue lesions due to injuries, and in both situations mitosis is stimulated.

One mutation is not sufficient for creation of cancer, only multiple mutations can cause degeneration of normal cell into a cancer cell. For malignant transformation one mutation is not enough, *a cascade of genetic events, one after the other, is necessary.*

Oncogenes can be brought into the host cell by viruses.

Uncontrolled cell division brings on gradual dedifferentiation. Dedifferentiated cells are often recognized and eliminated by the immune system unless it is weakened, such as due to HIV-infection. On the other side, cancer cells can express on their surfaces $CD95^+$ receptor, and binding of lymphocytes to such receptor causes the apoptosis and thereby weakening of immune system.

Proliferation of cancer cell leads to the creation of tumor. *Markedly dedifferentiated tumors are able to create metastases.* For that to happen, the cancer cells must get separated from their "mother" colony, i.e. be capable to migrate and break tissue barriers, penetrate into blood vessels, leave blood circulation in another organ by binding to the specific adhesive molecules of endothelium and penetration of blood vessel wall, and finally create a new colony in another organ.

Tumor growth, or metastases, requires adequate capillary network in order to get sufficient quantity of oxygen and nutrients. Angiogenesis is stimulated by mediators, or limited by inhibitors.

Energy needs of cancer cells are covered by glycolysis even with an adequate supply of O_2 so that one mol of glucose generates only 5% of energy that could be obtained via Krebs cycle. This results in hypoglycemia and acidosis. Hypoglycemia stimulates release of glucagons, adrenalin and glycocorticoids, which support breakdown of fats and proteins, and that leads to cachexia. Some cancer cells cause activation of coagulation, or fibrinolysis, production of abnormal antibodies, hormones, etc. that further disrupts homeostasis. Massive cancer cell death leads to the release of intracellular K^+ and hyperkalemia, and to breakdown of nucleic acids with hyperuricemia.

Cancer is a genetic disease on a somatic cell level. There are aberrations of various kinds on all chromosomes in solid tumors as well as in disseminated hematological malignancies. A majority of these are rare, some occur commonly, while some are found more frequently in certain kinds of tumors and represent "markers". Here is an attempt at *classification*:

1. **Single-gene cancer determinants**:
   - *single gene disorders with increased risk of malignant growth*, about 100 – 150 of them,
   - *genetic cancers*, such as bilateral retinoblastoma, familial melanoma, multiple endocrine adenomatosis, i.e. Zollinger-Ellison syndrome, Sipple syndrome,
   - pre-cancerous conditions:
     a) phacomatoses: neurofibromatosis, tuberous sclerosis, von Hippel-Lindau syndrome,
     b) polyposes syndromes : polyposis coli familiaris, Gardner syndrome,
     c) multiple exostoses,
     d) diseases of defective DNA repair mechanism: xeroderma pigmentosum, Bloom syndrome, ataxia teleangiectasia, Fanconi pancytopenia,
2. **Multifactorial predisposition toward cancer**, such as with breast cancer, stomach cancer, uterine cancer, leukemias,
3. **Association of chromosomal aberrations with increased risk of malignancy**:
   - Down syndrome, with leukemoid reactions, and myeloid leukemia,
   - Chromosomal Instability Syndrome,
   - Association of specific chromosomal aberrations with cancer, e.g. Philadelphia chromosome and chronic myeloid leukemia, reconstituted chromosome aberrations, reconstitution in the proximity of dominant oncogenes,
4. **Molecular oncogenesis**:
   - *oncogenes as triggers of AD disorders*,
   - *mutator-genes*, AR disorders: cancer cells are characterized by general genetic instability, with abnormal karyotypes, often of bizarre type, with multiple deletions, duplications, and chromosomal re-structuring,

and the responsibility for this lies with mutator-genes the function of which is to secure integrity of genetic information: their malfunction causes non-effective DNA replication or non-effective repair.

- *"oncogene viruses"* can cause cancer development in experimental animals, as was proven decades ago with the virus of Roux sarcoma in chickens.

After their entry into the cell, these RNA-viruses transcribe their RNA-genome with the help of reverse transcriptase into chromosomal DNA of the host, and so secure the replication of the virus.

Oncogene viruses play role in 15% of human cancers. RNA-oncogene viruses cause T-cell leukemia in adults (HTLV-1, HTLV-2) and Kaposi sarcoma. DNA-oncogene viruses cause cancer of uterine cervix (papilomavirus HPV16), nasopharyngeal cancer (Epstein-Barr virus), hepatocellular carcinoma in South-East Asia, and tropical Africa (hepatitis B virus).

There are additional genes in such viruses in all mammals, including man, called *protooncogenes, which turn into oncogenes in the course of preceding viral infection.* The main function of protooncogenes under physiologic circumstances is the regulation of cell cycle, cell proliferation and specific differentiation of normal cells. But also the *creation of solid cancer on oncogenes*, i.e. RAS oncogene is found in sarcomas, neuroblastoma, retinoblastoma, melanoma, lung cancer, cancer of urinary vesicle, breast cancer, but also leukemias and lymphomas.

SIS oncogene is found in osteosarcomas, fibrosarcomas, gliomas, and breast cancer, while ERB-B in squamous carcinoma, adenocarcinoma of salivary and mammary glands.

- *Tumor suppressive genes*, AR disorders: While the oncogenes trigger the start of cancerogenesis actively, tumor suppressive genes do so passively by being inactive. While oncogenes are effective even in heterozygote state, i.e. they are dominant genes, with tumor suppressive genes one normal allele is sufficient guardian against the development of cancerogenesis, i.e. they are recessive oncogenes.

Mutation of Gene TP53 is the most frequent genetic damage found in cancer. It is known as "guardian of genome". Product of gene TP53, i.e. protein p53, is active during the cell mitosis. It slows down the mitotic cycle before the beginning of S-phase so that the repair enzymes have enough time to repair any damage due to the mutation and thereby prevents a completion of mitosis that would allow transfer of damaged DNA to the daughter-cells.

The first malignant disease with a specific chromosomal aberration was chronic myelogenous leukemia. This disease is characterized by a long preleukemic phase, during which there is already a myelopoietic disturbance, but without any findings in blood. Dramatic turn into acute myeloid leukemia, i.e. myeloblastic crisis, can happen suddenly and unexpectedly. Typical cytological finding is a small eccentric "Philadelphia chromosome", which in adult type of this disease in found in 90% of patients, while it is absent in 80% of children.

Burkitt lymphoma is a common tumor in tropical Africa, predominantly of children. Specific chromosomal aberrations were found in cancer cells.

Acute lymphoblastic leukemias in children, acute promyeloid leukemia, non-Hodgkin lymphomas, are also characterized by specific chromosomal aberrations.

"Two hits hypothesis" is currently the leading theory of development of hereditary solid cancers. The examples are:

1. *Familial hereditary retinoblastoma* is a bilateral cancer of retina with incidence of 1:20,000, where the first hit is mutation of RB1 gene in gametes of parents: this is found in all cells of the children and is inherited as AD disorder with incomplete penetration; 50% of offsprings/heterozygotes has predisposition for retinoblastoma. For the creation of a cancer a "second hit" is necessary, and that is a mutation of the second RB1 gene in the target somatic cell of retina,
2. *Breast cancer* is inherited in 7% of cases,
3. *Li-Fraumeni syndrome*, AD disorder with incidence of 1:50,000, with high risk of development of cancer: by 30 years of age the

penetration is 50%, by 60 years it reaches 90%; patients get sarcomas of connective tissue, osteosarcomas, brain tumors, adrenocortical cancers, breast cancer,
4. *Wilms tumor* is the most common solid tumor of children with incidence of 1:10,000. It is diagnosed by the age of 30 months as an isolated disease, or a part of the following syndromes: WAGR (Wilms tumor, aniridia, urogenital anomalies, mental retardation), Denys-Drash syndrome (Wilms tumor, urogenital anomalies, glomerulonephropathy), Beckwith-Wiedeman syndrome (Wilms tumor, omphalocele, macroglossia, gigantism),
5. *Neurofibromatosis*, type 1 (von Recklinghausen disease) with incidence of 1:3,500, with high predisposition toward cancer: glioma of optic nerve, neurofibroma, astrocytoma, neurofibrosarcoma, osteosarcoma, Wilms tumor. There are multiple benign neurofibromas, bone anomalies, mental retardation, café-au-lait spots. Type 2 is AD disorder with 95% penetration, with incidence of 1:50,000, characterized by bilateral acoustic neurinomas with headaches, deafness, tinnitus, facial paralysis, mental disturbances,
6. *Familial adenomatous polyposis of colon* is AD disorder, with mucosa of colon covered by hundreds to thousands of polyps/adenomas, pre-cancerous, one of which invariably turns into cancer.

Chapter 19

> Man errs as long as he strives.
> *[Faust, x1805 – 1832]*
>
> Nothing is more damaging to a new truth than an old error.
> *[Proverbs in Prose]*
> Johann Wolfgang von Goethe, 1749 - 1832
>
> Do not veil the truth with falsehood, nor conceal the truth knowingly.
> Koran 2:42

PRE-CLINICAL VERSUS CLINICAL STUDIES

Stem cell transplantation has been used in clinical practice in its various forms for over 70 years, and enormous clinical experience has been accumulated in Germany, Switzerland, USSR, Peoples' Republic of China, etc., on the basis of which *certain facts have to be taken as "res ipsa loquitur"* today.

Since hundreds of thousands of patients have been treated by live cell transplantation, and millions of patients have been treated by lyophilized 'celltherapeutics'' or by quickly frozen 'celltherapeutics', and by cells preserved by other methods, and *every one of these various forms of cell transplantation was originally developed by testing in vitro and on experimental animals, there is no need to start every time from "point zero" by animal experimentation, when a new animal becomes a source of cell transplants.*

The entire field of cell biology has developed on the basic premise that all eukaryotic cells are built and function according to the same laws [67]. "Organospecificity", which means that the principal cells of the same organ (s) or tissue(s) are the same or almost the same in Nature, regardless of species of origin, is another 'res ipsa loquitur'. The entire development of cell therapy has been based on such essential data.

Likewise, US FDA *regulation of January 19, 2001 is treating all cell, tissue, and organ xenotransplants together, regardless of their animal source*. This US FDA regulation is tied to "Points to consider in human somatic cell therapy and gene therapy" of 1991, that legalized human fetal tissue transplantation in US and sanctioned the ongoing US FDA approved clinical trial in the treatment of IDDM by human fetal islet cells. So, US FDA *recognized many years ago that cell allo- and xenotransplantation follow the same biological rules*.

The review of respective medical literature in MEDLINE shows that different animals such as mice, rats, rabbits, dogs, guinea pigs, cows, pigs, horses, fish, chickens, even wild animals, have been used as a source of cell xenotransplants in the experiments with cell xenotransplantation as a treatment of various diseases. No one considered it necessary to re-prove the effectiveness of the respective cells of each animal species by starting the research from the ground up, i.e. *the concept of 'organospecificity' was tacitly accepted*.

It has been learned with islet cells that *even quite distant non-mammal species, such as fish and chickens, maintain a carbohydrate metabolism relatively close to that of humans* [37], and that *their insulin is practically the same as human* [188]. When the implanted islet cell xenotransplants from whatever animal source lower the level of blood sugar in an experimental models of diabetes mellitus, that represents sufficient proof about their effectiveness in view of what has been known from the previous experience with other members of the animal kingdom (and that includes human).

The immunological issues were largely resolved at RITAOMH and other research institutes of USSR while working with cell transplants of human, pig and cattle fetal origin, and the same rules were found to be applicable to those of rabbit fetal and neonatal origin, and in the author's opinion apply apparently to any other mammal or even vertebrate.

The above statement *does not apply to the organ xenotransplantation, where immunological problems remain formidable*.

Transmission of infections seems to be a real problem of cell transplantation today, with one solution only: *to use as a source of cell transplants only those members of the animal kingdom that do not represent any danger of transmission of infections to humans. Human cadavers do not qualify for this purpose too well*, while SPF (specific pathogen free) animals are an excellent source, although difficult to produce and thereby expensive.

In vitro tests and experimental studies on laboratory animals with cell transplants of rabbit origin were conducted at RITAOMH more than 17 years ago [79, 83, 85, 94, 109]. They followed similar studies done with bovine and porcine fetal cells and tissues, when cell xenotransplantation was launched in USSR in the 1980's and developed into an approved therapeutic method [73, 109, 183]. As far as porcine fetal and neonatal cells and tissues are concerned, extensive work was done by two other top centers: the Republic's Transplantology Center in Riga (today Latvia) and the Republic's Research Center of Endocrine and Metabolic Diseases in Kiev (now Ukraine). These were again just a continuation of similar studies at RITAOMH with human fetal tissues in the 1970's when cell allo-transplantation was developed into an approved therapeutic method [73, 109, 183].

Prior to our start of stem cell xenotransplant manufacturing, described in the section on "Manufacturing of stem cell xenotransplants", internal "pre-production testing" of "zero-series" of various stem cell transplants prepared from fetal and neonatal rabbits were carried out [191]. All other stem cell transplants listed [111] were similarly tested. Studies by BCRO were done solely to work out the details of the patented industrial technology of preparation of stem cell transplants, and not to carry out formal pre-clinical studies. Since over 5,000 patients have been treated during the period of 10 years by cell xenotransplants of rabbit neonatal and fetal origin by RITAOMH and IIBM/BCRO in Russia, and elsewhere (56 of them US patients treated in USA), and adequate reports are available, this would have been pointless [71, 75, 81, 82, 95, 97-100, 115].

After all, it is commonly known that *the value of experimental studies in the field of stem cell transplantation has been seriously questioned* since it has been observed, for example, that many of the animals do have a spontaneous return of function of their islets after Streptozotocine induced Diabetes Mellitus, which does not ever happen with diabetic patients [37]. Thus Russian and various foreign patients treated in Russia, US patients, treated in USA, patients from Qatar, treated in Qatar, Slovak patients treated in Slovakia during the development of the described in this book manufacturing method, have served as *"human volunteers", on whom stem cell transplants of rabbit origin were tested, or actually used for treatment in a standard clinical manner, without any ill effects.*

In the field of cell transplantation (whether allo- or xeno-), *the value of pre-clinical tests on laboratory animals can in no way be compared to the value of actual patient treatment*, and particularly when the patient treatment has been going on for as long as 25 years. Under these circumstances, the pre-clinical studies have become obsolete and immaterial, as the vast clinical experience can never be duplicated by any pre-clinical study. It is against any logic to start experimental work and clinical trials in countries such as Russia, where cell allo- and xeno-transplantation has been a standard clinical practice since 1984, or Germany where the same situation existed for five decades.

The rabbit insulin differs from the human by just two amino acids, and so should be as clinically effective as porcine used in human medicine [188]. The rabbits do not have enough blood so that they were never used commercially for the production of biologicals in general, while just the opposite applies to pigs.

RITAOMH scientists found out that the histology of adult and fetal rabbit tissues varied noticeably, particularly when considering the proportion of the exocrine to endocrine portion of pancreas, and of the quantity of collagen fibers. While the method of tissue culture for adult rabbit tissues did not differ in principle from the method developed and used successfully for bovine, porcine and human fetal source, the method of tissue culture for rabbit fetal tissues had to be changed, mainly by elimination of enzymatic dissolution of tissues. But the tissue cultures of both adult and fetal rabbit tissues were successful, and the cultures were actively producing insulin by RIA testing.

The adult rabbit tissues were used as cell xenotransplants at first, and in 1987 the first two patients with diabetes mellitus were so treated [85]. Subsequently RITAOMH switched to the fetal rabbit tissues in their clinical practice. Ultimately newborn rabbits were investigated by RITAOMH scientists as the animal source, purely for pragmatic reasons, since they were easier to obtain than fetuses, and since no difference was found in their characteristics, as compared with fetal rabbits, they were introduced into a clinical practice as an animal source for stem cell transplants of various endocrine organs [79, 83]. The progress of this work with cell transplants of rabbit origin was followed internally within RITAOMH [94], and was reported during USSR and international meetings, and published. *Whenever you see a reference in the "Bibliography" about stem cell xenotransplantation in Russian, it deals with xenotransplants of rabbit fetal or neonatal origin.*

Chapter 20

> There is nothing more difficult to take in hand, more perilous to conduct, or more uncertain in its success, than to take the lead in the introduction of a new order of things.
> Niccoló Machiavelli, 1469 – 1527, The Prince [1532]

ARTIFICIAL ORGANS AND BIO-PROSTHESES FOR RECONSTRUCTIVE SURGERY

At least the three decades old idea of replacing non-functioning organs and tissues of human body by artificial ones has come of age. Inability of organ transplantation to make a more substantial contribution to solving medical problems of seriously ill patients was probably one of the reasons for a medical science to vigorously turn toward artificial organs and tissues.

Various prosthetic materials used in reconstructive surgery can be improved in terms of lowering their immunogenicity and of the speed of healing by combining them with stem cell transplants.

Implantable artificial organs and tissues include all devices which substitute for an organ or tissue function and consist of three-dimensional synthetic matrix made from biodegradable bio-polymers, that serves as a template for live cells of an organ. They function primarily by repairing the patient's damaged organs and tissues, while leaving eventually no residual artificial material in the patient's body.

Bio-prostheses include nearly all available non-metallic prostheses used in surgery today and many not available yet. Some prostheses were found to be unusable because of serious healing problems or rejection reaction.

At the end of 1996 the first two US patents on artificial organs were granted. The number of medical reports in MEDLINE computerized medical database has steadily grown over the past years. The surge in the development of artificial organs and tissues is based on the progress in the field of stem cell transplantation and in the use of biodegradable biopolymers in medicine.

"Use of bio-degradable bio-polymers combined with stem cell transplants in medicine and surgery", is a project of two parts, closely related to each other:

A. The purpose of reconstructive surgery has been to correct the deformity, or tissue loss, with the best results, without causing additional damage to the patient's body.

   Whenever patient's own tissues could not be used for such purpose, and use of tissues from another human caused rejection, surgeons have been looking for alternative solutions. One of them was to use bio-compatible artificial materials: metals, ceramics, polymers.

   Over the time metals became the most important artificial material used in orthopedic surgery, and the same applies to ceramics in dentistry, and to polymers in plastic & reconstructive surgery.

   Use of metallic bone prostheses has been limited to the bone reconstruction. The main drawback of metals has been the need for their removal after they fulfilled their function. Thereby any long term problems due to the metal remaining in the body have been avoided.

   Ceramics, such as hydroxyapatite, tricalcium phosphate, aluminum oxide, or those containing glass or carbon fibers, have become more popular only lately, and so far have been used more externally than for implantation into internal environment of the body.

   Bio-polymers have been used in surgery for decades. Silicones, containing no carbon, were the first, and have remained the most popular. Then came poly-methylmetacrylates, used at the beginning as external prosthesis only. Next, polyethylens were discovered, that became the basis of poly-tetra-fluoroethylenes, containing only carbon, oxygen and fluor.

   The main problem with all above bio-polymers has been their recognition as foreign by the living body, and so their presence always triggered "foreign body reaction" by immune system of one type or another. Although no one has ever proved that biopolymers cause auto-immune diseases, it did not stop US courts from giving a multi-billion dollar judgment to the recipients of silicone breast implants in the past.

Discovery of polyurethanes caused a revolution because of their natural degradation, and eventual disappearance from the body.

Polymers are materials with a wide variety of mechanical and physical properties, readily molded into any desirable shape. Their mechanical properties are derived from their chemical composition and structure that can be easily manipulated. For example, polyethylene can be made with linear, branched, or cross-linked chains; short chains of low molecular weight are liquids that turn into viscous – waxy – plastic, and ultimately glass consistency, with increase of length of the chain.

The best solution to all problems with bio-compatible polymers appeared "bio-degradation", i.e. gradual disappearance of the prosthesis in the process of bio-destruction by phagocytosis. By combining various plastic materials in the production of final biopolymer, the bio-degradation is assured without a production of non-compatible disintegrating products. Further progress led some 30 years ago to the development of bio-polymers that not only biodegrade, but do so at a pre-determined time. It means that their bio-destruction can be pre-programmed.

Best bio-degradable bio-polymers consist of a capron fiber, modified by a type of acid treatment, and a co-polymer of vinylpyrrolidone and methylmetacrylate. Capron fiber serves as a filling material, while co-polymer of vinylpyrrolidone and methylmetacrylate as a binding material.

Over the last two decades, around 60 different products have been created from this type of bio-degradable bio-polymers. Several of them have been patented in many European countries and one in the US. They could be divided into five groups:

1. films for timed delivery of various medications: ophthalmologicals, nitroglycerine, anti-nicotine medication, medication for temporary suppression of alcohol intoxication,

2. implants for osteosynhesis, replacement of vertebral body or disc, covering of skull defects, filling of bone defects, external ear canal reconstruction, vascular prostheses, laryngeal prosthesis,
3. surgical adhesive tapes for securing surgical anastomosis of hollow internal organs such as intestines, for hemostasis during liver and kidney surgery, etc., and surgical sutures,
4. surgical glues, with a variety of options: such as with long term effect, for treatment of esophageal burns, injectable glues, etc.,
5. foam hydrogel, a water soluble bio-degradable bio-polymer mixture, usable as a filler of veins (bleeding esophageal varices), cavities, etc. More on this unique bio-polymer is included in section B bellow.

Clinical use of bio-degradable bio-polymers showed certain deficiencies, that were rectified by adding to the products during manufacturing process various antibiotics to help suppress infection locally, osteogenetic, chondro-genetic, or fibrogenetic additives, chemotherapeutica with local effect for cancer resection surgery, X-ray contrast substances, etc.

Binding of live cells, prepared for stem cell xeno-transplantation, to the bio-degradable bio-polymers represents the ultimate step in their development because it raises the level of bio-compatibility to presently un-attained levels. Improved bio-compatibility translates into much better and faster healing, with reduced possibility of treatment complications. This project will revolutionize reconstructive surgery in its entirety.

B. It is believed that stem cell transplantation will trigger a rejection reaction by the immune system. Many feel that immunosuppression is not the best way to deal with this problem because drugs used for this purpose are detrimental to the implanted cells. For several years another option has been researched: to protect implanted cells against immune system attack by mechanically shielding them inside a bio-polymer sponge with an opening large enough to permit passage of all biological substances from cell transplants into the recipient organism, but at the same time small enough to prohibit immune system cells and molecules to get to the transplanted cells. Such structure has been called an "artificial organ".

Several bio-polymers have been developed for that purpose. They all have failed to accomplish the task, because within 3 - 4 months the entire structure, consisting of bio-polymer and a cell transplant is surrounded by scar tissue, so that no biological substance produced by cell transplant can get into the recipient organism, thus the positive effect of cell transplant ends.

Bio-degradable 'foam hydrogel' mentioned above (under 5), can be programmed to bio-destruct much earlier than 3 - 4 months after its implantation, and thereby avoid encasement of an "artificial organ", and assure continuity of function. Creation of such an 'artificial organ' would increase number of implantation sites as well, invaluable for the overall therapeutic effect.

ADDENDUM

Here is a list of examples, by no means exhaustive, for clinical uses of "Live bio-degradable surgical prostheses and other tools" by different surgical specialties for various surgical procedures. In the following list numbers 1 - 5 after the name of surgical procedure are related to the above-described five groups of bio-degradable bio-polymers:

1 means "films",
2 "structured prostheses",
3 "adhesive tapes" and 'sutures",
4 "glues", and
5 "foam hydrogel".

GENERAL SURGERY
- prevention of local recurrence after cancer resections 3, 4
- treatment of ulcus cruris and other necrotic soft tissue defects 5
- treatment of non-healing wounds 1, 5
- treatment of post-irradiation defects of soft tissues 1, 5

THORACIC SURGERY
- sealing of lung parenchyma post partial resections 3, 4
- sealing of pleural surface to prevent adhesions 3, 4
- sealing of bronchus after lung resection 3, 4

CARDIOVASCULAR SURGERY
- sealing of vascular anastomosis 3, 4
- vascular prostheses 2, 4

ABDOMINAL SURGERY
- repair of extensive hernias 3, 4
- intestinal anastomosis 3, 4
- sealing of appendix stump 3, 4
- esophageal anastomosis 3, 4
- mucosal hemostasis in esophageal and gastric surgery 1, 4
- sealing of liver resection margins 3, 4
- endoscopic surgery of esophagus, stomach and duodenum 1, 4
- endoscopic hemostasis of esophageal, gastric or duodenal bleeding 1, 4, 5
- endoscopic treatment of acute esophageal burns 1
- endoscopic treatment of chronic proctitis and colitis 5
- anal sphincter reconstruction 5

UROLOGICAL SURGERY
- sealing of kidney resection margins 3, 4
- kidney transplantation 3, 4
- bladder sphincter reconstruction 5

GYNECOLOGICAL SURGERY
- myomectomy 3, 4
- uterine cervicoplasty 1, 4
- sealing of uterine wall post C-section 3, 4

ORTHOPEDIC SURGERY
- filling of bone cavities after bone excision 2
- replacement of bone auto-transplants in general 2
- fixation of bone grafts 2, (4)
- fixation of metallic prostheses 2, (4)
- cervical spine fusions 2
- lumbar vertebral fusions 2
- distal femoral or high tibial osteotomies 2
- humeral or radius/ulna osteotomies for congenital defects 2
- complex fractures of long bones 2 (with the exception of femoral neck)
- acetabular insufficiency 2, (4)

- surgery of Perthes disease 2
- surgery of chronic osteomyelitis 2, (1)
- foot arthrodesis 2, 4
- tendon sheath reconstruction 1, 3, 4
- surgery of pseudo-arthrosis 2, 4

NEUROSURGERY
- cranioplasties 2, (4)
- repair of depressed skull fractures 1, 4
- replacement of vertebral bodies and discs 2, (4)
- peripheral nerve suture 3, 4
- peripheral motor nerve auto-grafting 3, 4, 5

HEAD & NECK SURGERY
- reconstruction of larynx 2
- reconstruction of external auditory canal 2
- reconstruction of nasal synaechia post surgery 1, 3, 4
- reconstruction of floor of mouth post cancer resections 2, 3, 4

OPHTHALMOLOGICAL SURGERY
- corneal transplantation 1
- reconstruction of conjunctiva 1

MAXILLO-FACIAL SURGERY
- maxillary and zygomatic reconstruction 2, (4), (5)
- mandibular reconstruction 2, (4), (5)
- fracture of edentulous mandible 2
- fracture of facial bones 2, (4), (5)
- reconstruction of old naso-ethomoidal fracture 2, 4
- correction of fracture of frontal sinus

ORAL SURGERY
- dental extractions 2, (1)
- handling of delayed bleeding post dental extractions 1, 4
- infected socket post dental extractions 1, 4
- tumor excision 1, 3, 4

PLASTIC SURGERY
- correction of hemi-facial atrophy 2, 3, 5
- palate reconstruction 2, 3, 4

- reconstruction of tarsal plate of eyelid 2, 3, 5
- reconstruction of temporo-mandibular joint 2, 3, 5
- auricular reconstruction 2, 3, 4
- capsular contracture after breast augmentation 3, 4
- witch's chin after chin augmentation 3, 4
- capsular contracture after cheek augmentation 3, 4
- capsular contracture after calf implants 3, 4
- soft tissue filler 5

TRAUMATOLOGY AND MILITARY SURGERY
- prophylaxis of wound infections before or during transportation 1, 3

Part III

MANUFACTURING OF STEM CELL XENOTRANSPLANTATION

Chapter 21

> Indeed, what is there that does not appear marvelous when it comes to our knowledge for the first time? How many things, too, are looked upon as quite impossible until they have been actually effected?
> *Pliny the Elder, A.D. 23-79, Natural History*

PREPARATION AND MANUFACTURING OF STEM CELL XENOTRANSPLANTS

Stem cell transplantation is a procedure that is simple for the patients but complicated for those that prepare the transplants, i.e. if stem cell transplants are manufactured "lege artis", according to all rules.

The manufacturing stem cell transplants *requires a closed colony of the laboratory animals chosen to be the source for the preparation of stem cell xenotransplants,* and a production laboratory nearby, no more than 20 – 30 km (12 – 18 miles) away.

When setting up a new manufacturing facility for stem cell xenotransplants, the limiting factor is the closed colony of laboratory animals. For example, if you have chosen rabbits as the animal source, it is infinitely easier to locate the closed colony of rabbits first, and then build the manufacturing laboratory in the vicinity than the other way around.

If you decide to set up a new closed colony of rabbits, you must select a country or a region where there are several rabbit farms, and they are prosperous, as that is an indication that the ecology is suitable for rabbits. Then you build rabbit halls in accordance with AAALAC (American Association for Accreditation of Laboratory Animal Care) regulations, and buy rabbits from another well established closed colony to get started. *It takes a minimum of two years, or 25 generations, of careful observation before the rabbit colony could be designated "closed".*

Naturally if the rabbits do not do well, it takes much longer. If you want to avoid the serologic testing of all animals for every infectious disease occurring in the country or region as per epizootiologic data, you have to extend the period of observation to 3 years.

If one disregards the bureaucratic procedures for getting the necessary permits, the manufacturing laboratory is much less of a problem, as the sole complex matter is the appropriate air handling system. There are many companies specializing in building customized laboratories.

The author is about to describe the method of manufacturing individually prepared stem cell transplants for each patient to be implanted on a predetermined date, known as BCRO method, and incorporates all pertinent requirements of:

1. "PHS Guidelines on Infectious Disease Issues in Xenotransplantation", January 19, 2001, (Federal Register, Volume 66, pages 8120-1), that is the official version of the same regulation issued initially as a "Draft" on September 23, 1996 (available from Federal Register under 61FR49920),
2. decision of the German Supreme Court in case of 1 BvR420/97, issued on February 16, 2000,
3. EC Directives, in particular the Directive 2001/83/EC,
4. national laws of all Member States of European Union, and
5. US Patent (US patent Pending) 'Cell and Tissue Xenotransplants' and related know-how.

A manufacturing laboratory for preparation of stem cell transplants must be set-up, equipped and staffed in compliance with the laws of each country, and since such laws and regulations may not exist in many countries, then Directives of the European Union Council, US FDA regulations, or WHO advisories, and GMP (Good Manufacturing Practice) rules, should be adhered to instead.

In this book we describe a method of preparation of stem cell transplants from rabbit fetuses and newborns as the animal source. Nowadays, when everyone panics about the "Mad Cow Disease", it is important to stress that according to the world's medical literature, no transmission of any viral disease has been known to occur from rabbit to man. This was confirmed by the World Health Organization, the supervisory body for vaccine manufacturing in the whole world. Since vaccines are produced on cell cultures, and one of the most important is the culture of rabbit kidney cells, WHO follows the health status of laboratory rabbits worldwide very closely.

The natural barrier that has always existed in "Nature" has been largely preventing transmission of infections between species. *The more distant the species are, the stronger this barrier has been*; and this is the case between rabbit and man. In Mad Cow Disease such natural barrier was broken by man.

Coming from a well established closed colony, bred and raised in captivity with a minimal exposure to vectors of infectious agents, with documented lineages of at least 25 generations, the rabbit fetuses and newborns are remarkably free of any disease. Besides that, *rabbit is the sole laboratory animal in which no retroviruses have been identified* yet, despite the fact that theoretically they must be present in all mammals.

Preparation of stem cell transplants as "living systems" is a "biological" process rather than "biotechnological". "Biotechnological process" implies manufacturing of non-living substances by living cells, while "biological process" means manufacturing of live cells for various purposes, including cell transplantation.

Biotechnological products can be standardized to an acceptable degree, even though a certain inherent variability of production is unavoidable; production controls include not 100% reliable biological testing methods; and some deficiencies are not revealed by final testing.

Biological products cannot be standardized, as it is impossible to attain uniformity and consistency of stem cell transplants from one batch to the next. If an experienced tissue culture expert personally prepares ten tissue cultures from the same organ of the same animal source, at the same time, in the same laboratory in the same laminar flow box, nine of them grow perfectly, but the last one not so, i.e. it requires additional steps to reach the same level of quality as the remaining nine. No tissue culture expert can explain this phenomenon.

As long as we do not know what life is, it is impossible to standardize, control, and validate, the manufacturing of stem cell transplants.

Primary goals of manufacturing method are to *abolish immunogenicity* of stem cell transplants, or minimize it as much as possible, and *simultaneously prevent transmission of zoonoses* through implantation of stem cell transplants. It is accomplished by following steps of the described procedure, that is in accordance with the appropriate parts of 'PHS Guidelines on Infectious Issues in Xenotransplantation' of 1/19/2001 (Federal Register, Volume 66, No.19, pages 8120-1), as well as European Council Directive 2001/83/EC, which affirms the decision of German Supreme Court of 2/16/2000 in 1 BvR 420/97.

The key portion of the BCRO method of manufacturing of stem cell transplants is a unique procedure of primary tissue culture that actually is the same for stem cell xenotransplants as well as allotransplants.

While principles are firmly set, preparation of each stem cell transplant is not the same. *Each tissue culture is handled individually, like a "living being", i.e. tissue culture conditions are modified as required by the growth characteristics of cell colony, and cytological features of cultured cells observed in the native state.* The *daily "prescription for living conditions"* of each tissue culture is made by an experienced tissue culture expert. In other words, the procedures of primary tissue culture vary in details: know-how and years of experience are most important when an adjustment of utilized tissue culture conditions has to be made. The close daily observation of tissue culture prevents transmission of xenoses as well, because the tissue culture expert recognizes any cytopathic effects caused by the presence of pathogenic viruses upon an individual cell, or on growth characteristics of cell colony.

All the while the key point of US FDA Regulation of 1/19/ 2001 must be strictly observed. *The link between "scheduled" female rabbits from the closed colony*, identified by numbers given at birth, (source of all fetal and newborn rabbits used in manufacturing of stem cell transplants), and a *patient/recipient of a batch of stem cell transplants* necessary for treatment of his/her disease, identified by a code known only to the manufacturer, *must not be interrupted throughout the whole manufacturing cycle. It must be possible to re-trace the link at any time in the future.* This is accomplished by storing of samples each stem cell transplant, and via archiving of records. (It is valuable for liability protection, too).

BCRO method of primary tissue culture is *based on the creation of ideal growth conditions for one cell type of a tissue or an organ*, desirable for the therapeutic effect, *that are unfavorable at the same time for all other cell types of the same tissue or organ*, that are not only useless for therapeutic effect, but represent an "antigenic overload" as well, that triggers unnecessary and avoidable immune reactions.

The described method of stem cell transplant manufacturing secures non-immunogenicity of cell transplants, so that *immunosuppression is not required*, and by incorporating the pertinent requirements of "PHS Guidelines on Infectious Disease Issues in Xenotransplantation" of January 19, 2001 (Federal Register, Volume 66, Number 19, pages 8120 – 8121) it also assures to the greatest degree offered by modern science an absence of transmission of xenoses by cell xenotransplants from the animal donor to the human recipient/patient.

It was declared by the Ministry of Health of the largest country in the world already in 1984, that no immunosuppression is necessary if the stem cell transplants are prepared by a method of primary tissue culture [76]. Ample additional clinical evidence since then has further proven no clinically detectable immunogenicity after an implantation of stem cell transplants prepared by the described method, perfected over the past 12 years and worked out in detail for all cell types required for the treatment of patients. No genetic manipulations are used in the preparation of stem cell transplants by the described method.

Chapter 22

> One man with courage makes a majority.
> *Andrew Jackson, 1767 – 1845*
>
> Take calculated risks. That is quite different from being rash.
> *George Smith Patton, 1885 - 1945, letter to his son [1944]*

ANIMAL SOURCES FOR STEM CELL XENOTRANSPLANTS

"Because transplantation bypasses, in most of the patient's, usual protective physical and immunological barriers, transmission of known and/or unknown infectious agents to humans through xenografts may be facilitated." (US FDA regulation of January 19, 2001). The same concerns led to the ultimate selection of rabbits as the animal source for xenotransplantation in the described method. (They were selected also because they are abundant. The dissection of the fetal and newborn rabbits is technically much easier as compared with larger animals that have also been used as a source of stem cell transplants).

The lack of transmission of any infection by stem cell transplantation with fetal and newborn rabbits as the source of stem cell transplants has been, in author's clinical experience, the reason for the claim that the benefit/risk ratio of stem cell transplantation is very high.

Rabbits would be useless as a source of organ xenotransplants due to their small size but are an excellent source of stem cell xenotransplants for two key reasons:

A. It is a common knowledge in veterinary and human medicine that *none of the known viral diseases of rabbits are transmissible to man.*

As this is a major issue nowadays, let's elaborate on it, in particular on the transmission of retroviruses and prions.

No one argues the fact that there are rabbit retroviruses in nature, but the truth is that (and according to the following references), *they have not been recognized to this date*:

1. Murphy, FA, CM Fauquet, DHL Bishop, et al. **Virus Taxonomy,** (Sixth Report of the International Committee on Taxonomy of Viruses), Springer Verlag, Vienna - New York, 1995, Chapter: Families of Reverse-Transcribing Viruses, 23 - 42
2. the very recent updates (the above Committee meets every 5 years) [200]
3. Fauquet, CM, CR Pringle. Abbreviations for vertebrate virus species names, Arch Virology 1999; 144: 1865 – 1880 [201]
4. Murphy, AF, EPJ Gibbs, MC Horzinek, MJ Studdert. **Veterinary Virology,** Academic Press, San Diego, New York, London, 1999, 273 - 278 [202]

There are no viruses of the Genus Retroviridae that have been classified or taxonomically recognized in rabbits yet.

There are three articles by Bedigian, et al, published 24 years ago, that are considered by some to be the sole available proof of existence of retroviruses in rabbits. These three articles are apparently not recognized by the virological community, as no one has duplicated the findings of the authors in so many years. It should be pointed out that all three papers were written by the same authors working in the same laboratory, at the same time, and with their own WH/J strain of rabbits that served as a model for hereditary lymphosarcoma and immune hemolytic anemia associated with thymoma.

As per three papers by Bedigian, et al, no RNA-directed DNA polymerase was found in rabbit fetuses older that 10 days, (and in such early embryos the retroviruses may have a physiologic purpose, as the authors of the paper stated themselves), or in any normal cells of adult rabbits even from the artificially created strains of rabbits with high incidence of malignancy, such as WH/J strain.

On page 4694 of article #2, submitted for publication on the same day as article #1, the authors stated that "particles associated with RDDP (RNA-directed DNA polymerase) were detected in the extracts prepared from tumorous spleens, nodes, and kidneys, *but not in tissues of unaffected rabbits*", i.e. obviously of the same artificially created WH/J strain.

In the last paragraph, on pages 491-492 of article #1, authors wrote: "To date we have been unable, utilizing a wide range of mammalian cell lines, to demonstrate infection and replication of a rabbit oncornavirus." ..."The possibility exists that the viral information is defective and that a virus is therefore unable to replicate. A 2nd possibility may be that a permissive host has not yet been found that allows for the infection and replication of a rabbit type C RNA virus". And further on: "The role of the type C particles that appear in the early gestation is not clear. Their presence may be due to a hormonal influence early in gestation, or they may be involved in some normal physiological process such as information transfer from parent to offspring (see reference by Daniels, footnote # 2, page 4687)". The point here is that the authors found the RDDP reaction in the placenta and uterus *during the first 10 days of gestation only and not thereafter.*

Since the described method of manufacturing recommends the use of rabbit fetuses at 28 days of gestation, and the gestation of rabbits takes 30 - 31 days, the findings of Bedigian, et al are not pertinent at all.

There is a recent article by Maudru and Peden, in which the authors describe their exceptionally sensitive test for detection of RNA-dependent DNA polymerase activity. No one has identified such activity in rabbits even with such test. Also the authors state that their assay "can detect RNA-dependent DNA polymerase activity in DNA polymerases that are not retroviral reverse transcriptases (!)", thus "the usefulness of the PBRT assay to reveal the presence of low level of retrovirus in biological products or in patient material may be limited" (page 260).

One can understand the concern of some scientists in view of the discovery that porcine endogenous retrovirus is capable of infecting human cells *in vitro*, and that there is a possibility of mutations, or its recombinations with human retroviruses, that could create new pathogenic viruses. The fact remains that pigs were domesticated five millenia ago, and even after eating pork for 5,000 years, no human has been infected by any such virus yet, and it stays so as long as the 'pork-producing industry' continues to follow the ecologically sound principles, unlike what happened in the 'beef-producing industry', that caused the "Mad Cow Disease".

Even if, in the future, the rabbit retroviruses are found, it will not change the scientific fact that they are not infectious to humans or any other animal. Not even under extreme experimental conditions could hares be infected by the virus of haemorrhagic pneumonia of rabbits, and likewise the virus of the haemorhagic pneumonia of hares cannot be transmitted to rabbits, and so it is not surprising that humans or other animals could not be infected either [196].

At this moment there is no reason to think about prions in relation to rabbits. Since no one has come up with an idea to feed rabbits a food of animal origin, it is highly doubtful that any prions will ever be found in rabbits.

B. It is a scientific fact beyond any doubt that the *xenotransplantation between discordant species causes much less severe immunological reactions than xenotransplantation between concordant species*. Rabbits are phylogenetically distant from man, i.e. "discordant". That is probably, besides the procedure of preparation of stem cell transplants by the described method of tissue culture, a part of the reason why there is *no need for immunosuppression when stem cell transplants prepared by the described method are used for implantation in clinical practice*.

Many physicians feel that the immune reactions after stem cell xenotransplantation are not of importance anymore because of the availability of excellent and powerful immunosuppressants. The reality is that all immunosuppressants have multiple side effects and their chronic use leads to potentially life-threatening complications, and if they have to be used with stem cell xenotransplantation, then such treatment is fraught with a great risk and of limited value in everyday clinical practice. When stem cell xenotransplants are prepared by the described method, no immunosuppression is necessary, and stem cell transplantation is less dangerous than taking an aspirin. The ability to minimize immune reactions after stem cell xenotransplantation so that no immunosuppression is necessary in clinical practice is of crucial importance for the patient and for therapeutic success.

Chapter 23

The independent scientist who is worth the slightest consideration as a scientist has a consecration which comes entirely from within himself: a vocation which demands the possibility of supreme self-sacrifice.
Norbert Wiener, 1994 - 1964, The Human Use of Human Beings

CLOSED COLONY OF SOURCE ANIMALS

Fetal and newborn rabbits used for preparation of stem cell transplants in the described method have to originate from closed colony of rabbits, with documented lineages for over 3 years (>30 generations), bred and reared in captivity, and not exposed to vectors of infectious agents.

All rabbits have to be marked by an identification number for life that relates to their ancestors and to its genotype group.

In order to qualify as a source of fetal and newborn rabbits to be used for preparation of stem cell transplants, a closed colony has to be set up in accordance with guidelines of WHO and AAALAC, have an adequate surveillance program for infectious agents for over 3 years (if less than 3 years, then immunological assays for all known infections of rabbits have to be carried out, and their results must be negative), and live attenuated vaccines must not have been utilized for infection prevention.

Guidelines of WHO and AAALAC for closed colonies that are usually duplicated by the laws and regulations in individual countries, consist of:

1. *Criteria for animal admission*:
   New rabbits are admitted into the closed colony only from another closed colony that is proven to:

   - not contain animals with any sign of disease, infectious or non-infectious,

- contain only animals that are marked and identified for a minimum of 25 generations of ancestors,
- have documentation about the useful features of kept animals, and that of their ancestors,
- maintain acceptable nutritional and microclimactic conditions.

All new rabbits are placed under quarantine for 4 weeks, and if no sign of disease appears, then introduced into a closed colony.

2. ***Disease monitoring program***: Veterinary technicians observe rabbits daily. They watch for the amount of feed used, vitality, and the behavior of animals. If anything untoward is observed, the veterinarian is immediately called in to make a decision about the quarantine.

The rooms for quarantine are separate from the main rabbit pavilions. (Healthy animals transferred from other colonies are not mixed in the same quarantine room with diseased animals under observation).

After the transfer, in the quarantine room, specimens of blood for hematology, and possibly toxicology, nasal swab and feces specimen for microbiology, etc., are taken. No animal is ever returned from quarantine for diseased rabbits back to the colony. In case of death a full autopsy is carried out and specimens taken for bacteriological and toxicological testing.

Rabbit epizootiology of the country, or ecologic region of the country, has to be well studied, so that the disease monitoring program is targeted.

Every 6 months a nasal swab is obtained from randomly selected group of female rabbits, which is sent for a microbiological examination to the accredited veterinary laboratory.

3. ***Criteria for the isolation or elimination of diseased animals***: At the first sign of any disease the animal is quarantined, and from quarantine never ever returned back to the colony.

As a matter of policy, the use of antibiotics and other medications must be minimal. The organizational, zootechnical and nutritional regimen has to be set-up so that there is no need for a regular treatment by drugs.

4. *Criteria for health screening and surveillance of humans entering the facility*: Veterinary technicians in immediate contact with rabbits change before entering the rabbit hall completely from underwear up into work clothes and shoes. Upon departure, they change again into street clothes/shoes. Other people not working in the rabbit hall are prohibited from entering. All personnel undergo yearly physicals with chest x-rays, complete blood count and blood chemistry.

5. *Facility cleaning arrangements*: There must be a continuous cleaning of cages and rabbit halls. A scheme of cleaning of individual sectors has to be devised whereby the on-going programs are not interfered with. The empty space is mechanically cleansed by water under pressure, disinfected chemically and difficult to reach corners are cleaned and disinfected by propane flame. The quality of cleansing is controlled by regular collection of swabs from the surfaces critical from the viewpoint of contact with animals.

6. *The source and delivery of feed, water and supplies*: Feed must be made exclusively from components of plant origin. Although its composition is controlled by the manufacturer, it has to be re-checked in the closed colony by appropriate analytic procedures. Rabbit halls have to be connected to a source of drinking water for human consumption that fulfills all public health criteria, bacteriological and chemical.

Feed components for the entire colony must be documented. No recycled or rendered animal material must be used in the feed. All components of feed (peas, barley, dried grass, rye, etc.) have to be produced without chemical insecticides or herbicides and with only a minimal use of chemical fertilizers. A vitamin/ mineral mixture of prescribed combination, guaranteed by the manufacturer, must be added to the feed pellets. All feed should be from local production companies; imports are to be avoided.

7. *Measures to exclude arthropods and other animals*: Rabbit halls must be protected by mechanical barriers against insects and rodents.

8. ***Animal transportation***: There is no transportation of rabbits while in closed colony with the exception of being taken to the quarantine room for diseased animals. The quarantine rooms have similar technological, microclimactic and nutritional conditions as the main rabbit halls but are isolated and separate from rabbit halls. For the transportation of newborn rabbits, or pregnant female rabbits to be used as a source of rabbit fetuses to the manufacturing facility, see below.

9. ***Dead animal disposition***: Dead animals must be placed in transport cages that are moved out of the rabbit hall and handed to the transportation personnel in such a way that the transporttation personnel do not enter the interior of the rabbit hall at any time. Before any further use, the transport cages are mechanically cleaned and chemically disinfected.

Hormonal stimulation for impregnation must be avoided if fetuses/newborns are to be used for manufacturing of stem cell transplants.

Pregnant females deliver newborns in the delivery boxes filled with microbiologically verified straw.

The movement of rabbits is always s'one way' (i.e. 'all in - all out'). A necessary quantity of female rabbits is 'pre-scheduled' to deliver within 24 hours of the starting day of the primary organ cultures. On the next day, all newborns of these females are taken out of closed colony and transported to the manufacturing facility. The pregnant female(s) designated to be a source of rabbit fetuses for the production of the same batch of stem cell transplants are taken out of colony and transported to the manufacturing facility in the same fashion.

Transportation of newborn rabbits to the production facility is carried out in the closed boxes, in a passenger car. Newborn rabbits are taken out of their delivery boxes and immediately placed into the transportation boxes, which are opened only in the manufacturing facility by personnel attired in sterile gowns, with masks and sterile gloves.

Pregnant female rabbits, designated to be a source of rabbit fetuses, are removed from closed colony one to two days before delivery date and taken to the manufacturing laboratory in transport cages by car.

The distance from the closed colony to the manufacturing laboratory must not exceed 20 - 30 km (12 - 18 miles). Lengthy transportation can be extremely stressful for rabbits, as is evident during the autopsy, and disqualifies many of them as an animal source for stem cell transplantation.

No rabbit taken out of closed colony is ever returned back.

DOCUMENTATION

All age groups of rabbits in the colony are individually followed, insofar as the health and production usefulness is concerned. Identification numbers of each animal are interconnected with the system of dual evidence. Each animal has a record card on its cage which contains all data observed during its life. The same information is entered into the computerized data base, which also contains the genetic relationships of individual animals within the same generation and between generations. Notes of all visits by the veterinarian and all other medically important data, are entered in these records as well.

Chapter 24

Liberty is the possibility of doubting, the possibility of making a mistake, the possibility of searching and experimenting, the possibility of saying "No" to any authority ...
Ignazio Silone, 1900 – 1978, Essay in The God That Failed [1950]

SCREENING FOR INFECTIOUS AGENTS/INDIVIDUAL QUALIFICATION OF ANIMAL SOURCES

Screening for known infectious agents before and during manufacturing of stem cell transplants consists of:

1. continuous evaluation of health status of the entire closed colony of rabbits, all marked and identified by number since birth, with complete documentation,
2. continuous evaluation of all ancestors (for at least 3 generations) of "pre-scheduled" female rabbits, "sources" of all fetal and newborn rabbits needed for manufacturing of a batch of stem cell transplants, marked by a batch numbers,
3. continuous evaluation of health status of "pre-scheduled" pregnant female rabbits,
4. observation of health status of fetal and newborn rabbits,
5. daily macro- and micro- scopic evaluation of each primary tissue culture,
6. final assay of each stem cell transplant by:

    a. histologic evaluation, whereby bacteria can be identified as well,
    b. bacteriological testing,
    c. bacterial endotoxin test

The screening program relies on the following data:

a. in-depth knowledge of epizootiology of country (or ecologic region) of manufacture,
b. in countries with established rabbit farming, the pathogens are found in adult rabbits only (i.e. there are no pathogens in fetal and newborn rabbits that are used in the described method of preparation of stem cell transplants),
c. fetal rabbits are actually sterile,
d. no retroviruses have been found, to date, in rabbits,
e. there is no known transmission of viruses from rabbit to man.

Monitoring of closed colonies for infectious agents that are "not apparent clinically" is based on utilization of all adult female rabbits as "sentinel animals" for recognition of any new infectious agent or disease not known today, as per "PHS Guidelines on Infectious Disease Issues in Xenotransplantation" of January 19, 2001:

A. All adult female rabbits are examined by the doctor of veterinary medicine at the beginning of a breeding cycle, and every 6 months thereafter, and the following specimens are collected:

1. blood samples of serum and leukocytes, to be kept in liquid nitrogen for 5 years for future microbiological testing,
2. specimen for blood count and peripheral blood smear,
3. specimen of feces to test for parasites,
4. nasal swab for microbiological culture.

B. After death, all adult female rabbits are subjected to a full autopsy. Specimens of blood, liver, spleen, bone marrow, and brain, are obtained, and are stored for 5 years in liquid nitrogen. These specimens are used for future microbiological and other tests necessary for identification of viruses capable of recombination, complementation or pseudotyping, in an investtigation of new unexpected disease or of infectious agents that may not be apparent clinically today. The results of the autopsy are placed in the animal's health records and archived. If the autopsy reveals an infection pertinent to the health of the stem cell transplant's recipient, this finding is immediately communicated to a clinical center, where stem cell transplants originating from the fetuses and newborns delivered by this female rabbit were implanted in the named patient's body.

The daily evaluation of primary tissue cultures, macroscopically and under inverted microscope, and the final assessment of the quality of culture by a histological examination, also identifies a presence of microrganisms. Routine bacteriological cultures on fluid thioglycollate medium and soybean-casein digest medium, and a bacterial endotoxin test, are done for each stem cell transplant. In case of any suspicion of contamination, the respective stem cell transplant must be discarded without delay. In order to maintain their clinical effectiveness, stem cell transplants have to be shipped immediately after their release, as there is no time to make any extensive investigation and testing sufficient for making the decision whether to release the particular stem cell transplant for an implantation.

COLONY HEALTH MAINTENANCE AND SURVEILLANCE

The qualification of closed colony as a source of newborn and fetal rabbits for the preparation of stem cell transplants is based on the facts that:

- it fulfills all criteria of a closed colony, and
- an adequate surveillance program for infectious agents have been in place for at least 3 years.

Documentation of the colony health maintenance and surveillance program must be maintained for at least 5 years at the closed colony, the longer the better. All incidents that could have affected the colony health must be recorded, such as breaks in the environmental barriers, diseases outbreaks or sudden animal deaths.

INDIVIDUAL SOURCE ANIMAL SCREENING AND QUALIFICATION

The qualification of individual fetal and newborn rabbits as individual source animals for preparation of stem cell transplants are based on the facts that:

- they originate from a closed colony,

- they originate from documented pure lines,
- their health is documented,
- the health of their immediate ancestors is documented,
- the health of the colony they originate from is documented.

Chapter 25

He who would distinguish the true from the false must have an adequate idea of what is true and false.
Benedict Spinoza, 1632 – 1677, Ethics [1677]

PROCUREMENT OF STEM CELL XENOTRANSPLANTS

Procurement of stem cell transplants must be carried out under aseptic conditions in the manufacturing laboratory, following the GMP and GLP rules, with complete documentation.

The crucial link between the "scheduled" female rabbits from the closed colony as sources of fetal and newborn and rabbits used in the procurement of stem cell transplants, and a patient/recipient of the stem cell transplants necessary for the treatment (identified by a code), must not be interrupted throughout the entire production cycle. It is *accomplished in the following steps of manufacturing* of stem cell transplants by BCRO Method:

1. All stem cell transplants prepared for one specific named patient for a predetermined date of implantation are classified as a "batch".
2. All stem cell transplants in a batch are prepared from fetuses and newborns of "pre-scheduled" female rabbits only.
3. Each sterilized box (for transportation between rabbit colony and manufacturing laboratory) contains only one "pre-scheduled" female rabbit, to be used as source of fetuses, marked by identification number of that female rabbit. Or, each sterilized "small" transportation box contains only newborns of one pre-scheduled female rabbit, marked by

identification number of the female rabbit. All "small" boxes with rabbit newborns necessary for manufacturing a batch of stem cell transplants for one named patient are placed inside of one large cardboard.

4. All "source" animals are processed in groups. One "group" equals all fetuses of one female rabbit or all newborn rabbits from one small box, (i.e. from one female).
5. All euthanized animals of one group are placed in a metal container marked with an identification number of a female rabbit - the "source" of all fetal or newborn cadavers in the metal container.
6. A veterinary doctor/pathologist carries out a full autopsy, properly evaluates gross findings, and collects specimens for histological and microbiological testing, if necessary. *If there are any pathological findings, the source animal is discarded.* These findings are placed in the permanent record of each stem cell transplant, which also contains the summary of medical records of all female rabbits whose fetuses or newborns are used in the preparation of the batch of stem cell transplants for a specific patient.

If findings are normal during the autopsy, the veterinary doctor dissects all organ(s) and tissue(s) needed for the production of all stem cell transplants of a batch, and collects them in the Petri dishes, labeled with the:

   a. name of the stem cell transplant scheduled to be produced,
   b. sex of the recipient/patient which must be the same as the sex of all animal sources used for the manufacturing of stem cell transplants of placenta and adrenal cortex,
   c. identification number (s) of the female rabbits (s), and
   d. code of the patient/recipient of the batch of stem cell transplants under preparation.

7. After mechanical mincing by scalpel or scissors, the pre-determined quantity of tissue fragments of each organ or tissue is placed in the tissue culture flask, labeled with the name of stem cell transplant, and identification numbers of all female rabbits whose fetuses and newborns have been used in preparing the tissue culture in the respective culture flask, and the patient's code.

After the final step of the manufacturing process, collection of cultured tissue fragments into transportation vials occurs.

8. Each transportation vial contains the individualized treatment dose of one stem cell transplant of a batch. The vial must be properly labeled (see Chapter 28), including an identification number of stem cell transplant. This number is linked to all fetal and newborn rabbits used in the manufacturing of a stem cell transplant placed in that vial via the identification numbers of all female rabbits, "sources" of the same fetuses or newborns; and are linked to the:

    - details of the entire manufacture record,
    - histological verification of the organ or tissue origin of each stem cell transplant,
    - records of microbiological testing,
    - records of bacterial endotoxin test, and
    - records of other tests for quality control and validation.

On the last day of manufacturing of a batch of stem cell transplants for a named patient, three samples of supernatant of each stem cell transplant are taken:

- The first sample is kept by the manufacturer in liquid nitrogen for five years.
- The second sample is used for microbiological testing.
- The third sample is used for bacterial endotoxin testing.

Chapter 26

Everything that is hard to attain is easily assailed by the generality of men.
Ptolemy, 100 – 178, Tetrabiblos

Something is rotten in the state of Denmark.
William Shakespeare, 1564 – 1616, Hamlet

ARCHIVING OF MEDICAL RECORDS AND SPECIMENS FROM ANIMAL SOURCES

Archiving of records *allows a rapid and accurate linkage between*:

- medical records of a named recipient of stem cell transplants,
- release records of each stem cell transplant used for treatment,
- frozen specimens of last supernatant of tissue culture flasks of each stem cell transplant of a batch,
- records of autopsy of each female rabbit whose fetuses or newborns were used for preparation of stem cell transplants of the patient, and
- health data of the closed colony of rabbits that contain:

    1. Record cards posted on cages of each female rabbit, with identification number,
    2. Records of all incidents affecting the health of the colony (diseases, sudden death of rabbit(s), environmental breaks, etc.),
    3. Records of all closed colony health surveillance programs,
    4. All of the above are linked to the number of the stem cell transplant as it appears on its label.

Such recordkeeping is essential for the safety of stem cell transplantation as a treatment method, because it allows a public health investigation and containment of suspected new xenogeneic infection.

The following records must be kept for 50 years, as per US FDA regulations:

1. Record cards posted on the cage of each female rabbit of the closed colony. The cards contain the identification numbers, and written notes of all pertinent facts and observations of that female rabbit. The information is entered into the computerized data base as well, where genetic relationships of each animal within the same generation and between generations is documented.
2. Records of all incidents possibly affecting the health of the closed colony, such as disease outbreaks, sudden animal death, breaks in environment barriers, etc.
3. Documentation of the colony health maintenance and surveillance program, including standard operating procedures for the closed colony.
4. Results of autopsy of each deceased female rabbit.
5. Release records of each batch of stem cell transplants.

The above records are linked to the number of the stem cell transplant as appearing on its label.

For the purpose of retrospective public health investigations, the following samples of each batch of stem cell transplants are banked:

1. Samples of the last supernatant of each culture flask of each stem cell transplant, to be kept in liquid nitrogen for 5 years.
2. Blood samples from each female rabbit taken at the initiation of the breeding cycle and every 6 months thereafter, and consisting of five 0.5 cc aliquots of blood serum and plasma; and three aliquots of viable leukocytes, kept in liquid nitrogen for 5 years.
3. Paraffin-embedded, formalin-fixed and cryopreserved (in liquid nitrogen) specimens of spleen, liver, bone marrow and brain of each autopsied rabbit female.

Chapter 27

> He was a scholar, and a ripe and good one.
> Exceeding wise, fair-spoken, and persuading:
> Lofty and sour to them that loved him not;
> But, to those men who sought him sweet as summer.
> *William Shakespeare, 1674 – 1616, Henry VIII*

QUALITY CONTROL

The quality control unit is responsible for control of quality of the manufacturing of stem cell transplants. It must be located in a building separate from manufacturing and its laboratory must be a self-contained entity. The duties of "quality control" are:

1. Verify and approve conformance of actual production history of each batch, as documented by appropriate manufacturing records with established and approved written procedure protocols - with particular attention to the identity, strength, quality and purity of the final stem cell transplant.
2. Carry out inspections of the closed colony of rabbits for conformance with standard operating procedures of that facility.
3. Inspect the documentation of the environmental monitoring, the calibration and maintenance of the equipment of the manufacturing facility, the sterilization of equipment and supplies, and their conformance with written instructions.
4. Release or reject raw materials coming from reputable and regularly audited suppliers (e.g. tissue culture mediums, bovine fetal serums, washing solutions, antibiotics, antiseptics, etc.) by inspecting the certificates thereof, and by sampling and testing of same per written procedures.
5. Release or rejection of tissue culture supplies coming from reputable and regularly audited suppliers (e.g. Petri dishes, tissue culture flasks, vials, closures, containers, etc.) by inspecting the

certificates thereof, and by sampling and testing of same as per written procedures.
6. Release or rejection of packaging and labeling materials.
7. Inspect qualifications and training records of personnel, as well as records of their health examinations.
8. Ensure adequate collection, identification and segregation of laboratory samples - acute or those stored in liquid nitrogen.
9. Ensure accuracy of labeling and release records of released batches of stem cell transplants.
10. Evaluate results of tests of quality of stem cell transplants by histological examination of tissue cultures at the time of the release of stem cell transplants.
11. Evaluate results of bacterial sterility tests of stem cell transplants by inoculation of final supernatant of each culture flask onto fluid thioglycollate medium and soybean casein digest medium.
12. Evaluate results of bacterial endotoxin test.
13. Maintain a procedures book describing all responsibilities and procedures of the quality control unit.
14. Investigate all instances when the supervising tissue culture expert ordered a tissue culture discarded for any reason, and to keep a written record thereof.
15. Investigate all complaints from patients and physicians, particularly if they represent a serious adverse reaction, and to keep a written record thereof.
16. Review and approve validation protocols.

The manufacturing process for stem cell transplants is validated by:

1. Standardization of methods of quality control,
2. Standardization of the conditions of quality control within the rules of GMP,
3. Standardization of tests used for quality control,
4. Standardization of all laboratories facilities -both internal and external, and
5. Standardization of record-keeping.

Chapter 28

> People who know little are usually great talkers, while men who know much say little.
> *Jean Jacques Rousseau, 1712 – 1778, Du Contrat Social [1762]*

> He's a wonderful talker, who has the art of telling you nothing in a great harangue.
> *Molière, 1622 – 1673, Le Misanthrope [1666]*

RELEASE AND LABELING OF STEM CELL XENOTRANSPLANTS

Before the release of a batch of stem cell transplants, all documentation about manufacturing is checked by the quality control unit, especially the description of:

- all steps of the manufacturing process,
- all components, supplies, containers, closures, labels, used in the manufacturing,
- all post-manufacturing testing and sampling, including storage of the last supernatant of each tissue culture flask, and
- any and all other data required by GMP,

All such documents must be signed by the supervising tissue culture expert and co-signed by the manager.

On the batch release date, each transportation vial contains the full treatment dose of stem cell transplants of one organ or tissue of the batch (strength), and is labeled with:

a. name of stem cell transplant,
b. the patient's code (a + b = "identification"),
c. the number of the batch, and
d. the number of a stem cell transplant. The number is linked to:

All newborn and fetal rabbits used in its preparation via the identification number of all female rabbits; the sources of all fetuses/ newborns used (purity); and the records of the entire manufacturing process, histological and bacteriological testing, bacterial endotoxins, testing and other quality control unit data (quality).

All labeled vials of the batch are packed in the transportation box, on the top of which a final label is placed. The transportation box is then placed in a thermostatic container for transportation by a courier for implantation within the following 48 hours.

Labels placed on a box containing a batch of stem cell transplants to be used for the treatment of a specially named patient on the pre-determined date of implantation include the following data:

   a. Name and address of the laboratory that prepared a batch of stem cell xenotransplants,
   b. Name of each stem cell transplant in the batch, stating from which organ or tissue each stem cell transplant originate,
   c. Batch number,
   d. Patient's code,
   e. Identification codes of each stem cell transplant in the batch,
   f. Volume of each stem cell transplant of the batch (i.e. dosage),
   g. Description of supernatant,
   h. Release date,
   i. Statement: *Expiration date: 3 days from the release date, if maintained at room temperature at all times, but implantation within 48 hours strongly advised,*
   j. Statement: *Recommended storage temperature: 20° C",*
   k. Statement: *"Live cultured tissue fragments! NO PRESERVA-TIVES USED,*
   l. Statement: *Route of administration: implantation by specialized injection techniques as per enclosed instructions,*
   m. Statement: *HANDED TO THE PATIENT'S PHYSICIAN ONLY.*

The data on lines a, b, c, d, and e appear also on the label of the vial of each stem cell transplant of the batch:

   a. Name and address of laboratory that prepared a batch of stem cell xenotransplants,

b. Name of the actual stem cell transplant in the vial, that states from which organ or tissue the stem cell transplant originates,
c. Batch number,
d. Patient's code,
e. Identification code of the actual stem cell transplant in the vial.

A delivered batch of stem cell transplants is accompanied by the instructions about implantation sites for each stem cell transplant.

Part IV

USE OF STEM CELL XENOTRANSPLANTS IN HUMAN MEDICINE

Chapter 29

I see but one rule: to be clear. If I am not clear, all my world crumbles to nothing.
Stendhal, 1783 – 1842, Reply to Balzae

How marvelous is Man! How proud the word rings – Man!
Maxim Gorki, 1868 – 1936, Autobiography [1913]

THERAPEUTIC GOAL OF STEM CELL XENOTRANSPLANTATION

There are two types of clinical situations where stem cell transplantation has been utilized for treatment in its over 70-year long history. First, there are diseases with no known treatment, and second, there are diseases where standard treatment has been available, and was used to keep the illness under control for some time, but when it progressed to the stage when it stopped being effective, i.e. disease became untreatable, then stem cell transplantation was discovered, usually by the desperate patient, as a therapeutic modality. The examples of the first group are neurodegenerative disease, and nearly all genetic and chromosomal diseases, while a good example of the second group is diabetes mellitus and in particular its complications, e.g. retinopathy, nephropathy, polyneuropathy, and lower extremity arterial disease.

In patients of the first group the decision to select stem cell transplantation as treatment has been simple. There is no other therapy available, and since properly prepared stem cell transplants are 'safer that aspirin', stem cell transplantation was, or should have been, carried out soon after the diagnosis was made.

In the second group, the situation has been more complicated. The patient has usually continued one of the no longer effective therapies, without informing the stem cell transplantologist about it, and when there was an improvement, the physicians that oppose stem cell transplantation declared that the reason for the success has been a heretofore unknown benefit of the old therapy. Where there was a lack of success, stem cell transplantation was just "useless", without considering the possibility that the old therapy was detrimental to stem cell transplants. The patient's own opinion was ignored. As the patient's state of mind was usually dominated by negative emotions due to confusing information coming from various corners, the evaluation of the benefits of stem cell transplantation became a complicated matter.

This applies specifically to diabetes, since all patients with IDDM (insulin dependent diabetes mellitus) have to continue insulin injections even after stem cell transplantation, albeit at a lower dosage. It is better to limit the use of stem cell transplantation to the patients with complications of diabetes mellitus: nephropathy, retinopathy, lower extremity vascular disease, and polyneuropathy, etc., that had reached the stage of being otherwise un-treatable, i.e. where the patient had clearly recognized that even the best insulin treatment by the best diabetologist cannot stop the progression of serious, disabling and life-threatening diabetic complication(s).

It is a matter of good clinical judgment to avoid treatment of those 93% of diabetics who suffer from NIDDM (non-insulin dependent diabetes mellitus) until they develop diabetic complications. NIDDM is not a disease, but a label for multiplicity of abnormal conditions of sugar and lipid metabolism. Until the etiology of the metabolic malfunction in such patients can be found it is hard to treat them successfully with stem cell transplantation. *The exceptions are* MODY, *a mixed type1-2 diabetes mellitus, or diabetes mellitus type 2 due to an identified genetic cause.*

Unfortunately, as a matter of medical politics, children with recent onset of diabetes mellitus have not been permitted to be treated by stem cell transplantation by some regulatory agencies. In reality the only way to cure diabetes by stem cell transplantation, or postpone its progression, is by treating children with recent onset of IDDM by stem cell transplantation, and thereby prolong the period of their normal growth and development. This has been proven by our team in Russia, confirming the report by Benikova, et al from Ukraine [222]. See the subchapter on 'Diabetes Mellitus'.

The following rules on the patient selection for the treatment by stem cell transplantation apply when the patient is a diabetic with complications. US official statistics are utilized because similar data from other countries were not at the author's disposal.

Among diabetics with nephropathy those patients with stage III of diabetic nephropathy as per NIDDK staging [106] or "overt diabetic nephropathy" with loss of albumin and other proteins exceeding 200 micrograms per minute, i.e. "dipstick-positive proteinuria", and increased serum creatinine and BUN, and with early stage IV of diabetic nephropathy as per NIDDK staging [106], or "advanced diabetic nephropathy", with declining glomerular filtration rate, some hypertension, and noticeably increased serum creatinine and BUN, as a complication of insulin dependent diabetes mellitus (IDDM), *that have not responded to intensive insulin therapy, together with angiotensin converting enzyme (ACE) inhibitors*, are "ideal" candidates for stem cell transplantations.

In the US diabetes mellitus (DM) accounts for 35% of all new cases of end-stage renal disease (ESRD) [105]. In 1995, a total of 98,872 diabetics received a renal replacement therapy, and there were 27,851 new cases of diabetic ESRD.

NIDKK website states that 15.7 million of US population has diabetes mellitus [106], 7% of this number, it means approximately 1.1 million, suffers from IIDM [105], 30-50% of patients with IDDM would be expected to develop diabetic nephropathy after 40 years of DM [105]. It has been observed that incidence of proteinuria rises during the first 10 years of IDDM, and then begins to decline after about 15 years, so that apparently only a subset of patients with IDDM is susceptible to the development of renal disease [105]. As stated above, in DCCT intensive insulin therapy was associated with a 39% reduced risk of microalbuminuria and 54% reduced risk of macroalbuminuria. It is estimated that 20-30% of patients with DM has microalbuminuria (i.e. they are in stage II of diabetic nephropathy), and 20-30% of diabetics has macroalbuminuria (i.e. they are in stage III of diabetic nephropathy). In the Wisconsin study, in a group of IDDM patients, 21% had micro- and 21% had macro-albuminuria [105]. In IDDM, the incidence of persistent proteinuria reaches 25% after 15 years of DM [105]. Clinical proteinuria heralds a relentless decline of renal function leading to ESRD. Of IDDM patients at the Joslin Clinic in Boston, MA, 50% developed chronic renal failure after 10 years of persistent proteinuria [105]. Taking all of the above statistical data into consideration, it appears that approximately 12.5% of patients with IDDM should reach the stage V of ESRD, i.e.

about 137,000 patients. In absolute numbers, 27,851 diabetic patients developed end-stage renal disease in 1995. In 1995, a total of 98,872 diabetics underwent dialysis or kidney transplantation [106].

There are at least 137,000 IDDM patients within the US that should undergo stem cell transplantation as per the above statistics, which are rather old today.

Among diabetics with retinopathy, those patients with pre-proliferative stage of diabetic retinopathy as a complication of insulin dependent diabetes mellitus (IDDM), that have not responded to intensive insulin therapy for at least 6 months and photocoagulation of retina, are "ideal" candidates for stem cell transplantation by the clinical method described in this book.

Diabetic retinopathy is the leading cause of new cases of blindness of adults in the US (11% are due to diabetic retinopathy). In the Wisconsin Epidemiologic Study of Diabetic Retinopathy (WESDR) 97% of IIDM patients had evidence of retinopathy by 15 years of diabetes mellitus (DM). The most severe stage, proliferative diabetic retinopathy, was present in 30% of IDDM after 15 years of diabetes [105].

NIDKK website states that 15.7 million of US population has diabetes mellitus [106], 7% of this number, approximately 1.1 million, suffers from IIDM [105]. According to WESDR, 97% of this number will have retinopathy after 15 years of diabetes, and 30% will have proliferative diabetic retinopathy [105]. As per DCCT, 60% of these patients will be helped by the intensive insulin treatment [105]. In accordance with Diabetes Retinopathy Study (DRS), panretinal photocoagulation reduces the rate of severe loss of vision (visual acuity poorer than 5/200) by 50% [105]. As per WESDR data, around 45% of new patients with proliferative diabetic retinopathy develop DRS high-risk characteristics for severe loss of vision [105]. Based on the foregoing statistical data we estimate that there is in the US a population of around 150,000 IDDM patients with pre-proliferative retinopathy with DRS high-risk characteristics for severe loss of vision who have not responded positively to DCCT-type intensive insulin treatment and any form of retinal photocoagulation treatment.

As an example, the population of 150,000 IDDM patients in the US with pre-proliferative retinopathy with DRS high-risk characteristics for severe loss of vision, that recognized the futility of DCCT-type intensive insulin treatment, and retinal photocoagulation, in controlling the progression of their retinopathy, should seek stem cell transplantation treatment.

Among diabetics with lower extremity arterial disease those patients with a lower extremity arterial disease (LEAD) as a complication of insulin dependent diabetes mellitus (IDDM), that have not responded to intensive insulin therapy, and already underwent an unsuccessful revascularization surgery, or such surgery was contraindicated, or had an amputation, are "ideal" candidates for the described clinical method of stem cell transplantation.

In the US, more than 50% of all amputations occur in patients with DM, which amounts to 67,000 amputations a year in each of the years 1993 - 1995 [106]. The 4-year amputation incidence in WESDR cohort study was 2.2% for IDDM patients [105]. Between 9 - 20% of patients with DM had a second amputation (ipsi- or contra- lateral) within 12 months after the first one. Between 28 - 51% of diabetic amputees had an amputation of the contralateral lower extremity within 5 years [105]. The incidence of Lower extremity arterial disease (LEAD) in patients with DM was ~10 times higher than that of non-diabetics [105]. By the time LEAD becomes clinically manifest it may be too late to salvage an extremity [105].

NIDKK website states that 15.7 million of US population has diabetes mellitus [106]. 7% of this number, it means approximately 1.1 million, suffers from IIDM [105]. The full extent of diabetic foot problem in the US is unknown [105]. The annual incidence of foot ulcers in patients with DM is 2 - 3% with the prevalence of 4 - 10% [105]. In WESDR the incidence of foot ulcers in IDDM patients was 2.4% [105]. Foot ulcers precede 85% of non-traumatic amputations in patients with DM. Intermittent claudication was found in 9% of patients with DM [105]. Cumulative incidence of LEAD was 15% at 10 years after an initial diagnosis of DM and 45% after 20 years [105]. In DM patients LEAD is compounded by the presence of diabetic neuropathy and susceptibility to infection [105]. As per DCCT, none of these patients is significantly helped by the intensive insulin treatment [105]. In each of the years 1993 - 1995 as many as 67,000 amputations were due to diabetes mellitus. NIH statistics do not state the proportion of IDDM and NIDDM patients. Based on the foregoing statistical data, and on the 4-years' amputation incidence in IDDM patients of 2.2%, we estimate that in US there is a population of around 23,000 IDDM patients with diabetic major vasculopathy who have not responded positively to DCCT-type intensive insulin treatment, and revascularization surgery. Since one cannot wait until gangrene develops, we estimate that the prospective patient population in the US is around 9% of 1.1 million of patients with IDDM, which amounts to approximately 100,000.

So as an example, in the US there is a patient population of 100,000 IDDM patients with LEAD that recognized the futility of DCCT-type intensive insulin treatment, together with revascularization surgery, in controlling the progression of their lower extremity arterial disease, and should seek stem cell transplantation.

Among diabetics with polyneuropathy, those patients with otherwise untreatable severe diabetic polyneuropathy as a complication of insulin dependent diabetes mellitus (IDDM), that have not responded to intensive insulin therapy, and their pain became intractable despite the 'state-of-the-art' pain treatment, are "ideal" candidates for the described clinical method of stem cell transplantation.

Official US statistics show that the prevalence of any neuropathy with IDDM was 60%, of more severe forms 15%, and of very severe forms with intractable pain 6% [105]. Prevalence of distal polyneuropathy increased from 17% at 0 - 4 years of duration of DM to 50% at >15 years of duration of DM [105].

NIDDK website states that 15.7 million of US population has diabetes mellitus [106]. Approximately 7% of this number, approximately 1.1 million, suffers from IIDM [105]. Approximately 6% of this number suffers from severe forms of neuropathy. In Rochester, MN, Diabetic Neuropathy Study, the prevalence was 60% for any neuropathy, 47% for distal polyneuropathy, 34% for carpal tunnel syndrome, and 5% for autonomic neuropathy [105].

Although DCCT trial showed that in patients with IDDM who had no neuropathy at baseline, an intensive insulin treatment was associated with a 60% reduction in 5-year incidence of neuropathy [105], there is still about 40% of patients with severe diabetic neuropathy as a complication of IDDM remaining who should seek stem cell transplantation [36].

Based on the foregoing statistical data, we estimate that there is a population of around 55,000 IDDM patients in US with severe diabetic polyneuropathy who have not responded positively to DCCT-type intensive insulin treatment and intensive pain therapy, in controlling the progression of their neuropathy with intractable pain, who should seek stem cell transplantation.

As with any other untreatable disease, *stem cell transplantation should be carried out immediately after any one of the above diabetic complications was diagnosed.* This will be possible only after appropriate public education, and elimination of confusing media information.

There are abundant statistics to prove the effectiveness of stem cell transplantation as the treatment of choice for various complications of IDDM:

1. In patients with *diabetic nephropathy*, in whom the progression of nephropathy cannot be therapeutically controlled by intensive insulin treatment together with ACE inhibitors treatment, *the success rate* of stem cell transplantation *is 60%* in the experience of our Moscow team. In the earlier stages of diabetic nephropathy, the success rate would be higher.

   Although DCCT trial showed that in patients with IDDM who had no nephropathy at baseline, intensive insulin treatment was associated with a 39% reduced risk of microalbuminuria, and 54% reduced risk of macroalbuminuria [105], there is still about one half of patients with diabetic nephropathy as a complication of IDDM remaining for whom some other treatment is necessary: stem cell transplantation [36]. Between 20-30% of diabetics has stage II with microalbuminuria, i.e. "dipstick-negative", and 20-30% stage III of diabetic nephropathy with macroalbuminuria, or proteinuria, i.e. "dipstick-positive", which means loss of >500 mg of protein/day [105]. Many diabetologists doubt the optimistic conclusions of DCCT trial.

   IDDM patients with late stage IV and stage V diabetic nephropathy should not be accepted for treatment. Although the majority of patients will appreciate the improvement, as long as they will not get off the hemodialysis, the result will be classified by them as "failure".

   Since in the WESDR the risk of developing heart attack, stroke, diabetic nephropathy, and amputation, was higher in those with proliferative diabetic retinopathy as compared with those with no or minimal nonproliferative retinopathy at baseline [105], one has to expect that of the above described population of diabetic nephropathy patients, some will suffer from such diseases. Treating stem cell transplantologists should beware of this. Patients *suffering from more than one complication of IDDM should be considered individually and may not be accepted for treatment*, since it has been established that the presence of microalbuminuria in IDDM is associated with a nearly threefold risk of death from cardiovascular and renal disease [105], and that the risk of lower extremity amputation in diabetics with proteinuria is two to four times that of those without proteinuria, and that the relationship between diabetic nephropathy and retinopathy is well established [105]. The same applies to IDDM patients with diabetic nephropathy suffering also from other illnesses, not related to IDDM.

The criterion of effectiveness of the treatment by stem cell transplantation is the *termination of any further progression of diabetic nephropathy proven by an objective evaluation of results of a battery of standard tests of kidney function*. Whenever the tests show further deterioration of kidney function, that indicates a *re-activation of the disease process, stem cell transplantation must be carried out*.

2. In those patients with *diabetic retinopathy* in whom the progression of retinopathy cannot be therapeutically controlled by intensive insulin treatment and retinal laser treatment, in the experience of our team, *the success rate* of stem cell transplantation is 65%. In earlier stages of diabetic retinopathy the success rate would be higher.

Although Diabetes Control and Complications Trial (DCCT) showed that in patients with IDDM that had retinopathy at baseline, intensive insulin treatment was associated with a 54% reduction in progression of retinopathy, a 47% reduction in the incidence of preproliferative or proliferative retinopathy, and a 54% reduction in laser treatment [105], and panretinal photocoa-gulation reduced the rate of severe loss of vision by 50% as well [105], there is still about one half of patients with diabetic retinopathy as a complication of IDDM with DRS (Diabetes Retinopathy Study) characteristics for severe loss of vision remaining for whom some other treatment is necessary: stem cell transplantation [36]. Again, the results of DCCT trial have been questioned.

IDDM patients with proliferative retinopathy should be accepted only in early stages. Destroyed retina of a blind eye cannot be expected to return back to function after stem cell transplantation.

Since in the WESDR the risk of developing heart attack, stroke, diabetic nephropathy, and amputation, was higher in those with proliferative diabetic retinopathy as compared with those with no or minimal nonproliferative retinopathy at baseline [105], this should be considered in the treatment decision making process.

The criterion of effectiveness of the treatment by stem cell transplantation is the *termination of any further progression of diabetic retinopathy* proven by an evaluation of stereoscopic fundus photographs of seven standard photographic fields taken of each eye (as per WESDR). Whenever there is *an objective evidence of re-activation of the disease process, stem cell transplantation should be carried out without delay.*

3. In those patients with *diabetic lower extremity arterial disease* that have not responded positively to intensive insulin treatment as per DCCT, had an unsuccessful revascularization surgery, or such surgery was contraindicated, or had a previous amputation in the author's experience the *success rate* of stem cell transplanttation is 65%. Of course, in earlier stages of diabetic lower extremity arterial disease, the success rate would be higher.

Any diabetic with lower extremity arterial disease with progressively worsening intermittent claudication, or chronic leg ulcer, with positive clinical tests indicative of insufficient peripheral arterial circulation, that has been treated by DCCT-type intensive insulin treatment for more than 6 months, and underwent revascularization surgery, or such surgery was contra-indicated, or had a previous amputation, without a success insofar the control of progression of LEAD is concerned, should be treated by stem cell transplantation.

Although DCCT trial showed a beneficial trend of glycaemic control on lower extremity arterial disease in IDDM, this trend was not statistically significant [105], thus *diabetics with LEAD represent a particularly difficult group to treat*. It means that they should *be given stem cell transplantation without delay because the progress of their disease toward gangrene may be very rapid*.

Diabetics with lower extremity arterial disease *in the stage of gangrene, and smokers, should not be accepted* for treatment by stem cell transplantation.

Since the mortality rate for diabetes mellitus patients with LEAD are 2 - 3 times higher than in general population [105], and 3-year survival after amputation is less than 50% [105], the stem cell transplantologist should beware that many diabetics with LEAD *will suffer from advanced cardiovascular and other disease (s)*.

The criterion of effectiveness of the treatment by stem cell transplantation is the *termination of any further progression of diabetic lower extremity arterial disease* proven by an evaluation of objective standard clinical tests of peripheral arterial circulation. *In case of worsening*, i.e. Doppler study of peripheral pulses, or pre-gangrenous condition, *an immediate repetition of stem cell transplantation is required*.

4. In those diabetics with severe *diabetic polyneuropathy* with intractable pain, that have been treated by DCCT-type intensive insulin treatment for at least 6 months, together with an intensive pain treatment, without a success insofar the control of progression of neuropathy and alleviation of severe pain is concerned, in our experience the success rate of stem cell transplantation is 98%.

Any such patient should get stem cell transplantation treatment.

A special group of diabetics are those with autonomic neuropathy suffering from *impotence*. Of 5% of patients with autonomic neuropathy impotence was the most common problem, occurring in *13% of IDDM patients* [105].

Stem cell transplantologist should beware that *severe*

neuropathy can be a cause of other serious problems, e.g. it is a major contributing cause of lower extremity amputations [106].

The criterion of effectiveness of the treatment by stem cell transplantation is the *termination of any further progression of severe diabetic polyneuropathy proven by a complete or significant disappearance of pain for a period of 6 months*, as well as by standard objective clinical tests, and the subjective pain analog scale. *Upon the recurrence of pain, stem cell transplantation should be repeated.*

Stem cell transplantation is a unique therapeutic procedure due to the fact that stem cell transplants are individually prepared for a specific patient, and for a pre-determined date of implantation, so that stem cell transplants cannot be used by another patient, unless he is a "medical double" of the scheduled patient, i.e. his illness(es) is (are) very similar to the scheduled patient, and is prepared "to step in" when the first patient does not show up for treatment.

For that reason the patient expressing the interest in the treatment must be made aware that the batch of stem cell transplants necessary for the treatment is individually, i.e. "custom", prepared for each specific patient, and is "timed", i.e. prepared for a specific date of an implantation. Once the date of implantation was set and the production of the batch of stem cell transplants begun, the batch has to be either implanted on the scheduled date to that specific patient or discarded: *the full clinical effectiveness is guaranteed for 48 hours only since the release of the batch by the manufacturing laboratory.* A rigid policy of pre-payment of all the production costs by patients prior to the start of the preparation of stem cell transplants is mandatory [111]. Patient's financial involvement has been one proven way to minimize non-compliance and wasting of a very precious material.

Based on the author's years of clinical experience in treating patients in many countries, no serious risk and adverse reactions from stem cell xenotransplants (SCXT) is to be anticipated providing that the preparation of stem cell xenotransplants was "lege artis".

Chapter 30

> Common sense is not so common.
> *Voltaire, 1694 – 1778, Dictionnaire Philosophique [1764]*
>
> Men die but an idea does not.
> *Alan Jay Lerner, 1918 - , My Fair Lady [1978]*

GENERAL PRINCIPLES OF THERAPEUTIC APPLICATION

Stem cell transplantation is not a "magic shot" that will cure all ills. For the best results, the patients have to be selected. The selection criteria described in this book are based on the author's clinical experience with stem cell transplantation, and that was initially based on the study of the many references presented in this book, and discussions with authors of references, if possible.

The diagnostic procedures do not differ from those used in contemporary medicine, *but the evaluation of data is different*. Stem cell transplantologist must look at the patient *as "pathophysiologist"*, i.e. get a complete clinical picture of the function, and malfunction, of every organ system individually and of the whole body. Traditional diagnoses, particularly those that serve more as "labels", are of limited value in the field of stem cell transplantation.

It is not difficult to become a master of pathophysiologic diagnosis, just go back to your medical school textbooks on pathophysiology.

Once you mastered the art of pathophysiologic diagnosis, it becomes easy to select the appropriate stem cell transplants to be used for the treatment of your patient.

The author has always practiced the pathophysiologic approach in stem cell transplantation, i.e. patient receives stem cell transplants of all those organs or tissues required by the pathophysiologic diagnosis.

The current trend in the US, which has not gained much ground in the rest of the world, to treat by transplantation of hematopietic stem cells, or prepared in a laboratory "universal somatic stem cells", all diseases known to medicine, has not proven its value. As of this writing hundreds of patients have been treated by transplantation of hematopietic stem cells, or by transplantation of umbilical cord blood stem cell transplantation, i.e. "monotherapy", while over 5 million patients have been treated by the pathophysiologic approach to stem cell transplantation, i.e. "poly-therapy", over the period of over 70 years. (See additional discussion of this topic *in* Chapter 34.

We define stem cell transplantation as a surgical procedure, individualized for each patient in terms of selection of stem cell transplants in accordance with the pathophysiologic analysis of the malfunction of all organs and tissues of the patient, *details of preparation, dosage, and mode of implantation of stem cell transplants.* It has been not only the German school but also Russian school that calls for "polytherapy". It is easier to prescribe for every patient the transplantation of hematopoietic stem cells or of umbilical cord blood hematopietic stem cells. Transplantation of precursor stem cells of any and all damaged organs or tissues requires a careful and detailed diagnosis and in-depth knowledge of pathophysiology, applied to a specific patient. In the hands of a specialist, it is a very powerful therapeutic tool that becomes a waste if used without a proper knowledge.

The first step is to list all abnormalities uncovered during the diagnostic process. The next step requires a preliminary and logical analysis of the causative associations between various dysfunctions. The more knowledgeable and experienced the transplantologist is, the more detailed and treatment oriented his pathophysiological analysis will be. Everyone is familiar with the complicated scheme of relationships between various endocrine organs and their regulatory centers. Similar relationships of one-way or mutual synergism, or of antagonism, exist between pairs of organs or groups of organs and tissues, but they become apparent only when the overall functional balance is disturbed.

Based on clinical experience, the more frequent dysfunctional relationships between pairs of organs are, for example; those between liver and adrenal cortex, liver and adrenal medulla, thyroid and anterior lobe of pituitary, parathyroid and thyroid, etc. It has been observed that some organs are of key importance in analysis of pathophysiological relationships, i.e. thyroid, liver, adrenal cortex, sex glands, etc. [328].

Recommendations of stem cell transplants to be used for the treatment of a certain disease included in this book should be taken only as guidelines; they should not inhibit your clinical acumen and analytic abilities. After all, our profession is driven by a success in helping our patients.

Additional points for the selection of stem cell transplants to be used for an individual patient:

1. Any chronic disease disrupts the metabolic balance of an organism and the selection of stem cell transplants must include cell types that restore such balance.
2. A *hypofunction of any organ or* tissue should be treated *by stem cell transplants of the same organ or tissue*, while hyperfunction of an organ or tissue requires either stem cell transplants of *an antagonistic organ (s) or no stem cell transplants at all*.
3. For a regeneration of a function of damaged organ, stem cell transplant of the same organ alone is often not sufficient but stem cell transplants of the *synergistic organs or tissues* must be added [328].

The difficult part of stem cell transplantation takes place in the manufacturing laboratory, i.e. the patient does not see or experience the amount of effort and intellect that goes into the preparation of the individually and specifically prepared stem cell transplants. From the patient's viewpoint, stem cell transplantation is a very easy procedure, unless it requires a preliminary minor neurosurgical, orthopaedic, or reconstructive operation.

Each stem cell transplant is implanted separately, stem cell transplants of different organs or tissues are *never mixed in the same syringe* prior to the implantation.

The usual routes of implantation, summarized in the *Introduction*, become more meaningful from the description of ***implantation sites***.

2/3 of Adults have open umbilical vein

Of all the possible *implantation sites*, the liver is by far the best. It has been established beyond doubt that it is the most immunoprotective, i.e. it does not reject any foreign cells for reason (s) still unknown. But a direct intrahepatic implantation carries a definitive risk of intrahepatic haematoma.

The safer way of an intrahepatic transplantation is *the intraportal* one, when the cell transplants are *injected into portal vein, or one of its tributaries,* and in this way they get directly into "immunoprivileged" parenchyma of liver. A minor surgical procedure to re-open the obliterated umbilical vein is the easiest approach to accomplish intraportal implantation. In two thirds of adults, the umbilical vein is found not to be obliterated. The problem is that the obliterated umbilical vein can be re-opened only once. At RITAOMH attempts were made at leaving an indwelling catheter in the umbilical vein of a few patients to allow repeated implantation of stem cell transplants, but after a second implantation, four weeks later, the catheter invariably stopped functioning. All other intraportal approaches are technically more complicated, could not be repeated too many times either, and would have represented a drawback for a method of stem cell transplantation that was to become widespread (and thus had to be technically simple) by the order of the Ministry of Health of USSR in 1984.

The implantation *under the aponeurosis of the rectus abdominis muscle* was developed by RITAOMH as a practical alternative. The anatomical space under the aponeurosis of the rectus abdominis muscle is not considered "immunoprivileged" per se, but it is very closely connected with the portal venous system and peri-portal lymphatic channels. Thus an implantation of stem cell transplants in this space may serve the same purpose as direct intraportal implantation, and the procedure is safe, technically simple, and can be repeated as many times as necessary.

This is due to the existence of an accessory portal system of Sappey, i.e. veins occurring at the site of obliterated fetal circulation. These paraumbilical veins in the falciform and round ligaments are tributaries of the portal vein system. They join with the epigastric and internal mammary veins as well as with the azygos vein through the diaphragmatic veins of the systemic circulation. External part of this circulation is clearly visible around the umbilicus in patients with portal hypertension as "caput Medusae". The excellent drawings of Netter [160] equal the descriptions of authors of classical anatomy textbooks that follow.

"Lying in the free edge of the falciform ligament is the ligament teres, which is obliterated remains of the left umbilical vein of the fetus, and extends from the umbilicus to the notch on the inferior border of the liver. Here it runs in the floor of the fissure for the ligamentum teres to join the left branch of the portal vein at the left extremity of the porta hepatis. While the ligamentum teres is normally avascular, there are accompanying para-umbilical veins representing a potential collateral circulation between the portal vein and systemic venous system of the anterior abdominal wall [153]."

Other classical anatomy textbooks state: "...anastomoses between portal and systemic circulations, which may offer effective collateral circulation, are as follows: ...3/ At the umbilicus, veins running on the ligamentum teres to the left portal branch, connect with the epigastric veins; enlargement of these connections may produce varicosities of veins radiating from the umbilicus, the caput Medusae [151]."

"There are three specific locations where such porta-systemic anastomoses produce grossly dilated venous varicosities: ....around the umbilicus, the paraumbilical veins connect to tributaries of the epigastric veins, which drain into both superior and inferior venae cavae". The blood can flow in both directions in the portal system which "....is a consequence of the absence of valves in the portal system whereby blood can run retrogradely... [154]."

The epigastric veins are draining an area where cell transplants are implanted under aponeurosis of rectus abdominis muscle. "Nevertheless, under normal conditions along the length of the round ligament there is a venule, the paraumbilical vein, which originates in the abdominal wall, around the umbilicus, and runs toward the left branch of the portal vein. According to Wertheimer, it is connected with a newly formed vessel, the central umbilical vein, which is embedded completely in the round ligament....Accessory portal veins... are... 6/ Veins of the round ligament, originating in the abdominal wall, in the neighbohood of the umbilicus, and embedded in the round ligament. They follow the course of that ligament. Some of them terminate at the anterior border of liver, others along its longitudinal groove on the left [152]." (The round ligament and ligamentum teres is the same structure).

Nowadays, in the era of laparoscopic surgery, *an implantation into the greater omentum* has become quite popular [102], or *into epiploic flap*, [175], both of which are modifications of an intraportal implantation.

[handwritten at top: 6-8 wks to notice effects of Stem cells]

"Lymph vessels from the upper and anterior surface of the liver pass into the falciform ligament to join the lower parasternal nodes [153]." "The majority of nodes and node groups are clustered around or abut a prominent blood vessel or one of its branches [151]."

"Many superficial lymphatics from the upper part of the diaphragmatic surface of the liver run through the falciform ligament, turn upward along the superior epigastric vessels, and terminate in the parasternal lymph nodes [154]". The superior epigastric vessels run through the area where cell transplants are implanted by the described method superior to the umbilicus in the right and left subaponeurotic space above the rectus abdominis muscle.

The actual implantation procedures are described in the Chapter 38.

The *clinical effect of stem cell transplantation is delayed on average 6 – 8 weeks*. Since many patients are accustomed to an immediate "gratification", i.e. to feel the benefit of a medication within 10 – 20 minutes, they have to be explained that there is a "latency period" between the implantation and observation of the clinical effect. The actual length of such "*latent period*" varies from patient to patient but certain *general rules* have been observed:

1. The younger the patient is, the sooner clinical effect appears.
2. The more recent is the onset of the disease, the faster becomes apparent the therapeutic benefit of stem cell transplantation.
3. Metabolically active organs with excellent blood supply, especially endocrine glands, respond faster to stem cell transplantation than organs with slow metabolism.
4. In patients with dominant sympathetic division of autonomous nervous system, the clinical effect of stem cell transplantation appears faster than in those with a dominant parasympathetic division. *[handwritten margin: Sym vs psym]*
5. Symptoms of disturbed autonomous nervous system regulation disappear within 4 - 6 weeks.
6. Sclerotic changes of the old age delay the onset of the therapeutic effect, depending upon the extent and depth of tissue degeneration, and the delay of 4 to 6 months is to be expected [261].

Chapter 31

So long as the mother, Ignorance, lives, it is not safe for Science, the offspring, to divulge the hidden causes of things.
Johannes Kepler, 1571 – 1630, Somnium [1634]

CONCURRENT TREATMENT BY STEM CELL XENOTRANSPLANTATION AND PHARMACEUTICAL DRUGS OF CHEMICAL NATURE

Toxicity of chemical drugs for the entire body, or for certain organ systems, is investigated during the drug approval process by regulatory authorities, but such routine procedures do not include an investigation of the effect of individual drugs of chemical nature on the transplanted stem cells.

Under such circumstances, a warning to minimize the intake of drugs of chemical nature during at least 24 – 48 hours prior to stem cell transplantation and for 72 hours thereafter is logical.

The intake of essential drugs must continue, but all others, often prescribed by various physicians, that did not check the patient's "brown bag", can usually be stopped for a few days without any harm, if not permanently.

The toxicity of drugs of chemical nature for stem cell transplants is not the only matter of concern to stem cell transplantologists. Sometimes the interaction between stem cell transplants and essential drugs is of different nature, as for example, in type 1 diabetic that continues to take insulin while undergoing stem cell transplantation.

As with other diseases where there is a standard treatment, *in the treatment of diabetic complications, stem cell transplantation has to be carried out concurrently with the standard treatment of IDDM* the schedule of which is not altered.

As the transplanted cells do not begin their functioning, or their stimulation of patient's own cells does not start, until one to two months later, it is impossible to stop the ongoing insulinotherapy, even though there is most likely a competitive inhibition of the insulin production by the implanted β-cells of the pancreatic islands, or the "re-awakened" β-cells of the patient, and by the exogenous insulin. At the same time insulin, being a natural substance, is not toxic to the transplanted cells, and thus insulinotherapy can continue without any harm to the transplanted cells.

Logically there is hardly any additive effect between stem cell transplantation and insulinotherapy, on the contrary, there is some degree of *competitive inhibition*, but this is an unavoidable fact that has to be taken under scientific and statistical consideration in the evaluation of results.

The *concomitant insulinotherapy does not influence the level of serum C-peptide and/or the clinical course of already developed diabetic complications*, so that the measured changes of the clinical parameters after the stem cell transplantation can be safely ascribed to the beneficial effect of this treatment.

Chapter 32

Every man takes the limits of his own field of vision for the limits of the world.
Arthur Schopenhauer, 1788 – 1860, Studies in Pessimism [1857]

Intellect is invisible to the man who has none.
Arthur Schopenhauer, 1788 – 1860, Our relations to others

CONCURRENT TREATMENT BY STEM CELL XENOTRANSPLANTATION AND MEDICATIONS PREPARED BY BIOTECHNOLOGICAL METHODS

Extracts of cells of various tissues have been used therapeutically for over a century. Among those classified as cytokines, *lymphokines and other non-immunoglobulin secretions of activated lymphocytes, and monokines of activated monocytes*, have been studied extensively and used in clinical practice for overt 30 years. Their greatest advantage is an *exceptionally high activity even when used in extremely low concentrations*. A substance originally called *leukocyte dialysate (LcD)* belongs to this therapeutic group: it is a *unique immunomodulator*, very valuable because of its complex therapeutic effects.

The actions of leukocyte dialysate were recognized for the first time in 1942 when Karl Landsteiner (discoverer of human blood group antigens and antibodies, 1900) and M.V. Chase accomplished a transfer of the delayed hypersensitivity response of sensitized guinea pigs to the non-sensitized ones by transplanting live guinea pig leukocytes [223].

The same experiment was repeated in 1949 when H.S. Lawrence succeeded to transfer tuberculin hypersensitivity from sensitized donors to non-sensitized human volunteers [223]. Lawrence proved in 1955 that such property is retained also by a *purified leukocyte extract*; and named the effective component of such extract a *"**transfer factor**"* (TF) [224]. In those days, the claims of H.S. Lawrence about the transfer of ability to respond by delayed skin hypersensitivity via a soluble factor of molecular weight lower than 20,000 Da (daltones) were considered "quackery". The dominant theories of those times declared that all immune reactions, including delayed skin hypersensitivity, were dependent on antibodies (Ab) of a molecular weight at least 150,000 Da. In 1963, H.S. Lawrence discovered that the *ability to respond to an immunogen is retained by a leukocyte extract of molecular weight under 10,000 Da*.

In 1960, H.S. Lawrence proved that the final effect of TF results from *the action of many effector substances included in the leukocyte dialysate*, and introduced a term *dialysable leukocyte extract (DLE)*. DLE contains at least 200 components, the most abundant is *thymosin* [225, 226], and there is a wide spectrum of other biologically active substances, *all of molecular weight from 1,000 Da to 20,000 Da*, such as oligopeptides, nucleotides, serotonin, bradykinine, nicotine amide, prostaglandins, ascorbate, etc. One of them - with a molecular weight of only 3,000 Da - is an *antigen specific transfer factor* [227].

Dialyzable leukocyte extract causes the immune system of the recipient to respond to a new antigen as if the immune system have had a memory of previous encounters with that antigen: patient's "virgin" T-lymphocytes would have been already activated, clonal selection have taken place, even before the first exposure to this new antigen. So when the actual contact with the new antigen is made, a massive proliferation of memory and effector T-cells, as in a typical "secondary reaction", promptly develops.

Importantly, the molecule of dialyzable leukocyte extract is small, its molecular weight is low, so that *DLE is non-antigenic*, and does not cause any immune reaction in a recipient.

Even though the induction of cell-mediated immunity, i.e. antigen recognition, is dependent upon the identification of MHC of the individual, dialysable leukocyte extract acts as xenogeneic, it means that it ignores any species barriers in its effect, i.e. it is *"species non-specific"*.

The "transfer factor" has been *defined as the leukocyte dialysate capable to transfer the antigen-specific T-lymphocyte response* [228]. "Transfer factors" are molecules that *educate recipients to express cell-mediated immunity, and this effect is antigen-specific* [229].

Transfer factor exhibits *a broad range of biological activities*: increase of the E-rosette cell count, interferon (IFN) concentration, lymphokines production, antigen-triggered expression of IL-2 receptors on $CD4^+$ lymphocytes, of Ca^{++} influx into blood monocytes, as well as an accentuation of the delayed hypersensitivity skin reaction, etc.

Transfer factor is thermo-labile, and its *biological activity persists for months at temperature range from -20 °C to -70 °C*.

A hypothesis about the existence of transfer factor specificity for each antigen was postulated. The specificity of each transfer factor is based on the presence of at least 6 aminoacids in its structure. The structure of individual antigen-specific transfer factors varies in the same way as the binding of individual antigens on hypervariable regions of immunoglobulins G (IgG) [225].

MEDLINE lists over 1,100 scientific papers describing various uses of dialysable leukocyte extracts for immunotherapy, based on proven facts such as:

- *transfer of a specific immunity within 4 - 6 hours,*
- *long term duration of so transferred immunity,*
- *absence of an inter-species barrier,*
- *acceptance of transferred immune responses as "self",*
- *transfer of immunity by a peroral route.*

Since 1992, the transfer factor has been used successfully in clinical practice in the treatment of many diseases, usually in their advanced stages, when other therapies known to modern medicine failed, such as:

- *combined severe immunodeficiency, Wiscott-Aldrich syndrome, chronic mucocutaneous candidiasis, chronic fatigue syndrome, isolated T-cell defficiency,*
- herpes simplex, herpes zoster, including ocular herpes, mononucleosis, measles, varicella, progressive vaccinia, congenital cytomegalovirus infection,
- tuberculosis of lungs, tuberculosis of bone, sarcoidosis, leprosy, cutaneous leishmaniasis, cryptosporidiosis, cryptococcosis, coccidiomycosis, histoplasmosis,
- *AIDS, mycosis fungoides,*
- *bronchial asthma, chronic obstructive pulmonary disease, interstitial pneumonia,*

- *chronic hepatitis, Crohn's disease,* recurrent aphthous stomatitis,
- female chronic cystitis, chronic cystitis in children, chronic pyelonephritis,
- *agammaglobulinemia, hyperimmunoglobulinemia E, Waldenstrom's macroglobulinemia,*
- *epilepsy, autism, amyotrophic lateral sclerosis, multiple sclerosis, Alzheimer's disease, Guillain-Barre syndrome, subacute sclerosing panencephalitis,*
- chron, uveitis, *Behcet syndrome,* recurrent otitis media,
- psoriasis, discoid lupus erythematosus, lupus vulgaris, hereditary bullous epidermolysis; bullous pemphigoid, pemphigus vegetans, atopic dermatitis, alopetia areata, warts,
- papillomatosis of larynx,
- *metastatic cancer of lungs (all histological types), nasopharynx, bone, kidney, urinary bladder, prostate, liver, colon, uterine cervix, breast, head and neck, as well as osteogenic sarcoma, malignant melanoma in all stages, neuroblastoma, acute leukemia, Hodgkin's disease, Burkitt lymphoma,*
- juvenile rheumatoid arthritis, adult rheumatoid arthritis.

In all of the diseases which are italicized, stem cell transplantation is, or should be, used in the treatment along with transfer factor.

About 30% of publications deals with the use of transfer factor for the treatment of malignancies. The logic behind it has been the concept of F. McFarlane Burnet, presented in 1960, and of L. Thomas of 1970, of host immune surveillance, according to which, the immune system recognizes and destroys frequently developing immunogenic tumor cells.

Cell-mediated immunity is the most important host response for the control of growth of antigenic tumor cells. Humoral immunity has not been found to be of much value for cancer therapy up until now. T-cells are responsible for direct killing of cancer cells and for activation of other components of the immune system. Natural killer (NK) cells apparently play a significant role in this process as well, but up until now they have remained an enigma to the medical science.

Dialysable leukocyte extract lowers the content of DNA and RNA in cancer cells, and diminishes their protein synthesis. DLE also triggers differentiation of hematopoietic stem cells that explains its benefit in cancer patients treated by irradiation and chemotherapy.

It is not quite clear at this time why the immune surveillance fails in the first place, by allowing growth and spread of cancerous cells, originating from the malignant transformation of a normal cell. The idea to use transfer factor has been based on its ability to transfer the antigen specific T-cell response from a donor to a patient with cancerous cells, stimulating patient's own T-cells to act more efficiently.

As all cancer cells of a patient are of monoclonal origin, i.e. they originate from a single transformed cell, at least in the earlier stages of cancer growth, the therapeutically most effective type of dialysable leukocyte extract, a transfer factor, is the one prepared from the patient's own cancerous cells, or white blood cells, if the cancer cells from the biopsy or surgical resection specimen are not available. This is what our group has researched and is available as *individually for each patient prepared dialysable leukocyte extracts*.

At the beginning, most dialysable leukocytes extracts used in research and clinical practice were of human origin, which made the *process of preparation* of DLE's lengthy, inefficient and expensive. After the lack of inter-species barriers was proven beyond any doubt, the donors of DLE became livestock and pigs.

Our group has used rabbits as donors of lymphocytes for variety of reasons: absence of recognizable retroviruses, i.e. rabbit is the sole laboratory animal today that is so distinguished, absence of slow viral infections, fast reproduction cycles with numerous fetuses from each pregnancy, ease of manipulation during the production process and during the collection of blood and tissue specimens of spleen, lymphnodes, so it is obvious that there is a full compatibility between stem cell xenotransplants of rabbit origin and transfer factor of rabbit origin.

Chapter 33

It is not enough to have a good mind. The main thing is to use it well.

The first precept was never to accept a thing as true until I know it as such without a single doubt.
René Descartes, 1596 - 1650, Le Discours de la Méthode [1637]

TREATMENT OF IATROGENIC DISEASES BY STEM CELL XENOTRANSPLANTATION

New practitioners of stem cell transplantation ask why so many patients receive the stem cell transplants of hypothalamus and adrenal cortex? The reason is a *malfunction of hypothalamus – adrenal cortex – peripheral endocrine gland axis* that is very common in patients living in the modern fast world due to two causes:

1. modern medicine prescribes cortisone for many diseases, for an excessive length of time, and chronic cortisone intake suppresses the function of the adrenal cortex,
2. chronic stress triggers an excessive secretion of adrenaline and cortisol from the respective cells of adrenal medulla and cortex, and that brings on a state of chronic exhaustion of cortisol-producing cells of adrenal cortex.

In both situations stem cell transplantation treatment of the patient suffering either from chronic bronchial asthma treated by cortisone for 15 years, or from "manager syndrome" for 10 years, must include a support of hypothalamus - adrenal cortex - peripheral endocrine gland axis in order to get a good clinical result. Another example is secondary amenorrhea and infertility after the many years' use of contraceptives, when it is necessary to - restart the functioning of the same axis of hypothalamus - adrenal cortex - ovary. The regeneration of various neurons damaged by the use of various "home-made" street drugs requires stem cell transplantation as well.

Chapter 34

The facts will eventually test all our theories, and they form, after all, the only impartial jury to which we can appeal.
Jean Louis Rodolphe Agassiz, 1807 - 1873, Geological Sketches [1870]

New opinions are always suspected, and usually opposed, without any other reason but because they are not already common.
John Locke, 1632 - 1704. Essay Concerning Human Understanding [1690]

MONO- VS. POLY-THERAPY BY STEM CELL XENOTRANSPLANTATION

This discussion was *begun in Chapter* 30.

Here the explanation of the concept of *simultaneous implantation of various cell transplants in accordance with the pathophysiology of the treated disease of each individual patient, is offered*, i.e. the basis of the described clinical approach to the stem cell transplantation. It is gradually gaining ground in the US under a term "composite grafts" [23-26, 181].

If we take diabetes mellitus as an example to explain this concept, there is a difference between the treatment of a patient with an early IDDM, soon after the sudden onset in childhood, and of the patient with a chronic IDDM with complications. In an *early IDDM*, the repeated implantation of cell transplants of Langerhans islets of pancreas alone is probably sufficient for the disease control. In the old IDDM, when secondary organs and tissues of the patient have become exhausted by an over-load of having to compensate for malfunction of the diseased organ or tissue for many years, these secondary damaged organs or tissues have to be treated by an implantation of appropriate stem cell transplants along with stem cells of the islets of pancreas: hypothalamus, liver, adrenal cortex, stomach/intestine (i.e. "peripancreatic block"), placenta.

Placenta good for damaged vascular system

When the clinical picture shows clear pathological changes of the retinopathy, nephropathy, etc. due to advanced stages of IDDM, it is hard to conceive that there are no pathological changes of the regulatory organ, i.e. *hypothalamus*; of the key organ of metabolism, i.e. *liver*; or of the organ that copes with a chronic metabolic stress, i.e. *adrenal cortex*; and that these organs do not require a direct stimulation by the stem cell transplants of the same organs.

The reasoning behind an implantation of "*peripancreatic block*" is to transplant:

1. the tissues with the greatest supply of *stem* cells of the pancreatic islets,
2. the GALT (gut-associated lymphoid tissue) and MALT (mucosa-associated lymphoid tissue), intimately involved in the auto-immune pathogenesis of IDDM,
3. other cells involved in the paracrine regulation of function of the Langerhans islets.

Placenta has been known as the source of cells capable to induce the repair of the damaged vascular system and is added for all diabetic patients with microangiopathic complications.

Undoubtedly, we are dealing with an "empirical science" here, based on observation of hundreds of thousands of patients by experienced physicians over many decades. But the foundation of this intellectual process have been solid scientific facts about the structure and function of the living body. At the same time, we have to be humble and acknowledge that the field of the stem cell transplantation is virtually at the "beginning of the road".

There are two schools of thought in stem cell transplantation today. The classical school, followed by the author, and developed originally by the founders of cell therapy, calls for an implantation of cell transplants of all those organs and tissues that have been damaged or malfunction as a result of a disease(s) of a particular patient. Only in a very early stage of a disease is an implantation of only one stem cell transplant of a primarily damaged organ or tissue (so called "monotherapy") sufficient to repair the damage. The newer school of thought has called for "monotherapy" in every case, but lately the need to co-transplant other cell transplants along with the primary one has been widely discussed in the Anglophone literature.

Hypothalamic-pituitary system participates closely in the regulation of insulin secretion. Stress increases the activity of this system, and that applies to the stress of metabolic derangement of decompensated IDDM as well. IDDM-induced pathological responses of hypothalamic-pituitary system cause changes in the secretion of hypothalamic release factors and pituitary tropic hormones that in turn lead to hormonal changes in the periphery, and those trigger further metabolic dysfunction, and the vicious circle is closed. On the basis of the above, *a theory on the pathogenesis of diabetic angiopathies* has evolved: DM-induced abnormal carbohydrate and lipid metabolism triggers a stress reaction, that includes sudden severe changes of level of various hormones, and such hormonal changes cause damage to blood vessels over a long time. Abnormal utilization of glucose by the cells of an organism leads to a *compensatory increased activity of hypothalamic – pituitary - adrenal axis*, as a result of which there is an *increased secretion of insulin antagonists*: glucagon, somatotropin, cortisol, and other contra-insulin hormones, all of which play a role in the mechanism of development of secondary complications of diabetes mellitus [138, 139, 140].

This theory appears more logical and correct than the newer one implicating a lack of C-peptide as the cause of microangiopathic complications of IDDM, because it is based on well-known facts of physiology. No one has proved that C-peptide has any physiologic function in the body yet [67, 149]. The recently proposed and tried addition of C-peptide to insulin as a treatment of diabetic microangiopathy does not seem logical. There probably are some other factors in the various cells of the Langerhans islets of pancreas that may play a part in the development of diabetic microangiopathy, but to try to isolate them and use them as a part of treatment seems implausible.

Another leading theory proclaims that the extensive irreversible damage of organism and development of secondary lesions after years, or decades of disturbed metabolism in diabetes mellitus relates largely to the severity and chronicity of hyperglycaemia. It has been the basis of the DCCT approach to the treatment of DM. The NIH statistics of 50% decrease of incidence of microangiopathic complications of IDDM appear convincing, but not to many US practicing diabetologists. Besides that, the rigid maintenance of blood sugar level bordering on hypoglycemia makes the everyday living very hard for the patients.

Two distinct mechanisms of the development of complications of diabetes mellitus have been proposed by this theory:

1. *Protein glycosylation*: Irreversible binding of glucose to free amino groups of proteins creates "advanced glycation end products" in proportion to the degree of hyperglycaemia. This inactivates the function of certain proteins, and causes cross-linking of others. The cross-linking of proteins allegedly contributes to the thickening of the basement membrane, so typical of diabetes mellitus. "Advanced glycation end products" are bound to cell membrane receptors that support collagen accumulation in the basal membrane of endothelium. Collagen fibers subjected to glycosylation, cause thickening of basal membranes with blockage of passage through endothelial wall, and narrowing of lumen, i.e. *microangiopathy*. Clinically it appears as retinopathy, nephropathy (Kimmelstiel-Wilson syndrome, glomerulosclerosis), etc.

   Nephropathy causes hypertension, which along with increased VLDL and increased blood clotting, triggers *macroangiopathies*: myocardial infarction, CVA, peripheral arterial disease with gangrenes.

2. *Polyol pathway*: Hyperglycaemia *increases the uptake of glucose by tissues not dependent on insulin via a variety of metabolic pathways*, of which the polyol pathway is the best known. Such an augmentation of sorbitol (polyol) pathway of glucose metabolism via activation of aldose reductase leads to *accumulation of sorbitol* (sugar alcohol or polyol) *that cannot pass through cell membrane, accumulates in cell and causes intracellular edema.* The resulting *blockage takes place also in the blood vessel walls* of retina, kidneys, aorta, and peripheral nerves, with resulting swelling, hypoxia, and metabolic impairment of these structures, a very plausible pathogenesis of diabetic microangiopathy. Drugs that inhibit aldose reductase prevent the development of cataracts, retinal damage, peripheral neuropathy, and early functional derangement of kidneys.

An accumulation of sorbitol in the lens of the eye causes water retention that lowers the transparency of lens and thereby causes *cataract*. An accumulation of sorbitol in Schwann cells and neurons disrupts energy flow in axons, causing *polyneuropathy*, especially affecting autonomous nervous system, sensation, and reflexes.

Due to insufficient glucose intake and extracellular hyperosmolality, the cells are losing water and their function suffers. For example, in lymphocytes this dehydration leads to creation of superoxides, lowered defense capabilities, and *predisposition toward infections* in diabetics.

Hyperglycemia supports production of various plasma proteins and thereby increased blood viscosity and blood clotting, with increased risk of *thromboembolism* [164].

Let's consider the *atherosclerotic coronary heart disease*, the major cause of death among adults with diabetes mellitus. Cerebrovascular accidents, peripheral arterial disease with obstructions, and other major vasculopathies, are also common with diabetes mellitus. The extent and severity of atherosclerotic lesions in large- and medium-sized arteries are increased in long-standing diabetes mellitus, and their development is accelerated.

The multiplicity of pathogenetic factors responsible for atherosclerosis with diabetes mellitus is the best argument in favor of described method of "targeted poly- therapy" over the "monotherapy":

1. hypertension is present in one-half of diabetes mellitus patients for no obvious reason,
2. glycosylated LDL (low density lipoproteins) do not readily bind to the LDL receptor in the liver, thereby LDL-cholesterol remains in the lumen of blood vessels available for atheroma development,
3. there is an enhanced turnover of glycosylated HDL (high density lipoprotein), thereby decreasing its protection against atherosclerosis,
4. there is cross-linking of glycosylated proteins in the arterial wall,
5. defect of lipoprotein lipase in diabetics leads to an impaired lipolysis of chylomicrons, that are atherogenic,
6. platelet aggregation and synthesis of thromboxane A2 is increased in diabetics,
7. sorbitol accumulation in the cells of arterial walls could be atherogenic [164].

These seven pathogenetic factors are tied to hypothalamus (No. 1), adrenal cortex (Nos. 1 and 5), liver (Nos. 2, 3, 5, and 7), placenta (Nos. 1, 4, and 6), peripancreatic block (No. 1), our recommended co-stem cell transplants along with islets of pancreas.

Niehans stated that endocrine glands are under control of the central regulator, and have a reciprocal influence on one another, so that consequently cell transplantation treatment of any endocrine disease must almost always be of a polyglandular type. As the organism does not store hormones, but produces only the quantities necessary for the momentary needs, treatment by hormones is only a temporary form of therapy and does not ever lead to a cure. In addition, over a course of time, an atrophy of the primary endocrine gland due to competitive inhibition ensues, and thereby a cessation of the function of its cells [18].

In the treatment of IDDM with complications, we recommend using stem cell xenotransplants of pancreatic islets, "co-transplants" liver, "peripancreatic block", adrenal cortex, placenta and hypothalamus.

Liver: Liver is a key organ of metabolism, and that applies also to the metabolism of a majority of hormones. So the high incidence of diabetic hepatopathy is not surprising. In liver biopsies of 100 consecutive patients undergoing surgery for morbid obesity, all those with diabetes had some steatosis of liver, and in 42% the steatosis was severe. Increased liver intake of saturated fatty acids is caused by lipolysis, secondary to the deficit of insulin, and a compensatory action of cortisol. Liver fibrosis was found in 81% of diabetics, and cirrhosis in 10% of diabetics [105]. In autopsy materials, the cirrhosis of liver is found at least twice as often in diabetic than in nondiabetics. In clinical studies of patients with chronic liver disease, such as steatosis, fibrosis, cirhosis, chronic active hepatitis, the prevalence of diabetes ranges from 10 to 75% [105]. Hepatomegaly is present in 100% of patients with diabetic ketoacidosis.

Fetal liver was found to have a positive trophic effect on fetal pancreas when separately prepared tissue fragments of both organs were implanted next to each other. It elaborated factor(s) that promote engrafment and/or function of co-transplanted fetal pancreas [181]. The time interval between transplantation and normoglycemia was shorter in the recipients of composite fetal liver/fetal pancreas grafts. There are several mediators that could be responsible for these paracrine effects. Insulin-like growth factor (IGF-1) is elaborated by fetal liver, and it increases replication, insulin synthesis and islets' growth in culture, induces neovascularization as well, that may be important for islet differentiation. Simultaneous intramuscular injection of IGF-1 with fetal islet transplantation increases the overall success rate, and decreases the quantity of islets needed for normoglycemia [26]. The addition of IGF-1 to the culture of islets was found to be beneficial [27]. Perhaps some other factor released by fetal hepatocytes may protect the islet cells, such as IGF-2, [23, 25, 46] or somatomedins, acting in a paracrine manner [27, 162].

After transplantation to the adult liver, epithelial progenitor cells from adult pancreas differentiate into hepatocytes, express liver-specific proteins, and become fully integrated into the liver parenchyma. Apparently adult liver and pancreas retain common progenitor cells that upon activation, proliferate and differentiate along a specific foregut epithelial cell lineage. The same applies to the adult tissues of the brain, bone mesenchyme, and bronchial epithelium [24, 159].

Intrahepatic transplantation of islets causes a modification of structure and function of hepatocytes surrounding the islets. These new, hepatocyte-like cells, contain in their cytoplasm typical insulin granules, i.e. they are hybrids, that developed as a result of paracrine influence of islet cells [131].

Liver has the potential to immunologically protect other simultaneously transplanted organs from the same donor. Severity of allograft rejection can be reduced by simultaneous intrasplenic transplantation of isolated liver cells from the same donor [42].

Transplantation of unmodified fetal liver cells into allogeneic recipients results in stable multilineage chimerism with donor-specific tolerance, due to the presence of pluripotent hematopoietic stem cell in the fetal liver, capable of engrafment in allogeneic adult recipients [6].

Liver and gut are organized stem cell lineage systems, with three compartments: a *slow cycling stem cell compartment*, with cells expressing a fetal phenotype and responding slowly to injury; an *amplification compartment*, with cells of intermediate phenotype rapidly proliferating in response to regeneration stimuli or acute injuries; and a *terminal differentiation compartment* in which cells increasingly differentiate and gradually lose their ability to divide [22].

Stomach/intestine, a "peripancreatic block": Physiological abnormalities associated with diabetes have been described in every part of the digestive tract where measurements can be made [105]. Prevalence of gallstones, peptic ulcer, diverticultitis, irritable bowel syndrome, undiagnosed frequent abdominal pain, constipation, etc., has been found by the National Health Interview Survey (NHIS) in 1989 significantly higher in diabetics than nondiabetics [105]. In 32% of all hospitalizations of diabetics there was at least one digestive disease diagnosis [105]. They result from autonomic neuropathy, diabetic microangiopathy, electrolyte imbalances secondary to uncontrolled diabetes, altered levels of insulin and glucagon causing depression of gastrointestinal mobility and secretion, and increased susceptibility to gastrointestinal infections.

Diabetic gastropathy occurs in 28% of patients with IDDM. There is an association between DM and constipation. Secretory abnormalities of exocrine pancreas are common in diabetics, for example 73% had diminished carbohydrate output to secretin administration. Exocrine pancreatic atrophy is probably caused by insulin deficiency [105]. The diagnosis of chronic pancreatitis was found in a high percentage of hospital discharges with diabetes [105]. Prevalence of celiac disease in IDDM patients has varied from 1.1% to 11%. In reverse, 5.4% of patients with celiac disease has also IDDM [105].

Here is a reason for using "peripancreatic block" in the stem cell transplantation treatment of complications of diabetes mellitus:

1. *Undifferentiated epithelium in the duodenal anlage is stimulated by the overlying mesenchyme to grow and differentiate into mature pancreas* with acinar, endocrine and ductal structures. In the *first, early, undifferentiated stage*, endoderm evaginates as the starting step of the chain of morphogenetic events; at that time among the pancreatic cell differentiation genes only endocrine ones, for insulin and glucagons, are expressed. In the *second stage*, epithelial branching with a formation of primitive ducts, and differentiation and separation of islet cells from the epithelium, and from the basement membrane, takes place. In the *third stage*, acinar cells form with enzyme carrying zymogen granules. The purity of the islets suggests that the lineage of most or all of the original epithelial cells was channeled toward the endocrine phenotype so that it appears that the *default path for growth of embryonic pancreatic epithelium is to form islets*. Islet formation requires no specific embryonic signals, and neither presence of ducts nor mesenchyme nor acini [28].

In the endocrine portion of human or animal fetal pancreas, a proliferation of respective precursor stem cells, and their further differentiation into a new generation of islet cells, takes place. In the fetal pancreas a large quantity of β-cells is present outside of Langerhans islands, and this status persists partially even after birth, and there are also many *acinar-islet complexes* present, which have been thought of as another important source of pancreatic stem cells [124, 125]. This is the reason why mechanical separation of pancreatic islets in fetal donors is useless for manufacturing.

In the adult organism stem cells can re-activate too. As examples of activation of respective stem cells can serve the adult urinary bladder epithelium induced by fetal urogenital sinus mesenchyme to form prostatic glandular tissue, adult mammary tissue induced by fetal salivary mesenchyme to produce salivary gland tissue, or adult pancreatic duct epithelium directed by fetal mesenchyme toward islet cytodifferentiation [29].

2. *Inclusion of stem cell transplants from peripancreatic lymph nodes with islet cell transplants provides a high degree of protection from autoimmune β-cell destruction*: recipient rats became chimeric for a donor auto-regulatory T cell population from the peripancreatic lymph nodes, capable to suppress the autoimmune state. In diabetic patients that are not lymphopenic, the number of autoregulatory cells required to abrogate auto-immunity may be quite small and difficult to detect macroscopically [41].

The human gastrointestinal tract contains as much lymphoid tissue as the spleen does. The mucosal T cell population is composed of both $CD4^+$ and $CD8^+$ cells, with the former being twice as numerous as the latter, just as in peripheral blood. Dome cells of the lymphoid aggregate, just below the epithelium, are rich in APC's, i.e. cells capable of antigen presentation following exposure to antigens via oral feeding *in vivo* [108].

The lining of gastro-intestinal tract has a specific function of absorbing a food from the environment into the organism, and it excludes unwanted factors from it, such as microrganisms, etc. *The principal protective tools* are the *GALT* (gut-associated lymphoid tissue) and *MALT* ('mucosa-associated lymphoid tissue'). *In the jejunum there are 20 intra-epithelial lymphocytes per 100 epithelial cells, mostly T-lymphocytes.* Antigen from the food is presented by APC's to the lymphocytes of GALT and MALT, and that leads to a lymphoid cell division. Dividing lymphoblasts travel with antigens via regional lymphatics to the mesenteric lymph nodes, where further cell division takes place, and here the activated lymphocytes acquire the ability to "home" to the gut. Subsequently they enter blood via intestinal lymphatics and thoracic duct. Immunoblasts ultimately extravasate through high endothelial venules in the gut following the 'homing' principle [163].

Antigens administered directly to the gastrointestinal tract frequently elicit a local antibody response in the intestinal lamina propria, while at the same time produce a *state of systemic tolerance* that manifests itself as *a diminished response to the same antigen if it is administered in immunogenic form elsewhere in the body* (split tolerance) [165]. Orally administered antigens induce tolerance to themselves by a variety of mechanisms. High doses of antigen can cause anergy or deletion due to clonal exhaustion. Low doses can induce priming of T cells in the gut, primarily $CD4^+$ cells: T_H2 cells produce cytokines, such as IL-10, and T_H3 cells produce TGFβ, that in turn inhibits the proliferation and functioning of B cells, cytotoxic T cells and NK cells, and also inhibits cytokine production in lymphocytes, and antagonizes the effects of TNF. Although the induction of mucosal T_H2 and T_H3 is antigen specific, the suppressive activity of TGFβ is not. Thus the *induction of oral tolerance to one antigen is able to suppress the immune response to a second, associated antigen* [165, 166].

Oral unresponsiveness may be due to induction of antigen-specific suppressor T cells in Payer's patches, or due to the presence of antigen-nonspecific suppresor cells, or due to clonal inhibition (or clonal anergy) resulting from a direct effect of antigens on B or T cells in mucosal follicles [108]. The mucosal system elaborates suppressor cells that interact with ubiquitous antigens and down-regulate responses not only in the mucosal but also in systemic lymphoid tissue. This could be *the reason for tolerance of cell xenotransplants prepared from organs and tissues of domestic animals used as a food by humans, particularly when also a variety of animal organs from many different animal species are consumed by the population,* as is typical in Europe, China, and many other countries.

3. *The liver and exocrine pancreas* may have a modulating if not causal role in the development of DM for various regulatory

reasons. There is a hypothesis about independent insulin-regulating mechanism of the gastrointestinal tract, in which the key role is played by the hormones and peptides of the stomach and duodenum, functioning simultaneously with those of pancreas [74, 105]. *The same neuropeptides produced by hypothalamic neurons are produced in the pancreatic islets by the neuroendocrine cells from the upper portion of the gastrointestinal tract: they function in the paracrine manner*, presumably influencing the function of the pancreatic islets [155, 162] (see under description of "duodenal anlage" above).

Somatostatin is a neuropeptide synthetized by *hypothalamic neurons, δ-cells of islets of pancreas, and by the mucosa of the gastrointestinal tract*. It is a *powerful inhibitor of GH release* by blocking the stimulation of the hypothalamic GHRH (growth hormone releasing hormone), and TSH (thyroid stimulating hormone) [155, 162, 163].

Somatostatin *suppresses secretion of insulin*, as well as the exocrine secretion of the pancreas [163]. In decompensated IDDM the hypersecretion of somatostatin takes place, even at rest. In subcompensated IDDM with ketoacidosis, the secretion of somatostatin goes up 250% after physical load. The strongest stimulus for secretion of somatostatin is insulin induced hypoglycemia, however. There is *a direct correlation between increased secretion of somatostatin and labile course of diabetes mellitus* that leads to increased sensitivity of peripheral tissues to endogenous somatostatin.

Somatostatin stimulates glucagon-secreting α-cells of islets, and increases activity of enzymes involved in insulin breakdown.

Increased somatostatin in IDDM causes an augmentation of sorbitol (polyol) pathway of glucose metabolism, which leads to accumulation of sorbitol in cell membranes, as described above [164].

Somatomedins are produced in many tissues in response to GH, particularly in the liver. Without them GH cannot carry out its growth-promoting functions. (*See further discussion below under Hypothalamus*).

Gastrin is a group of 7 peptides, produced by *modified cells of the mucosa of the pre-pyloric portion of stomach and duodenum, as well as δ -cells of pancreas*, after gastric stimulation by food, or after stimulation of vagus nerve. *C-terminal portion of gastrin and octapeptid of cholecystokinin* are found in the brain in high concentrations, as well as in the cerebrospinal fluid. Besides other actions, gastrin stimulates secretion of insulin [74].

Increased serum levels of gastrin are found in diabetics after 8 - 19 years' duration of disease. After stem cell transplantation, serum levels of gastrin drop to normal [70].

There is a *correlation between the lowered serum level of gastrin and improvement of symptoms of diabetic polyneuropathy after stem cell transplantation* [70, 74].

Glucagon is produced by α-cells of Langerhans islands, which represent 75% of the cells of the islet. Since insulin and glucagon have an opposite effect on the liver, and since glucose suppresses secretion of glucagon, a theory was proposed that carbohydrate homeostasis is controlled by a molar relationship of insulin/glucagon rather than by a concentration of each of these two hormones individually [140].

Glucagon can impair glucose tolerance only when there is an absolute lack of insulin, as is the case with IDDM. In diabetes mellitus, glucagon worsens the effect of insulin deficit. In decompensated diabetes mellitus, the glucagon secretion triggered by food intake causes an additional rise of hyperglycaemia after a meal [141]. In patients with decompensated IDDM the level of glucagon is 4 - 5 times, and in compensated IDDM 2 - 3 times, above the normal level. The level of glucagon in severe labile forms of IDDM grows accordingly. When an exogenous glucagon is injected in the amount that would increase its concentration to a level usually found in diabetics with metabolic decompensation, a significant rise of blood flow through kidneys and, in parallel, of glomerular filtration, takes place. Glucagon increases the ejection volume of the heart. As glucagon breaks down in kidneys, there is higher level of glucagon in uremia. After islet cell transplantation, the concentration of glucagon drops to the normal level, or is significantly decreased, depending upon the level of compensation of IDDM [142]. Glucagon increases production of ketone bodies from fatty acid progenitors [141].

There is a correlation between an increased level of glucagon and higher rates of autonomous neuropathy [141].

Subcutaneous implantation of pieces of **placenta**, i.e. "Filatov treatment", has been a treatment that countless millions of patients have taken ever since it was described by Russian opthalmologist Filatov. As he was developing the transplantation of cornea, and the clinical results were not satisfactory, regardless of what he tried, at some point he decided to implant subcutaneously to the patient/recipient at the time of corneal transplantation also pieces of human placenta. Suddenly his corneal transplantation results dramatically improved. He became obsessed with placental implantation, and this method of treatment became known world-wide. Oddly, the modern medicine, as well as regulatory agencies, has totally ignored this therapeutic method. No official statistics exist about the results, but there are no condemnations of this therapeutic method either. School of cell therapy has used placenta as a part of the therapeutic combination for a variety of conditions, for reasons that "were so obvious", that there are not too many publications explaining them.

In 58-cell human blastocyst of the human conceptus, the outer cells, destined to produce trophoblasts of the placenta, cannot be distinguished from the inner cells, destined to form the embryo. In 107-cell human blastocyst, 8 embryo-producing cells are surrounded by 99 trophoblastic cells. This completely explains the reason for frequent use of tissue fragments of the placenta by the school of cell therapy. The absolutely unique metabolic, endocrine, and immunological properties of trophoblasts, *that are the same cells as the "embryonic stem cells"* from which the entire human being can be "built", also makes them the "universal stem cells" [110].

Placenta is the largest endocrine organ of any organism. It produces:

1. chorionic gonadotropin (only in human and primates), with the biological activity of luteinizing hormone (LH), produced principally in the syncytiotrophoblast, with an important paracrine assistance of cytotrophoblasts,
2. placental lactogen, combining lactogenic and potent growth hormone-like bioactivity, structurally very similar to growth hormone (GH), produced by syncytiotrophoblast alone,
3. chorionic adrenocorticotropin, with an ACTH-like biological activity,
4. chorionic thyrotropin,
5. parathyroid hormone-related protein, with the biologic activity of parathyroid hormone, produced by cytotrophoblasts,
6. hypothalamic-like-releasing hormones: for each known hypothalamic-releasing hormone there is an analog produced in placenta, i.e.

- gonadotropin-releasing hormone (GRH), present in cytotrophoblasts only,
- corticotropin-releasing hormone CRH), present in trophoblast, amnion, chorion, and decidua,
- thyrotropin-releasing hormone (TRH),
- growth hormone-releasing hormone (GHRH), present in cytotrophoblasts,
- inhibin, which inhibits action of pituitary FSH, present in syncytiotrophoblast,

7. estrogens: estradiol and estriol, produced in enormous amounts exclusively by syncytiotrophoblasts,
8. progesterone, produced in large amounts in syncytiotrophoblast [110].

Amnion produces vasoactive peptides: endothelin-1, potent vasoconstrictor, and parathyroid hormone-related protein, vasorelaxant, thus perhaps serving as a modulator of chorionic blood vessel tone and blood flow [110].

Pregnancy is an immunoprotected state. The fetus, only half matched to the mother, is a partial allograft, yet it is not rejected [40]. Clinical evidence for depressed cell immunity during pregnancy is indisputable. Class I and class II MHC antigens are absent from trophoblasts at all stages of gestation in human and other mammalian species [108, 110]. In mice, low levels of class I MHC antigens present at the conception disappear in the cytotrophoblasts, i.e. in Langhans cells, the germinal cells or cellular precursors of the syncytiotrophoblast, and secretory cells, by the time of implantation [110]. The extravillous cytotrophoblasts transcribes the non-classic class I HLA-G gene, not expressed on any other human cell type, and synthetize a unique class I HLA-G protein, most likely involved in the invasion of trophoblast [110]. Both trophoblasts and decidua probably produce agents that suppress lymphocyte immune responses [110]. But the changes in T cell morphology and function are inconsistent, and the same applies to B cells [108]. During murine pregnancy there is a weakening of T_H1 responses and strengthening of T_H2 responses.

The trophoblast is capable of phagocytosis, and secretes cytokines associated with macrophages, thus could be a part of macrophage-like tissues distributed throughout the body. In the fetal portion of the placenta the actively phagocytic Hofbauer cells are found [110].

Placenta cells increase the capillary collateral network by stimulating the development of collateral buds. They dilate the blood vessels and thus improve circulation of the blood throughout the organism. They have a hypotensive and a strong diuretic effect. The placenta of the very early fetus is rich in cells with pituitary-like phenotype while the placenta of the mature fetus acts more in the manner of cells of the sex glands [18]. In stem cell transplantation, *placenta assures the nutrition of fetal cells* [18].

Adrenals: Adrenal cortex is essential to life. In adulthood it comprises 80 - 90 % of the weight of adrenals. It consists of outer zona glomerulosa, where mineralocorticoids are produced, middle zona fasciculata, in which glucocorticoids are produced, and inner zona reticularis, where androgens are produced. The hormones of adrenal cortex play a key role in the metabolism of proteins, carbohydrates and fats, and water and electrolytes. They modulate the tissue response to injury or infection. Stress reaction is largely dependent on the adrenals: vasodilatation, increased oxidation, increased basal metabolic rate, increase blood pressure, bradycardia, hyperthermia, increased body strength, resistance to infection, etc., are all important in the 'fight or flight' response [162].

Glucocorticoids are insulin antagonists via:

1. their direct action on insulin-sensitive tissues:

    a) they stimulate gluconeogenesis by increased proteolysis,
    b) they decrease glucose intake by lowering the affinity of insulin to insulin receptors in muscle and fatty tissues,

2. their indirect action by potentiating the action of other diabetogenic hormones, such as glucagon and somatostatin; while increased level of glucagon, somatostatin, or cortison, alone, causes only slight hyperglycaemia, in decompensated IDDM the combined effect of increased levels of all contra-insulin hormones multiplies on a geometric scale. As an example, cortisol alone has only weak influence on glucose production, but it enhances the short-term effect of increased glucagon level on liver into a sustained one, that leads to prolonged hyperproduction of glucose.

Cortisol is required for the storage of glucose as glycogen, maintenance of plasma glucose level, and for survival during prolonged fasting. It blocks the suppressive effect of insulin on hepatic glucose output. Cortisol favors glucose output by the liver, whereas insulin inhibits it. The net result of cortisol excess is a rise in plasma glucose concentration and a compensatory increase in plasma insulin levels. When the rise in insulin is insufficient, diabetes mellitus can develop, or, if already present, greatly deteriorate.

Glucocorticoids increase the concentration of blood cholesterol, fatty acids, triglycerides and LDL lipoproteins, and this explains why their increased level in IDDM contributes to an increased incidence of vascular complications with severe, labile course of the disease. In addition, cortisol affects CNS function by modulating perceptual and emotional functioning, skeletal metabolism by a decrease of bone formation, hematopoiesis, muscle function by positive inotropic effect, renal function by water retention and hyponatremia. Cortisol supports vascular responsiveness that is important for the maintenance of normal blood pressure. So *cortisol is catabolic, antianabolic, and diabetogenic hormone* [162].

Cortisol is required for survival of "stressed" organism. Patients with serious illnesses, or with hypoglycemia, secrete extra cortisol: *the higher the cortisol level, the higher the mortality*. Activation of cell-mediated immunity increases ACTH and cortisol release: a *significant feedback relationship exists between immune and endocrine systems*. Cortisol prevents the proliferation of thymus-derived lymphocytes, thus blocking the entire cell-mediated immunity; decreases the production of T_H1 cytokine, while sparing T_H2 responses; induces the production of TGFβ, that inhibits immune response; and reduces the process of inflammation. Adrenal cortex synthesizes Il-1 and Il-6 that are potent stimulators of adrenal corticosteroid production, via CRH (corticotropin-releasing hormone) [162, 166]. Adrenal cortical cells may provide local steroid secretion to protect other cell types from rejection [181].

Aldosterone sustains extracellular fluid volume by conservation of sodium, and deficiency of aldosterone produces a critical negative sodium balance, with hypovolemia and hypotension. It also prevents an overload of potassium by accelerating its excretion. The juxtaglomerular cells of kidneys and the zona glomerulosa form a feedback system for maintenance of extracellular fluid volume [162].

Fetal adrenals are the largest organ of the fetus. At term, the weight of the fetal adrenals approximates the weight of the adult adrenals. *Relative to body weight, the human fetal adrenals are 25 times larger* than those of the adult. More than 85% of the fetal adrenal gland is composed of the peculiar fetal zone, not found in the adult adrenals. Near term, the daily fetal adrenal steroid production is 8 - 10 times higher than that in resting adults [110].

Hypothalamus acts as an integration center controlling the autonomous, endocrine and behavioral responses, essential for the survival of the individual animal, and of the species: water balance, thermoregulation, food intake, aggression, reproductive functions, sleep-wake cycle [167]. It is the oldest part of the diencephalon, called "central gray matter", *closely connected with the frontal lobe of the cerebrum, limbic system, thalamus, basal ganglia, brain stem, eyes, and pituitary,* the "master" of the autonomous nervous system, regulating almost all internal body functions, including that of immune system, homeostasis, as well as motivations, and emotions. Electric stimulation of hypothalamus will cause hyperglycaemia, among many other internal changes [156]. By puncturing the mid-brain of a rabbit, Claude Bernard succeeded in inducing diabetes mellitus, i.e. "diabetic puncture". Lesions of tuber cinereum cause diabetes mellitus as well [18].

Within the hypothalamus there are multiple non-distinct clusters of cells, sometimes called *hypothalamic nuclei*. Two of them are well defined: *supraoptic and paraventricular nuclei* produce two peptide hormones, i.e. ADH and oxytocin, that are stored in the posterior lobe of the pituitary, and released as necessary [161].

Neurosecretory cells *within the medial basal hypothalamus*, i.e. 'hypophysiotropic area', produce *six neurohormones, called "releasing factors"*, that control the synthesis and secretion of six hormones of the anterior pituitary, which they enter via a unique portal venous circulation [67, 162]. Hypothalamus is a central relay station for collecting and integrating signals from different sources and funneling them into the pituitary. The output of pituitary hormones responds to changes in autonomic nervous system activity. *Anterior pituitary lies outside of blood-brain barrier, but its hormones can penetrate through blood-brain-barrier via retrograde flow of pituitary portal veins, or via fenestrated cells of the capillaries that bathe hypothalamic neurons* [162].

Growth hormone (GH) is a protein hormone with anabolic effects. Growth-promoting effect of GH requires participation of other peptides; such as, somatomedins, that resemble pro-insulin in structure. They are called insulin growth factors (IGF). *IGF-1 has 50% and IGF-2 has 70% aminoacid homology with A and B chains of insulin.* They are produced by many tissues in response to GH. They work as endocrine hormones as well as in paracrine fashion. (*See also above under "peripancreatic block"*).

Under normal conditions the secretion and actions of GH and insulin are metabolically coordinated. But under pathologic conditions the insulin-antagonistic nature of GH becomes apparent: by stimulation of lipolysis, and inhibition of glucose uptake, the actions of GH are diabetogenic [162].

Corticotropin-releasing hormone (CRH) - adrenocorticotropic hormone (ACTH) - cortisol axis is central to the integrated responses to stress, which involves multiple hormones: ACTH, catecholamines, ADH, angiotensin, glucagon, growth hormone. CRH-secreting cells are regulated by many different nerve impulses, with a participation of several neurotransmitters: norepinehrine, serotonine, acetylcholine, dopamine, and GABA. Via a negative feedback control system, in response to CRH, the ACTH is released, and ACTH in turn stimulates cortisol production. Hypothalamic - pituitary - gonadal axis is essential for a reproductive process in both males and females. GRH (gonadotropin- releasing hormone) stimulates synthesis and secretion of both FSH and LH that in turn control the function of granulosa and luteal cells of the ovary, and of the Leyding cells and Sertoli's cells of the testis [67, 155, 167].

The control of the immune system by the central nervous system is accepted today. Most lymphoid tissues receive direct sympathetic innervation. The nervous system controls output of various hormones, in particular corticosteroids, GH, thyroxine and adrenaline that in turn affect the immune system. Il-1 and Il-6 are produced by neurons and glial cells, predominantly of hypothalamus, and by pituitary cells [165].

Chapter 35

How glorious it is, but how painful it is also, to be exceptional in this world!
Alfred de Musset, 1810 - 1857, La Merle Blanc [1842]

DESCRIPTION OF VARIOUS STEM CELL XENOTRANSPLANTS

LANGERHANS ISLETS OF PANCREAS
Organ culture, individual cells and cell clusters, islet cells with granules, estimated 80% of total B cells (β), 10% A (α), D and PP cells, and 10% other cells, including stem cells.

ADRENAL CORTEX
Organ culture, 70% of total cells are of the fetal layer, which include stem cells, 20% of zona fasciculata, 10% of zona glomerularis (percentages estimated), cells round, polyhedral or pyramidal, without granules.

PITUITARY GLAND
Organ culture of anterior lobe of the gland, some cells are with granules (chromophils), others without (chromophobes). Occasional glial cells (pituicytes) can be found.

THYROID
Organ culture containing follicles with colloid, round or cubical cells, less than 5% of total are somewhat larger C cells with granules. Some parathyroid cells can be found: small chief cells with some granules and rare large oxyphil cells.

OVARY
Organ culture consisting predominately of follicular (granulosa) cells of the primordial follicle.

TESTIS
Organ culture consisting predominately of smaller interstitial Leydig cells, larger Sertoli cells and spermatogenic epithelium.

PROSTATE
Organ culture consisting largely of granular cells originating from seminal vesicles, tuboalveolar glandular structures, and some smooth muscle fibers.

STOMACH/INTESTINE, i.e. *"peripanceatic block"*
Organ culture, primarily consisting of cuboidal stem cells, round parietal cells and granular zymogenic cells of stomach, pancreatic stem cells, and of intestinal absorbtive cells with brush border, all originating in the mucosa, with a component of lymphoid cells.

LIVER
Organ culture, individual cells or cell clusters, 90% hepatocytes, the remainder consists of hepatic and hematopoietic stem cells, endothelial cells and some Kupffer cells.

THYMUS
Organ culture consisting predominately of lymphocytes (T- and B-) and epithelial reticular stellate cells.

KIDNEY
Organ culture, primarily of the cortical layer, consisting of round podocytes, larger round to cuboidal cells of convoluted tubules, with and without brush border.

HEART MYOBLASTS
Organ culture, individual cells or cell clusters, fusiform cells with central nuclei.

MUSCLE MYOBLAST
Organ culture, individual cells or cell clusters, fusiform cells with peripheral nuclei, with some stem cells, a tendency toward syncytial arrangement.

SPLEEN
Organ culture, network of reticular tissue with lymphoid cell and macrophages, arranged in Billroth cords, with thoroughly washed off blood elements, some flattened sinusoidal endothelial cells.

LYMPH NODES
Organ culture, network of reticular cells with lymphoid cells and macrophages, partially arranged in medullary cords and sinuses.

LUNG
Organ culture, dispersed cell clusters of terminal and respiratory bronchioli and of alveolar system, estimated 30% of alveolar cells, 30% of endothelial cells, 30% of interstitial cells and 10% of macrophages.

PANCREAS
(Even at the fetal stage 85% of the mass of pancreas is that of an exocrine gland. This preparation fulfills that function). Organ culture, typical serous cells with granules, some disassociated acinar arrangement, and centroacinar (stem?) cells, and cells of the Langerhans islets.

MESENCHYME
Abundant amorphous ground substance, mostly of hyaluronic acid, pluripotential fibroblasts.

PLACENTA
Organ culture, dispersed cytotrophoblast cells from both fetal and maternal portion, with a few chorionic villi, decidual cells, endothelial cells.

CARTILAGE
Organ culture, prepared from hyaline cartilage, with extracellular matrix with type II collagen, and chondroblasts, also of attached perichondrium with type I collagen and numerous fibroblasts.

BONE
Organ culture, prepared from cancellous portion of long bones, with multiple osteoblasts from endosteum, also with some haematopoietic stem cells of bone marrow.

HYPOTHALAMUS/THALAMUS
Organ culture, individual cells and cell clusters, of multipolar smaller neurons of the autonomous nervous system variety, with an abundance of glial cells.

BASAL GANGLIA
Organ culture, individual cells and cell clusters, of multipolar neurons and abundant glial cells.

CEREBELLUM
Organ culture, individual cells and cell clusters, consisting of Purkinje cells and very small neurons, with an abundance of glial cells.

CEREBRAL CORTEX
Organ culture, individual cells or cell clusters, consisting of a variety of neurons, including those of pyramidal shape, with an abundance of glial cells.

(Periventricular) MEDULLA ALBA OF BRAIN
Organ culture, occasional small neurons, some of them stem cells, glial cells, fragments of axons.

BRAIN STEM
Organ culture, individual cells or cell clusters, consisting of a variety of neurons, usually of smaller size and abundant glial cells.

CEREBRUM
Organ culture, individual cells or cell clusters, consisting of a great variety of neurons, some of them stem cells, with abundant glial cells.

PINEAL GLAND
Organ culture, individual cells or cell clusters, consisting of melatonin producing pinealocytes and astrocytes.

Stem cell transplants of any of the 200 types of cells can be manufactured. In addition, artificial organs with a bio-polymer base and any of the stem cell xenotransplants can be prepared. The same applies to biologically enhanced bio-degradable bio-polymer materials for reconstructive surgery, such as bio-degradable bio-polymers used together with an osteogenetic combination of stem cell xenotransplants, foam hydrogel used together with a chondrogenetic combination of stem cell xenotransplants, foam hydrogel used together with a soft tissue combination of stem cell xenotransplants.

Chapter 36

> Where the telescope ends, the microscope begins. Which of the two has the grander view?
> *Victor Hugo, 1802-1885, Les Miserables [1862]*

> Experience, the universal Mother of Scinces.
> *Miguel de Cervantes, 1547-1616, Don Quijoté de la Mancha*

INDICATIONS/CONTRA-INDICATIONS

During the last over 70 years physicians have utilized stem cell transplantation as treatment of many diseases, whenever they recognized that the patient needs a *direct stimulation of regeneration, i.e. repair* of the damaged cells or tissues of various organs, or an *outright transplantation of precursor stem cells* to replace the dead or non-functioning cells. Certain diseases or groups of diseases have been treated by stem cell transplantation more than the others, and so more clinical experience has been accumulated or more scientific papers written. There are many publications about the neurotransplantation for Parkinson's disease, although only a few patients have been so treated and the reported results have been outright poor. Very few reports have been written about the treatment of immune system diseases by stem cell transplantation until very recently, and too few patients treated, although there is strong reason to believe that stem cell transplantation is the best immunostimulant available to the medicine today, capable to restore even the immune function in the pre-terminal AIDS patients. Very few reports have been written about the treatment of aging disease, although millions of patients have been treated for this indication.

The list of indications that follows is rather arbitrary, as well as comments on the patient selection. Both the physician and the patient must realize that scar tissue cannot be "turned back" to become a functioning original healthy tissue again, and stem cell xeno-transplantation cannot accomplish it either.

Diabetes Mellitus: Juvenile and adult patients should be accepted for treatment by stem cell transplantation only when they have already developed complications of diabetes, such as:

a. *Retinopathy*: all patients in the pre-proliferative stage should be accepted, while those in the proliferative stage may be refused, it all depends on the details of the clinical situation, and the patient's determination, but it is really pointless to treat patients that are blind already.

b. *Nephropathy*: only patients in the pre-uremic stage should be accepted, i.e. patients with various degrees of proteinuria, micro- or macro-albuminuria, but with acceptable creatinine clerance.

c. *Polyneuropathy*: all patients are accepted.

d. *Peripheral arterial disease*: patients with gangrene of their lower extremity are not accepted, while all patients in pre-gangrenous stage must be accepted.

(Patient selection for treatment of diabetic complications is covered extensively in the Chapter 29.

Children and juveniles: all patients are accepted, preferably in the acute stage, i.e. as soon after the onset of the disease as possible, as well as all patients with "brittle diabetes" of children.

Pregnant women with a history of diabetic fetopathy, or women with infertility due to diabetes mellitus: all patients are accepted, but they must be treated before the pregnancy commences, or during the 12th to 16th week of pregnancy.

Insulin-independent Diabetes Mellitus (type 2): Obese patients with type 2 diabetes mellitus should be refused, and that presents a dilemma for the treating physician when such patient develops a diabetic complication, and it is progressing fast. Obese patients with type 2 diabetes and complications can be accepted if they were adequately prepared by a proper metabolic treatment, and their weight loss had become apparent.

Hypoendocrinopathies other than diabetes mellitus: Only those adult patients that no longer respond to a standard hormone replacement therapy are accepted. This usually applies to autoimmune diseases: Hashimoto's thyroiditis, Addison's disease, etc. All children are accepted as they usually suffer from genetic diseases, and there is no alternative treatment.

Premature ovarian failure: All patients that no longer respond to a standard hormone replacement therapy are accepted, i.e. approximately one half of such patients.

Male hypogonadism: All patients are accepted, as there is no other treatment available, but the treatment has to be carried out in cooperation with infertility clinic.

Myocardial infarction: If the patient in the acute stage brought to the center of invasive cardiology and the center has an established stem cell transplantation program, all patients should have a coronary catheterization, stent placement, followed in selected patients by intracoronary implantation of stem cell transplants.

If no treatment is given in the acute stage, then a standard kind of implantation of stem cell transplants should be carried out four weeks later.

Patients in the acute stage of cerebrovascular accident will hopefully be treated in the same way in the near future. Today a neurosurgical operation has to be carried out as described in Chapter 55.

Hypofunction of the immune system: All patients are accepted, as well as children with inborn hypofunction of the immune system of any etiology, for whom there is no alternative treatment.

Autoimmune diseases: All patients in whom the standard treatment no longer works are accepted.

Some chronic diseases of the digestive system (*see Chapter 57*): All patients in whom the routine treatment no longer works are accepted.

Aging disease: All patients over the age of 45 are accepted.

Non-healing fractures and other non-healing bone diseases: All patients are accepted, unless they have a "florid" osteomyelitis which requires an aggressive antibiotic treatment. This usually happens, when the orthopedic surgeon has "run out of solutions". The same applies to all other diseases with non-healing bone destruction.

Mental retardation: All patients are accepted as there is no alternative therapy. The treatment has to be started as soon as possible after the diagnosis is made, and that should be made as soon as possible after birth.

Genetic, chromosomal, and other inborn diseases: All patients are accepted as there is no other treatment. After a possibility of such diagnosis is suggested, stem cell transplantation must be started without delay, and repeated every 4 months, even if the exact diagnosis has not been established yet.

After there is a suspicion of the brain damage in the newborn, a CT scan of the brain must be made without delay. Whenever there is a periventricular leukomalacia found (often combined with intraventricular bleeding), stem cell transplantation should be started immediately, and repeated every 4 months. Time must not be wasted for the establishment of an exact diagnosis.

CONTRA-INDICATIONS

Terminal stage of a chronic disease is an absolute contraindication. Moribund patients laying in a vegetable position for years must not be treated with stem cell transplantation. The same does not apply to patients in recent coma, as the reported experience of F. Schmid with treatment of apallic syndrome in children, and our own experience with the treatment of recently comatose patients by intrathecal implantation of stem cell transplants proves beyond a doubt [95].

All temporary contraindications, such as:

- acute infection,
- untreated chronic infection,
- uncontrollable severe hypertension,
- uncontrollable severe allergic status,
- severe acute exhaustion, can be removed by appropriate medical treatment.

Acute infections are a problem with small children with genetic and chromosomal diseases coming in for the stem cell transplantation treatment from a distance, because they frequently get upper respiratory infection during travel. Since the parents often do not have the time to wait for the intercurrent infection to run its course, there is a pressure on the physician to take an action. In the author's experience, if the patient is not toxic, and does not have excessively high fever, the injection of an appropriate antibiotic permits that stem cell transplantation be carried out after a few hours without any ill consequences for the patient or implanted stem cell transplants.

Untreated chronic infection is notoriously troublesome in conjunction with stem cell transplantation. There are hardly any adult patients without a hidden "silent" chronic infection somewhere in the body, and the same applies to many children as well. It happens infrequently only, but certain patients do get a flare-up of their dormant chronic inflammation in the immediate post-SCT course.

It is mandatory to ask every patient about any non-symptomatic chronic infections during the history taking, and then check the current status of such chronic inflammations, and complete an appropriate treatment *before the start of preparation of the batch of stem cell transplants for the patient treatment.*

Acute exhaustion is a major issue with some patients suffering from "manager syndrome" that consider stem cell transplantation a quick way to "re-charge their batteries". If a patient cannot stay at full rest for 3 days, without a cell phone, and with a minimum of visitors, and then be prepared for another 7 days of decreased activity, i.e. to follow the post-SCT instructions, it is better not to accept such patient for stem cell transplantation treatment.

Chapter 37

Man is so made that he can only find relaxation from one kind of labor by taking up another.
Anatole France, 1844 - 1924, The Crime of Sylvestre Bonnard [1881]

PATIENT'S PREPARATION FOR STEM CELL XENOTRANSPLANTATION

A proper preparation of the patient for stem cell transplantation is mandatory. The patient has to be brought into as good a metabolic state as possible by standard therapeutic means, i.e. to carry out stem cell transplantation, while for example, the diabetic patient is in the state of ketosis, hyperosmolality or prolonged hypoglycaemia, is probably minimally effective and should be done only as a last resort. Patient must also be detoxified, which means in particular the treatment of the gastrointestinal tract: forgotten nowadays, treatments by digestive enzymes, bacterial symbionts, enema(s), as well as dietary modifications (high fiber diets, etc.), are necessary. Oral fluids must be forced for 24 hours before the treatment unless otherwise contraindicated. Patient must receive an optimum dosage of vitamins and minerals for 4 weeks prior to stem cell transplantation. Patient's body must be free of any medications that are not absolutely necessary at the time of transplantation. Patient must not drink any alcohol for 48 hours before stem cell transplantation and substantially cut down on smoking. There must be no exposure to x-ray, or any other form of electromagnetic energy for 3 days prior to stem cell transplantation. Patients must have no vaccinations or any serum therapy for 4 weeks before stem cell transplantation.

After stem cell transplantation, these precautions and additional therapeutic measures must be prolonged for another 4 weeks.

The summary of the patient preparation:

1. Stabilization of the metabolic state of the patient, by hospitalization if necessary, etc., so that the patient's clinical condition will be compensated as well as possible before stem cell transplantation,

2. Detoxification of the gastrointestinal tract by increase of fiber in the diet, by increase of high carbohydrates so that up to 60% of caloric intake would be from this food group, digestive enzymes, bacterial symbionts, etc., for 4 weeks, including enemas if constipated, particularly 2 days before cell transplantation,

3. Forcing of oral fluids for 24 hours, unless contraindicated,

4. Intake of optimum dosage of multi-vitamins/minerals for 4 weeks,

5. Discontinuance of non-essential medications (including "street" drugs) for 7 days,

6. Avoidance of exposure to x-rays, or any other form of electromagnetic energy for 3 days,

7. Avoidance of vaccinations or serum therapy for 4 weeks prior to stem cell transplantation,

8. Mild to moderate daily physical activity,

9. No alcohol for 3 days, elimination of or a diminution of smoking.

Chapter 38

The real scientist...is ready to bear privation and, if need be, starvation rather than let anyone dictate to him which direction his work must take.
Albert Szent-Györgyi, 1893-1990, Science Needs Freedom [1943]

TREATMENT PROCEDURE

All stem cell transplants prepared for the named (actually "coded") patient are implanted at the same time under sterile conditions in the minor operating room. Standard precautions must be used for the care of patients, e.g. appropriate hand washing, use of barrier precautions, care in the use and disposal of needles and other sharp instruments, proper procedures for handling and disinfection/sterilization of medical instruments and disposal of potentially infectious waste in order to minimize transmission of nosocomial pathogens or possible xenogeneic infections. No additional infection control or isolation precautions have to be employed in view of lack of transmission of xenogeneic infections in many years of our clinical experience and since no immunosuppression is used.

The procedure is preferably carried out in the morning after the patient had a small breakfast.

Space requirements: minor operating room or aseptic procedure room with adjacent aseptic preparation room where stem cell transplants are loaded from the transportation vials into the implantation syringes.

Personnel requirement: one physician/surgeon to carry out stem cell transplantation, one senior laboratory technician to load stem cell transplants from transportation vials to implantation syringes, and nursing staff.

Supplies: 18 GA 3″ epidural anesthesia (or liver biopsy) needles with blunt end and opening on the side for subaponeurotic and intrathecal implantation, 18 GA 2" needles for deep gluteal epifascial implantation, 18 GA 2" needles for drawing of stem cell transplants from the transportation vials into syringes, 5 cm^3 Luer-Lock syringes for implantation, 70% alcohol, Betadin tincture, 1% Xylocaine (without Epinephrine), sterile physiological solution, tuberculine syringes with 30 GA needles, 4x4 gauze, small window drapes, small regular drapes, Band-Aids, 3 metal trays, surgical greens + hats + masks + boots + sterile gloves.

Procedure:

- Put on greens, hat and shoe covers, and surgical mask.
- In the preparation room, load stem cell transplants into Luer-Lock syringes.
- Take out all transportation vials from the package, check the label on each vial, shake each one thoroughly, and then line them up on the "Implantation Scheme" that you received with stem cell transplants from the manufacturer.
- Prepare as many 5 cm^3 Luer-Lock syringes, 18 GA 2" needles, for drawing, and 18 GA implantation needles as there are transportation vials. Note that implantation needles for subaponeurotic and intrathecal implantation are the same, while implantation needles for deep epifascial gluteal implantation are ordinary 18 GA 2" ones.
- Cover a surgical tray on wheels with a sterile drape. Place stickers with the visible name of stem cell transplants on the drape in the same way as displayed on the "Implantation Scheme".
- Put on sterile gloves.
- Ask your assistant to take the first vial with stem cell transplant, shake it thoroughly, open the screwed on top. Take a Luer-Lock syringe, attach 18 GA drawing needle, and draw the contents of the vial into syringe. Note that transportation vial have a peculiar bottom with a sharp narrow end where clusters of stem cell transplants often get stuck. If that has happened, have your assistant put the top back on and repeat vigorous shaking. If even that does not solve the problem, then dislodge the clustered "glued on" cells at the bottom with the tip of drawing needle.
- Express the drawn in air and place the filled up syringe on its designated place (by a sticker) on the surgical drape.
- Repeat the same procedure with all vials containing stem cell transplants manufactured for the patient identified by a code on a

label of each transportation vial.
- Then wheel the surgical tray into the treatment room.

Subaponeurotic implantation:

With a patient in supine position prep the upper abdomen, umbo, and area just below belly button, with Betadin soap and solution three times, like for an abdominal surgery. Select a spot approximately ½" superiorly and ½" laterally from umbo, and carry out intradermal anesthesia of those tiny skin areas with 1% xylocaine in tuberculin or 1 cc syringe, and do so bilaterally.

Attach 18 GA epidural anesthesia needle to a Luer-Lock syringe containing stem cell transplant that is marked on the "Implantation Scheme" to go RIGHT UP. Note that the epidural anesthesia needle has a blunt end, and its opening is on the side. Line up the needle so that the flat side of the end with the opening is parallel with the wings on the Luer-Lock syringe; that will help you during the implantation to be always oriented about the position of the opening of the needle.

Take the syringe with attached needle in your hand in such a way that the opening of the needle is parallel with and facing the abdominal skin of the patient. Then turn your hand in such a way that the syringe with attached needle is at the right angle to the abdominal skin at the point marked with the "wheel" from your intradermal anesthesia right to and up from the belly button. Then pierce the skin with enough force to push the tip of needle into subcutaneous tissue. Beware that it is hard to pierce the skin with such a blunt needle: do not be afraid to use adequate force to penetrate the skin. Holding the syringe with the needle at a right angle to the skin makes the skin penetration easier.

After the skin penetration, change the direction of the syringe with needle into oblique and direct it to the right side of the patient's body and upward toward the axilla. Advance the needle tip, and then probe with the needle tip the surface of the aponeurosis of rectus abdominis muscle. In some patients the aponeurosis may be weak, and hard to palpate: ask the patient to push down like for a bowel movement, whereupon aponeurosis of rectus abdominis muscle becomes hard and palpable with the tip of the needle. Making sure that the needle opening is parallel to, and facing, the surface of the aponeurosis of rectus abdominis muscle, palpate its surface, and if the needle tip is touching it, pierce the aponeurosis by a jolt like when penetrating the wall of the vein during i.v. injection.

After penetration of aponeurosis, aspirate and then inject the contents of the syringe, not too fast, not too slow.

After you injected the entire contents of the syringe, separate the Luer-Lock syringe from the needle, and attach to it the syringe with 1% xylocaine. Inject 0.2. cc of xylocaine to implant the cells that remained in the implantation needle.

Withdraw the needle from under the aponeurosis back into the subcutaneous space, but do not pull it out of subcutaneous space (!). Re-attach the Luer-Lock syringe that contains the next stem cell transplant marked on the "Implantation Scheme" to go RIGHT DOWN.

Change the direction of the needle/syringe into oblique going to the right side of the patient and downward toward the groin. Advance the needle tip and probe with the needle tip for the surface of the aponeurosis of rectus abdominis muscle. Making sure that the needle opening is parallel to and facing the surface of the aponeurosis of rectus abdominis muscle, palpate its surface, and if the needle tip is touching it, pierce the aponeurosis by a jolt like when penetrating the wall of the vein during i.v. injection. After the penetration of aponeurosis, aspirate and then inject the contents of the syringe, not too fast, not too slow. Then withdraw the syringe with needle.

Repeat the above steps on the left side of the patient's body always following the "Implantation Scheme". Apply band-aids to the skin puncture points.

Gluteal implantation:

After subaponeurotic implantations, ask the patient to turn into a prone position and carry out a surgical scrub of upper gluteal regions bilaterally with Betadine soap and solution three times.

Technique of deep epifascial implantations is the same as that of deep subcutaneous injections. Implant all pre-prepared stem cell transplants in accordance with the 'Implantation Scheme'. Cover the puncture marks with Band-Aids.

Intrathecal implantation:

Depending upon the therapeutic indication, it can be done either utilizing a lumbar puncture or a ventricular tap technique, as described bellow:

a. Technique via lumbar puncture: Using 18 GA lumbar puncture needle carry out a standard lumbar puncture. Allow 5 cc of cerebrospinal fluid to drain out, and then implant the contents of the syringe pre-filled with the stem cell transplant as per "Implantation Scheme". If two different stem cell transplants are to be implanted, wait 3 – 5 minutes after the first implantation, drain again 5 cc of cerebrospinal fluid, and then implant the contents of the second syringe pre-filled with the second stem cell transplant as per "Implantation Scheme". Apply Band-Aid to the skin puncture site. Place the patient in a supine position without any pillow for 24 hours as is routinely done after the lumbar puncture.

b. Technique via ventricular tap: In the operating room, with the patient awake, local anesthesia is carried out for incision of skin and soft tissues overlying the area of the Burr hole to be made. After skin incision, which is extended deeply to the level of skull, Burr hole is made. Dura mater is exposed, and 18 GA ventricular tap needle inserted into Cornu Ammonis of the lateral ventricle of the brain. After draining 5 cc of cerebrospinal fluid the contents of the syringe with stem cell transplant as per "Implantation Scheme" are implanted. If another stem cell transplant is to be implanted, wait 10 minutes, again drain 5 cc of cerebrospinal fluid and then implant the contents of another syringe with stem cell transplant as per "Implantation scheme".

Observe dura mater for possible signs of intra-cerebral hematoma for 10 minutes, secure hemostasis of dura mater, bone margins, and suture the soft tissues and skin.

Treatment has to be repeated every 9 - 36 months. The exact timing is determined, usually *on clinical grounds, by the respective specialist* observing a recurrence of the progression of the complication. There does appear, however, to be *some degree of cumulative effect* as the next stem cell transplantation often gives a better and longer lasting result than the previous one.

Chapter 39

> The strongest of all warriors are these two – Time and Patience.
> Leo Nikolaevich Tolstoi, 1828 - 1910, War and Peace [1865 - 1869]

> Important principles may and must be inflexible.
> Abraham Lincoln, 1809 - 1865, Public address, Washington, D.C. [1865]

POST-STEM CELL XENTRANSPLANTATION PRECAUTIONS AND PATIENT MONITORING

Each patient will have to observe following precautions after stem cell transplantation:

1. rest for 48 hours, which does not mean a complete bed rest, sitting in a sofa chair is sufficient,
2. continue with a healthy life style for at least one month, if not forever,
3. avoidance of any activities for 10 days, in particular those during which body temperature is raised, i.e. sport, intense exercise, active sex, cleaning of the garage, work in the garden, etc. are not permitted,
4. avoidance of alcohol, "street" drugs, intake of non-essential medications, smoking, etc. for 2 months,
5. avoidance of exposure to electromagnetic energy (sunbathing, x-rays, etc.) for 2 months,
6. use of high potency multi-vitamins/minerals for at least one month,
7. avoidance of any vaccination or serum therapy for one month.

Observing the schedule of post-treatment visits, 24 hours, 7 days, one month, 3 months, 6 months, 9 months, and 12 months after transplanttation, is mandatory.

In case of symptoms of acute infection with fever, call your treating physician immediately, so that a proper treatment can be started without delay, as such an infection, if left untreated, during the first 6 weeks after transplantation, could jeopardize the survival of the stem cell transplants.

Description of observations and measurements after the stem cell transplantation treatment can be found at the end of the respective chapters or subchapters in the section on "Clinical treatment by stem cell xentransplantation".

Chapter 40

A journey of a thousand miles must begin with a single step.
Lao-tzu, c. 604-c. 531 B.C., *The Way of Lao-tzu*

A people without history is like the wind on the buffalo grass.
Sioux saying

PATIENT'S PRE- AND POST-TREATMENT INSTRUCTIONS

Here is a sample of an instruction sheet.

PATIENT INSTRUCTIONS – STEM CELL TRANSPLANTATION

Dear Mr. - Mrs. - Miss_____

You have decided to undergo a stem cell transplantation as a treatment of your disease(s). It is one of the newest therapeutic modalities of modern medicine, and for that reason, prior experiences of yours or those around you that you trust may not be adequate to prepare you psychologically for such treatment so that you would cooperate and do all that is necessary to make sure that this treatment gives you the maximum benefit possible. It is mandatory to follow these instructions; otherwise such therapeutic efforts may be wasted. *If you feel that you cannot follow these, rather simple, instructions it is better for you to change your mind about receiving stem cell transplantation.*

This method of treatment is remarkably free of any significant complications, appears quite simple from the patient's viewpoint, 'just a few, somewhat unpleasant injections', and *thus patients are very prone not to take it seriously*, that much more that it can be carried out, as is commonly done, on an outpatient basis. This leads many patients, especially the 'go-getters', that 'do not have time to waste on themselves', to ignore these instructions, *particularly when the post-treatment symptoms are very mild*, as is usually the case.

It is normal to have some degree of 'reaction' after stem cell transplantation during the first 10 days after the treatment. The symptoms of this reaction resemble a 'flu': malaise, weakness, lack of energy, 'not feeling well', change of an appetite, even a slight fever up to 98.8 °F (37.2 °C), discomfort and some swelling in an area of injections (remember that each stem cell transplant is injected in 5 cc of the culture medium), etc., can be observed. But this 'reaction' is usually too mild to remind the patient that such treatment was just administered and that certain strict, although very simple, instructions have to be followed.

Before stem cell transplantation a patient must:

- *for at least 3 days prior* to the transplantation, slow down and lead a 'regular' healthy lifestyle, without overwork, parties, excessive physical activity, etc., as acute exhaustion is a contraindication to this form of treatment,
- *during the last 7 days prior* to the transplantation, 'detoxify' the organism: avoid any alcohol and 'street drugs', minimize smoking, avoid intake of any non-essential drugs and medications, increase the intake of water (particularly during the last 24 hours),
- *during the last 4 weeks prior* to the transplantation, 'regularize' the function of the digestive system, that is the greatest source of toxins for most sedentary people with gastrointestinal malfunctions: increase the un-cooked fiber in diet, increase the proportion of high carbohydrates in diet up to 60%, if necessary use digestive enzymes, bacterial symbionts, etc., and if constipated, use laxatives, (enema 48 hours prior to the treatment is strongly advised to those chronically constipated),
- *during the 4 weeks prior* to the transplantation, use the high potency multi-vitamins/minerals,
- *during the 4 weeks prior* to the transplantation, avoid any vaccination or serum therapy,
- *during the last 3 days prior* to the transplantation, avoid sunbathing, and any other exposure to electromagnetic energy (microwave ovens, x-rays, etc.),

- in case of symptoms of an acute infection with a fever, such as pharyngitis, bronchitis, urinary tract infection, gastroenteririts, etc., call your treating physician immediately so that a proper treatment can be started without delay. Such an acute infection, if left untreated, would be a contraindication for transplantation, that means that stem cell transplants, "custom" prepared specifically for each patient, would be wasted, as the clinical efficiency of stem cell transplants is uncertain beyond 7 days from the release date.

Besides these general instructions for certain diseases, there are additional ones for: diabetes mellitus, autoimmune diseases and immune deficiencies, diseases of digestive system and liver, etc. If your treating physician forgot to discuss them with you, do not hesitate to ask for them.

After stem cell transplantation patient must:

- *rest for 48 hours*, not necessarily in bed, sitting in a sofa chair is adequate,
- continue with a healthy life style *for at least 1 month*,
- *for 10 days* avoid any activity, during which body temperature is raised, it means sport, intense exercise, active sex, cleaning of the garage, work in the garden, etc. are not allowed,
- avoid alcohol, 'street' drugs, intake of non-essential medications, smoking, etc., *for 2 months*,
- avoid exposure to electromagnetic energy (sunbathing, x-rays, etc.) *for 2 months*,
- use high potency multi-vitamins/minerals *for at least 1 month*,
- avoid any vaccination or serum therapy *for 1 month*;
- follow religiously the schedule of post-treatment visits, *24 hours, 7 days, 1 month, 3 months, 6 months, 9 months and 12 months after transplantation*;
- *in case of symptoms of acute infection with* fever call your treating physician immediately, so that a proper treatment can be started without delay, as such an infection, if left untreated, during the first 6 weeks after transplantation, could jeopardize the survival of stem cell transplants.

Besides these general instructions, there are additional ones for each patient specific to their diagnosis(es). If your treating physician would forget to discuss them with you, please, do not hesitate to ask for them.

Chapter 41

The diagnosis of disease is often easy, often difficult, and often impossible.
Peter Mere Latham, 1789 - 1875, Collected Works

SURVEILLANCE FOR POSSIBLE TRANSMISSION OF XENO-ZOONOSES

Surveillance of Xenotransplant Recipient

Every patient/recipient of stem cell xenotransplants should undergo a surveillance for 5 years in order to monitor the possible introduction and propagation of xenogeneic infections into a general population. All documentation of this surveillance must be kept by the treating physician, entered also into the computerized data base, if possible, which documentation allows a prompt retrieval, and linkage of the medical records of the recipient to the records of manufacture of stem cell xenotransplants, and of source animals. *The link of treating physician to the manufacturer is via the patient's code.*

During the scheduled office visits, every recipient of stem cell xenotransplants must be evaluated also for adverse clinical events potentially associated with xenogeneic infections. Careful attention must be paid to acute infectious episodes that under usual circumstances in the general population are never etiologically identified. When the source of a significant illness in a stem cell xenotransplants recipient remains unidentified after standard diagnostic procedures, more testing of samples of body fluids and tissues is carried out under the supervision of the hospital infectious disease specialist. Appropriate isolation precautions may be recommended until a suspected xenogeneic infection has been proven and resolved or ruled out in the recipient.

Archiving of acute and convalescent sera obtained in association with acute unexplained illness may be recommended by the infectious disease specialist, which would permit retrospective study and etiologic diagnosis of the clinical episode.

All adverse events after stem cell xenotransplantation must be recorded, even if most likely related to the patient's chronic illness, or representing a concomitant illness. The date of discovery, or of the office visit when found out, of the adverse event and the time relationship to stem cell xenotransplantation must be noted, classified as mild, moderate and severe, and as serious and non-serious, and their duration noted. Action taken and outcome must be recorded.

Deaths and other serious adverse events must be especially watched for. A narrative report must be obtained of each case describing the following: nature and intensity of event; the clinical course leading to an event, timing relevant to stem cell xenotransplantation; relevant laboratory measurements; countermeasures; post-mortem findings; investigator's opinion on causality, as well as relevant concomitant/ previous illnesses and relevant concomitant/previous medications.

As the adverse events have been non-existent in our experience, they all must be individually analyzed in detail if they would occur.

In the US, biological specimens will have to be collected and archived from each stem cell xenotransplants recipient to allow retrospective investigation of possible xenogeneic infections, marked for "public health investigative purposes". Each set of biological specimens consists of five 0.5cc aliquots of citrated anticoagulated plasma, two aliquots of viable leukocytes (1×10^7) and blood mononuclear cells. Two sets should be obtained before and after stem cell xenotransplantation, another set should be obtained one month, and 6 months after the transplantation. Subsequently a set should be obtained yearly twice, and then every 5 years thereafter until the death of the recipient. At the autopsy, recipient's snap-frozen samples stored at -70 °C, paraffin embedded tissue, and tissue suitable for electron microscopy must be collected from stem cell xenotransplant implantation site and all major organs involved in the pathophysiology of the disease, as determined to be the cause of death. All these specimens must be archived for 50 years for "potential public health use" as per US FDA requirements.

In case that it would become known or suspected that xenogeneic agents were present in stem cell xenotransplants, an active surveillance of the recipient is instituted by collecting specimens of blood serum, peripheral blood mononuclear cells and tissue at frequent intervals. Assays for the detection of classes of viruses known to establish persistent latent infection (herpesviruses, retroviruses, etc.) would be used, along with co-cultivation of cells coupled with appropriate detection assays. The purpose is to detect sentinel human infections prior to their dissemination in general population. Testing of archived biological specimens would be conducted alongside epidemiologic investigation to assess potential public health significance of the infection.

In the process of obtaining an informed consent, the treating physician must inform stem cell xenotransplant recipients of the responsibility to educate his/her close contacts of the possibility, however distant, of the emergence of xenogeneic infections from the source animal species, without causing at the same time an undue alarm and panic. Most importantly the physician must educate stem cell xenotransplant recipient that whenever they or their close contacts develop any significant unexplained illness, they must promptly inform their physician that treated them by stem cell xenotransplantation.

Health Care Records

Three cross-referenced record systems should be maintained by the stem cell transplantologist:

a. *Institutional Xenotransplantation Record* that documents all stem cell xenotransplantation procedures: the treating physician, the source animals for stem cell xenotransplants and their procurement facility, the date of procedure and what kinds of stem cell xenotransplants were used, the xenotransplant recipient, and a summary of the recipient's clinical course, close contacts, and the health care workers associated with each procedure.

b. *Xenotransplantation Nosocomial Health Exposure Log*, which documents the dates, involved persons, and nature of all nosocomial exposures associated with a protocol for stem cell xenotransplantation and which potentially pose a risk of transmission of xenogeneic infections.

c. *Individual Xenotransplant Recipient Health Records*, that document each patient's clinical course, the results of post-stem cell xenotransplantation surveillance studies and contain a summary of the results of the screening assays performed on female rabbits of the colony and of the health status of newborn rabbits (see above) from which stem cell xenotransplant was obtained.

These records must be always current and accurately cross-referenced for an easy investigation of adverse events.

Chapter 42

> Politics ruins the character.
> *[Berlin Tägliche Rundschau x1881]*
>
> He who has thumb on the purse has the power.
> *[Speech to North German Reichstag, x1867]*
> Otto von Bismarck, 1815 – 1898

SURVEILLANCE FOR POSSIBLE IMMUNOLOGICAL REACTIONS AFTER STEM CELL TRANSPLANTATION

There are many published medical reports on hundreds of patients showing that *changes of laboratory parameters of the immune system function after stem cell transplantation,* using the pre-SCT levels as a baseline, *are minimal and statistically not significant.*

The repeated implantation of cell transplants should greatly increase the risk of allergic and immunologic reactions, yet the clinical practice is refuting such expectations. In 264 patients who underwent between one and 12 cell therapy treatment antibody levels against sheep erythrocytes and organ specific antibodies against fetal sheep liver were measured. (The cell therapy preparations were prepared from sheep fetuses). In 54 new patients that have never received cell therapy, and thus served as a control group, antibodies against sheep erythrocytes and sheep fetal liver were found in more than one half. Titers of 1:32 were classified as non-specific and 1:64 as border-line. In only 11% of patients from the group that received between one and 7 cell therapy treatments there were significant titers of antibodies against sheep erythrocytes and sheep fetal liver in the range from 1:128 to 1:256, but clinically no significant reactions were observed. An immune tolerance through MALT and

GALT or low immunogenicity of cell therapy preparations explain the observations [263].

If cell therapy preparations prepared without any special technology of primary tissue culture cause such minimal immunological reactions it is not surprising that when stem cell transplants have been prepared "lege artis", such as by the method described in this book, there are no immune reactions whatsoever.

Until we learn what life is (and many philosophers believe that it will never happen) and thus can explain many aspects of the function of the living body, we have to be satisfied with the fact that implantation of stem cell transplants prepared by the 'state-of-art' method does not cause clinically apparent immune reactions.

Stem cell transplantologist can prove this fact by getting the following battery of immunological tests, a minimum of *48 hours before SCT*, and after SCT once a month three times, and subsequently every 3 months until satisfied that there is no reaction:

 i. total lymphocytes
 ii. T-lymphocytes ($CD3^+$)
 iii. T-helpers ($CD4^+$)
 iv. T-suppressors ($CD8^+$) and CD4/CD8
 v. NK (CD16)
 vi. B-lymphocytes (CD22 and CD19)
 vii. serum IGG, IGA, IGM
 viii. serum complement (CH50).

The use of immunosuppression has been one of the main reasons why the success rate of cell transplantation has been so low in the US.

Long-term immunosuppression is not only dangerous to the patients, it is detrimental to stem cell transplants, because these are very young cells, enormously sensitive to any toxin, and immunosuppressants are highly toxic indeed.

Chapter 43

Let these describe the undescribable.
Lord Byron, 1788 – 1824, Childe Harold's Pilgrimage [1812]

The will to do, the soul to dare.
Sir Walter Scott, 1771 – 1832, The Lady of the Lake [1810]

MECHANISM OF ACTION

The mechanism of action of cell transplantation is hypothetical. There are a few published but rather exceptional reports of autopsy findings where the implanted cell xenotransplants were found surviving at the implantation site (brain, under the kidney capsule). There are published data of animal experimentation with histological proof of survival of implanted cells at the implantation site [72].

But the authors of the most authoritative book on cell transplantation in the treatment of diabetes mellitus [109] feel that the majority of the clinical effect is *a result of direct stimulation of patient's own cells and tissues by the transplanted cells, rather than the functioning of transplanted cells themselves.* The cell therapy publications state that all implanted cells disappear very quickly from the implantation site, and the greatest portion of them ends up within 2 - 3 days in the organ or tissue "where the respective cell belongs", i.c. in all organs and tissues of the patient malfunctioning as a result of a disease, treated by the implantation of cells or tissue fragments of each such mal-functioning organ or tissue, following the rules of "organospecificity" [95, 108, 116 - 119].

This hypothesis is supported now by the recent US publications dealing with "homing" [19 - 21, 179, 180]. If transplanted cells and tissues exert their effect mostly by direct stimulation of the corresponding malfunctioning organs and tissues of the patients, to which they are "homed", the question is raised what is the basis of such direct stimulation: outright metabolic influence, paracrine regulatory effect, messenger function, etc.

Let's look at the specific example, that of complications of IDDM. In case of complications of IDDM the answer is very difficult because of our lack of understanding of the cause of the microangiopathic changes underlying diabetic complications. *It is not a result of lack of insulin.* On the contrary, there is *a hypothesis that exogenous insulin is the cause of microangiopathic complications of IDDM* [15]. Lately it has been believed that lack of C-peptide is the cause of microcirculatory pathology [16, 149].

We think, together with Alexis Carrell, that the *problem of IDDM is not only a lack of insulin* (Carrel: "Insulin does not cure a diabetic "[18]), but also *the lack of some heretofore unknown factors produced by other cells of the Langerhans islets, besides α- and β-cells. But, and most importantly, the chronic insufficiency of various factors* normally produced by various cells of Langerhans islets *places great undue demands on the regulatory system of the metabolism of carbohydrates and lipids, primarily the "hypothalamic/ pituitary - adrenal axis", and on the liver* as the key organ of metabolism. This is forcing compensatory steps by all these organs that after a certain period of time lead to an *overload, and eventually an exhaustion,* of these organs. The appearance of complications of IDDM is the signal that the system is starting to break down.

Hypothesis on the lack of immune response with BCRO system of stem cell transplantation
After many discussions with deceased F. Schmid [184] and several Russian scientists, a hypothesis developed about the lack of overt immune response after cell transplantation.

A few introductory remarks ought to be made first. Prior to the start of our IIBM project on stem cell transplantation in Russia, RITAOMH used a "monotherapy" only, i.e. in the treatment of complications of IDDM they used only islet cell transplants and not a combination of cell transplants of various organs, as developed by the German cell therapy school, and adopted by BCRO, and thereby IIBM, from its inception. This was contrary to the past experience in USSR.

After Prof. Filatov, the father of the implantation of placenta fragments for therapeutic purposes, a treatment that has been taken by some 20 millions patients worldwide for over 80 years, opened up the field of cell transplantation in the USSR, a lot of work was done in this area there.

Interestingly enough, although there was a deep animosity between Germany and USSR between WW1 and WW2, and thereafter, and contacts were minimal, cell transplantation was flourishing in USSR, and was following essentially the same principles as in Germany/ Switzerland, and that included the use of combinations of cell transplants, i.e. "polytherapy" rather than "monotherapy".

The new leadership of RITAOMH in the 1970's began to pay more attention to English than German literature and got 'swayed' away from traditions, and toward 'monotherapy'. But the older generation of Russian physicians remembered the works of the followers of Prof. Filatov: Prof. Tushnov in 1920's – 1930's, Research Institute of Metabolic and Endocrine Disorders of the Ministry of Health of Russian Federation in Moscow, under the direction of Prof. Kazakov, in 1930's, Prof. Rumi'antsev in 1950's, and others, and so IIBM found a lot of intellectual cooperation and fertile ground for re-introducing German/Swiss/Soviet concepts of the use of combinations of cell transplants [328].

The hypothesis of our team has been, that it is indeed the *combination of stem cell xenotransplants, the sources of which are many individual fetal rabbits*, that is partly responsible for the *diminution of the immune response to stem cell transplantation*. It evolved logically from an everyday clinical observation of hundreds of children treated by stem cell transplantation for various untreatable chromosomal and genetic diseases every 4 months, with *transplants of human fetal origin prepared by IIBM without a tissue culture, by a special technique, that included cryopresevation* [37], *with no immune reactions whatsoever despite a complete lack of immunosuppression.*

Multiple discussions were carried out with scientists at RITAOMH, that used only cultured cell transplants, mostly of animal fetal origin, in their clinical practice, and who were amazed by such an absolute lack of immune reactions with non-cultured allo-transplants. Not only that there were no immune reactions in children treated by cell transplantation every 4 months, on the contrary the deficiencies of their immune system function were corrected [144, 145].

Many of these treatments were carried out at the Central Clinical Hospital in Moscow, the same hospital used by President Yeltsin, where rules were extremely strict, and thus a large team, that included an anesthesiologist, had to be in attendance at every cell transplantation that we carried out there. One year later the hospital changed this rule, since it was recognized that no reaction ever took place after the treatment, and so the attendance of an anesthesiologist, ready for re-animation, was terminated.

Our experience is in agreement with reports that *cell transplantation from multiple donors has resulted in induction of tolerance in experimental models* [181]. *When small number of islets from multiple histoincompatible donors are combined into one graft, then islets of each donor induce only a minimal immune response, that significantly prolongs their survival, and the clinical effect is substantially improved without increasing the overall immunogenicity* [182]. The above stated facts together with the growing body of US literature about the *diminished immune reaction as a result of "co-transplantation"*, i.e. simultaneous use of tissue fragments of more than one organ or tissue for stem cell xenotransplantation [6, 23 - 27] gives strong support to this hypothesis.

Chapter 44

The cautious seldom err.
Confucius, 551 – 479 B.C., The Confucian Analects

COMPLICATIONS

In the author's personal experience with stem cell transplantation, in approximately 5,000 patients, excluding patients involved in clinical trials, that included both allo- and xeno-transplantation, there were only three complications: all involved diabetic patients with complications, and all three were low grade infections/granulomas at one of the implantation sites. In all three patients the low grade infection developed at one of the subponeurotic sites, while all remaining subaponeurotic implantations were without any problem, and there were no signs of inflammation at the gluteal sites of implantation. The source of infection at the subaponeurotic sites were three different types of stem cell transplants. In one case, allo-transplants were used, in two cases xeno-transplants. Bacterial culture alters I & D showed no growth, i.e. the granulomas were sterile. In other words all three cases of low grade infection appeared purely accidental.

It was remarkable that the clinical effect of implantation was not destroyed by the infection/inflammation; on the contrary the benefit of stem cell transplantation was complete in all three patients, similar to patients that had no post-SCT infection.

The author is obliged to discuss the allergic/immunologic reactions in a textbook, but since none have ever been observed, despite the fact that no immunosuppression or any form of treatment to prevent immune reactions was ever given to the patients as pre-medication, the question is posed what to write? If stem cell transplants are prepared properly, i.e. according to all rules, or "lege artis", then the fear of untoward reactions could be abandoned. Countless letters to prospective patients were written with a statement that stem cell transplantation is 'safer than aspirin providing that stem cell transplants are prepared properly', i.e. in accordance with the rules described in this book, and not a single time has such written statement haunted us.

Part V

CLINICAL TREATMENT BY STEM CELL XENOTRANSPLANTATION

Chapter 45

All essential knowledge relates to existence, or only such knowledge as has an essential relationship to existence is essential knowledge.
Sören Kierkegaard, 1813 – 1855 [Concluding Unscientific Postscript]

GENETIC DISEASES

Approximately one out of 50 newborns has a serious congenital disease, one out of 100 a single gene disorder, and one out of 200 a chromosomal abnormality. Approximately 30% of hospitalization of children is due to prenatal conditions, most of them genetic. Approximately 33% of perinatal mortality is due to genetic causes: in 30% of cases the cause is direct, while in 45% indirect. An official website of the government of the British Columbia shows that at the age of 25 at least one out of 20 individuals suffers from a serious disease due to a dominant genetic cause, and as many as 60% of people will suffer of a serious disease due to a dominant genetic cause during their lifetime.

With rare exceptions, the genetic diseases have no treatment. The prenatal and early postnatal diagnosis can, in some diseases, prevent damage due to faulty genes by giving an opportunity to institute preventive measures soon after birth. In all instances where such diagnostic measures are not available yet, the future of such patient entirely depends on stem cell transplantation.

There is an experience in clinical treatment by stem cell transplantation in some diseases, but frequently not at all, particularly in very rare genetic diseases. Since animal models for 99.9% of genetic diseases do not exist, and the value of such models for evaluation of stem cell transplantation has always been suspect, there is only one way to handle such patients: propose to the parents or guardians to treat the patient once by stem cell transplantation. Since stem cell transplantation is *safer* than taking aspirin, providing that cell transplants were prepared "*lege artis*", such an approach is not harmful to the patient. If there is no response, then stem cell transplantation is not repeated. If there is a positive response, then stem cell transplantation is carried out every 3 to 4 months.

Every genetic disease is potentially treatable by stem cell transplantation. The problem is the selection of stem cell transplants to be used for treatment of patients with very rare diseases, where current medicine has too few or no data available. The more is known about the genetic disease, and the earlier after birth the stem cell transplantation treatment begins, the greater is the chance of success. At this moment the problem is a lack of education of parents of handicapped children, with resulting in delayed start of therapy.

Single gene abnormalities are characterized by an *inheritance of simple mendelian type*. A certain phenotype is dominant if manifested even in heterozygote, and recessive if manifested in homozygote but not in heterozygote. They are infrequent, and among them is an unknown number of 'contiguous gene syndromes'. They are due to point mutations that cause a change in the specific gene product, i.e. *a structural or quantitative modification of synthesis of a polypeptide chain*.

Total incidence of pathologic phenotypes in population is 0.6 – 0.8%. *Approximately 25% of pathologic phenotypes of mendelian type is obvious already at birth, and as much as 90% by the end of puberty.* In more than one half of cases only one organ system is malformed or malfunctioning. Approximately 57% of single gene disorders shortens lifespan, and 69% reduces reproductive ability. Majority of so stricken struggle with defects that limit their schooling or work choices, mainly due to CNS damage.

Autosomal dominant (AD) type of inheritance is *the most common*. Variable expressivity and penetration of pathologic gene is typical. Usually, it is due to neomutations which *code non-enzyme protein*, with the exception of porphyria, where each of 6 dominant forms is caused by a deficit of activity of one of series of enzymes involved in heme synthesis. Hereditary angioedema, and deficit of antithrombine, are likewise caused by enzymatic defect.

In the lists of genetic diseases, those *marked with * are described in other parts of this book*.

List of diseases with AD type of inheritance, and their incidence

Disease	Incidence
Familiar combined hyperlipidemia*	1:70 - 350
Familiar hypercholesterolemia (heterozygotes)*	1:500
Dominant otosclerosis	1:1,000
Neurofibromatosis	1:2,500
Noonan syndrome*	1:2,500
Hereditary spherocytosis	1:5,000
Dentinogenesis imperfecta	1:10,000
Polyposis of colon*	1:10,000
Marfan syndrome	1:25,000-50,000
Achondroplasia*	1:50,000
Sturge-Weber syndrome	1:50,000
Cornelia-de-Lange syndrome	1:50000
Tuberous sclerosis	1:100,000
Acute intermittent porphyria*	1:100,000

Neurofibromatosis, or von Recklinghausen disease, with "café-au-lait" hyperpigmented spots, soft fibromas of skin, and multiple neurinomas along peripheral and cranial nerves, neurofibromas in the bone, intestines, endocrine glands, etc., often causes compression syndromes. Stem cell transplantation of *diencephalon, liver, placenta, hypothalamus, medulla alba of brain, basal ganglia*, is advised.

Tuberous sclerosis, or Bourneville-Pringle disease, is clinically characterized by a triad: mental retardation, epilepsy, adenoma sebaceum on the nose and cheeks, and "café-au-lait" depigmented skin areas. Cachectic nanism with progeria facies due to the loss of subcutaneous fat, and premature graying of sparse hair, becomes obvious from 2nd to 4th year of life. There is a progressive mental retardation, intracranial calcifications, sensori-neural deafness, retinitis pigmentosa, with a 'salt and pepper' appearance of retina, optic nerve atrophy, and photosensitive dermatitis. Besides that there are skeletal abnormalities with disproportionately large hands and feet and flexion contractures of large joints. Patients survive until adulthood. Stem cell transplantation of *placenta, liver, bone marrow, adrenal cortex, mesenchyme, exocrine pancreas, retina*, is recommended.

Cornelia-de-Lange syndrome, is clinically characterized by a typical facies, short stature, microcephaly, micromelia, severe mental retardation and speech delay, and normal life span.

Our own experience with the treatment of an 8-year old boy with Cornelia-de-Lange syndrome, with pronounced psychomotor delay at the level of imbecility, speech delay, seizures, severe myopic astigmatism, by human fetal cell transplantation of *brain cortex, medulla alba of brain, frontal lobe of brain, mesencephalon, diencephalon*, was positive as the patient's height increased by 2.5 cm in 4 months, and the speech progressed to the level of speaking in phrases. The 2nd cell transplantation carried out 4 months later brought on another 2.5 cm growth in height and 1.0 kg in weight, and noticeable improvement of self-care abilities. It should be noted that the treatment of this patient by cell transplantation began very late. Treatment took place at the Endocrinology Research Center of Russian Academy of Medical Sciences in Moscow.

Autosomal recessive (AR) type of inheritance occurs in genetic diseases expressed in children but parents/heterozygotes are phenotypically disease-free. AR diseases are often associated with inbreeding, and also among people living for generations in secluded areas, and so are limited to certain populations: cystic fibrosis in Caucasians, sickle cell anemia among blacks, Tay-Sachs disease among Ashkenazy Jews, etc.

Wilson's disease, AR disorder of copper metabolism, causes an accumulation of copper in liver, CNS, eye, kidney, heart, and skeleton. 40 to 60 % of copper is absorbed in the stomach and upper duodenum. In liver the copper is built into ceruloplasmin and enters systemic circulation. One molecule of ceruloplasmin binds 6 – 7 atoms of copper. Copper is important for oxidation of plasma Fe^{2+}. ATP-ase in the liver binds copper and removes copper ions into the bile. There is a lowered output of ceruloplasmin and thereby decreased elimination of copper through bile, and incorporation of copper into ceruloplasmin. As a result, toxic free copper accumulates in the liver and other organs, and by binding with proteins, especially SH- groups, it supports the production of O_2-radicals and lipid peroxidation.

Clinical symptoms start between 10 and 25 years of age, when chronic active hepatitis develops, that progresses into cirrhosis with hepatosplenomegaly and ascites. Defective copper pump in the liver leads to an accumulation of copper in other tissues, such as basal ganglia of brain, where it causes neuronal degeneration, with Parkinsonism-like clinical picture, and a variety of nerve, neuromuscular, and psychic disturbances. Copper accumulates also in erythrocytes, causing hemolytic anemia, and in kidneys. Copper deposits in the cornea are seen as golden or green Kayser-Fleischer ring. Free copper can be removed by penicillamine that chelates copper into urine, or by chelation therapy. Stem cell trans-plantation of *liver, retina, optic nerve, placenta, exocrine pancreas, intestine*, is recommended.

List of diseases with AR type of inheritance, their incidence, and relation to populations

Interstinal lactase deficit	1:10	in Caucasians
Thalassemias*		very high in Mediterranean, African and Asian populations
Familia dysautonomy	1:100	Jews
Dubin-Johnson syndrome	1:1,300	Iranian Jews
Cystic fibrosis*	1:2,000	Caucasians
Gaucher disease type 1*	1:2,000	US Jews
Tay-Sachs disease*	1:3,000	US Jews
A1 antitrypsin deficit*	1:3,500	
Congenital hypothyreosis*	1:4,000	
Cystinuria*	1:7,000	
Phenylketonuria*	1:10,000	
Congenital adrenogenital syndrome*	1:10,000	
Alkaptonuria*	1:19,000	
Hartnup syndrome	1:2,4000	
Wilson's disease	1:50,000	
Galactosemia*	1:60,000	
Cystinosis*	1:100,000	
Laurence-Moon-Biedl syndrome	1:100,000	
Maple-syrup-disease	1:160,000	
Xeroderma pigmentosum*	1:250,000	
Russell-Silver syndrome		

***Familial dysautonomy**,* or Riley-Day syndrome, has onset in infancy, with progressive degeneration of peripheral autonomous, motor and sensory nerves, and of CNS. Defect of swallowing reflex is observed first, followed by diminution of pain sensation and corneal reflex, dysarthria, ataxia, disturbed temperature control, hyperhidrosis, excessive salivation, cardiovascular dysregulation, and taste defect. Death occurs during the 2nd decade from lung infections.

***Russell-Silver syndrome**,* has onset in utero with growth retardation, that continues postnatally. There is an absolute lack of interest in food and eating. Head is of normal size, face is small and triangular, with a weak narrow chin, and there is a general asymmetry of the entire body with a hypotrophic right or left side, with resulting uneven length of extremities, clinodactyly of the 5th finger.

Our experience with treatment of a patient with Russell-Silver syndrome by human fetal cell transplantation was negative as 7 ½ years old male with oligophrenia at the level of debility, and severe seizure disorder, had two seizures after *cell transplantation of brain cortex, medulla alba of brain, temporal lobe of brain, frontal lobe of brain*, and so any further treatment was stopped as this was quite unusual in our experience with treatment by cell transplantation in children with genetic diseases. On the other side, the height and weight of the patients increased over the next 3 months, and overall there was a clinical improvement. The patient was hospitalized at the Endocrinology Research Center of the Russian Academy of Medical Sciences in Moscow.

X-linked recessive (XR) type of inheritance occurs predominantly in males, because in men with XY configuration of sex chromosomes one pathologic gene on dominant chromosome X suffices for phenotypic expression. Classically, a pathologic gene transfers from the asymptomatic mother/ carrier to 50% of her sons and to 50% daughters/ asymptomatic carriers. Transfer from father to son is impossible, because father transfers to son chromosome Y.

List of more common XR disorders:

Addison's disease*
Agammaglobulinemia – type Burton, and Swiss type
Color blindness red/green
Muscular dystrophy Becker*
Muscle dystrophy Duchenne*
Diabetes insipidus renalis*
Fabry's disease*
Hemofilia A and B*
Mucopolysaccharidoses*
Hunter's syndrome (MPS type II)*
Lesch-Nyhan syndrome*
Lowe's oculocerebrorenal syndrome*
Gangliosidoses*
Menkes' disease
Non-spherocytic hemolytic anemia due to G6PD deficit
X-linked mental retardations*

Familial hyperuricemia
Ocular albinism, types I and II*
Syndrome of testicular feminization

Menkes' disease, XR disorder of copper metabolism with incidence of 1:50,000 of newborn boys, is due to a defective ATP-ase that binds copper, and removes copper ions from cells. There is an accumulation of copper in the intestine and other tissues, but *not in the liver*. It affects CNS, connective tissue and vascular system, and is fatal in infancy. There is a typical facies with full cheeks and fish-like mouth, microgenia, flat nose with short philtrum, minimal eyebrows, depigmented kinky hair 'stiff like steel shavings', microcephaly, mental retardation, seizures. Serum level of copper, and ceruloplasmin, are low. The activity of copper dependent enzymes: SOD and cytochrome oxidase is low [230].

X-linked dominant type of inheritance occurs mostly *in females*, but when it happens in males, the course of disease is much more severe and usually lethal. Transfer from father to son is impossible because father transfers to son chromosome Y. Such disorders are rare.

Hereditary hypophosphatemic vitamin-D resistant rachitis, with a decreased reabsorption of phosphorus in proximal tubule of kidneys, and hypophosphatemia, decreased mineralization of bones, with bony defects, and retarded growth, is rare.

Others, such as Aarskog syndrome, Incontinentio pigmenti, Ornitintranscarbamylase deficiency, are all very rare.

Y-linked *genetic disorders* are unknown except for those causing *infertility*, since the sole gene on chromosome Y is 'testis determining factor' that determines the male sex.

Syndromes of defective DNA repair mechanism, also known as *syndromes of spontaneous chromosomal instability*.

Essential biological prerequisite for normal prenatal and postnatal development is the ability of organism to maintain a structural integrity of DNA, carry out DNA synthesis exactly, and continuously remove or repair changes of DNA caused by mutations and environmental cancerogens. Several diseases with defective DNA repair processes have been identified, with resulting hypersensitivity to various damaging factors, i.e. radiation of variable wavelength from UV to X-rays. In these cases there is a *continuous 'spontaneous' disruption of structural integrity of chromosomes* (that explains the name *'syndromes of spontaneous chromosome* instability), *chomosomal tears and breaks*, with eventual imperfect reconstruction of chromosomes, the consequence of which is a *higher incidence of malignancy*.

The following 5 diseases are the most common of such syndromes.

Xeroderma pigmentosum is AR disorder with incidence 1:250,000. Hypersensitivity to sun rays is the main abnormality. In 80 – 90 % of patients there is a faulty repair of DNA damaged by UV radiation, in remaining cases a defect of post-replication DNA repair after UV-radiation. Photosensitivity and photophobia appear between 6 months and 3 years of life. In the 1st stage, there is a pronounced erythema after sun exposure with subsequent diffuse pigmentation. In the 2nd poikilo-dermic stage, lentigo-like pigmentations, skin atrophy, teleangiectasias, angiomas, ectropion, develop. In the 3rd precancerous stage tensile skin atrophy, senile keratoses, flat ulcers, appear. In the 4th cancerous stage various skin cancers develop. Two thirds of patients die by the age of 20 from cancers or secondary infections.

Fanconi syndrome, or Syndrome of Fanconi anemia, is AR disorder with incidence of 1:350,000 newborns, characterized by progressive panmyelophthisis. Besides pancytopenia, in 50% of patients there is a short stature, anomalies of radius and thumb, and microcephaly, in 20% mental retardation, in 7% deafness. Leukemias and other cancers develop frequently. Patients die young from bleeding disorders, infections, and other complications of panmyelophthisis.

Ataxia-teleangiectasia, or Louis-Bar syndrome, is AR disorder with incidence 1:40,000 to 1:100,000 of newborns. Oculocutaneous teleangiectasias appear in the first year of life, first on conjunctivas, later on the cheeks next to the nose, on auricles, gingivas, and elsewhere. When infant starts to walk, ataxia appears, and becomes progressively worse. Later on choreoathetosis, intentional tremor, dysarthria, are observed. At the age of 6 months recurrent respiratory infections begin, which become frequent between 3 and 8 years of age, often leading to bronchiectases, and such clinical cause leads to a suspicion of immunodeficiency disorder. Cancer development is frequent. There is a lack of IgA and IgE, decreased cell immunity, and increased level of α-fetoprotein due to liver damage. Lifespan is shortened due to pathology of brain and lungs, as well as due to cancer.

Bloom syndrome is AR disorder with incidence 1:100,000 newborns, most common in Ashkenazy Jews. In the 1st year of life, a typical teleangiectatic erythema of butterfly shape appears on the face that exacerbates following sun exposure. Growth delay begins already in utero. There is immunodeficiency with B-cells malfunction and recurrent infections. Cancer is frequent and is the main cause of death at a young age.

Cockayne syndrome is a rare AR disorder with hypersensitivity to UV radiation and to chemical carcinogens.

Unstable trinucleotide repeats, one of the newest discoveries in genetics, are the cause of ***Syndrome of fragile chromosome X type A***, also known as Martin-Bell syndrome, a single gene disorder with an incidence of 1:250 in males, and 1:2,000 in females, the *second most frequent specific cause of mental retardation after Down syndrome*. The fragile chromo-some X is found in males in 5 – 40% of cells, in females less often. Male patients are tall, have a long face with prominent mandible, long auricles which stick out laterally, and large testes. Mental retardation is accompanied in 10% of cases with epilepsy. Diagnosis is possible after 2 – 3 years of age.

Enzymopathies, or inborn errors of metabolism is another way to group *single gene disorders*, and is more pragmatic for a medical practitioner.

Metabolism consists of multiple biochemical steps, each one catalyzed by a specific enzyme. Any change of sequence of purine and pyrimidine bases in DNA causes a change of sequence of aminoacids in the protein portion of an enzyme that leads to a malfunction of the affected enzyme. There is a subsequent blockage in the metabolic pathway the outcome of which is that the substrate A, which should enter into a biochemical reaction with the enzyme X as catalyst to create a substance B, but has not done so due to the defect of enzyme X, has accumulated in the cell instead. The result of such accumulation can be:

- substrate A by its sheer volume 'crowds out' all cell components, as is the case with 'storage diseases', such as glycogenoses, lipidoses,

- substrate A becomes toxic in higher concentration, or solidifies because of low solubility, and thereby becomes harmful, i.e. cystine in cystinuria, uric acid in gout,
- entry of substrate A into alternative metabolic pathway with enzyme Z as a catalyst creates a harmful metabolite E, as in phenylketonuria,
- inhibition of metabolism of another enzyme Y, or of transport protein necessary for carrying other substances, such as substrate C,
- a lack of substance B, the product of the original biochemical reaction, i.e. in glycogenosis there is a lack of glucose; a lack of substance B can also raise the turnover of other enzymatic reactions, or it can disrupt a feedback mechanisms, such as when the lack of 21-hydroxylase stimulates secretion of ACTH-releasing factor from hypothalamus, and thereby of ACTH, and that then leads to an increased secretion of various precursors of cortisol, with resulting *adrenogenital syndrome.*

In order to elucidate the preceding explanation, look at the metabolic pathway A→B→C→D→E→F→G and assume that there is a deficiency of an enzyme that converts C into D. That reduces the production of D, E, F, and finally of G, the end product, but increases the level of C, later on also of B, and perhaps even A. If C, B, or A, are toxic in high concentrations, or can be converted to toxic compounds by other metabolic pathways, a pathological condition will develop, a disease, and often premature death.

Because of their enormous importance, the enzymes are produced in excessive quantities, and for that reason, enzymopathies are clinically apparent only in homozygotes where both alleles are abnormal.

A lack of an amino acid, due to poor nutrition, defect of transport protein, or defect of production of urea, cause serious disturbances as a rule. An excess of aminoacids is usually harmful as well.

Phenylketonuria (PKU), AR disorder with incidence 1:10,000, is caused by a diminished activity of phenylalaninhydroxylase, an enzyme that turns L-phenylalanine into tyrosine in the liver. Abnormal concentration of phenylalanine causes damage of cells of developing CNS that leads to severe mental retardation and seizures. When plasma concentration of phenylalanine reaches certain level, it starts to break down via secondary pathways, mostly to pyruvate, that appears in urine, and inhibits transport of other amino acids so that they cannot enter brain cells in sufficient quantities. Lack of melanine, produced from tyrosine, disrupts pigmentation and triggers photosensitivity. Onset is at birth, blond hair, blue eyes, eczema and typical mouse odor of urine, are typical clinical findings. Screening eliminates most of such patients as candidates for stem cell transplantation as they stay well by following a strict non-phenylalanine diet.

But in a malignant form of phenylketonuria with defective synthesis of tetrahydropterine (BH4), a co-factor of phenylalaninehydroxylase, that causes deficit of hydroxylation of phenylalanine, tyrosine and trypto-phan, and thereby a decreased production of neurotransmitters dopamine, noradrenaline, and serotonine, not even strict diet can prevent CNS damage, unless the patient received missing neurotransmitters, i.e. DOPA, 5-hydroxytryptophan, and BH4. In these 2 – 3 % of patients with PKU stem cell transplantation has to be considered.

Alkaptonuria, also known as ochronosis, AR disorder with incidence of 1:10,000 to 1:100,000, is due to a lack of homogentisate-1-2-dioxygenase, that leads to an accumulation of homogentisic acid in the organism, a normal product of metabolism of phenylalanine and tyrosine. The elimination of homogentisic acid causes dark color of urine. Onset is at birth. Deposits of excess of ochronotic pigment in various connective tissues: sclera, cartilage, tendons, intima of larger vessels, endocardium, lungs, tympanic membrane, etc., are typical clinical signs. There is an increased incidence of kidney and prostatic stones, starting in childhood, and disabling arthropathy of spine and large joints, appearing after 20 years of age, that make a timely treatment of this disease by stem cell transplantation mandatory.

Albinism, oculo-cutaneous, or ocular, is a group of genetic disorders of melanocyte system of eye and skin, mostly AR, but also XR, or AD, with an inborn lack or paucity of pigment melanine in skin, hair, eyes, that leads to white skin, red iris, photophobia, nystagmus and decreased vision. The onset is at birth.

Hyperglycinemia due to faulty propionyl-CoA-carboxylase, *Hyperoxaluria, Maple sirup disease* with defects of multiple enzymes for decarboxylation of valine, leucine, isoleucine, *Homocystinuria, Cystinosis* due to transport defect, *Hyperprolinemia* caused by faulty prolindehydrogenase, which is also also the cause of *Alport syndrome*, are other enzymopathies involving amino acids.

A lack of carbohydrates occurs in the following genetic disorders.

Galactosemia, AR disorder of galactose metabolism with incidence of 1:62,000, is divided into three types.

In Type I, or classical galactosemia, defect of galactose-1-phosphaturidyltransferase blocks a conversion of galactose to glucose. The accumulation of toxic galactose becomes apparent from the moment that newborn ingests milk for the first time. There is an immediate vomiting, unwillingness to drink, diarrhea, hypoglycaemic attacks, and subsequently cachexia, icterus, hepatomegaly, cataracts, seizures, and mental retardation develop. Screening for enzymes in erythrocytes and trophoblast, prevents death, but even galactose-free diet cannot stop long term complications, i.e. poor growth, neurologic and speech abnormalities, mental retardation, so that stem cell transplantation should be strongly considered.

Types II and III are due to absence of different enzymes. Type III is a major problem, because insufficient intake of galactose leads to an insufficient production of UDP-galactose, and that causes already in the 2nd year of life severe mental retardation and sensori-neural deafness, since galactose is an essential structural component of the brain.

Hereditary fructose intolerance, is due to a defect of fructose-1-P-aldolase; splitting of fructose from fruits is blocked, and fructose-1-phosphate accumulates, which triggers in the liver an inhibition of activity of fructose-1,6-P_2-aldolase, that in turn causes hepatogenic hypoglycemia, and can cause acute liver failure, or cirrhosis.

Glycogenoses: Glucose is stored in muscles and liver as glycogen. Its breakdown generates glucose that can be used in liver or in other organs. If splitting of glycogen is blocked, it accumulates and *hypoglycemia* develops. The cause is various enzymatic defects, and each is responsible for a different type of glycogenosis:

> Type Ia, named after von Gierke, with locus in the liver,
> Type Ib due to defect of microsomal glucose-6-phosphate-translocase,
> Type II, named after Pompe, with anorexia, hepatomegaly, muscle dystrophy, cardiomegaly and respiratory muscle weakness, death in the 1st year of life,
> Type III, the most common, named after Forbes and Cori, with locus in the liver,

Type IV, named after Anderson, where an abnormal form of glycogen is stored in brain, heart and peripheral muscles, and liver, with liver failure, and death already in childhood,
Type V, named after McArdle, with locus in peripheral muscles,
Type VI, named after Hers, with locus in the liver,
Type VII, named after Tarui, in which skeletal muscle glucose cannot be used for energy,
Type VIII, named after Huijing, with locus in the liver.

Lesch-Nyhan syndrome, XR disorder, a hypoxanthine-guanine-phosphoribosyltransferase deficiency, '*children's gout*', causes a premature appearance of gout with urolithiasis and pronounced brain dysfunction, e.g. choreoathetosis, paralysis of cranial nerves, mental retardation with self-mutilation.

Hyperhomocysteinemias, caused by an absence of cystathionine-β-synthase (CBS) and 5,10-methylene-tetrahydrofolate-reductase, lead to an accumulation of homocystein, an important lipid-independent factor of atherosclerosis, which due to its toxic effects causes:

1. direct damage of endothel,
2. changes of oxidation/reduction in blood vessel wall,
3. disturbance of thrombin/antithrombin system in favor of thrombogenesis.

In clinical practice it causes a premature arteriosclerosis and its complications, as well as spina bifida, and pathologic pregnancies.

Severe hyperhomocysteinemia is the 'classical' *homocystinuria*, AR disorder, with an incidence of 1:130,000, with onset at 2 – 30 years of life, where a lack of the same cystathionine-β-synthase(CBS) causes:

- lens dislocation, myopia,
- marfanoid tall habitus with long fingers, osteoporosis, spine deformities,
- mental retardation, psychiatric disorders, seizures, EEG abnormalities,
- arterial and venous thrombosis [234].

For treatment of **single gene disorders**, particularly when not sure of the exact nature, the stem cell transplantation of *liver, mesenchyme, adrenal cortex, placenta, brain cortex, medulla alba of brain, cardiomyoblasts*, is recommended.

Lysosomal enzymopathies, is a group of inborn errors of metabolism, so named because the accumulation of complex macromolecules, resulting from a failure of normal degradation due to a defect of a specific enzyme, takes place in lysosomes. They are known also as *'Lysosomal storage diseases'*. Lysosomes are cell organelles that contain an abundance of *acid hydrolases*, which degrade proteins, nucleic acids, glycoproteins, acid mucopolysaccharides, glycogen, glycolipids, lipids, *and peroxidase*. In majority of these diseases the basic dysfunction is the genetically caused failure of synthesis of active forms of specific hydrolases in ribosomes, or of their protein activators.

Genetic heterogeneity, involvement of multiple organ systems, and great clinical variability, is characteristic for lysosomal enzymopathies. Many of them are *genetic diseases of connective tissue*. See also chapter 56.

Clinically there is a big difference *between enzymopathies causing abnormal metabolism of small molecules*, i.e. aminoacids, and those causing *abnormal metabolism of large molecules*, i.e. glycosaminoglycans, sphingolipids, glycolipids, glycogen. In the first case the metabolism of mother can compensate the metabolic derangement of fetus, so that the abnormality becomes noticeable only after birth, while in the second case, the abnormality becomes apparent already in utero.

Lysosomal storage begins in early fetal stage, but clinical manifestation starts during the first 2 years of life, or later. Clinical course is of variable severity, usually with progressive *CNS malfunction, dysostosis multiplex*, i.e. dolichocephalia, ovoid vertebrae with hypoplasia, hypoplastic pelvis, flat acetabulum, wide diaphyses of long bones, wide ribs, abnormalities of metacarpal bones, as well as deafness, visual impairment, *hepatosplenomegaly*, skin abnormalities. A fatal outcome is common.

There are over 30 known lysosomal storage diseases. With the exception of XR disorders of Fabry's disease and Hunter syndrome (MPS II), all remaining are AR disorders. The following three groups are based *on the type of macromolecules accumulated in lysosomes*:

A. **Mucopolysaccharidoses** *always* include a *serious skeletal dysplasia*:

- *Hurler syndrome*, type IH, or 'Gargoylism', due to a defect of α-L-iduronidase, is diagnosed before the 2nd year; there is a typical facies like on antique water-fountains, dysostotic

macrocephaly, kyphoscoliosis, nanism, early cataract, corneal opacities, hepatosplenomegaly, and mental retardation; death before 10 years of life,
- *Scheie syndrome*, type IS, due to a defect of α-L-iduronidase, is diagnosed later; there are cataracts, normal intellect, and normal lifespan,
- *Hunter syndrome*, type II, due to a deficit of iduronate-2-sulphatase, is diagnosed before the 4th year; clinical findings are somewhat similar as in Hurler syndrome, but much milder: a lesser degree of mental retardation, nanism; there are no cataracts, corneal opacities, or skeletal deformities; death before 15 years of life,
- *Sanfillipo syndrome*, type III, due to a deficit of heparan-N-sulphatase in type A, α-N-acetyl-D-glucosaminidase in type B, α-glucosamine-N-acetyltransferase in type C, N-acetyl-glucosamin-6-sulphatase in type D, is diagnosed after the 2nd year; there is progressive dementia, nanism, disturbed behavior with aggressivity, some hepatomegaly, hypertrichosis, but no other physical abnormalities,
- *Morquio syndrome*, type IV, due to a defect of galactose-6-sulphatase in type A, or of α-galactosidase in type B, causes a nanism of various degree, cataract, thin dental enamel, progressive spine deformities, death in adulthood,
- *Maroteux-Lamy syndrome*, type VI, due to a deficit of N-acetylgalactosamine-4-sulphatase, causes a nanism of various degree, monster-like facies, typical kyphoscoliosis, corneal opacity, cardiopulmonary insufficiency, hepato-splenomegaly; intellect is normal, and lifespan nearly normal,
- *Sly syndrome*, type VII, due to a defect of β-glucuronidase, can be present at birth as a fatal hydrops fetalis, or it appears in infancy as mental retardation, minor skeletal deformities, or it becomes apparent in teens as a moderate mental retardation.

Cell transplantation of *various parts of brain, eye, placenta, liver, mesenchyme, cartilage, osteoblasts, peripheral myoblasts*, has brought only temporary improvements and retardation of progress of the disease. The lack of lysosomal enzymes can be positively influenced only for a short time, and incompletely. But this statement is based on clinical experience of treating such patients too late. If the treatment starts immediately after birth then the evaluation of possibilities of stem cell trans-plantation can begin.

B. **Oligosaccharidoses** are characterized by a disturbance of saccharide metabolism in glycoproteins and glycolipids, due to which there is an excessive accumulation of oligosaccharides in tissues and body fluids, and their excessive elimination in urine. *Glycoproteinoses* are the most common among oligosaccha-ridoses:

- *Mucolipidosis* Type I, or 'Pseudo-Hurler polydystrophy', and Types II – III – IV, or 'Sialidoses', are due to a defect of N-acetylglusosamino-1-phosphotransferase,
- *Glycoproteinsialidosis*, known as 'cherry-red-spot-myoclonus syndrome',
- *Aspartylglucosaminouria*, a L-aspartylamido-β-N-GlcNAc-aminohydrolase defect,
- *Fucosidosis*, due to a defect of α-L-fucosidase;
- *Mannosidosis*, due to a defect of α-D-mannosidase.

Aspartylglucosaminouria, appears between 1 and 5 years of age, with mental retardation, speech impairment, cataracts, hepatomegaly, and the same bone deformities as in mucopolysaccharidoses.

Fucosidosis, is diagnosed in infancy by Hurler-like phenotype, muscle hypotonia, slowly developing spastic tetraplegia and decerebration rigidity, frequent respiratory infections, hyperhidrosis, cardiomegaly; death before 6 years of age.

Mannosidosis, becomes apparent between 1 and 3 years of age, with Hurler-like phenotype, muscle hypotonia, hepatosplenomegaly, cataracts, bone abnormalities, frequent respiratory infections, vacuolised lymphocytes.

C. **Lipidoses**:

- *Farber's diseases*, or ceramidosis,
- *Krabbe disease*, or globoid leukodystrophy,
- *Gaucher disease*, types 1 – 2 – 3,
- *Metachromatic leukodystrophy*,
- *Neimann-Pick disease*, or sphingomyelin, or cholesterol, lipidoses,
- *Fabry's disease*, glycosphingolipidosis, or angiokeratoma corporis diffusum,
- G_{MI} *gangliosidoses*, types 1 – 2 – 3, due to a defect of β-D-galastosidase,

G_{M2} gangliosidoses, and variants, due to deficits of hexosaminidase A that splits N-acetylgalactosamine off sugar chains attached to the complex lipids called gangliosides; the variant B is Tay-Sachs disease,
- *Wolman disease,* due to a deficit of acid lipase,
- *Neuronal ceroidlipofuscinoses,* infantile, juvenile, adult.

Gaucher disease, is a defect of lysosomal β-glucosecerebrosidase, as a result of which glucosecerebrosid accumulates in spleen, liver, and bone marrow in Gaucher cells. There is hypersplenism with thrombocytopenia, spontaneous fractures, pneumonias, cor pulmonale. There are 3 types:

- *infantile* type, onset by 3 months of age, with massive hepatosplenomegaly, dysphagia, digestive malfunction, cachexia, mental retardation, muscle hypertonia, opisthotonus, strabism, normal retina,
- *juvenile* type,
- *adult* type, onset at the age of 20, with massive splenomegaly, some hepatomegaly, hypersplenism with leukopenia, hemorrhagic diathesis, Perthes disease, bone pain.

Stem cell transplantation of *liver, cardiomyoblasts, peripheral myoblasts, exocrine pancreas, intestine,* is advised.

Our study of infantile type Gaucher's disease was carried out at the Research Center of Pediatrics of the Russian Academy of Medical Sciences, and reported at the 1st Symposium on Transplantation of Human Fetal tissues in Moscow, December 4 – 7, 1995, under the title: "Treatment of Gaucher disease in children with the help of human fetal tissues". The report deals with 6 children, from 6 to 13 years of age, 3 girls, and 3 boys, treated by infusions of human fetal hepatocytes. Diagnosis was confirmed in all 6 children by bone marrow biopsy and finding of typical cells filled with glucocerebroside. In two children a cytogenetic study to uncover the defect of glucocerebrosidase was done. The diagnosis was proven in all 6 children by DNA study to find a specific Gaucher's disease allele. One child underwent splenectomy at the age of 4.

All children showed growth retardation, frequent intercurrent infections, bone lesions, hepatosplenomegaly, slight anemia, and thrombocytopenia.

During the first round of treatment, every child received 5 *infusions of human fetal hepatocytes*, one week apart. In one female patient fever and hallucinations appeared after the 4th infusion, which resolved in 3 days, and so no further treatment was given. Interestingly, this patient had the best clinical result of the whole group, i.e. decrease of size of liver and spleen by 6 cm, so that further treatment was not needed. The second round of treatment began 4 months later, and consisted of 3 infusions, 7 – 12 days apart. Subsequently infusions were carried as necessary, every 6 – 8 weeks.

In one male patient signs of intrahepatic type of portal hypertension developed, and so further treatment was stopped: the result was not as good as in the remainder of the group, but there was an increased growth rate and subjective improvement.

There was a dramatic decrease of hepatosplenomegaly in 5 of 6 children during 6 months of treatment, but after the termination of infusions the hepatosplenomegaly re-appeared. Bone pain disappeared in all 6 patients. X-ray findings remained unchanged. There was a marked growth spurt, physical development, and decreased frequency of intercurrent infections.

Gaucher's disease is one of those where the exact nature of enzymatic defect has been known for some time, and the missing enzyme is commercially available for treatment. The sole problem is the enormous cost of such medication, prohibitive in most countries. The purpose of this study was to find an alternative, more affordable treatment.

Farber's disease, with reddish subcutaneous lumps, swelling and rigidity of extremities, dysphonia, fever, sometimes also with CNS and cardiopulmonary symptomatology.

Krabbe disease, starting in infancy as a slowly progressing encephalitis-like condition, cerebral degeneration with spasms.

Metachromatic leukodystrophy, where the deficit of arylsulfatase A, and its variants causes demyelination, and storage of myelin breakdown products in CNS, liver and kidneys. Onset is in early childhood. There is muscle hypertonia, hyper-reflexia, delayed gross motor development, *and eventually* muscle atrophy of lower extremities, ataxia, dysarthria, progressive mental retardation, rigidity, blindness, deafness, loss of speech, total loss of contact with the world; death between 2 and 6 years of life. There are also very rare juvenile and adult forms with chronic clinical course over many years. Stem cell transplantation of *liver, placenta, intestine, exocrine pancreas, adrenal cortex, mesenchyme, spinal cord, peripheral myoblasts,* is advised.

Niemann-Pick disease, is an accumulation of sphingomyelin and cholesterol in lysozymes, that becomes apparent at different age of the patient, with food refusal, vomiting, hepatosplenomegaly, mental retardation, red spots on retinal macula, muscle hypotonia, psychomotor delay. Four types are clinically recognized:

- type A (80% of cases), a defect of sphingomyelinase, has onset at 6 months of age, with severe developmental delay, hepatosplenomegaly, macular degeneration with blindness, death before 2 years of age,
- type B, a defect of sphingomyelinase, is a storage disease without CNS involvement,
- Type C, a defect of protein, very important in intracellular transportation and distribution of cholesterol, with onset in the 2nd year of life, is the most common, with progressive gross motor and mental retardation, death between 3 and 6 years of life,
- Type D with onset in middle childhood and survival until 20 years of life.

Fabry's disease, begins in teens, or early twenties, with diffuse teleangiectasias, diarrhea, kidney disorders, lower leg edema, corneal opacities, burning pain in fingers and toes. Stem cell transplantation of *mesenchyme, placenta, liver*, is advised.

Gangliosidoses, various defects of hexoseaminidase and its activator, or defects of β-galactosidase, cause an accumulation of gangliosides that results in very serious brain dysfunction and death in childhood. They begin at 6 months of age, with psychomotor delay, blindness, nystagmus, decerebration state, mental retardation, macrocephaly, seizures. There are a few variants:

- G_{M1} Gangliosidosis, or 'Pseudo-Hurler syndrome', with muscle hypotonia, delayed motor development, neurologic defects, skeletal abnormalities,
- G_{M2} Gangliosidosis, with mental retardation, typical red spots on retinal macula, macroglossia, hepatosplenomegaly, limitation of

joint motion, gross facial features, lymphocyte vacuoles,

A variant B is *Tay-Sachs disease*, where non-degraded lipid gangliosides accumulate in lysosomes, leading to cell death. Phenotypically there are severe neurological signs and symptoms, blindness, mental retardation, death in childhood.

A variant O is *Sandhoff syndrome*, where non-degraded lipid gangliosides accumulate in brain, with progressive mental breakdown.

Stem cell transplantation of *liver, placenta, mesenchyme, adrenal cortex*, is advised.

Wolman's disease, a defect of acid lipase leads to pathologic accumulation of cholesterol esthers, begins with vomiting, steatorhea, hepatosplenomegaly, liver cirrhosis, adrenal calcification, and causes death in the first 4 months due to cachexia; there is no CNS involvement; vacuolized lymphocytes are typical [231, 234].

Peroxisomal enzymopathies, AR disorders with exception of adrenoleukodystrophies, that are XR disorders, are named after peroxisomes, cell organelles found in all cells with the exception of erythrocytes. Peroxisomes produce oxidases, which in turn generate hydrogen peroxide that is then reduced by catalase into water. Peroxisome enzymes fulfill multiple essential functions for the cell: synthesis of plasmalogel, dolichol, and cholesterol, β-oxidation of long fatty acids, production of hydrogen peroxide, degradation of all active kinds of oxygen, superoxide, etc. Since these enzymes are of *vital importance for metabolism of lipids, particularly those in CNS*, many of peroxisome disorders present a clinical picture of progressive psycho-motor dysfunction.

Combination of craniofacial dysmorphism, i.e. high prominent forehead, wide fontanelles and cranial sutures, epicanthus, auricle deformities, gothic palate, *with neurological findings*, such as psychomotor retardation, hypotonia, absent or minimal reflexes, deafness, degenera-tion of white matter, abnormal EEG, etc. and *with ophthalmological findings*, such as cataract, chorioretinopathy, optic nerve dysplasia, and *hepatomegaly* with fibrosis/cirrhosis, short extremities, as well as the *laboratory finding of a lack of peroxisomes and lamellar inclusions in hepatocytes*, point to the diagnosis of peroxisomal enzymopathy.

Among these very rare disease a few are somewhat more common:

- *Adrenoleukodystrophy*, neonatal, infantile, adolescent, or adult, characterized by adrenal gland dysfunction and generalized demyelination of CNS, invariably fatal,
- *Zellweger syndrome*, or cerebro-hepato-renal syndrome, due to a deficiency of pipecolate oxidase,
- *Refsum disease*, or Phytanic Acid Storage Disease,
- *Hyperoxaluria*, types I and II, characterized by severe nephrolithiasis, and kidney failure,
- *Chondrodysplasia punctata*, rhizomelic type, characterized by pug nose, marked shortening of proximal limbs, death in infancy.

Zellweger syndrome, or cerebro-hepato-renal syndrome, is a very rare disorder, diagnosed at birth or early infancy, with typical facies: hypertelorism, flat nose, full cheeks, hypognathia, and extreme muscle hypotonia, areflexia, weak swallowing and suction reflexes, minimal gross motor development, mental retardation, hepatomegaly [230].

Refsum disease, a deficiency of phytanic acid α-oxidase, leads to a blockage of the breakdown of phytanic acid that accumulates, and is progressively built into myelin, which causes polyneuropathies. It begins between 2 and 20 years of age, with night blindness, paresthesias, ataxia, pareses, painful attacks [230, 234].

Stem cell transplantation of *cartilage, mesenchyme, liver, kidney, medulla alba of brain, brain cortex, diencephalon, retina, optic nerve*, is advised.

Mitochondrial genetic diseases

The most important function of mitochondrias, cytoplasmatic organelles with double membranes, is the production of energy necessary for cell metabolism by creation of ATP via oxidative phosphorylation system, or OXPHOS. Oxidative phosphorylation is carried out by five complexes of 'respiratory chain cascade', that are complexes of polypeptide enzymes located in the intermembraneous space in continuity with inner mitochondrial membrane. The first four complexes represent the respiratory chain proper and the 5th complex is that of ATP-synthase. The number of mitochondrias in cytoplasm is commensurate to the energetic needs of the cell.

Mitochondrias contain also DNA organized into a separate genetic system, which is 10 – 20 times more vulnerable to mutations in comparison with nuclear DNA, but due to multiple copies of mitochondrial DNA in majority of mammal cells the impact of each mutation is substantially reduced.

OXPHOS processes are controlled to a great degree by nuclear genes, and *mutation of nuclear genes and mitochondrial genes cause mitochondrial genetic diseases with autosomal inheritance.*

Typical property of mitochondrial DNA is its *exclusive transfer from mother*, and for that reason is this type of inheritance called '*maternal cytoplasmatic*'. Only females can carry mutant gene from generation to generation.

During mitosis the segregation of mitochondrial genetic material is *by a pure chance* and thereby *even minimal genotypic changes can cause major phenotypic changes*, i.e. there is a 'threshold effect'.

In summary, *mitochondrial genetic diseases are characterized by*:

- maternal type of inheritance,
- segregation of mitochondrias during mitosis with 'treshold effect',
- signs of OXPHOS malfunction in those organs where it is of vital importance, and where mitochondrias are abundant, such as CNS, peripheral muscles, (including extraocular), heart muscle fibers, including those of the conductive system of the heart, liver and kidneys, deafness, retinitis pigmentosa, optic nerve atrophy,
- laboratory findings in muscle biopsy of 'ragged red fibers (RRF)', abnormal paracrystallic inclusions, abnormal mitochondrias, and of lactic acidosis.

The basic difference between mitochondrial inheritance and X-linked dominant inheritance is that in the first group of diseases there is no transfer from father, and in the second group there is a pre-dominant incidence in female patients.

Clinically these diseases are *extremely important in newborns and infants*, where they sometimes *masquerade as Reye Syndrome, or Sudden Infant Death Syndrome. In early stages the neuromuscular signs are present only in minority of patients. Diagnosis is difficult until signs of multiple organ involvement become apparent*, i.e. simultaneous appearance of hepatomegaly and liver dysfunction, and malfunction of CNS, i.e. dementia, myoclonus, seizures, mental retardation, of kidneys, i.e. Fanconi syndrome, aminoaciduria, heart, including arrhythmias, of hematopoietic system, and growth retardation. Extreme variability of clinical picture and course is typical for mitochondrial diseases: unusual combination of symptoms & signs, early onset with rapidly progressive course, involving organs with seemingly no relationship from the viewpoint of embryology and biological functions.

Here is a brief description of some mitochondrial genetic diseases:

- *Kearns-Sayre syndrome* begins before 20 years of age, with a typical 'sleepy facies' due to ophthalmoplegia, atypical retinitis pigmentosa, mitochondrial myopathy, cardiomyopathy with a pacemaker requiring arrhythmia, cerebellar syndrome, kyphoscoliosis, hyperlordosis, dry 'pellagra-like' skin, high protein concentration in CSF.

- *Leigh disease*, a neurodegenerative multisystem disease with great variability of clinical findings, starts before 2 years of age, with optic nerve atrophy, ophthalmoplegia, retinal degeneration, respiratory malfunction, ataxia, seizures, psychomotor retardation, typical findings on MRI of brain, and lactic acidosis. Myopathy is non-specific, and liver and heart are involved only occasionally. There is a sudden and unexpected worsening of clinical picture and metabolic parameters after infections. General condition is serious, the disease is fatal by 5 years of age.

- *Leber hereditary optic nerve neuropathy*, acute or subacute painless loss of central vision caused by bilateral atrophy of optic nerve, begins between 12 and 30 years of age, with typical retinal findings; it is *a common cause of bilateral blindness of adolescents and young adults*.

- *Myoclonic epilepsy with ragged red fibers*, starts in late childhood to early adulthood, with characteristic progressive myoclonic epilepsy, slowly progressive dementia, deafness, ataxia, mitochondrial myopathy with RRF.

- *Mitochondrial encephalomyelopathy*, commences between 5 and 15 years of age, when in a previously perfectly normal child *suddenly a cerebrovascular accident-like state* develops with infarcts of brain cortex or subcortex proven by CT scan or MRI, which then subsides within hours or days. During the next episode of a CVA-like status additional neurological findings appear: ventricular dilatation, cortical atrophy, basal ganglia calcification. There is always mitochondrial myopathy.

- *Pearson syndrome with OXPHOS malfunction* involves predominantly hematopietic stem cells in bone marrow: serious macrocytic anemia, requiring repeated blood transfusions, with variable degree of neutropenia and thrombocytopenia that appear already in early childhood. Marked variability of clinical findings and course is typical for this condition. Patients can die in early stage or a spontaneous improvement of pancytopenia is possible. Later on, a malfunction of additional organs becomes apparent, caused by defects of OXPHOS. There is growth retardation, progressive neurological disorders, mitochondrial myopathy, pancreatic malfunction, and lactic acidosis [230].

As treatment of all mitochondrial genetic diseases stem cell transplantation of *cardiomyoblasts, peripheral myoblasts, liver, placenta, intestine, mesenchyme, exocrine pancreas*, is recommended, along with supplementation of enzymes of the respiratory chain, and neuro-muscular chain by Coliacron, a combination of succinate-dehydrogenase, NAD-kinase, acetyl-CoA-synthetase, and glutaminsynthetase, and high oral intake of γ-linoleic acid and vitamin E for mitochondrial double membrane regeneration.

There are about 2,000 known genetic diseases, and many variants thereof, and only a few of them have any known treatment. Some of them have been treated with stem cell transplantation with success, but many others, particularly the rare ones, have not, because no one has attempted to do it, or at least no medical report has been written about it.

Since stem cell transplantation is indeed safe, there is no harm to use it to treat an infant with a newly diagnosed genetic disease. There are only two possible outcomes: either there will be an improvement, or there will be no change in the condition of the patient. Unfortunately a physician can learn about the benefit of stem cell transplantation for the treatment of that specific child with a rare genetic disease only by trial and error. There is no harm in trying in such case. If parents make a decision to treat their child, then stem cell transplantation must be carried out without delay [230].

Chapter 46

There can be no progress (real, that is, moral) except in the individual and by the individual himself.
Charles Baudelaire, 1821 – 1867 [Mon Coeur Misà Nu, 1887]

Science is the search for truth – it is not a game in which one tries to beat his opponent, to do harm to others.
Linus Carl Pauling, 1901 – 1994, [No More War! 1958]

CHROMOSOMAL DISEASES

Treatment of chromosomal aberrations has been one of the major success stories of stem cell transplantation. They result from *mutations that alter number of chromosomes* or their *structure*.

Depending upon the type of stricken chromosome, location of damage caused by mutation, and its extent, chromosomal aberrations present themselves in the phenotype.

When chromatin is lost or gained in the process of re-arrangement, it is said to be unbalanced. *Unbalanced re-arrangements* are generally associated with developmental delay or intellectual impairment, birth defects or nanism, whereas *balanced re-arrangements* often have no effect on physical or intellectual development.

Structural chromosome re-arrangements that are *present at conception affect every cell* and are called constitutional. Re-arrangements that *occur during later development affect only a portion of cells and result in mosaicism*. Structural re-arrangements that occur after birth are called acquired, and may cause cancer by altering cell cycle regulation.

Chromosomal abnormalities due to structural aberrations make up a significant portion of chromosomal genetic diseases. At birth, structural re-arrangements, both balanced and unbalanced, were found in *1:400 of infants*.

If a balanced structural re-arrangement is inherited, there is a low risk for physical or mental impairment. However, *when the abnormality is de novo, when parents have normal karyotypes, the risk for genetic disease is increased* even when the re-arrangement is balanced.

In *numerical aberrations* the number of chromosomes differs from the normal diploid number of 46. *Every human has a certain number of polyploid cells even under normal conditions*, i.e. cells with doubled, tripled, or quadrupled number of chromosomes. The classical example is megakaryocytes. Some cells, i.e. thrombocytes, erythrocytes, squamous epithelial cells, have no nucleus, i.e. are nulliploid. Aneuploidia means decreased or increased number of chromosomes by one or 2.

Chromosomal aberrations are very frequent in humans, the younger the fetus, the higher the incidence. It is estimated that in aborted embryos or fetuses of the 1st trimester approximately 50% would be found with chromosomal aberrations, or that serious chromosomal aberrations would be encountered in 25% of all pregnancies. In very early spontaneous abortions the incidence of chromosomal aberrations is 60%, in non-live births 4 – 6%, and in live births 0.6%. Fetuses with polyploidia, the most serious chromosomal aberration, are practically never born live, and if born live, they never survive. Overall incidence of chromosomal aberrations in live births is approximately 1.7%.

Today, medicine knows syndromes of complete trisomy, partial trisomy or monosomy for each of 22 autosomal chromosomes, in some cases in more that one chromosome. The overall incidence of autosomal chromosomal aberrations is *1:400 of live births*.

NUMERICAL CHROMOSOMAL ABERRATIONS:

- *Abnormal number of autosomal chromosomes is the most frequent lethal factor*, i.e. cause of the fetal death. *Only the monosomies of chromosomes 21 and 22 have ever been born live* of all possible complete monosomies. On the other side *trisomies* of chromosomes *7, 8, 9, 10, 13, 14, 18, 21, 22, were born live.*

- The number of types of *sex-chromosome mosaicism* is relatively large. Abnormalities are in numbers or structures. Incidence of serious sex-chromosome aberrations in live-born boys is 1:400, and in newborn girls 1:650.

A. Autosomal chromosomal aberrations

Trisomy 21, Down syndrome or mongolism, is the most frequent and best known chromosomal disorder with incidence of 1:700 live births. It is a disorder of the whole body involving primarily abnormalities of physical and mental development, with an added insult of marked weakness of the immune system:

1. Somatic, gross motor, intellectual and mental development, are lagging behind norms, and more so with each passing day after birth,
2. Nanism, hypothyreoidism, and adrenal insufficiency, are the result of endocrine abnormalities,
3. Dysproportionate growth of face and cranium, not noticeable at birth, becomes more obvious with age as a result of cranial growth delays; brain growth is slowed down dyspropotionately as well: occipital and parietal lobes lag behind more than the other parts, but actually the cerebellum is the most affected,
4. Mongoloid physiognomy becomes more noticeable with age,
5. Delayed development of all mesenchymal structures causes immune system deficiency,
6. There is no direct relationship between the degree of visible chromosomal damage and the delay of intellectual development,
7. Nanism begins in infancy but becomes most pronounced during puberty.

Typical clinical findings are psychomotor retardation, growth delay, muscle hypotonia, joint hypermobility, as well as brachycephalia with flat occiput, dysplastic auricles, wide, flat facies, mongoloid slant of eyes with epicanthus, Bruschfield corneal spots, button nose with a wide root, open mouth with macroglossia and lingua scrotalis, gothic palate, dental anomalies, pectus carinatum, absence of ribs, congenital heart defects, umbilical hernia, gastrointestinal stenoses, short and wide fingers, brachymesophalangia and clinodactyly of little fingers, and atypical dermatoglyphics.

There is an increased incidence of leukemias and immunological defects. At autopsy of adult Down syndrome patients, morphological and histochemical changes typical of Alzheimer disease are found in the brain.

Lifespan is shortened, but in absence of congenital heart defects and serious immunological deficiencies, Down syndrome patients can live up to 60 years of age.

There is no reproductive ability in complete trisomy 21, but patients with mosaic forms of trisomy 21 can be fertile and have normal offsprings.

The older the mother, the higher is the incidence of trisomy 21 and all other chromosomal aberrations [95, 185, 187, 197, 198, 235 - 240].

Therapeutic principles:

1. regulation of endocrine balance, in particular hypothyroidism and lowered function of glucocorticoid portion of adrenal cortex,
2. elimination of ever increasing delay in brain development,
3. correction of immune system deficiency,
4. repair of defects of supportive tissues of the body,
5. total rehabilitation of all body systems, by physiotherapy, active exercise, speech therapy, occupational therapy, and all educational tools available,
6. avoidance of therapeutic nihilism.

Correct nutrition, including yoghurt made by Acidophilus species, and mega-vitamin/mineral supplementation, are mandatory, in particular of vitamins A, B1 and B6. Enzymotherapy should be routinely used, in particular if the quality of nutrition lags.

Ultrafiltrates of animal fetal brain tissue should be given orally, or in suppositories, once a week between stem cell transplantation treatments.

A majority of patients, with a suspicion of hypothyroidism, even though the laboratory tests of thyroid function are within limits of normal, have to receive minimal doses of thyroid hormone.

Depending upon the experience of the treating physicians, Down syndrome patients may be given Phosphatidylcholine, Choline bitartrate, or Centrophenoxine, for a neurotransmitter function augmentation. Piracetam has been shown to raise tryptophan levels in Down syndrome patients and the same applies to 5-hydroxytryptophan.

Since the brain is the most damaged organ, stem cell transplantation treatment is begun with implantation of *brain cortex, diencephalon, mesencephalon, and hypothalamus*. Subsequently, in every 4 months repeated implantations, cell transplants of *spinal cord, cerebellum, occipital lobe of brain, temporal lobe of brain, frontal lobe of brain, and parietal lobe of brain*, are selected as clinically necessary.

In addition to cell transplants of various parts of brain:

- cell transplants of *thymus and adrenal cortex* are advised for immune deficiency,
- cell transplants of *cartilage and placenta* for achondroplasia-like condition,
- cell transplants of *thyroid and liver* should be given once between 6th and 10th year of age,
- cell transplants of *adrenal cortex and ovary* to girls should be given *once* between 6th and 10th year of life,
- cell transplants of *adrenal cortex and testis* to boys should be given *once* between 8th and 10th year of life,
- cell transplants of *cardiomyoblasts, liver, lung*, for heart defects,
- cell transplants of *intestine, exocrine pancreas, liver*, for gastrointestinal damage,
- cell transplants of *placenta, lens, corpus vitreum*, for early cataract.

Standard medical textbooks state that genetic and chromosomal diseases have no known treatment, with rare exceptions. In reality, there have been many publications from the university hospitals of Germany, USSR/Russia, Spain, and USA prior to 1957, etc., that report on the success in the *treatment of many genetic and chromosomal diseases by a complex therapeutic protocol based on stem cell transplantation*, so that therapeutic nihilism is not justified whatsoever.

Down syndrome has been a shining example. Schmid published data about his personal treatment of over 3,000 children with Down syndrome, whereby 25% of his patients were able to attend regular schools [95].

Published data prove the statistically significant improvement in height, skull circumference, index of brain volume, IQ and mental development, motor development. Among untreated children with Down syndrome 50 – 60% dies during the first 5 years of life due to intercurrent infections and cardiac failure, while the mortality of children treated in accordance with the described protocol is the same as in normal children. *Typical features of Down syndrome become less pronounced with each subsequent stem cell transplantation treatment, and immune system deficiency is completely corrected.* In all such cases stem cell transplantation has been carried out at an early age, or as soon as possible after the diagnosis was established. The earlier in life stem cell transplantation was carried out, the better was the outcome, while beyond certain age any such treatment was of questionable benefit: for example, to start stem cell transplantation for a child with Down syndrome beyond the age of 4 years was found to be of minor to minimal therapeutic benefit.

Our own published study of the first 83 patients with Down syndrome in which we evaluated mental and psychological functions showed the following [241].

The percentage of younger Down syndrome children (up to 3.5 years of age) with mental development index of over 50 points increased from 17% before the 1st SCT, to 58% after the 1st SCT, and to 71% after the 2nd SCT.

The IQ in the older children (4 - 9 years of age) moved after two cell transplantations from the 25 to 49 points-range to 50 - 69 points-range, and the difference was statistically significant.

A decreased hyperactivity, improvement of impaired concentration, lessened stereotypia and behavioral inertia, and improved speech expressivity, were observed already after the 1st cell transplantation, and the difference was statistically significant.

Volume of auditory/visual memory, productivity of thinking in categories, acoustic gnosis, and optic/spatial gnosis, were improved, but not significantly.

After cell transplantation, there was an improvement in motor area, particularly in fine coordinated movements, and in self-care habits, that were not psychometrically tested.

There was an absence of paroxysmal activity on EEG [241].

Patients under 4 years of age were treated by human fetal transplantation of *brain cortex, mesencephalon, diencephalon, and parietal lobe of brain*, while patients older than 4 years of age received also cell transplants of *frontal lobe of brain* and *occipital lobe of brain*.

After the publication of the report, the Down syndrome project in Moscow continued, and altogether 350 patients were treated.

Immune system deficiency of Down syndrome can be completely corrected. In our study of two age-matched groups of patients with

Down syndrome, carried out at the pediatric hospital specialized in genetic and chromosomal aberrations in Moscow, one group of 6 Down syndrome patients was treated every 6 months altogether three times by transplantation of human fetal cells of *medulla alba of brain, brain cortex, and cerebellum*, and the other group of 7 received implantation of saline. Height and weight, head circumference, psychological evaluation, laboratory tests: CBC, serum proteins, calcium, phosphorus, SGOT, SGPT, alkaline phosphatase, and immunoglobulins, were measured. Already after 6 months, just before the 2nd cell transplantation, we had to re-evaluate the situation as 3 of 7 children in the control group were dead due to infections, while in the treated group all children were well. In the controlled group there was an increase of IgG and a marked decrease of IgA and IgM. In the treated group there was a mild decrease of IgG and an increase of IgA and IgM.

The decreases of IgA from 166 to 85, and IgM from 140 to 74, in the control group, were signs of immune system deficiency responsible for the death of 3 out of 7 infants, while the marked increase of IgG from 459 to 872 might have been an expression of recurrent infections.

The transplantation of human fetal cells apparently stimulated the immune system, as the levels of IgA increased from 68 to 83, and of IgM from 101 to 111, and that of IgG decreased from 551 to 463, which may be an indication of lesser frequency and severity of bacterial infections. A markedly improved immune system function in treated patients was a result of one treatment by stem cell transplantation only, and in that treatment only fetal cells of three parts of brain were implanted and no cells of immune system organs whatsoever [144, 145].

Trisomy 13, or Patau syndrome, with incidence 1:4,000-10,000, is a highly lethal disorder with 86% of patients dying before reaching the 1st year of life. Psychic and somatic development is very retarded, there is marked failure to thrive, microcephaly and arhinencephaly, with anophthalmia, iris coloboma, dysplastic auricles, cleft lip and palate, as well as deafness, kidney anomalies, congenital heart defects, polydactyly, nail changes, and abnormal dermatoglyphics.

Trisomy 18, or Edwards syndrome, with incidence 1:7,500, four times more frequent in females, with substantially shortened lifespan. There is severe psychomotor retardation, dolichocephalia with bulging occiput and neck kyphosis, wide fontanelles and cranial sutures, dysplastic, low-placed auricles, hypertelorism with high eyebrows, micrognathia, short sternum, congenital heart defects, Meckel's diverticulum, U-shaped kidneys, campodactylia, hip dysplasia, pes equinovarus, protruding calcaneus, abnormal dermatoglyphics, etc.

B. Sex chromosome aberrations

They are in comparison with autosomal chromosome aberrations more variable and much less dangerous to the patient's life and health. Main phenotypic features are anomalies of external and internal genitalia and related defects of reproduction. The larger the number of extra chromosomes X is, the more pronounced is mental retardation, i.e. *patients with supernumerary chromosme X are frequently found among mentally retarded.*

Monosomy X, or Turner syndrome, with incidence 1:4,000 in live born girls, causes primary hypogonadism with gonadal dysgenesis, and from that resulting delayed puberty and primary amenorrhea, frequently also mental retardation, low stature, pterygium colli that has developed from cutis laxa, short neck with low hair line on nape of neck, low placed auricles, pectus carinatum with lateral placement of nipples, temporary congenital lymphedema of hands and feet, congenital anomalies of heart and large vessels, mainly coarctation of aorta and aortic stenosis, cubiti valgi, multiple pigmentary nevi, etc. Habitus is feminine and estimated 99% of all conceptions with karyotype 45,XO are miscarried. Some Turner syndrome patients can get pregnant, but the outcome is usually unfavorable. Stem cell transplantation of *ovary, placenta, adrenal cortex, and pituitary*, is recommended.

Our own experience with treatment of 9 years old patient with Turner's syndrome, hypothyroidism, speech delay, with height 112.0 cm, weight 18.0 kg, increased TSH, by cell transplantation of human fetal *ovary, adrenal cortex, diencephalon, anterior lobe of pituitary, thyroid*, was positive, as height increased 2 cm in 3 ½ months, weight one kg, overall activity increased, speech cleared, appetite improved, TSH became normal. After the 2nd cell transplantation again the height increased by 2.0 cm within 4 months, weight another 1.0 kg, and the overall impression was that of noticeable improvement. The patient was hospitalized at the Endocrinology Research Center of the Russian Academy of Medical Sciences.

Noonan syndrome, 46,XY configuration, or male gonadal dysgenesis, has the same symptoms as Turner's syndrome, infantilism, nanism, hypoplasia and dystopia of testis, lymphangiectastic edemas, no hair on the body, delayed bone development and skeletal abnormalities on hands. The findings become worse with age. Urinary 17-ketosteroids are decreased, and the gonadotropin level is low. Treatment is by cell transplantation of *adrenal cortex, placenta, hypothalamus, testis*, every 6 months, and additionally by cortisol, and gonadotropin.

Klinefelter syndrome, 47,XXY configuration, is relatively frequent chromosomal aberration in males with incidence 1:1,000 of live born boys. Patients are tall, eunuchoid, with small, soft testicles, their secondary sex characteristics, i.e. facial hair, pubic hair, gynaecomastia, osteoporosis, varicose veins, are frequently more feminine than masculine, but the overall habitus is masculine. As a result of testicular dysgenesis, there is azoospermia and infertility. These patients are frequently in psychiatric institutions. There is higher concentration of gonadotropins in urine, while levels of 17-ketosteroids are decreased.

***Trisomy X*, or XXX syndrome**, with incidence of 1:1,000 in live born girls. There is mental retardation, while malfunction of sex glands is present only in 49% of patients.

XYY syndrome with incidence 1:1,000 in live born boys. There is tall stature, often mental retardation, and tendency toward aggressive behavior and criminal activity.

There are no reports of treatment of *Intersex states* by stem cell transplantations:

- XY-female with sex reversal,
- XX-male with sex reversal,
- True hermaphroditism,
- Swyer syndrome, in females with XY sex chromosome configuration, with gonadal dysgenesis and sexual infantilism,
- Morris syndrome, or testicular feminization syndrome, or syndrome of androgen insensitivity, XR disorder, in females with karyotype XY,
- Overzier syndrome, or agonadism, in females with XY configuration.

STRUCTURAL CHROMOSOME ABERRATIONS

Partial monosomy 5p-, or 'cri du chat' syndrome, with incidence 1:50,000 to 1:100,000, was so named because of a typical cry of infants resembling a cat.

Children are born prematurely, are hypotrophic, with microcephaly, round moon facies, i.e. cranium is small, face is large, with hypertelorism, epicanthus, anti-mongoloid slant of eyes, gothic palate, mandibular hypoplasia, low placed auricles, and abnormal EEG. Stem cell transplantation of *diencephalon, placenta, medulla alba of brain, and additional CNS cell transplants* according to the dominant clinical findings, is advised.

Partial monosomy 4p-, or Wolf syndrome, with prenatal hypotrophy, microcephaly with severe CNS malfunction, frequent cranial asymmetry, cleft lip, skeletal deformities, dysmorphic U-shaped kidneys, hypoplasia of kidneys, congenital heart defects, abnormal genitals, is fatal in childhood. Stem cell transplantation of *thalamus, frontal lobe of brain, medulla alba of brain, temporal lobe of brain, mesencephalon, and partietal lobe of brain, placenta*, is recommended.

Deletion of long arm of chromosome 15, *Willi Prader syndrome*, or *Angelmann syndrome*, is treated by an implantation of stem cell transplants of *hypothalamus, adrenal cortex, gonads, placenta*. We treated, in Italy, a 6 years old female with a typical *Angelmann syndrome*, with mental retardation, speech delay, attacks of laugh, spasticity of extremities, and hypotonia of trunk, ataxia, one time only, but despite the positive response the parents did not continue with treatment, and were lost to a follow-up. When the treatment of genetic diseases starts too late, even though the parents are forewarned not to expect much, the results are seldom impressive.

Clinical protocol for treatment of genetic and chromosomal diseases by stem cell transplantation:

1. The diagnosis of the genetic, chromosomal or congenital, diseases has to be as complete as possible.
2. Any attempt to treat such patients by stem cell transplantation must be carried out immediately upon any suspicion that patient suffers from genetic or chromosomal disease, and quick diagnostic confirmation. The later will the treatment begin, the lesser will be the success rate.
3. SCT treatment has to be repeated at least every 3 - 4 months until no further improvement is observed. Any benefit of stem cell transplantation for impaired CNS function after the first 3 years of age is questionable.
4. Treatment is a complex one; besides biological treatment, it includes non-specific and specific metabolic stimulation, and

rehabilitation measures. Partial treatment, i.e. omission of certain therapies recommended here, may be actually harmful in the long term. After the patient reached 4 years of age any such therapeutic errors cannot be corrected.
5. It is nearly impossible to anticipate the success of stem cell transplantation for the treatment of genetic and chromosomal diseases. The crucial decision is whether to continue with the treatment after the first stem cell transplantation. The decision to continue has to be made by parents and physicians together!

Clinical parameters to be followed in patients before and after stem cell transplantation, and the frequency:

General: once a month, or as necessary:

    i. growth chart (height and weight, head circumference) every 3months
    ii. measurement of body proportions once every 3 months
    iii. complete neurological examination once every 3 months
    iv. x-rays of skull every 6 months, and of chest as necessary
    v. CT scan or MRI of brain, and other organs, as necessary
    vi. total body x-rays
    vii. chromosomal evaluation
    viii. urine and blood enzyme studies for enzymopathies
    ix. blood and urine metabolic screen for aminoacids
    x. complete blood count, urinalysis
    xi. SMA 12
    xii. blood smear, reticulocyte count
    xiii. serum calcium, phosphorus and magnesium
    xiv. blood glucose, glucose tolerance test, if necessary
    xv. blood lead level
    xvi. prothrombin time, partial thromboplastin time
    xvii. blood clotting time, bleeding time, clot retraction time
    xviii. serum alkaline phosphatase
    xix. muscle enzymes: creatine kinase, LDH
    xx. serum iron and ferritin
    xxi. bone marrow examination
    xxii. cerebrospinal fluid examination
    xxiii. ultrasound of brain, liver, kidneys, and other organs
    xxiv. EKG
    xxv. TORCH screen (toxoplasmosis, rubella, cytomegalovirus, herpes)
    xxvi. urine culture for virus and other microorganisms

Only tests pertinent for the treated disease are to be carried out.

Immunological: once a month x3, then every 3months:

    i. total lymphocytes
    ii. T-lymphocytes (CD3$^+$)
    iii. T-helpers (CD4$^+$)
    iv. T-suppressors (CD8$^+$) and CD4/CD8
    v. NK (CD16)
    vi. B-lymphocytes (CD22 and CD19)
    vii. serum IgG, IgA, IgM
    viii. serum complement (CH50)

Special: once every 4 month, or as clinically indicated, choice of tests according to diagnosis:

    i. intravenous pyelogram
    ii. angiograms
    iii. urine electrophoresis
    iv. 24 hour urine for sodium
    v. 24 hour urine for phosphorus
    vi. urinary 17-ketosteroids, 17 hydroxysteroids, pregnanetriol, 17- hydroxyprogesterone
    vii. serum renin level
    viii. EEG if necessary
    ix. ophthalmological examination if necessary
    x. blood & urine for galactose and fructose
    xi. biopsy of liver, gonads, muscles, lymphnodes, spleen aspiration for enzymes
    xii. vaginogram
    xiii. hemoglobin electrophoresis
    xiv. plasma von Willebrand factor, level of factor VIII and IX
    xv. stool for trypsin and chymotrypsin, and fat content
    xvi. spirometry
    xvii. quantitative pilocarpine iontophoresis sweat test
    xviii. plasma level of phenylalanin and tyrosine
    xix. water deprivation test
    xx. urinary mucopolysacharides
    xxi. dystrophin by immunoblotting
    xxii. electromyography
    xxiii. nerve conduction velocity

Only tests pertinent to the treated disease are to be done.

Frequency of office visits: 4 weeks and 48 hours before stem cell xenotransplantation, 24 hours after, and then once a week for the first month after stem cell xenotransplantation, once a month thereafter.

CASE HISTORY

A white female, born in November 1989, with a Down syndrome, was treated by Prof. Schmid by cell therapy at the age of 12 months, and started to follow his protocol of supportive treatment, which included homeopathic doses of thyroid extract, Cerebrolysin, and multivitamins/minerals, in addition to various forms of rehabilitation.

The patient did not have any congenital heart or gastrointestinal disease, nor any thyroid abnormalities. Her hearing and vision appeared normal. The cell therapy was repeated one year later.

With the recommendation of Prof. Schmid, this patient was treated by our team using cell transplantation in Moscow on March 10, 1993 in front the cameras of 'CBS-60 Minutes'. The parents of this patient (as well as ourselves) were too naive and trusted the unscrupulous 'CBS-60 Minutes' staff. We were betrayed and grossly abused by Mike Wallace. Responses of the patient's parents and ours to one question were pasted to a completely different question, and the whole matter of treatment of Down syndrome by cell transplantation was misrepresented and ridiculed.

The next treatment of this patient by cell transplantation was carried out by our team in Moscow in March 1994. In addition to physical and neurological examinations, and necessary laboratory tests, prior to this treatment the patient underwent an evaluation by our pediatric clinical psychologist. (This was not done in March 1993 due to all the havoc with CBS-60 Minutes). The patient's IQ was 63. The baseline levels of impairment of various parameters, such as hyperactivity, concentration, behavioral inertia and stereotypia, expressive speech, articulation, auditory/verbal memory, optic/spatial gnosis, acoustic gnosis, and categorical thinking, were established, while recognizing that this patient had had quite competent treatment already, thus these were not true 'baseline' data. Another difficulty was the language barrier.

In March 1995 this patient was treated by Prof. Schmid by cell transplantation.

Subsequently the patient underwent a psychological evaluation by a US pediatric psychologist, and parents showed us the report when in April 1996, they brought their daughter to Moscow for another cell transplantation. The psychologist did not find any significant abnormalities, and did not realize that their daughter had Down syndrome, as the parents told us with great excitement.

Prior to her treatment of April 1996, the patient underwent another evaluation by our pediatric clinical psychologist. IQ was 78. Hyperactivity, concentration, behavioral inertia, expressive speech, and articulation, were significantly improved. Auditory/verbal memory, optic/spatial gnosis, acoustic gnosis, categorical thinking, were improved as well, but not to a significant degree. Fine coordinated actions were significantly improved, as well as self-care habits.

All these years the protocol of supportive therapy of Prof. Schmid was followed as well.

Note: Cell transplantation was continued by the parents of this patient despite all of the media attacks, and sensation seeking, because they recognized the benefit of this treatment for the improvement of the condition of their daughter. At the age of 6 hardly anyone could somatically recognize that this girl had a Down syndrome. Actually she was very attractive. She was attending regular school and able to scholastically compete with other children. Her only real deficiency was in the area of abstract thinking. Her vocabulary was below the level of her classmates, and one could expect difficulty in mathematics in the future.

No one could tell these parents that Down syndrome cannot be successfully treated.

Chapter 47

> In the fields of observation, chance favors only the mind that is prepared.
> *Louis Pasteur, 1822 – 1895, [The Life of Pasteur 1927]*
>
> A man of genius makes no mistakes. His errors are volitional and are portals of discovery.
> *James Joyce, 1882 – 1941, [Ulysses 1922]*

NEONATAL AND PERINATAL DISEASES

Based on our own clinical experience, *when a newborn has a low Apgar score of 3 or less, a CT scan of the brain should be done at the age of 2 weeks, and if a 'periventricular malacia' is found, stem cell transplantation should be carried out immediately, and repeated every 3 – 4 months.* The report on our clinical research project that ran between 1995 and 1997 in the Russian Research Center for Obstetrics, Gynaecology and Perinatology of the Russian Academy of Medical Sciences in Moscow, was presented at the 1st Symposium on Human Fetal Tissue Transplantation in Moscow, December 4 – 7, 1995, under the title "Possibilities and perspectives of use of transplantation of human fetal tissues in treatment of CNS disorders in newborns". The report included several case histories.

Naturally when the newborn is found at the age of 2 weeks to have 'periventricular malacia' and stem cell transplantation treatment is started without delay it is hard to defend your therapeutic strategy because no one can predict the severity of clinical symptoms and signs in this future 'cerebral palsy' patient. If modern morals and ethics demand a resuscitation of every newborn and extraordinary intensive care to keep such newborns alive, then medicine must also assure that such newborns get a chance to be more than just permanent wards of chronic care hospitals.

The earlier in life stem cell transplantation is carried out, immediately after the diagnosis was established, even *in utero*, the better the outcome is, because stem cell transplantation cannot repair scar tissue.

As explained in the preceding chapters of this book, at such an early age there is no need to implant stem cell transplants directly into the brain, a deep subcutaneous implantation is adequate, because 'homing', is most active at an early age. 'Homing", as explained elsewhere in this book, attracts brain stem cells into the damaged parts of patient's brain. In other words in any case of brain damage caused by events *in utero*, or during birth, treatment by stem cell transplantation should start immediately. Beyond a certain age any such treatment is much less effective, definitely so after reaching the 4th year of life.

Once the child is diagnosed with a 'cerebral palsy' later on in life, any treatment, including stem cell transplantation, will have noticeably lesser effect. Parents of 'cerebral palsy' children spend enormous amount of time and money seeking treatment at the time when it is already too late. This is tragic in particular for children with severe brain damage laying in a vegetable state in the chronic care hospitals.

Handicapped individuals represent the challenge for our modern society and medicine. The best solution requires a coordination of efforts between medicine and special education, psychology, exercise, sport, speech therapy, social sciences, etc., otherwise an optimal result cannot be attained.

Handicapped individuals suffer from the effects of antropometric, gross motor, psychosocial and intellectual developmental faults. A complex therapy can be optimal only when it takes all these factors into consideration, and thereby the entire persona of the handicapped patient. Focusing only on some aspects, i.e. motor disturbances, or seizure disorders, etc., rather than on all aspects, may actually harm the patient, and after 3 years of life such damage may not be correctible. The first 4 years of life represent the period of brain development when the plasticity of brain gives incomparably better therapeutic possibilities than later on in life.

The first step is to obtain a complete diagnosis of the handicapped patient:

- antropometric data; length, weight, and body proportions, at birth and at the present,
- evaluation of the skull; overall shape, measurement of circumference, CT scan or MRI study,
- developmental analysis of gross motor and fine motor function;

coordination, eating/drinking/feeding, mental status, intellectual performance, social abilities,
- neurological examination,
- bone age,
- EEG
- any other examinations and tests as necessary.

A great majority of handicapped belongs into *six etiopathogenetic groups*:

1. ***Inborn errors of metabolism, or enzymopathies***,
   Discussion on *inborn error of metabolism, lysosomal enzymopathies, peroxisomal enzymopathies*, and *other genetic developmental disorders, autosomal dominant, autosomal recessive, and X-linked*, is in the chapter 45.

2. ***Chromosomal diseases***,
   Chromosomal diseases are discussed in the respective chapter.

3. ***Disorders due to environmental factors***:
   - *prenatal damage to pregnant mother*; nicotine, alcohol, drugs, anti-epilepsy drugs, cytostatica, radiation, toxins, blood group incompatibilities, infections by toxoplasmosis, syphilis, rubella, cytomegalovirus, or other viruses,
   - *birth damage*: prematurity, umbilical cord pathology, prolonged delivery, difficult delivery, anoxia, prolonged hypoxia, forceps delivery,
   - *post-natal damage*: encephalitis, meningitis, enteritis, subdural hematoma, anesthetic complications, angiography complications, CNS trauma, seizure disorders, athyreosis, hypo- and hypercalcemia, hypoglycemia.

4. ***Disorders due to multiple factors***,
   Anencephaly, hydraencephaly, arhinencephaly, porenecephaly, microcephaly, hydrocephalus, cleft lip and palate, spina bifida, dysmorphic syndromes.

5. ***Cerebral palsy***,
   - *hypertonic* forms: spastic mono-, di-, tri-, tetra-plegia, spastic hemiplegia,
   - *hypotonic* forms: 'floppy infant syndrome', various muscle hypotonias,
   - *dystonic* forms: swings between hyper- and hypo-tonia,

- *dyskinetic* forms: chorea, athetosis, choreoathetosis (side-by-side, or back and forth swings from chorea to athetosis), clumsiness,
- *ataxia*: cerebellar ataxia, cerebro-spinal ataxia,
- *mixed* forms with sensory defects, trophic disturbances, intellect deficiencies, minor mental retardation.

6. **Minimal brain damage**.
   Minimal brain damage: learning disorders, such as dyslexia, written expression disorder, speech defects, etc.

Therapeutic guidelines

The human brain is the sole organ which continues its 'fetal' development after birth, i.e. maturation and differentiation. This *makes CNS very vulnerable to noxious stimuli but offers unique therapeutic possibilities.* This 'treatment window' of the first 3, maximum 4 years of life, must be taken advantage of, as losing this therapeutic opportunity means lost chances forever.

Let's list the basic facts:

1. The number of neurons is final at birth.
2. Despite that the brain of a newborn weighs only 350 gm, while at the end of somatic growth it weighs 1,250 gm, although the number of neurons is unchanged.
3. Without any increase in the number of neurons, the brain volume, i.e. weight, increases three and a half times, a result of development of secondary neuronal structures.
4. The main growth of brain volume, around ¾ of postnatal brain growth takes place in the first three years after birth.

In CNS disturbances we are dealing therapeutically with three basic problems:
   a. neuronal deficit,
   b. inhibitions of maturation and differentiation of neuropile,
   c. destructive processes.

The main source of mental handicaps is an inhibition of maturation of central nervous system.

Neuron can be therapeutically influenced by:

- non-specific metabolic stimulation,
- specific metabolic stimulation,
- biologic structural substitution,
- peripheral training.

Non-specific metabolic stimulation is usually accomplished by improved blood circulation and that is hardly attained in early childhood by any currently available medications. Only optimal nutrition is of therapeutic value.

Specific metabolic stimulation can be assisted by:

- Pyritinol (Pyrithioxin), vitamin B6 derivative, improves glucose utilization and protein synthesis in CNS via an initial increase of the membrane permeability, followed by a rise in cytoplasmatic metabolism; therapeutic indications are deficit of short-term memory, concentration, learning ability, seizure disorders, all hypotonic disorders, i.e. Down syndrome, hypotonic cerebral palsy, and loss of vitality,
- Piracetam (Noortrop), γ-amino-butyric acid, augments synapse function; therapeutic indications are depression, slowness, lack of initiative, concentration lack, hypodynamic cerebral palsy and Down syndrome,
- Centrophenoxin, a product of synthesis of p-Chlorphenoxyacetic acid and aminoalcohol, increases spontaneous activity, dissolves lipofuscin, stimulates metabolism of glial cells, and prevents premature aging process in Down syndrome,
- Nicotinic acid derivatives improve peripheral blood flow,
- Membrane activators contain neurotransmitters, vitamins and minerals improve performance of cell membranes, and that is important for treatment of inborn errors of metabolism, premature aging, Down syndrome, athyreosis.

Peripheral training means a *'functional training of neurons from the periphery'*. A *certain sequence of functions, that the neuron is not yet by itself capable to carry out, is passively triggered, and repeatedly so, in order to 'pave the way' for such sequence*. CNS differentiation processes that, due to functional deficiencies, cannot take place, are passively enabled in this way. The value of peripheral training can be appreciated when a comparison of treatment results is made between institutionalized handicapped children and those taken care of by their parents at home. The first three steps of the complex therapeutic protocol are the same at an institution or at home, but the *continuous peripheral training by parents makes enormous difference in the outcome. Stem cell transplants are the most valuable 'building blocks' but they atrophy by non-use or mis-use.*

There are many suitable methods of peripheral neuronal training: various physiotherapeutic methods, including any form of active exercise available, gymnastics, rhythmic training, swimming, etc., behavior therapy, psychotherapy, occupational therapy, speech therapy, visual training, acoustic training, etc.

Biologic Structural substitution by stem cell transplantation

Non-existent cells cannot be replaced. The purpose of transplanted stem cells is to augment the maturation process of secondary structures of central nervous system: dendrites, axons, myelin, and synapses. In order for stem cell transplantation to perform its task two conditions are mandatory:

- *there must be a need for stem cells in the corresponding organ of the recipient due to a defect, deficiency, or disease,*
- in order to be built into the damaged organ, stem cell transplants *must possess the corresponding organ-specific structure.*

As stated repeatedly, the therapeutic success is much higher when stem cell transplantation is begun as early as possible, definitely before the 4th year of life, and is a part of a complex therapeutic protocol as outlined in this chapter. Stem cell transplantation must continue every 3 to 4 months as long as there is an objective proof of further improvement, and *parents are the best judges of the progress made by their child.*

The general principles for the selection of stem cell transplants to be used for treatment varies between the various etiopathogenetic groups:

1. In *inborn errors of metabolism* stem cell transplants of cells or tissues with the highest metabolic turnover should be used, i.e. *liver, brain, myocard*, because these organs are usually much more damaged than organs with low metabolism. In addition, the *adrenal cortex, placenta, and mesenchyme*, are frequently used.

    In *immune deficiencies* stem cell transplants of *thymus, bone marrow, mesenchyme and liver*, are recommended.

2. Among *chromosomal disorders* there is a plenty of clinical

experience with treatment of Down syndrome. As brain tissues are the most affected, stem cell transplants of various parts of the brain must be given every 4 months, i.e. *cortex of brain, occipital lobe of brain, temporal lobe of brain, and deeper parts of brain: diencephalon, mesencephalon, cerebellum, hypothalamus*.

Since an immune deficiency is always present in Down syndrome, an implantation of *thymus* may be considered. During the pre-puberty period *adrenal cortex* may be added, and during the pubertal rapid growth spurt also *thyroid and liver*.

In '*cri-du-chat*' *syndrome* only the first two or three stem cell transplantations are of any benefit. Microcephaly can hardly be positively influenced.

In *sex chromosomal disorders* the best experience has been with Turner syndrome, where stem cell transplantation of *hypothalamus, adrenal cortex, ovary*, will often trigger a dramatic growth spurt.

3. Cerebral palsy

The most common problem is that parents think of, or learn of, stem cell transplantation after their child is older than 4 years, so that a prudent practitioner of stem cell transplantation does not accept the patient. Actually there are *some forms of cerebral palsy when some improvement is possible even after 4 years of age*, and those will be described here, but in general the expectations must be low. If treatment is contemplated, them stem cell transplants of *brain cortex, medulla alba of brain, thalamus, mesencephalon, cerebellum, and spinal cord*, are recommended.

In *spastic* forms the fixed spasticity not responding to an intensive gymnastic training cannot be improved by stem cell transplantation, only the overall health and mental abilities can.

In *dyskinetic* forms, i.e. choreo-athetosis, and *ataxic* forms, some improvement by stem cell transplantation is possible *up to 10 years of age*. For dyskinetic forms stem cell transplants of *diencephalon, basal ganglia, hypothalamus, thalamus, cerebellum, temporal lobe of brain, frontal lobe of brain*, are advised. For *ataxic* forms, that are due to damage to cerebellum or spinal cord, stem cell transplants *of spinal cord, cerebellum, mesencephalon, occipital lobe of brain*, are recommended.

Hypotonic forms can sometimes respond to stem cell transplantation after 4 years of age, and the only way to find out is by trying it once, as is many times the case in the field of stem cell transplantation, in particular when one deals with a rare disease where there is an insufficient prior clinical experience, whether personal or from reports by other practitioners. For hypotonic forms stem cell transplants of *spinal cord, occipital lobe of brain, cerebellum, mesencephalon, peripheral myoblasts*, are recommended [260].

A 2 year old girl developed, at age of 10 months, a high fever followed by a paralysis of deglutition muscles. She was hospitalized several times with a diagnosis of profound brain damage, and no one offered any treatment. The patient could not walk, talk, eat, focus, and salivated profusely. She was fed through a gastrostomy tube. EEG showed generalized extensive damage. It was impossible to decide if the condition was the result of toxoplasmosis that mother acquired at 4 months' of pregnancy or encephalitis at 10 months of age. In June 1986 she received cell transplantation of *basal ganglia and brain stem*. Four months later the child began to eat by mouth and two months later her feeding tube was removed and gastrostomy closed. Salivation stopped, and the patient became more alive. In December 1986, cell transplantation of *frontal lobe of brain and cerebellum* was carried out. Six weeks later the child began standing without assistance and began to walk around holding onto things. She was making sounds for the first time in her life, and became animated. In June 1987, she received cell transplantation of *medulla alba of brain, thalamus and temporal lobe of brain*. Subsequently patient began to walk without assistance, spoke two-syllable words, became sociable, and her growth curve appeared normal. Last EEG in May 1987, showed a moderate improvement of EEG pattern [289].

Clinical protocol for treatment of patients with neonatal, perinatal, and infantile disorders by stem cell transplantation

1. The cause of mental retardation is unknown in 80% of cases, so do not waste the time to start the treatment by looking for a complete diagnosis.

2. Any attempt to treat patients with mental retardation by stem cell transplantation must be carried out immediately upon any suspicion that serious brain damage occurred. The later begins the treatment the lesser will be the success rate. Any birth trauma, or asphyxia, jaundice, meningitis, seizures, hyper- or hypo-tonia, areflexia, in any newborn, requires CT scan to check for periventricular leukomalacia no later than at two weeks of age.
3. Treatment has to be repeated at least every 4 months until no further improvement is observed. Any benefit of stem cell transplantation for an improvement of CNS function beyond 4 years of age is questionable.
4. Treatment is a complex one, besides biological treatment, it includes non-specific and specific metabolic stimulation, and rehabilitation measures. Partial treatment, i.e. omission of certain therapies recommended here, may be actually harmful in the long term. After the patient reached 4 years of age any such therapeutic errors cannot be corrected.
5. As etiology is usually unknown, it is nearly impossible to anticipate the success of stem cell transplantation for the treatment of mental retardation. The crucial is the decision whether to continue with the treatment after the first stem cell transplantation. The decision has to be made by parents and physicians together!

Clinical parameters to be followed in patients before and after stem cell transplantation, and the frequency:

General: once a month, or as necessary:

 i. growth chart (height and weight, head circumference) every 3 months,
 ii. measurement of body proportions once every 3 months,
 iii. complete neurological examination every 3months,
 iv. x-rays of skull every 6months,
 v. CT scan or MRI of brain,
 vi. bone age by x-rays every 6months,
 vii. chromosomal evaluation as necessary,
 viii. urine & blood enzyme studies for enzymopathies,
 ix. blood & urine metabolic screen for aminoacids,
 x. T3, T4, TSH by radioimmunoassay,
 xi. growth hormone level,
 xii. muscle enzymes: creatine kinase, LDH,

xiii. serum calcium, phosphorus and magnesium,
xiv. blood glucose,
xv. blood lead level,
xvi. cerebrospinal fluid examination,
xvii. ultrasound of the brain,
xviii. visual acuity assessment,
xix. auditory assessment,
xx. complete blood count, urinalysis, SMA 12,
xxi. blood clotting if necessary,
xxii. TORCH screen (toxoplasmosis, rubella, cytomegalovirus, herpes),
xxiii. urine culture for virus and other microorganisms.

Immunological: once a month x3, then every 3months:

i. total lymphocytes,
ii. T-lymphocytes ($CD3^+$),
iii. T-helpers ($CD4^+$),
iv. T-suppressors ($CD8^+$) and CD4/CD8,
v. NK (CD16),
vi. B-lymphocytes (CD22 and CD19),
vii. serum IgG, IgA, IgM,
viii. serum complement (CH50).

Special: once every 4 months, or as clinically indicated:

i. Denver Developmental Screening Test-R
ii. Developmental Screening Inventory
iii. Early Intervention Developmental Profile
iv. Psychological testing
v. Bayley Scales of Infant Development
vi. Stanford-Binet Intelligence Scale
vii. Wechsler Preschool and Primary Scale of Intelligence
viii. Wechsler Intelligence Scale for Children-R

Other:

ix. EEG if necessary
x. ophthalmological examination if necessary

Frequency of office visits: 4 weeks and 48 hours before stem cell xenotransplantation, 24 hours after and then once a week for the first month after stem cell xenotransplantation, once a month thereafter.

Chapter 48

> But where are the snows of yesteryear?
> François Villon, 1431 – 1465, [Ballade des Dames du Temps]

> Prolong human life only where you can shorten its miseries.
> Stanislaw Jerzy Lec, 1909 – 1966, [More Unkempt Thoughts, 1968]

AGING DISEASE

If medical textbooks include such topic at all, aging is declared a natural process, there is no 'aging disease', and there is no reason for any R&D as there is nothing that you can do about aging anyway.

World Health Organization Study Group on Aging and Working Capacity met in Helsinki, Finland, in 1991, and analyzed all issues thoroughly, i.e. demographics, aging workforce, ratio of retired people to the working population, physiological changes with age, age and work performance, mortality, morbidity, disability, and advised governments on problems in this area, but no time whatsoever was devoted to discussion on how to influence aging by therapeutic means. The message to the aging population world over was clear: the very moment you stop working you are becoming a financial burden on governments, so why talk about any therapies for the aging-related diseases that would require even more funds.

Approximately 80% of 5 million patients treated by cell transplantation/cell therapy worldwide during the last 70 years have done so because they suffered from 'aging disease'. Their decision was based on their instincts and intuition, and in total disregard of official statements about a lack of acceptable research protocols to prove the value of any therapy in slowing down the aging process. The medical profession may ridicule it, but many of their patients wish to do something about it, but *'not to add years to life, but life to years'*.

The percentage of older people is growing and not only in 'highly developed' countries, but also in those labeled as 'developing'. In our life, after a developmental phase, or a period of maturation, and a period of maturity, comes inevitably a period of regression. Motor, psychological/social, and intellectual skills are acquired during the developmental phase, utilized during maturity, and then gradually lost during the regression period: abilities acquired last are lost first.

The goal of medicine should be not only to find out why aging takes place, but also discovering therapeutic and other means to *preserve the vitality of aging organism for as many years to come as possible, and perhaps until the limit of our life, that is allegedly 120 years.*

The causes of aging disease are hypothetical because it is impossible to run a longitudinal study on the vitality in man. Framingham study ran for 20 years but that is not long enough for study on vitality and aging. Many healthy controls have to be found to establish a baseline of 'healthy aging' and they are largely not available. There is a considerable variation in the lifestyle of controls, thereby limiting accuracy of the 'baseline healthy aging parameters'. Our empirical knowledge, based on the treatment of millions of patients spread over 70 years, compensates greatly for this deficiency of science.

Vitality measures an ability of one's organism to realize all vital functions in physical, mental and spiritual spheres. It is an optimal performance of capacities existing in an individual. *'Devitalization'* means a loss of vitality due to aging and other diseases. *'Revitalization'* means a re-establishment of lost functions, while *'rejuvenation'* goes beyond that limit, as it means improvements in one's total biological capabilities, or lowering of one's biological age. Some are critical of the term 'rejuvenation' but the author met people who accomplished that. It requires a complex therapeutic approach, i.e. more than stem cell transplantation, and a belief that it can be done.

Biological age refers to functional capacities of an organism corresponding to the respective stage of an individual's lifespan. There were several attempts to develop a system of assessment of biological age simple enough to be useful in everyday clinical practice, such as that proposed by Ries, that includes an evaluation of [254]:

- cardiovascular system, i.e. blood pressure, vital lung capacity, partial pressure of arterial oxygen, Ruffier functional index,

- sense organs, and psyche, i.e. visual acuity, audiogram, color-word-test by Stroop, reading ability, speed of movement,
- locomotor system, i.e. power of hand muscles, hand dynamometer, tendon extension in degrees,
- dental status, i.e. number of decayed, missing, and filled teeth [254].

What are the *leading symptoms of 'devitalization'*?
- lack of initiative,
- lack of activity,
- rapid exhaustion,
- reduced physical capabilities,
- reduced psychological responses,
- reduced alcohol tolerance,
- loss of ambition,
- reduced self-confidence,
- dullness, despair,
- lack of concentration,
- impaired memory,
- insomnia,
- depression.

For the sake of an early diagnosis, and ability to evaluate the results of therapy, *more detailed lists of 'devitalization' symptoms and signs'* were devised, such as the one by Schmid [95].

'Personality':
- loss of initiative,
- lack of vigor,
- emotional 'emptiness',
- lack of inspirations,
- feeling of insecurity,
- egocentric behavior,
- inability to act,
- loss of sanity,

'Gross motor abilities':
- rigid posture,
- unsteady gait,
- shuffling walk,
- reduced walking distance,
- difficulties to climb stairs,

- walking with walking aids.

'Fine motor abilities/Coordination':
- reduced mimicry,
- reduced gestures,
- tremor,
- shakiness,
- unsteady grip,
- restlessness.

'Social behavior/Psyche':
- discontent,
- self-reproach,
- loss of interpersonal relationships,
- fear of living,
- desire to live like a hermit,
- loss of interest in sports, politics, acquaintances, environment, hobbies.

'Intellectual performance':
- impaired comprehension,
- impaired intellectual grasp,
- memory disturbances,
- loss of short-term memory,
- 'senseless' mistakes,
- reduced concentration,
- reduced vocabulary,
- loss of contemplation,
- taciturnity,
- monotonous stereotypes,
- loss of orientation abilities.

'Physical regression':
- skin atrophy,
- vascular sclerosis,
- cerebral sclerosis,
- aged heart,
- pulmonary emphysema,
- digestive disorders,
- impotence,
- menopause,

- old-age diabetes,
- liver disorder,
- immune deficiency.

A physician *cannot treat aging related diseases, or for that matter many other diseases in an aging individual, without an anti-aging treatment.* On the other hand, one cannot seriously talk about the 'revitalization' or 'rejuvenation' therapies, or a treatment of aging disease, without a 'state-of-the-art' diagnosis of any and all diseases that the patient suffers from, and their successful treatment, because otherwise any attempt at 'revitalization' will fail.

There are not too many individuals over 40 years old in the western world today that are perfectly healthy physically, mentally and spiritually, and thus do not require treatment of 'aging disease'. *The earlier in life the revitalization program is begun, the better the results are.* The best time *to start is between 40 and 50 years of age.* The later the revitalization program commences, the more aggressive the therapeutic approach has to be, i.e. various simultaneous therapies, and in shorter time intervals.

Gianoli reports on the treatment of 531 of his own patients by cell transplantation with a success rate of 75%. The therapeutic effect lasted 8 – 12 months and never more than 24 months [258].

The Merck Manual of Geriatrics [242] defines the '*usual aging*' as 'changes due to the combined effects of the aging process and of disease and adverse environmental and lifestyle factors', while '*successful aging*' as 'changes due solely to the aging process, uncomplicated by damage from environment, lifestyle, or disease'. These excellent definitions that acknowledge the possibility of 'aging successfully' stem from the growing acceptance of the rights of the aging population to live a full and complete life rather than to die in a hurry right after the retirement.

In reality the 'usual aging' should be classified as an '*aging disease*', and all diseases related to aging should be clearly described as such. Scientists agree that genetically we are programmed to live 120 years. In reality, we live on average less than 80 years in the civilized world. But there are some societies with simple lifestyle where people frequently live much longer than that.

The 'successful aging process', that should lead to our graceful demise at the age of 120 years, is disrupted in principle by three factors: *severe illness, severe trauma, or 'usual aging', i.e. 'aging disease'*. The first two factors are self-explanatory: severe disease or severe trauma can destroy even the healthiest individual. But what about the 'aging disease'? Here are some well established facts:

1. The rate of age-related decline in the function of every organ of the body varies greatly, so that people become less alike as they age,
2. Within any organism the functions of different organs decline at different rates,
3. Each one of us has at least one weak organ or organ system.
4. Different people age at different rates.

There are two major types of 'aging diseases': those that are *accidental or random*, and those that are programmed. We seem to age 'by accident' and 'by design': it is not only that the stresses and strains and traumas of everyday life set off processes which make us grow old, there is some internal mechanism that limits our lifespan. Our evolutionary, biological, purpose is fulfilled once we have passed on our genes, and have protected our children until they can protect themselves. Once that happened, around the age of 40, we begin to notice the aging process.

Before that time our bodies have been in a state of *dynamic equilibrium, constantly renewing, rebuilding, and replacing every cell in the body by cells of equal quality*. Now our *physiological functions begin to decline*. Our *ability to adapt to, and survive in a changing environment, declines*. All over the body, *the structure of tissues becomes disorganized*.

More fat is deposited, numbers of key cells of each organ or tissue decrease. Individual cells increase in size, but diminish in number, by almost one-third. Connective tissue between cells, muscle fibers, and bones enlarges and becomes less elastic.

Myocardium and the heart valves lose gradually their elasticity and strength, although the left ventricular wall thickens as a result of myocardial hypertrophy and increased quantity of fibrous tissue.

As the heart grows weaker, the blood vessels become more rigid due to changes in the amount and nature of elastin and collagen in their walls, and calcium deposits, as well as clogged with fatty atheromas of atherosclerosis, blood pressure rises.

In the kidneys, the number of functioning nephrons decreases 30 - 40 % between ages 25 and 85, with the related loss of renal mass, particularly of the cortical layer. This leads to a reduced renal blood flow, glomerular filtration rate and performance of tubular system.

The vital capacity of the lungs decreases, while the residual volume increases. The gas distribution irregularities and decreased compliance of the lungs cause lowered arterial oxygen tension. The diameter of chest wall increases, and the flexibility decreases. The maximum breathing capacity decreases steadily: in 80's it is one half as compared with 30's. From the age of 55 on the respiratory muscles begin to weaken.

The motility of digestive system is affected by aging process first, before the digestion of food and absorption. This leads to constipation, incontinence and diverticulosis, which become a cause of many problems with digestion and absorption of nutrients. Production of all digestive enzymes declines. Liver weight and its blood flow decrease.

The skin wrinkles, sags, and grows less elastic and dry. Healing takes longer. The hair thins and turns gray. Nail growth slows down.

Loss of muscle cells and disorganization of muscle tissue cause a progressive reduction in muscle strength. Half of muscle mass and of maximum isometric contraction force is lost between ages of 30 and 75. Joints deteriorate. Bones become weaker as more minerals are lost than are replaced.

Blood flow to the brain is reduced. Most of lost nerve cells are not replaced. Connections between nerve cells are substantially diminished. The gross motor and fine motor abilities and coordination deteriorate. Psychometrically, reaction time slows down, learning takes longer, and memory fades, in particular the recent one. The social skills and intellectual abilities of young years slip away. There are changes of personality.

Vision deteriorates as the lens and other parts of the eye become less transparent. Vision dims as a result of decreased adaptation to low light and darkness. Senses of taste, touch, smell and hearing grow weaker.

Menopause appears in women, and loss of sexual potency in men.

When it comes to the treatment of 'aging disease' the opinions vary. This is due to the lack of a single hypothesis able to explain all aspects of aging processes. According to the Merck Manual of Geriatrics [242] there are *six such hypotheses.*

Experts have always believed in a complex approach to the treatment of aging disease, i.e. ***stem cell transplantation alone is not sufficient***. It has to start with lifestyle adjustments, correct nutrition, regular active exercise, proper handling of stress along with spiritual immersion. Normalization of function of all organ systems has to be attained by all means of orthodox and alternative medicine, all the while the elimination of toxins should be foremost on the mind of treating professionals. The two most important parts of the complex therapeutic approach are stem cell transplantation for direct stimulation of regeneration and – along with electromagnetic therapy – for securing the optimum performance of regulatory systems of the body.

Female patients should receive, as a minimum, stem cell transplants of *ovaries, placenta, adrenal cortex, hypothalamus, mesenchyme, spleen*; while male patients should receive stem cell transplants of *testes, placenta, adrenal cortex, liver, hypothalamus, frontal lobe of brain*. Other stem cell transplants, necessary for the treatment of any other disease(s) that the patient suffers from, which have a negative influence on aging disease, are added.

Gross motor disturbances require also stem cell transplants of *brain cortex, medulla alba of brain, spinal cord*, and

- if rigid posture dominates, then also *diencephalon, basal ganglia*,
- if insteady gait dominates, then also *cerebellum*.

Fine motor disturbances require also stem cell transplantation of *thalamus, diencephalon, basal ganglia, cerebellum*, and if decreased mimicry, and reduced gestures dominate then also *temporal lobe of brain, and frontal lobe of brain in female* patients.

Disturbed coordination requires also stem cell transplantation of *thalamus, diencephalon, basal ganglia, and cerebellum*.

Reduced initiative also requires stem cell transplants of *thalamus, hypothalamus, and frontal lobe of brain in female patients*.

Memory loss also requires stem cell transplants of *temporal lobe of brain, and frontal lobe of brain in female patients*.

Reduced intellect also requires stem cell transplants of *brain cortex, medulla alba of brain, and thalamus*.

Arteriosclerosis also requires stem cell transplants of *placenta, artery, mesenchyme*, while *cerebral arteriosclerosis* requires stem cell transplants of *placenta, artery, and medulla alba of brain*.

Senile heart requires also stem cell transplants of *placenta, and artery.*

Impaired liver function requires also stem cell transplants of *stomach/ intestine.*

Gout requires also stem cell transplants of *kidney.*

Senile lungs require also stem cell transplants of *lungs, and mesenchyme.*

Osteoarthrosis also requires stem cell transplants of *cartilage, bone marrow, parathyroids, and mesenchyme.*

Immune deficiency requires also stem cell transplants of *thymus, and spleen in male patients.*

Wolf specialized for decades in the treatment of patients with brain atrophy due to aging by various modifications of timing and dosage of cell transplantation of *placenta and frontal lobe of brain only*, sometimes including hypothalamus. He repeated such implantations every 4 weeks for 3 to 6 months in a new patient until there was a definitive improvement in the clinical status, and then the patient received the same treatment one to four times a year. In those instances when the patient' condition became worse; he re-started the initial treatment schedule of implantation of above cell transplants every four weeks [243].

Menopause is the most significant period of life for women since it is the time of the greatest vulnerability, physical, mental and spiritual. Many educated women postpone this period into their later years by hormone replacement therapy today. It can be accomplished, yet hormone replacement therapy cannot replace stem cell transplantation. The center of regulation of sexual glands is in diencephalon, close to the centers for autonomous nervous system regulation and the centers for a variety of psychic functions. These three centers work closely together, and influence each other. Amenorrhea due to prolonged stress is not a rare occurrence, and the same applies to the premature menstrual bleeding due to fright, or psychic disturbances, or autonomous nervous system changes, or due to disorders of the sex glands regulation system. On the other hand, it is possible to improve menopausal malfunctions through psychotherapy, or by sedatives of autonomous nervous system.

Back in 1957, Bernhard reported on his success in treatment of menopause by cell transplantation of *diencephalon, anterior lobe of pituitary, ovary, and placenta*, in 98 patients with a natural menopause, in 49 patients with premature menopause, and 27 patients with artificial menopause, and stressed that the effect of cell transplantation is not due to a hormone replacement.

Lehmacher treated 6 patients with artificial menopause after a complete hysterectomy, and bilateral total oophorectomy, with cell transplantation of *ovary and placenta* with 100% success rate. None of these patients showed any estrogen effect on vaginal mucosa smear because cell transplantation does not work by stimulating ovaries to produce estrogen and progesterone. These patients were an excellent example because they did not have ovaries for production of estrogen and progesterone.

A preliminary report describing findings in the first 11 patients of a double blind study that included 40 patients, one half of which received cell transplantation of *diencephalon, anterior lobe of pituitary, placenta and ovary*, while the second half a placebo, states that cell transplantation did significantly improve the difficulties of menopausal patients, although no changes of FSH or 17-β-estradiol were observed, and cell transplants had no hormonal effect whatsoever. Cell transplants of diencephalon, anterior pituitary, ovary and placenta, balance out the autonomous nervous system regulatory circuits [313].

Clinical protocol for treatment of patients with aging disease by stem cell transplantation

1. A patient with 'aging disease' needs an improvement of biological functions in their entirety (i.e. 'vitality'): physical, mental and spiritual. As an example, to attend to a physical fitness of a deeply senile patient without an improvement of the mental state is not a therapeutic goal,
2. A follow-up requires a measurement of described parameters but also an evaluation of the 'vitality', which is to some degree a matter of the personal judgment of the patient,
3. The more advanced are the symptoms and signs of aging disease the more thorough must be the diagnosis of malfunctions of all organ systems and the more attentive the after-care,
4. The regenerative ability of an organism is diminishing with age, thus the 'aging disease' should be treated early, and repeatedly. The older is the patient at the time of the first treatment, the more frequent should be the treatment, i.e. in 50 years' old patients every 3 years, while in 70 years' old every year. But, as long as

there is some regeneration potential left, and the patient is not in the terminal stage of some disease(s), stem cell transplantation should not be refused.

A proper preparation of the patient for stem cell transplantation is mandatory. A patient has to be brought into as compensated metabolic state as possible by standard therapeutic means, i.e. to carry out stem cell transplantation while the patient is in the state of severe malnutrition, dehydration, depression, etc. is probably minimally effective and should be done only as a last resort.

Parameters to be followed in patients before and after stem cell xenotransplantation, and the frequency:

Physical:
  i. complete blood count, urinalysis, every month
  ii. creatinine clearance every 3months
  iii. serum alkaline phosphatase every 3 months
  iv. serum cholesterol: total, LDL, HDL, and triglycerides, every month
  v. fasting blood sugar every month
  vi. serum calcium and phosphorus every 3 months
  vii. blood pressure every month
  viii. exercise EKG testing every 3 months
  ix. spirometry every 3months
  x. serum estrogen, progesterone or testosterone, every 6 months
  xi. serum FSH and LH every 6 months
  xii. visual acuity every 6 months
  xiii. audiogram every 6 months
  xiv. bone density every 6 months (females only, males only if indicated)

Immunological: once a month x3, then every 3 months:
  i. total lymphocytes
  ii. T-lymphocytes (CD3$^+$)
  iii. T-helpers (CD4$^+$)
  iv. T-suppressors (CD8$^+$)   and CD4/CD8
  v. NK (CD16)
  vi. B-lymphocytes (CD22 and CD19)
  vii. serum IgG, IgA, IgM
  viii. serum complement (CH50)

Neuropsychological evaluation: every 6 months or, at least once a year:
  i. personality: loss of initiative, loss of drive, loss of affection, loss of imagination, general insecurity, easy tiredness, unmotivated

depression, despair, loneliness, egocentrism, inability to act, loss of 'soundness of mind', loss of attention span,
  ii. gross motor: impairment of posture, gait, and balance,
  iii. fine motor function and coordination: poverty of mimicry and gesticulation, tremor, restlessness, impairment of grasping of objects,
  iv. social: sullenness, self-reproach/self-accusation, loss of interest in intersocial relations, loss of interest in politics, sport, friends, hobbies, surroundings, fear of life,
  v. intellect: impairment of comprehension of new ideas, impairment of thought, decrease of concentration, loss of thoughtfulness, monosyllabism, monotone stereotypes, loss of recent memory, decrease of vocabulary, loss of orientation ability, speech impairment, impairment of abstract thinking, impairment of judgment.

Various scales can be used as well, such as:
  i. Mini-Mental State Examination form (MMSE),
  ii. Hamilton Depression Scale or Yesavage Geriatric Depression Scale,
  iii. Sandoz Clinical Assesment - Geriatrics (SCAG), and others.

Frequency of office visits: 4 weeks and 48 hours before stem cell xenotransplantation, 24 hours after, and then once a week for the first month after stem xenotransplantation, once a month thereafter.

CASE HISTORY:

A white female patient, born in 1940, developed an early menopause at the age of 34. At the age of 36, the patient started the hormone replacement therapy of estrogen/progesteron in a program that simulated a menstrual cycle. At the age of 41, she was found to have a mitral valve prolapse, the therapy of which required an avoidance of caffeine and other stimulants, and a regular exercise, but no drugs.

She has been a sportive type all her life, thus besides the appearance, and the subjective evaluation of the mental faculties, the patient has been able to use her physical performance to judge her aging process.

In 1989 she observed some lowering of physical stamina, and on physician's advice took a cell transplantation consisting of injection of 9 (nine) various transplants, the primary purpose of which was to support the hormonal system stressed and strained by the premature ovarian failure. Her physician was of the opinion that the hormone replacement therapy did not sufficiently control the generalized hormonal imbalance of the premature menopause.

Prior to cell transplantation her tests showed a normal complete blood count, a normal blood chemistry, a normal cholesterol and triglycerides, normal exercise EKG; while blood estrogen, progesteron, FSH and LH were all at menopausal level, visual acuity showed a minimal presbyopia, and audiogram was within normal limits.

Neurological examination was normal, posture and gait was normal, balance was unimpaired, mimicry and gesticulation was vivid, there was no tremor, the grasping of objects was unimpaired.

The psychological evaluation of personality showed normal initiative, normal drive, normal affection, normal imagination, "sound mind", normal attention span, lack of depression, absence of insecurity. The psychological evaluation of intellect showed normal thought process, no impairment of comprehension of new ideas, normal concentration, normal memory, normal orientation, normal speech, normal judgment, no impairment of abstract thinking. Patient showed no loss of interest in friends, hobbies, surrounding, politics, etc., continued to be very sociable, and be the "life of the party". The sexual functioning was normal, libido not diminished.

In 1993, the patient received the 2nd cell transplantation of *ovary, placenta, hypothalamus, liver, adrenal cortex, cardiomyoblasts, cartilage, and spleen*, by our team in Moscow. The indication was to maintain the status quo insofar physical, mental and spiritual functions was concerned.

Prior to the treatment, her tests showed a normal complete blood count, a normal blood chemistry, a normal cholesterol and triglycerides, normal exercise EKG; while her blood estrogen, progesteron, FSH and LH were at menopausal level. All other examinations, visual, auditory, neurological and psychological were normal.

In 1995, the patient had an episode of high blood pressure following an attack by a dog, but the blood pressure went back to normal with just sedatives.

Subsequent to that, in 1995, the patient received 3rd cell transplantation of the same 8 transplants by our team in Moscow again. The indication was to maintain the status quo insofar physical, mental and spiritual functions.

Prior to the treatment, her tests showed the same findings as always before, and all her examination showed no change as compared with the previous ones.

In 1998, the patient received 4th transplantation of 10 different stem cell transplants; all those received before, with addition of *frontal lobe of brain, bone*, of our manufacturing. The indication was to maintain the status quo. All tests and examinations showed no change.

In March 2000, the measurement of bone density of the whole body revealed values characteristic for a woman of 40 years of age, i.e. 20 years less than the age of the patient.

In October 2001, patient underwent 5th stem cell transplantation of the same 8 transplants of our manufacturing as before.

Note: The above write-up proves the difficulty of presenting a case history of a patient where the indication for stem cell transplantation is primarily a 'disease of aging', even though there are usually some other indications as well, in this case a premature menopause. When you read it, it seems like time has stopped. All that various physicians or psychologists can state that the standard examinations used are within limits of normal. That's the whole point. The chronological aging clock is "ticking" the way it should, while the biological aging clock appears to have slowed down so that the aging becomes inconspicuous.

How to state medically that a woman of 62 looks, moves, acts, behaves, thinks, etc. like a 40 year old, and that no one wants to believe her true age. The human life in its physical, mental and spiritual aspects just cannot be measured. It appears possible to slow down the aging process. And not only seemingly 'ageless' movie stars that you see in the movies or on your TV screens can accomplish it.

But it is not only a result of stem cell transplantations every 3 years or so. Everyone knows that there is no cosmetic surgical procedure for the 'lifting' of aging body.

This patient has had a proper nutrition, that she prepared herself most of the time from ecologically sound fresh ingredients, ate a lot of cheese made of raw milk, drank regularly wine without additives and preservatives, but also plenty of real spring water, but no 'soft drinks'. She exercised regularly, had no problem going through a 60 minutes' aerobics/total body fitness class with fit women and men who could be her children or grandchildren. She was mentally active, not long ago finished a supervision of a construction of a new house that she has never done before in her life, and she has kept her spirits up.

Chapter 49

It is the lone worker who makes the first advance in a subject: the details may be worked out by a team, but the prime idea is due to the enterprise, thought and perception of an individual.
Alexander Fleming, 1881 – 1955 [Address at Edinburgh University, 1951]

Leave no stone unturned.
Euripides, c. 486 – 406 B.C., [Heraclidae, c. 428 B.C.]

ENDOCRINE DISEASES

Hormones are responsible for homeostasis of internal milieu of organism, regulation of metabolism, adaptation to stress. Their deficiency causes endocrine diseases. Hormones are produced by endocrine glands but also by specialized cells in brain, kidneys, gastrointestinal tract, lungs, etc.

Deficiency of hormones has been historically the first indication for cell transplantation. The same is not true about the excessive production of hormones: hyperfunction of any endocrine gland is an indication for stem cell transplantation only in the case when an antagonist of the hormone is known, and is produced by a specific cell type, that is then used for cell transplantation treatment. For illustration, although several antagonists of thyroid hormones are known, as well as cell types producing them, they affect Graves, or Basedow, disease only to a limited degree. The same applies to Cushing's syndrome.

Because of complex interrelationships of endocrine glands, and their control by hypothalamus/pituitary gland, it is very rare that a specific patient gets cell transplantation of a single type of cell: *cell transplants of all related glands, and of hypothalamus and pituitary, are implanted*, too.

From chemical viewpoint, hormones can be:

1. polypeptides and proteins, produced on ribosomes as pre-

prohormones first: after removal of a 'signal peptide' a prohormone is created, which then, after the next biochemical step, becomes a hormone,
2. steroids,
3. low-molecular amines (catecholamines, thyroid hormones).

Hormones do not influence cell functions directly, only through secondary intracellular signals. Active hormone is secreted into blood and taken by protein carrier to the target cells of the respective tissue, to *the first messenger* that accepts from the multiplicity of data only what is pertinent. This selection of data is possible via specific receptors on the cell surface, macromolecules with a high affinity to the given hormone and capability to communicate with the hormone. Connection of hormone with its specific receptor creates 'hormonal system' that enables entry of the hormone into the cell, i.e. internalization. Thereby a cascade of secondary effects is triggered, including the creation of intracellular *'second messengers'*, which could be:

- activation of membrane adenylatecyclase by the complex 'hormone-receptor',
- creation of cyclic AMP from ATP by adenylatecyclase,
- activation of proteinkinases (phosphokinases), that catalyse phosphorylation of various proteins, mainly enzymes, and thereby activate them as well.

Many peptide hormones utilize cyclic adenosinmonophosphate (cAMP) as a 'second messenger', such as ACTH, luteotropin (LH), thyreotropin (TSH), prolactin, somatotropin, portion of releasing hormones (RH) and release inhibiting hormones (RIH), glucagons, parathormone, calcitonin, ADH, gastrin, secretin, oxytocin, adenosine, serotonin, dopamine, histamine, and prostaglandins. Cyclic guanosin-monophosphate (cGMP) is a 'second messenger' for atrial natriumuretic factor, and nitric oxide (NO). The same hormone may, depending upon the target cell and receptor, cause production of various 'second messengers'.

The remaining molecular mechanisms take place in the cell nucleus that secures and regulates the expression of respective target genes. This is carried out via *third messengers*, or 'transcription factors', the proteins bound to the specific DNA sequences in the regulatory portion of such genes, and causing stimulation or suppression of the gene expression. The result is the realization of respective metabolic response, specific for the effect of the hormone in the respective target organ.

Hormones regulate and direct the function of organs. Stimulation (or inhibition) of their release is controlled by specific factors. Hormones act upon the hormone producing cell itself via *autocrine* effect, or upon the neighboring cells via *paracrine* effect through mediators or neurotransmitters, or upon distant target cells in other organs via *endocrine* effect. Hormones must not be inactivated before reaching their target cells. In target cells, hormones are bound to receptors and trigger intracellular signal transduction to accomplish their effect.

Hormonal disorders can be *caused* by:

- erroneous synthesis or activation of hormones due to enzymatic disorder,
- faulty production of protein, that is the actual hormone, or pre-hormone, or protein carrier of hormones, or a macromolecule of specific receptor,
- decreased number of receptors,
- lowered receptor affinity toward respective hormone,
- limited connection with intracellular signaling chain.

It can be due to a single gene defect.

Lowered hormonal effect can be due to its *accumulation or disturbed release*. Sometimes the lack of activation of endocrine gland leads to insufficient production of hormones for the body needs, or the hormone producing cells are not sensitive to the stimuli, or the quantity of hormone producing cells is not adequate due to hypoplasia, or aplasia.

An inactivation, or a breakdown of hormones, that is too fast, can also be the cause of insufficient level of a hormone. When a hormone is bound to the plasma proteins then the duration of effectiveness depends upon the proportion of bound hormone. *Hormones bound to protein are not active, but they also avoid any breakdown.*

Some hormones must be converted to the active form at the periphery. If such conversion is not possible, because of enzymatic defect, the hormone remains inactive. Finally, hormone can be inactive due to the lack of sensitivity of target organs, i.e. there is a defective hormone receptor, or intracellular transport, or complete malfunctioning of target cells or organs.

The cause of increased hormonal effect can be an abnormally high level of release of hormone. This can be due to excessive stimulation, increased sensitivity, or too large quantity of hormone producing cells, i.e. in hyperplasia, adenomas, etc. Occasionally an ectopic production of hormones by cancer cells is the cause. Sometimes the problem is too slow breakdown or inactivation of hormones, as in liver or kidney failure. In other cases the hypersensitivity of target organs to a specific hormone, increased intracellular transport, or hyperfunction of hormone sensitive cells, is cause.

Hormones are usually *components of regulatory circuits*. Disturbance of one unit of regulatory circuit leads to characteristic changes of other units of the circuit.

In endocrine system a regulatory circuit with negative feedback dominates since the production of a hormone of the target endocrine gland in the periphery usually lowers a release of the hormone from the regulatory gland via reduction of stimulatory factors.

Regulatory circuits with positive feedback, i.e. when hormones of the target endocrine gland in the periphery lead to increase of stimuli, and thereby support of their own release, are rare and usually only temporary.

Release of hormones not dependent upon pituitary gland is regulated by those parameters that are influenced by the respective hormone. A hormone acts upon the target organ and its function, then leads to limitations of stimuli necessary for the release of the same hormone, i.e. regulatory circuit with negative feedback. Let's take a secretion of insulin as an example. An increase of blood glucose stimulates the release of insulin, the effect of which upon target organs, i.e. liver, lowers the blood glucose via increased glycolysis, gluconeogenesis inhibition, and glycogen production. On the other hand, the excessive release of insulin, not commensurate to the plasma glucose concentration, leads to hypoglycemia. In case of disturbance of the endocrine gland the plasma level of the respective hormone is lowered and thereby also its effect. Insufficient β-cell count leads to hyperglycemia.

Release of hormones is directed by hypothalamus and pituitary: 'Releasing hormones' are produced in hypothalamus and cause the release of respective tropins in pituitary. In turn, tropins stimulate the release of the respective hormone at the periphery. The hormone at the periphery, and to some degree also its effects, suppress the release of releasing hormones in hypothalamus and of tropins in the pituitary. *Decreased release of the peripheral hormone can be due to the disturbance of the function of hypothalamus, pituitary, or the peripheral endocrine gland.*

Stem cell transplantation takes a vastly different approach to the treatment of endocrine diseases as compared with the use of individual hormones:

1. hormones are produced, and released by, organism as necessary, there is no storage of active hormones,
2. hormones have only short-term effect, while transplanted cells have long-term therapeutic benefit,
3. hormone replacement therapy is a treatment for life, without possibility of cure,
4. long-term hormone replacement therapy suppresses the respective endocrine gland, and cause atrophy and loss of function of the gland.

Somatotropin, growth hormone, is produced in the anterior lobe of pituitary. It inhibits intake of glucose into muscle and fatty cells, supports lipolysis, gluconeogenesis, collagen synthesis, erythropoietin synthesis. It also stimulates resorption of calcium and phosphorus in the intestine, as well as excretion of calcium through kidneys. It supports bone growth before closure of epiphyses, and thereby also height, and growth of soft tissues, and stimulates proliferation of T-cells, IL-2, 'killer' cells, macrophages, and thereby the entire immune system.

The release of somatotropin is stimulated by growth hormone releasing factor, and inhibited by somatostatin, from hypothalamus.

Excess of somatotropin is usually due to pituitary adenoma, and causes acromegaly.

Insufficient release of somatotropin before the closure of epiphyseal ossification centers leads to pituitary nanismus, while *later on in life it cannot be easily detected but has to be watched for in case of immune system weakness in elderly.*

Various forms of *endocrine nanism* are disorders of the axis hypothalamus - anterior lobe of pituitary – adrenal cortex – gonads.

Nanismus, or dwarfism, was historically one of the first indications for cell transplantation. In the first two years of life, cell transplants necessary for treatment are selected according to the etiology summarized below. Between the 3rd and 8th year of life, *diencephalon, hypothalamus, anterior lobe of pituitary, and thyroid,* has to be implanted as well, and after the 8th year of life, *adrenal cortex and gonads*.

Pituitary nanism due to the isolated deficit of growth hormone, or somatotropin, an AR disorder, (but can be also AD or XR), is a 'nearly' proportional nanism with normal sexual development, with delayed development of facial skeleton, delayed permanent dentition, progeric facies, typical voice, hair and nail abnormalities, hypoglycemia, etc. It can be due to any mis-step along the pathway from the release of neurotransmitters by neurons of brain cortex and suprahypothalamic region, that stimulate the release of growth hormone releasing factor (GHRF), or somatoliberine, from hypothalamus, and that in turn stimulates respective cells of anterior lobe of pituitary to secrete the growth hormone. Finally, growth hormone stimulates the receptors of multiple tissues, mostly liver, where Insulin-like Growth Factors IGF-I (somatomedin C) and IGF-II (somatomedin A) mediate the activity of growth hormone. Today testing permits us to differentiate the cause of nanism as being of pituitary or of receptor origin.

Laron nanism is an AR disorder occurring in Jews, with accentuated nanism, abnormal facial expression, high-pitch voice, small external genitalia, but normal reproductive ability, acromicria, and trunk obesity, delayed dentition, and closure of major fontanelle. Failure of response of membrane receptors to the growth hormone is the cause [233].

Other forms of ***nanism***, and its etiology are:

1. ***proportionate***:
    - hereditary, e.g. familial, constitutional, progeria, pseudo-hypoparathyreoidism, etc.,
    - metabolic: *renal*, i.e. Debre-de Toni-Fanconi syndrome, phosphate diabetes, vitamin-D-resistant rachitis, or *intestinal*, i.e. megacolon, pancreatic fibrosis, or *hepatic*, i.e. glycogenoses, mucopolysaccharidoses, cystinosis, *lysosomal storage disease*.

2. ***nearly proportionate***:

    - *neuro-endocrine*, i.e. hypothyreosis, adrenal, dysgenital, or *dyscerebral*, e.g. Down syndrome, microcephaly, Laurence-Moon-Biedl syndrome, etc.,
    - hypoxemic, i.e. cardiac, pulmonary, anemic.

3. ***disproportionate***:

    - defective bone growth: chondrodystrophy, achondroplasia, osteogenesis imperfecta, chondroectodermal dysplasia, Morquio disease, Hurler disease, Sanfilippo disease, marble bone disease, dysostosis cleidocranialis, etc.

Our own experience in the treatment of familial and constitutional nanismus, without any deficit of growth hormone, by human fetal cell transplantation in 11 patients at the Endocrinology Research Center of the Russian Academy of Medical Sciences, was positive. Our patients were from 4 to 15 years of age, 7 males, and 4 females. With the exception of slightly higher TSH in 2 patients, the hormonal testing was normal in all patients. Cell transplantation of *hypothalamus, entire pituitary, thyroid*, was carried out for patients up until 8 years of age, and after that age also cell transplants of *gonads and adrenal cortex* was implanted. Four patients also received the 2nd cell transplantation. Within 3 months of cell transplantation, the height of all patients increased by 2.0 to 2.5 cm, but the response was not as pronounced as typically seen in the proportionate nanismus due to growth hormone deficiency.

Diencephalon/hypothalamus system is involved in many disturbances of growth, weight loss, obesity, and, therefore, stem cell transplantation of such cells should be considered in various affections of brain [271, 272, 273]. One of those is post-partum **Sheehan syndrome**, that often appears silently, and leads to a variety of 'hormone' problems without any effective treatment. Stem cell transplantation of *diencephalon, adrenal cortex, ovary, placenta, liver, and intestine*, is recommended. Another is '***anorexia neurosa***', *or* '***bulimia***', where stem cell transplants of *diencephalon, hypothalamus, anterior lobe of pituitary, adrenal cortex, gonads*, should be considered 'when everything else fails'.

Anorexia nervosa is a very hard to treat condition, so it is of no surprise that cell transplantation was tested as a treatment of such patients. A wife/husband team developed a therapeutic program which included all steps known and described, but after a proper preparation of patient it was a cell transplantation of *thymus, spleen, placenta, ovaries, diencephalon, liver, stomach/intestine, exocrine pancreas,* and *thyroid*, that made the difference. The report is based on an experience with the first 10 patients, all of them 'failures' of the previous therapeutic attempts, two of them are described in case histories in detail.

Overall, when compared with published data about 54 patients treated by traditional methods, the 10 reported patients spent 10 days in outpatient preparatory phase, then 5 – 10 days as in-patients, during which time they received cell transplantation, and 32 – 50 days in the follow-up ambulatory care, while those 54 patients spent 32 – 749 days in outpatient preparatory phase, then 6 – 175 days as in-patients, and 28 – 630 days in the follow-up ambulatory care. It seems apparent that cell transplantation makes the difference [296].

Even the treatment of **obesity** can be assisted by stem cell transplantation in motivated patients by implanting *diencephalon, hypothalamus, and entire pituitary gland including infundibulum*. Many young females develop obesity during the first pregnancy, that is not responsive to diet and exercise. Here the regeneration of the entire endocrine system should be carried out by stem cell transplantation of *diencephalon, hypothalamus, entite pituitary including infundibulum, thyroid, adrenal cortex, ovary, and placenta*.

Antidiuretic hormone, ADH, or vasopressin, is produced in nucleus supraopticus and paraventricularis of hypothalamus, and is transported through axons of the hormone producing neurons into the posterior lobe of pituitary. ADH influences channels for H_2O in distal tubules and collecting tubules of kidneys and supports water reabsorption. It stimulates also reabsorption of Na^+ and urea, and in high concentrations causing vasoconstriction.

Lack of ADH can be genetic, i.e. **diabetes insipidus**, or due to autoimmune destruction of ADH producing neurons, or any other hypothalamic damage. Stem cell transplantation of *hypothalamus, entire pituitary including infundibulum, kidney, and placenta*, is advised.

In **renal diabetes insipidus** there is a defect of channels for water, and thereby of concentration ability of kidneys, as for example, with low levels of K^+, excess of Ca^{++}, or inflammation of renal medulla.

Our study of treatment of *central diabetes insipidus* in children by transplantation of human fetal cells of *diencephalon, pituitary, kidney, hypothalamus*, was carried out at Endocrinology Research Center of Russian Academy of Sciences and included 5 children, of 3 to 15 years of age, 3 females, and 2 males. Three patients suffered from autonomous nervous system disorder with hypotonia and two female patients from chronic pyelonephritis. Two patients had atopic dermatitis. One female patient, nearly 16 years old, received cell transplantation three times, and her dose of ADH decreased after the 1st cell transplantation from 6 drops to 1 – 2 drops, and has remained the same for over 18 months, her headaches disappeared completely, as well as dysmenorhea. Another female patient, 11 years old, had cell transplantation twice, her dose of ADH decreased to 1 – 2 drops a day, thirst and polyuria disappeared, headaches were less frequent. In all three remaining patients the ADH dose was substantially decreased, headaches less pronounced or disappeared.

Insulin and Diabetes Mellitus

In the April of 1994 issue of Bulletin of Experimental Biology and Medicine, Vol. 117, an official journal of the Russian Academy of Medical Sciences, there are two summary articles about 16 years of Soviet, Russian, and our clinical experience in the treatment of over 3,000 patients with type 1 diabetes mellitus, and type ½, with complications: retinopathy, nephropathy, polyneuropathy, and peripheral arterial disease, as *described in detail in chapter* 29. The average success rate was 60 – 80%, depending upon the type of complication and the stage of its development. Duration of the effect was 9 – 18 months, and longer after subsequent treatments. The rate of complications decreased significantly in the treatment of diabetic women during pregnancy and has nearly eliminated the fetal death due to diabetes of mother [146, 147].

Diabetes mellitus (DM) is a disease with enormous variability of its clinical and biochemical features. The much less common *type 1 of DM (IDDM)* is substantially better clinically defined than the *type 2 of DM (NIDDM)*. The incidence and prevalence of DM, with its life-threatening and crippling complications, has been growing worldwide with such a speed that one could speak of an 'epidemic'. Several new therapeutic approaches have been developed in an attempt to solve this problem. New methods of intensive insulinotherapy, that try to simulate normal functioning of pancreatic β-cells, improve the physician's ability to maintain the relationship between levels of insulin and blood glucose. For optimal insulinotherapy, automatic systems of insulin delivery were introduced, of sophisticated closed type, permitting imitation of physiological feedback (used in situations of 'clinical crises'), and of simpler open type. But the transplantologic methods of treatment appear the most promising, since only in this way the normal physiology can be restored [17].

Full correction of carbohydrate metabolism in patients with IDDM can be accomplished by the *organ transplantation of pancreas*. The great risk of such surgical procedure, i.e. transplant rejection, destruction of transplant by enzymatic activity of the exocrine portion, leading to the creation of vascular shunts, and thrombosis of vascular anastomoses, etc., and the need for life endangering continuous high dosage immunosuppression afterward, has limited the indication of this operation to those instances where also a life-saving kidney transplantation is carried out [120]. As a rule, *at that stage, the complications of DM, the main cause of death of such patients, have become severe and irreversible* [121].

Stem cell transplantation permits normalization of carbohydrate metabolism and prevention of development of late complications of DM at a much earlier stage of the disease. *The advantages of this therapeutic approach* are:

1. from the patient's viewpoint the treatment is simple, and carries a minimal risk, regardless of route of implantation used,
2. there is a great variety of animal sources of stem cell xeno-transplants available,
3. immunosuppression can be avoided [121, 122].

A comparison of treatment of diabetes mellitus by stem cell transplantation and insulin can be summarized as follows:

1. insulin cannot cure diabetes mellitus,
2. insulin cannot prevent disabling, often life threatening, complications of diabetes mellitus,
3. even the optimal insulinotherapy cannot stop relentless progress of diabetic complications, only stem cell transplantation can,
4. but stem cell transplantation cannot replace insulinotherapy yet: it must be used simultaneously with insulinotherapy.

As the clinical experience of the past four decades have shown *only stem cell transplantation can stop the relentless progress of the complications of diabetes mellitus once they start*. This implies that the transplanted cells of all organs and tissues involved in carbohydrate metabolism trigger, directly or indirectly, the production of those endocrine or paracrine hormones that prevent the microangiopathic changes, the basis of all diabetic complications.

Carrel stated that *insulin does not cure diabetes*, and diabetes cannot be overcome until medical science succeeds to regenerate or replace islet cells, i.e. not only β-cells. Regeneration of islet cells is a more efficient way of treating diabetes mellitus than giving the patients daily injections of insulin. This statement is still valid today, even after the DCCT trial in the US. Insulin prevents death of a new diabetic but cannot stop the development of diabetic complications, severely disabling, and often fatal after years of suffering. The cause of all diabetic complications is still unknown but is probably due to *the lack of other, still unknown, hormones produced by various cells of Langerhans islets of pancreas, or by different cells of various organs of the regulatory system of carbohydrate and lipid metabolism.*

Only stem cell transplantation can treat diabetic complications with success. *Before the introduction of primary tissue culture into the preparation of cell xenotransplants* the success rate of treatment of diabetes was minimal. It was believed that human fetal cell transplantation solves this problem, but US FDA approved clinical trials of the late 1980's by HANA Biologicals failed as well. It is clear that the primary tissue culture method of preparation of stem cell transplants it the key to success.

Stem cell transplantation can successfully treat complications of diabetes mellitus. In 1978 the first IDDM patient with retinopathy and nephropathy was treated in Moscow: this female patient remained insulin-independent for over 21 years.

In summary, *the success rate of treatment by stem cell transplantation*, described in detail in the chapter 29, for patients in the:

- pre-proliferative stage of diabetic retinopathy has been 65%
- pre-azotemic stage of diabetic nephropathy 65%
- any stage of diabetic poly-neuropathy 98%
- pre-obstructive stage of diabetic vasculopathy 65%
- clinically un-controllable children's 'brittle diabetes' 90%.

Part of the reason for such a high success rate has been that *no immunosuppression had to be used for treatment* when stem cell transplants are prepared by the *method described in Part III* 'Manufacture of stem cell xenotransplants'. Additionally, well known side-effects, the specific problem of immunosuppression in diabetics is that it causes an increased metabolic demand on β-cells of pancreatic islets so that their capacity to produce insulin may be exhausted. This deleterious effect is much greater for islet cell transplants than for organ transplants of the pancreas.

Diabetes mellitus is a heterogenous group of diseases with one common finding, that of *hyperglycemia*, responsible for polyuria, polydipsia, weight loss, polyphagia, and complications, i.e. retinopathy with potential loss of sight, nephropathy leading to kidney failure, polyneuropathy with intractable pain, lower extremity arterial disease with crural ulcers, gangrene requiring amputations, autonomous neuropathy with gastrointestinal, genitourinary, cardiovascular abnormalities, and sexual dysfunction. There is an increased incidence of atherosclerosis in coronary, brain and peripheral arteries, and hypertension. Glucose reacts with hemoglobin HbA to create HbA1c, and increased concentration of HbA1c proves that hyperglycemia has been present for many months. HbA1c has a higher affinity to oxygen than HbA, and does not easily release oxygen at the periphery.

Pathologic anatomy

Absolute mass of the endocrine portion of pancreas in late human fetus is 300 mg, which represents about 10% of total weight of pancreas. In children the mass of the endocrine portion grows to 450 mg, which represents only 7% of the total weight of pancreas, however. In adulthood the weight of endocrine portion reaches 1,500 mg, but that represents only 2% of the total weight of pancreas [73, p.103].

At least four endocrine cell types with specific granules are currently recognized in the Langerhans islands of pancreas. *A(α) cells* produce glucagon, are localized in the periphery of the islets, and appear first during the embryonic development. *B(β) cells* produce insulin, including pro-insulin and C-peptide, and are localized in the center of islets. *D(δ) cells* produce somatostatin, are localized paracentrally in association with A cells, and appear second during the embryonic development. *PP (or F) cells* produce Pancreatic Polypeptide, that possibly suppresses enzyme production and gallbladder contraction, are localized in the periphery of the islets but also scattered outside of islets, and are the last to appear. Additional cell types have been described on the basis of their electron-dense secretory granules, but no peptide hormones have been attributed to them yet [163, pp. 1997-1999].

Two types of islets are recognized: *β-cell rich*, scattered throughout the gland, and *PP-cell rich*, restricted to the posterior lobe of pancreas.

In an autopsy study, the weight of a whole pancreas in healthy subjects was 1,395 mg, while in IDDM it was 413 mg, and in NIDDM 1,449 mg.

The loss of endocrine tissue observed in IDDM was almost completely restricted to the PP-cells-poor anterior lobe of pancreas, where it reached 81%. Here B cells were practically absent, but the 'atrophic islets' still contained numerous A, D, and PP cells. In the PP cells-rich posterior lobe the decrease of total endocrine tissue was not significant. Here many islets contained a few B cells. The mass of A, D, and PP cells, and the ratio of D to A cells were the same in IDDM and normal controls. In NIDDM the mass of A cells was increased but, the mass of B, D, and PP cells was the same as in healthy controls. Outside the islets in three out of four cases rare B cells still could be identified, usually between the acinar cells. The proportion of D-cells was increased 3.5 times in IDDM[168].

In another autopsy study of IIDM patients dying within a year of the onset of symptoms, three populations of islets were recognized: the majority of islets were B cell deficient, but contained a normal complement of A, D, and PP cells; some islets were affected by insulinitis, particularly those that still contained B cells; and some islets were totally unaffected by the disease. Aberrant expression of class II MHC was demonstrated on the great majority of B cells in IDDM of recent onset. Such abnormalities of MHC expression are unique to IDDM, and precede the start of the insulinitis in a given islet [163, pp. 2000-2001].

There is a general agreement that in order to attain insulin-independence after cell transplantation, a certain minimum quantity of islets has to be transplanted: about 350,000 [136]. This has been proven by cases of auto-transplantation of pancreatic islets [137]. In allo-transplantation such number of islets can be obtained only from adult cadavers, and in these situations the severe rejection reaction is unavoidable, unless massive immunosuppression would be used. The better alternative is a stem cell xenotransplantation.

Pathogenetically it is often hard to determine if the development of disease is due to autoimmune destruction of β-cells of Langerhans islands of pancreas with resultant deficit of insulin or resistance to insulin by target cells. Even though there are excellent clinical guides for separating various causes of hyperglycemia, in the case of a specific patient all such processes are at work and it is hard to decide which one, or both working together, are the primary causes.

Absolute majority of diabetics falls into two categories:

- type 1 diabetes mellitus, also known as insulin-dependent (IDDM),

- type 2 diabetes mellitus, also known as insulin-independent (NIDDM).

Diabetes mellitus type 1, formerly known as *juvenile diabetes mellitus*, is either due to autoimmune mechanism or is idiopathic. Autoimmunity is the favored way to explain pathogenesis of DM Type 1. Destruction of β-cells of Langerhans islands of pancreas is due to cell-based autoimmune process. It reaches such a magnitude that there is an absolute paucity of endogenous insulin so that patient's life is dependent on a continuous supply of exogenous insulin. The autoimmune pathogenesis is proven by a typical infiltration of Langerhans islands by various immunocytes in the early stages and finding of the following markers:

- Islet cell auto-antibodies identifiable years before onset of the disease,
- Glutamic acid decarboxylase auto-antibodies,
- Insulin auto-antibodies,
- Tyrosinephosphatases 1A-2 and 1A-2β auto-antibodies.

Such markers are found in 85 – 90% of newly diagnosed patients, while their incidence in general population is only 5%.

The course of autoimmune destruction of β-cells of Langerhans islands of pancreas is variable. In some patients, especially infants and children, it can be very fast, in others, such as adults, it can be slow. While in children and adolescents a ketoacidosis can be the first evidence of disease, in adults the remaining still functioning β-cells respond to the body needs for years before exogenous insulin has to become a part of treatment program.

There can be some genetic and exogenous predispositions to cell-mediated autoimmune destruction of β-cells. It is believed that *only a tendency toward diabetes in inherited*, not the disease itself.

Among genetic predispositions, the most important is *a strong association with HLA-system*: 95% of Caucasian patients with IDDM have a haplotype HLA-DR3 or HLA-DR4, while the number for general population is only 50%. These haplotypes are of global nature, and other autoimmune diseases are in distinct association with the same haplotypes. Genes coding antigens HLA-DQ, especially DQ2-DQ8, are connected with the highest risk for IDDM.

In summary, although the majority of IDDM patients carry predisposing HLA-alleles, not all such carriers will become diabetics. At the same time, the presence of protective HLA-alleles is a guarantee of protection against diabetes mellitus. It appears that predisposing or protective role of HLA-alleles is becoming less important with the age of patient at the time the first clinical symptoms and signs of the disease appear.

Environmental predispositions are obesity, lack of breastfeeding, viral infections by rubeola, coxsackie, enteroviruses, chemical toxins, i.e. rat poison, nitrosamines from smoked food, etc., increased load on β-cells, i.e. prolonged hyperglycemia, hormones, such as during pregnancy or puberty, ethnic factors, etc.

Latent autoimmune DM of adults, LADA: Many patients were classified as NIDDM when in reality they had a late-in-life occurring and slowly developing IDDM. This type is now called LADA. Autoantibodies proving autoimmune insulinitis are present except with varying frequency of different types. There is different frequency and ratio between predisposing and protective HLA-alleles. The course of disease is milder and slower and the same applies to the aggressivity of destructive process of insulinitis. The same applies to biochemical findings.

Diabetes mellitus type 2, previously known as *diabetes of old age*, represents 80 – 90% cases of diabetes mellitus worldwide, and is characterized by a combination of resistance toward the effects of insulin by target cells at the periphery and insufficient compensatory response in terms of its secretion by β-cells. Degree of hyperglycemia is sufficient for causing pathologic and functional changes in various target tissues while patient is completely asymptomatic and that applies to micro- and macro- angiopathic complications. These patients do not need insulin to survive. The basis of diabetes is not a destruction of β-cells by an autoimmune process, so that there are no such markers to be found in the patient's body, and there is *no association with HLA-system*.

It has been proven that the lowered sensitivity to insulin is due to genetic predisposition. Lowered sensitivity to insulin affects predominantly glucose metabolism, while metabolism of fats and proteins function normally: in NIDDM there is high level hyperglycemia but without disturbed fatty metabolism, i.e. lack of ketoacidosis. There is an increased concentration of fatty acids in blood, and decreased consumption of glucose in muscle and fatty tissues. The insulin resistance leads to increased release of insulin. The subsequent down-regulation of receptor causes further increase of resistance, and a 'vicious circle' is closed. The majority of patients are obese, which is the result of a separate genetic predisposition, excessive intake of highly caloric food, lack of physical activity, emotional psychic stress, and aging.

Diabetes mellitus can be due to increased secretion of antagonists of insulin: somatotropin, as seen in acromegaly, glucocorticoids, as found in Cushing's disease, or stress in steroid diabetes, adrenalin, due to stress, progesterons and choriomammotropin as happens in gestation diabetes mellitus, ACTH, thyroid hormones, glucagons. Insulin antagonists gain upper hand when blood glucose levels drop.

The first and most important one, in particular in acute situations, is *glucagon* made by α-cells of Langerhans islands, released in response to falling levels of blood glucose. It binds glucagon receptors in the hepatocytes, the only glucagons receptors in the body, and stimulates the liver to:

1. increase the rates of glycogenolysis,
2. decrease the rate of glycogen synthesis,
3. decrease the rates of glycolysis,
4. increase the rates of gluconeogenesis,
5. decrease the rates of fatty acid synthesis.

Adrenaline is released from adrenal medulla in response to signals from the brain triggered by falling blood glucose levels. Adrenaline has different effect after binding to its receptors in different cells:

1. In muscle, as there is no glucose-6-phosphatase there, adrenaline will trigger the use of glucose-6-phosphate for glycolysis, but not as a source of glucose, so that muscle glycogen cannot be a source of glucose for blood, and for brain.
2. In adipose tissue adrenaline activates lipase, which hydrolyzes triacylglycerides and thereby activates fat, so that fatty acids are released for use as fuel substrates in order to conserve levels of blood glucose.
3. In the liver, adrenaline activates breakdown of glycogen and inhibition of fatty acid synthesis, thus shutting down fat anabolism.

Cortisol is also an insulin antagonist.

In type I diabetes mellitus the insulin antagonists have usually an upper hand. In type II diabetes mellitus the defect lies in the insulin signaling pathway so that the binding of insulin cannot elicit the usual anabolic responses, or the rapid clearance of glucose from blood.

Genetic disturbance of insulin effect is rare. Mutations of gene for human insulin receptor cause:

- *leprechaunism* with intrauterine growth retardation, failure to thrive, facial dysmorpia, acanthosis nigricans, lipoatrophy, hyperinsulinism, postprandial hyperglycemia with hypoglycemia on empty stomach, death already in infancy;
- *Rabson-Mendelhall syndrome* with short stature, acanthosis nigricans, dental and nail anomalies, oversized penis, mental retardation, hyperplasia of pineal gland.

Insulin-resistant lipoatrophic diabetes is due to post-receptor signal transmission defects.

Gestation diabetes mellitus occurs in 4% of pregnancies, but disappears after delivery, but sometimes it may take years to do so.

Biochemistry and physiology of insulin

Under normal circumstances, insulin is produced as a *linear polypeptide* pre-proinsulin first, with a signal sequence at N-terminus that facilitates its movement into the lumen of endoplasmic reticulum. In endoplasmic reticulum this *signal sequence is removed* and a much shorter proinsulin is generated. *Proinsulin molecule is bent and disulfide bridges are created* between the side chains of neighboring amino acids. Eventually proinsulin is *selectively cleaved and its one portion, C-peptide, is released* whereby a proinsulin becomes a mature insulin.

Following food ingestion, a glucose concentration begins to rise in blood; *glucose enters β-cells of Langerhans islands, and triggers a depolarization event, a rise in intracellular calcium, and release of insulin from insulin granules within β-cells*. Level of insulin in blood rises. Insulin interacts with insulin receptors on the surface of striated muscle cells and adipose cells, which generally show the strongest responses to insulin of all cells. An increased uptake of glucose by stimulated cells is carried out by a glucose transporter GLUT 4 that enables a facilitated diffusion for glucose. *Additionally, insulin*:

1. increases the rate of glycolysis,
2. increases the rate of glycogen synthesis,
3. decreases the rate of glycogen breakdown,
4. decreases rates of gluconeogenesis,

5. increases the rate of synthesis of fatty acids and triacylglycerides,
6. decreases breakdown of triacylglycerides,
7. increases the rate of protein synthesis.

Overall metabolic effect of insulin is the promotion of anabolism, while suppressing catabolism of glycogen and fat.

In diabetes mellitus, the fat is used as a principal fuel with deleterious consequences for cells, and the body in general. In absence of insulin that stops β-oxidation from going into overdrive, an enormous quantity of triacylglycerides breaks down in adipose tissue due to unopposed adrenaline stimulation, and that leads to an excessive β-oxidation and enormous rates of ketone bodies synthesis in the liver. Ensuing ketonemia causes metabolic acidosis, and a drop of tissue pH. *Hyperglycemia with ketonemia dehydrate cells*, with loss of water and electrolytes, hypotension, diabetic coma, and kidney failure.

Treatment of diabetes mellitus and its complications by stem cell transplantation

Indications. *There are 3 main indications:*

- Diabetes Mellitus, types 1 and mixed 1/2, particularly with complications, such as:

    a. Diabetic Retinopathy,
    b. Diabetic Nephropathy,
    c. Diabetic Polyneuropathy,
    d. Diabetic Lower Extremity Arterial Disease.

- Brittle Diabetes Mellitus in children; and
- Diabetes Mellitus in pregnancy, or diabetes mellitus as a cause of female infertility and habitual pregnancy loss.

The key stem cell transplant for the treatment of diabetic complications is *Langerhans islands of pancreas*, the co-transplants used in the described clinical system are stem cell transplants of *liver, adrenal cortex, stomach/intestine* (peripancreatic block), *placenta and hypothalamus.* Sometimes, *anterior lobe of pituitary, parathyroid, gonads*, may be added [328].

When patient suffers from a 'pure' *type 2 DM, or NIDDM, the implantation of islet cells of pancreas, is often meaningless*, but an addition of cell transplant of *intestine* may be considered.

The sooner the patient receives stem cell transplantation after the diagnosis of diabetic complication was established; the better will be the success rate of such therapy.

In the US, the sole criterion of success of stem cell transplantation in the treatment of diabetes mellitus has been a complete insulin-independence. Factors such as a *stabilization of the course of DM or a prevention of further progression of secondary complications of DM* have been disregarded. The first US attempts at fetal allo-transplantation of non-cultured pancreatic islets were reported in 1976, and were unsuccessful.

In the USSR the first fetal allo-transplantation of cultured pancreatic islets was carried out at RITAOMH in 1978, and was successful. *The criterion of success was a prevention of further progression of diabetic complications in the treated patient for 2 years.* In reality the patient was insulin-independent for the next 21 years.

Since the insulin-independence was obtained only rarely, and even then it was only temporary, *the new criteria of success after cell transplantation became the increase of serum C-peptide, or appearance of C-peptide in serum of the initially C-peptide-negative patient, and the lowering of dose of exogenous insulin.* Pronounced chronic IDDM, 3 - 5 years after onset, is accompanied by an absolute insulin deficiency, with absence of C-peptide in serum, even after glucose stimulation. The *criterion of rejection* is a recurrence of hyperglycaemia and lowering of serum C-peptide level [135]. However, the serum C-peptide never goes above the lower level of normal, even after allo-transplantation, and thus cannot explain the beneficial clinical effect of stem cell transplantation over a longer time, e.g. for over one year. On the other hand, in the instances where C-peptide level reached normal or near normal level after cell transplantation, patients were clinically not insulin-independent. So the level of serum c-peptide is only a partial criterion of success.

In the USSR and CIS (Commonwealth of Independent States) the key criterion of success has been *an arrest of further progression of microangiopathic complication of IDDM.*

In a study of 100 IDDM patients treated by xenotransplantation of islet cells, in 100% of patients there was a clinical evidence of damaged structure and function of the capillary network of lower extremities, in 74 % vasomotor abnormalities, and 41.2% of patients were found to have a diabetic retinopathy. During the follow-up after 3 weeks, and after 3 months - 4 years after the procedure, in 74% of patients there was a stabilization of the hemodynamic status of lower extremities, in 18% there was an improvement and in 8% worsening. Stabilization of retinal pathologic changes was observed in 70.4%, improvement in 24.7% and worsening in 4.9% of patients. In 34.1% there was an improvement of visual acuity, in 60% stabilization, and in 5.9% worsening [68].

In a study of 55 IDDM patients the vascular condition of lower extremities was evaluated by rheovasography, and capillaroscopy, the eyegrounds by direct and inverted opthalmoscopy, and the kidney function by laboratory tests. In 80% of patients there was a vasomotor abnormality, and in 100% there were abnormal capillaroscopic findings: 30% of patients were in the 1st and 70% in the 2nd stage. After cell xenotransplantation with a follow up for one year in 73% stabilization was observed, in 22% an improvement, and in 5% worsening. Ophthalmologically in 43% of patients an improvement and in 57% a stabilization was observed. In 20% of patients visual acuity improved, in the remaining 80% it stayed the same. 24-hour proteinuria dropped from 1.8 gm/l to 1.2 gm/l [84].

Of the 85 IDDM patients, 41% were found to have a diabetic retinopathy: 1st stage in 11, 2nd stage (pre-proliferative) in 21, and 3rd stage (proliferative) in 3 patients. All 3 patients with stage 3 and one patient with stage 2 had to be removed from the study because of increased severity of their diabetic nephropathy. Follow-up examinations were 24 hours, 2 - 3 weeks, 3, 6, 9 months, up to 4 years, after allo- and/or xeno-transplantation of islet cells. In 58 - 86% there was a gradual improvement of retinal pathologic changes over 3 - 9 months, and in 24% of patients in stage 1, there was a complete regression of retinopathy. Following intercurrent diseases in 6% of patients a worsening occurred over the period of 1 - 2 years. Visual acuity increased in 34.1%, stabilization in 59.4% and worsening in 6.5% of patients [88].

In another study of 100 patients with moderate and severe diabetes mellitus, from 18 to 60 years of age, in 72 there were abnormal rheovasographic findings, and in all 100 there were abnormal capillaroscopic findings: in 25 of the 1st and in 75 of the 2nd stage. Follow up was 3 weeks, 3, 6, 9, and 12 months and up to 3 years after transplantation of islet cells. In 74% of patients there was a gradual stabilization, in 10% an improvement, and in 3 worsening [89].

In *our own study, 106 patients with IDDM* were treated by transplantation of cultured islet cells (CT) of newborn rabbits. All patients selected for CT suffered of severe IIDM, with labile course, quick progression of the disease, and diabetic complications.

All patients were divided into two groups. 73 patients of the 1st group, 48 males and 25 females, underwent intramuscular CT. Their age was from 18 to 57 years, with a median of 35.4 years. Duration of diabetes was from 6 to 35 years, with a median of 17.4 years. Labile course of the disease was noted in 76.8% of patients, i.e. in 41.1% there were frequent (1 - 4 times a day), and in 35.7% less frequent (1 - 2 times a week) episodes of hypoglycemia. In 69.9% of patients there was a secondary ketoacidosis. The majority of patients were admitted in the state of sub- or fully decompensated carbohydrate metabolism, with the median blood sugar of 11.7 ± 1.4 Mmol/l, the daily dose of insulin ranged from 18 to 96 U., with a median of 51.3 ± 15.4 U.

33 patients of the 2nd group, 24 males and 9 females, underwent intraportal CT. Their age was from 7 to 55 years, with a median of 32.6 years, duration of diabetes was from 7 to 25 years. Labile course of the disease was noted in 87.9% of patients, in 27.4% there were frequent and in 60.6% less frequent hypoglycaemic episodes. In 81.8% of patients there was ketoacidosis. The majority of patients were admitted in the state of sub- and de- compensated carbohydrate metabolism. The median blood sugar was 11.6 ± 1.0 Mmol/l. The daily dose of insulin ranged from 18 to 60 U., with a median of 49 ± 9.7 U.

Frequency of IDDM complications is listed in Table 1.

Cultures of pancreatic islet cells of newborn rabbits were used for the transplantation. The rabbit insulin is close in sequencing of aminoacids to the human insulin. Pancreatic islet cells were prepared by tissue culture of 11-days duration. For intramuscular transplantation floating or mixed fraction was used, while for intraportal the attached fraction.

Intramuscular transplantation of cultures of pancreatic islet cells was carried out under local anesthesia into the subaponeurotic space of the right rectus abdominis muscle above umbilicus through a large-bore needle.

TABLE 1
Frequency of IDDM complications

IDDMComplication	Group #1 No. of patients	I.M. XT %	Group #2 No. of patients	Intraportal XT %
Polyneuropathy	68	93.1	31	93.9
Peripheral arterial disease	68	93.1	31	93.9
Retinopathy and of these *	57	78	28	84.9
Proliferative Retinopathy	22	30.1	12	36.4
Nephropathy	50	68.5	19	57.8

* *Of all patients with retinopathy, we separately report on those with proliferative retinopathy.*

Intraportal transplantation of cultures of pancreatic islet cells was carried out under local anesthesia by exposing the umbilical vein, its dilatation, followed by catheterization of the portal vein. Implantation of cultures was carried out after preliminary intraportal injection of 5,000 U of heparin along with intra-operative control of the intra-portal pressure.

Lowering of hyperglycemia was observed post-transplantation, most commonly after 7 - 10 days. But in 6 recipients of the 1st group (8.2%) and 12 of 2nd group (36.4%), there were minor hypoglycaemic episodes during the first 1 - 2 days. Apparently the cause of hypoglycaemia was the release of insulin from implanted β-cells damaged during transplantation. In 23 cases of the 1st group (31.5%) and 2 cases of the 2nd group (6.0%) the lowering of hyperglycemia occurred only after 1 - 2 months.

Lowering of glycaemia required a decrease of the dose of exogenous insulin.

Changes of glycemia in the recipients of CT are shown in Table 2.

Another serious criterion for an evaluation of carbohydrate metabolism of the recipients after the CT are the dynamic changes of glycosylated hemoglobin HbA_{1c} (see Table 3).

The optimal regimen of insulinotherapy was established before cell transplantation. After transplantation, all patients were maintained on the same types of insulin, and as much as possible, with the same frequency. This makes the interpretation of changes in the need for exogenous insulin after CT much easier, as seen in Table 4.

Table 2
Changes of glycemia

Implantation site	Median Glycemia (Mmol / l)					
	Pre XT	Post XT				
		14 days	1 month	3 months	6 months	10-12 months
Group #1 I.M. XT	11.7 ±1.4	10.8 ±0.9	8.5 ±0.9*	8.7 ±0.9*	9.1 ±1.1*	10.9 ±1
Group #2 Intraportal XT	11.6 ±1.0	10.8 ±0.9	8.9 ±0.8	8.1 ±0.2	8 ±0.3**	9.2 ±0.6**

* $P < 0.05$ in comparison with initial value
** $P <$ in comparison to the 1st group

Table 3
Changes of HbA$_{1c}$

Implantation site	Pre-XT	Post XT		
		3 months	6 months	10-12 months
Group #1 I.M. XT	13.8 ±1	9.2 ±0.6*	9.5 ±0.1*	10.2 ±0.4*
Group #2 Intraportal XT	12.9 ±1.5	8.3 ±0.2*	8.4 ±0.3*	8.7 ±0.9*

* $P < 0.05$ in comparison with initial value
** $P < 0.05$ in comparison to the 1st group

Table 4
Changes of dosage of exogenous insulin after CT

Implantation site	Pre-XT	Post XT				
		14 days	1 month	3 months	6 months	10-12 months
Group #1 IM	51.3 ±15.4	49.9 ±13.7	41.2 ±13.2*	40.1 ±13.0*	41.8 ±13.3*	47.4 ±14.1
Group #2 Intraportal XT	49.3 ±9.7	40.3 ±9.4	33 ±9.0*	26.3 ±6.9**	25.7 ±6.2**	37.1 ±10.4**
%	100	81.7	66.9	53.3	52.1	75.2

* $P < 0.05$ in comparison with initial value
** $P < 0.05$ in comparison to the 1st group

The pain syndrome of distal polyneuropathy substantially decreased after CT. In 35 out of 43 recipients (81.4%) of the 1st group, followed up for 3 months after transplantation, the pain in lower extremities either substantially decreased or disappeared. After 6 months such effect was maintained in 74.2% of followed patients and after 10 - 12 months in 50%. In the 2nd group the percentage of such patients was higher, therefore 3 months post-transplantation 87.8% of the recipient had no pain, and after 10 - 12 months 76.1%.

All parameters reflecting status of blood flow in patients with diabetic arterial disease of lower extremities of both groups significantly differed from parameters of the control group ($p<0.01$). The half-time of disappearance of the isotope from the tissue depot was increased 1.5 times; tissue circulation was substantially lowered at rest, and in particular was decreased almost 3 times with exercise leading to ischemia. After CT the half-time disappearance of Tc99M from the tissue depot decreased and tissue circulation increased. In comparison with initial parameters the changes were statistically significant ($p<0.05$). The most pronounced parameters were obtained by measuring blood flow with exercise leading to ischaemia in the recipients of the 1st group. There were no statistically significant differences between the patients of both groups.

Evaluation of concentration of serum C-peptide showed that in 29 out of 56 recipients (51.8%) of the 1st group and 18 out of 33 recipients of the 2nd group (54.5%), the initial level of C-peptide was zero; they were C-peptide negative. All measurements below the sensitivity level of the method were so interpreted. In all initially C-peptide-negative recipients of the 1st group the concentration of C-peptide remained below the sensitivity level of the method, and out of 18 initially C-peptide-negative patients of the 2nd group in 5 only did the level of C-peptide not reach over the sensitivity limit of the method (see Table 5).

In cases of intraportal CT a one-time determination of concentration of hormones in the portal and hepatic veins permits objective evaluation of the functional activity of the transplants. In the angiographic operating room the catheterization of hepatic vein was carried out and simultaneous collection of blood specimens from portal and hepatic veins was done. Subsequently, 20 ml of 20% glucose was injected into portal vein and blood was collected 1, 5, 15, 30, and 60 minutes afterward. The data are shown in the Table 6.

In this study there were 27 repeated CT's, in 19 cases intramuscular and in 3 intraportal, and 5 cases of third intraportal transplantation. *Indications were the worsening of general condition of patients, with decompensation of carbohydrate metabolism, increased dosage of exogenous insulin, re-*

appearance of symptoms of the secondary complications. In 18 cases the previous transplantation was an allotransplantation of human fetal islet cells. *By comparison, the results of allo- and xenotransplantation of cultured islet cells were in principle the same, with the exception of the need in exogenous insulin: 18 - 22% of the initial dose after xenotransplntation as compared with 20 - 60% after allotransplantation.*

Table 5
C-peptide levels

Implantation site	Initial Value of C-Peptide	Pre-XT	Post XT 14 Days	Post XT 1 Month	Post XT 3-6 Months
Control Group of Healthy Donors N = 20		0.266 ±0.07			
Group #1 I.M. XT	C-peptide + N = 27	0.108 ±0.08*	0.163 ±0.03**	0.166 ±0.05**	0.152 ±0.03**
Group #2 Intraportal XT	C-peptide - N = 13	-	0.111 ±0.03	0.173 ±0.02	0.158 ±0.04
	C-peptide + N = 15	0.115 ±0.06*	0.281 ±0.09**	0.18 ±0.04**	0.188 ±0.07**

* $Pk < 0.01$ in comparison with control group
** $P < 0.05$ in comparison with initial value

Table 6
Concentration of hormones in portal and hepatic veins

TIME	Portal Vein			Hepatic Vein		
	Insulin U/ml	C-peptide pmol/l	Glucagon picog/l	Insulin U/min	C-peptide pmol/l	Glucagon picog/l
Start	4.9 ±0.6	0.12 ±0.04	187.3 ±18.2	6.1 ±1.0^	0.21 ±0.08^	187.7 ±26.2
1 min	4.2 ±0.5	0.13 ±0.07	176.9 ±22.5	9.1 ±1.3*^	1.2 ±0.46*^	195.4 ±19.8
5 min	4.2 ±0.8	0.12 ±0.1	140.1 ±18.0*	5.5 ±0.9^	0.15 +0.08	176.9 ±20.9
15 min	4.6 ±0.6	0.11 ±0.09	156.8 ±15.9	2.3 ±0.04*	0.12 ±0.03	218.4 ±32.7
30 min	2.6 ±0.03*	0.1 ±0.02	202.2 ±24.1	3.9 ±0.5*	0.11 ±10.05	226.5 ±27.8
60 min	3.5 ±0.5	0.11 ±0.03	198.3 ±29.3	1.5 ±0.1*	0.12 ±0.07	166.4 ±13.8

* $P < 0.05$ in comparison with starting value
^ $P < 0.05$ in comparison with portal vein value

The obtained results show that repeated CT's from newborn rabbits permit prolongation of compensation of diabetes, and that it is preferable to carry it out prior to the return of unfavorable laboratory findings.

The evaluation of parameters of cellular immunity showed that T lymphocyte count in the recipients of the 1st group was on the first day decreased to the level of parameters of control group of healthy blood donors (1227 ± 260/μl), on the 7 - 10th day further normalization took place, and on 14 - 20th day the T-lymphocyte count again increased to the initial higher level (1668 ± 294/μl), in comparison with the control group. Activation index was higher during the entire study, which was the same situation as at the beginning. The findings in the 2nd group were in principle the same as in the 1st group. The T-lymphocyte count was somewhat higher at 14 - 20 days after transplantation (2115 ± 209/μl), but the *difference was not statistically significant.*

In the evaluation of humoral immunity, the B-lymphocyte count in the recipients of the 1st group was lower than in the control group during the entire study, but in the recipients of the 2nd group the B-lymphocyte count was higher, reaching 925±59/μl after 14 - 20 days, which was twice as high as in the control group ($p<0.05$), and more than 4-times as high as before transplantation ($p<0.05$). Concentration of IgA, IgG, IgM, remained the same in both groups for the duration of the study, and *was on the same level as that of the control group.*

In addition to the standard tests, antigen-specific methods of evaluation of immune status were used. The studied parameters showed that there were no obvious changes of the immune status of the recipients, which prove a satisfactory elimination of class II MHC surface antigen carrying 'passenger cells' during the process of the cultivation of pancreatic islet cells of newborn rabbits. *No statistically significant differences in the cellular immunity were found between various implantation sites* [71].

Up to 80% of children with *therapeutically uncontrollable 'brittle' diabetes* of children had already developed typical diabetic complications by the time of their referral for stem cell transplantation, and such patients *benefit from such therapy in 81% of cases.* A group of 86 children and juveniles with otherwise clinically uncontrollable 'brittle' diabetes was treated by transplantation of human and animal fetal tissues. Thirteen patients received cell transplantation twice and one patient three times. In summary, 81 ± 6% transplantations had good result, and not a single one harmed the patient. The main benefit was the clinical compensation of diabetic state. On admission, only 6 children had normal HbA_{1c}, 12 children higher HbA_{1c}, and all others were in the state of decompensation, i.e. HbA_{1c} from 10.2% to 15.9%. Already 7 to 15 days after cell transplantation a median HbA_{1c} was lowered to 8.25 ± 0.43%, and 3 months after cell transplantation to 5.69 ± 0.40%, and then began to rise to 8.10 ± 1.00% at 6 months, to 9.29 ± 0.92% at 9 months, and 11.89 ± 1.56% at 12 months after cell transplantation. In terms of clinical compensation, on admission only 10 ± 2% of patients were compensated, while 3 months after cell transplantation it was 94 ± 3%, at 6 months 75 ± 6%, at 12 months 70 ± 7%, and at 18 months after cell transplantation 54 ± 8% of children were compensated. Most importantly, 76% of patients were discharged with one insulin injection a day, which in this age group is extremely important for compliance.

Average level of C-peptide on admission was 0.51 ± 0.32 µg, two weeks after cell transplantation it was 3 times higher, and three months after cell transplantation 4.4 times higher. At 12 months after cell transplantation the level of C-peptide returned to the original level. The higher the level of C-peptide at the beginning, the better the result of cell transplantation, which proves the high probability that cell transplantation stimulated endogenous production of insulin in some patients.

The effect of cell transplantation disappeared 10 – 14 months post-treatment.

A detailed diagnostic effort revealed that *81 out of 86 patients already had a clinical evidence of diabetic complications*, such as diabetic microangiopathies, i.e. retinopathy, nephropathy, and hepatopathy, diffuse lipodystrophy, encephalopathy, lipoid necrobiosis, and the incidence and severity of all complications significantly improved during 12 months after cell transplantation.

The clinical status of all 14 patients that served as controls became worse during 6 – 15 months of observation [222].

Our own study of treatment by cell transplantation of 35 children with insulin-dependent diabetes mellitus, carried out by the 1st Republic Pediatric Hospital of Ministry of Health Care of Russian Federation, was reported at the 1st Symposium on Transplantation of Human Fetal Tissues in Moscow, December 4 – 7, 1995, under the title: "Experience with transplantation of cultured β-cells to children with insulin-dependent diabetes mellitus at the 1st Republican Pediatric Hospital."

Cell transplantation of solely β-cells of islets of pancreas was carried out. All 6 children with recently diagnosed IDDM became insulin independent within 3 weeks, and remained so for 4 – 8 months. Remarkably, all basic parameters of cell and humoral immunity were within normal limits during this time. The clinical status of all other patients substantially improved but not to the point of insulin-independence, which was due to low dosage of transplanted β-cells, and mono-therapy by β-cell of islets of pancreas alone.

Based on the enormous past experience with human fetal cell transplantation with absence of reactions of any sort, there was no need to lower the dosage of cell transplants for safety reasons. Monotherapy by β-cell of islets of pancreas alone is sufficient only for patients with recent IDDM, but not at the later stage, in particular when the autoimmune process is still active: here cell transplants of various immune organs and tissues are necessary to inhibit the autoimmune destruction of patient's islet cells.

Unknown number of children with recent onset of diabetes mellitus have been treated successfully with stem cell transplantation: there have been some cures, and in other patients at least a delay in the onset of diabetic condition. *If one could postpone the onset of child's diabetes by one or more years, it would be of tremendous value because of well known deleterious effect of diabetic condition on growth and development of such children.*

When a *female diabetic* has been under treatment for *infertility* for over a year without a success, stem cell transplantation should be strongly considered. If *a female diabetic has had 2 – 3 miscarriages*, stem cell transplantation is indicated. When *a pregnant diabetic delivered a baby with a diabetic fetal distress syndrome*, stem cell transplantation should be carried out before her next pregnancy, or even during her next pregnancy, between 12th and 16th week.

A method of *retrobulbar implantation* of cell transplants of β-cells of islets of pancreas developed by Fedorov Ophthalmological Institute in Moscow was reported on at the 1st Symposium on Human Fetal Tissue Transplantation in Moscow, December 4 – 7, 1995, under the title: "Retrobulbar transplantation of cultures of islet cells to patients with diabetic retinopathy". Our International Institute of Biological Medicine provided cell transplants for this treatment. Analysis of observations of 40 patients with diabetic retinopathy over 3 years showed in 76% of cases of pre-proliferative retinopathy a remarkable improvement, consisting of resorption and decrease of frequency of recurrent hemorrhage, and in 47% of cases of proliferative diabetic retinopathy an improvement in aggressivity of the proliferative process and diffuse neovascularization, all accompanied by a noticeably better visual acuity.

Retrobulbar implantation of cultured cell transplants of retina developed by International Institute of Biological Medicine was carried out by the Fedorov Ophthalmological Institute as treatment for *retinitis pigmentosa*.

Immunological reactions after stem cell xenotransplantation

There are a few reports on the changes of immune parameters after xenotransplantation of cultured islet cells [48, 66, 69, 92, 93]. The fact that IDDM is an autoimmune disease, the basis of which is selective destruction of β-cells, caused by the development of the cellular and humoral immune reaction, has made the analysis of generally rather subtle laboratory immunological findings after cell xenotransplantation quite complex. In testing of IDDM patients, changes in ratios and function of immunocompetent cells on one side, and appearance of circulating antibodies to the antigens of patient's own β-cells on the other side, have been seen. In the early stages of IDDM, autoantibodies, reversal of $CD4^+/CD8^+$ ratio, as well as activated T-lymphocytes, are present. In the chronic stage of the disease, as β-cells are gradually destroyed, autoantibodies to the antigens of patient's own β-cells disappear, and the main findings during the entire course of the disease are abnormal relationships (and ratios) of various subpopulations of immunocompetent cells. At the same time these abnormal relationships are quite heterogenous, i.e. $CD4^+/CD8^+$ ratio is sometimes in favor of T-helpers, sometimes in favor of T-suppressors, probably depending upon the stage of the disease. A possibility cannot be ruled out that the immune response to the exogenous insulin, or the metabolic crises during the chronic course of IDDM, play part.

After stem cell transplantation there is an activation of both cellular and humoral immunity. The immune reactions are most pronounced on 7th – 10th day treatment. Some authors claim that cellular immune reactions peak 2 days after, while humoral reactions 14 days post-transplantation. T-helpers dominate the immune response, and the whole picture is that of a delayed hypersensitivity reaction. Increased level of proliferative and metabolic activity of lymphocytes (2.5x) is observed on

7 - 10th day, and lasts 7 days. There is an increased activity of macrophages. Sometimes the T-lymphocyte count is increased, while the B-lymphocyte count remains the same. Occasionally on 7th day the index of leukocyte migration inhibition is decreased. The changes of immunoglobulin level after cell xenotransplantation are variable and statistically insignificant [48, 66, 69, 92, 93].

A group of 55 patients was followed before and after an allotransplantation of islet cells, and total T and B cell count, $CD4^+$ and $CD8^+$, circulating immune complexes, IgG, IgA, IgM, were measured. Before the procedure a decreased phagocyte activity of white blood cells, a generalized immune deficit, and an increased level of circulating immune complexes, were observed. After islet tissue transplantation there was a decrease of $CD8^+$ and increase of $CD4^+$, their ratio < 1, and an increase of IgM [69].

In a study of 157 xenotransplantations of islet cells, before the procedure 70.1% of IDDM patients had laboratory evidence of immune deficit, while after islet cell xenotransplantation the immune deficit was only 22.5%. With NIDDM patients the numbers were 79% and 18%, respectively. In patients with normal $CD4^+$ and $CD8^+$ before the procedure, these parameters remained normal even after islet cell xenotransplantation, but their ratio changed in favor of $CD4^+$. In IDDM patients with low T lymphocytes before the procedure, the T cell count normalized one month after xenotransplantation, but the ratio was in favor of $CD4^+$. In IDDM patients with low B lymphocytes before the procedure, the B cell count became normal one month after xenotransplantation as well. All other immune parameters: IgG, IgA, IgM, circulating immune complexes, and phagocytosis index, were within limits of normal both before and after the procedure in both IDDM and NIDDM patients [66].

In another study 7 IDDM patients were treated by allo- or xeno- transplantation of islet cells and the level of islet cell surface antibodies was continuously measured. No association between the level of islet cell surface antibodies and allo- or xeno- transplantation, age, duration of diabetes, was observed. One half of patients had an increase of autoantibodies with a peak two weeks after the procedure, while the second half showed no response [92].

In 61 diabetics treated with xenotransplantation of islet cells, levels of IgG, IgA, and IgM, were measured before and 3 - 5 days, 3 months and 10 - 12 months after the procedure. There was an increase of immunoglobulins after xenotransplantation, but the rises were not statistically significant. In patients with increased immunoglobulins before the procedure, their level decreased after xenotransplantation [93].

Cellular immunity: T lymphocyte count decreased on the 1st day post-CT to the level of healthy controls, then on 14 – 20th returned to the initial level, as compared with healthy controls. Activation index of T lymphocyte was higher than in healthy controls initially as well as during the entire follow-up after CT. There were no differences between the 1st and the 2nd group: the 1st group had subaponeurotic implantation, while the 2nd group intraportal implantation of islet cell transplants.

Humoral immunity: In the 1st group B-lymphocyte count was lower than in healthy controls during the entire study, while in the 2nd group it was 14 – 20 days after CT twice as high as in controls ($p<0.05$), and four times higher than before CT ($p<0.05$).

Concentration of IgG, IgM, IgA, remained the same in both groups for the duration of follow-up after CT, and was the same as in healthy controls.

Conclusions:

1. There were no obvious and statistically significant changes of the immune status of patients after CT when stem cell transplants were prepared by a BCRO method of primary tissue culture from fetal/newborn rabbits.
2. There were no obvious changes of the immune status of patients after stem cell xenotransplantation as compared with cell allo-transplantation.
3. No statistically significant differences in cellular immunity were found between I.M. and intra-portal implantation sites after stem cell xenotransplantation [48].

Reactivation of IDDM after SCT

A unique problem with diabetes mellitus is the recurrence of the original disease process in the transplanted islets. IDDM patients have antibodies directed toward several β-cell products, including insulin. There is also a prevalence of insulin-specific T cells in islet cell infiltrates. These insulin-specific T cells are capable of adoptive transfer of diabetes mellitus, i.e. they can destroy β-cells *in vivo* in two different animal systems [56, 165]. In this respect, the islet cell xenotransplant, particularly a discordant one, could be expected to be relatively immune to recurrence of disease, since the membrane antigens which would form the target of an immune insulinitis are quite dissimilar to those which were the targets of the original disease process [37].

Theoretically, the islet xenotransplant are largely protected from autoimmune processes. The xenogeneic islets may have a special utility in stem cell transplantation to patients with diabetes mellitus suffering from anautoimmune islet destruction. The resistance of the cell xenotransplants to autoimmune recurrence as a late cause of graft failure seems well established in a number of models. The mechanism of the long term functional tolerance is not known, but the phenomenon of humoral adaptation, whereby all xenotransplants in residence for prolonged periods of time appear to be resistant to rejection after such a long time may play a part [63].

In February 1999, Bio-Cellular Research Organization LLC, filed four Investigational New Drug applications with US FDA for the treatment of advanced stages of the life threatening and severely disabling complications of IDDM (Insulin Dependent Diabetes Mellitus) by own method of cell transplantation, described in this book:

- Diabetic retinopathy
- Diabetic nephropathy
- Diabetic polyneuropathy
- Diabetic lower extremity arterial disease

Incidence

It is interesting to see, in 'one' country, the magnitude of problems with 'one' serious disease that is treatable by stem cell transplantation with a great success.

According to the National Institutes of Health data as of April 1, 1998:

- As many as 15.7 million of people in the US (~6%) had diabetes mellitus, of which 7% suffered from insulin-dependent diabetes mellitus ('IDDM'), i.e. 1.1. million, and the rest from other types, mostly insulin-independent diabetes mellitus (NIDDM),
- Diabetic retinopathy is the leading cause of new cases of blindness of adults in the US, after 15 years of diabetes 97% of

IDDM, 80% of insulin treated NIDDM, and 55% of non-insulin treated NIDDM patients will have retinopathy, of which number approximately one third will develop the stage of proliferative retinopathy leading to blindness,
- Diabetic nephropathy, the leading cause of end-stage kidney disease in the US requiring hemodialysis or kidney transplant-ation, takes place in 35% of all diabetics, after 15 years 25% of diabetics will have protein in urine, and of those 50% of IDDM and 11% of NIDDM patients will be on hemodialysis within 10 years,
- Diabetic polyneuropathy will develop after 15 years in 30 – 70% of diabetics, equally in IDDM and NIDDM patients,
- Diabetic lower extremity arterial disease has been the cause of one half of all leg amputations in US,
- Diabetes mellitus is the 7th leading cause of death in the US with 200,000 deaths reported each year,
- Diabetics have much higher incidence of heart disease, at an earlier age, and with fatal prognosis, than non-diabetics,
- Diabetics have 2.5 times higher risk of stroke than non-diabetics,
- Many digestive diseases, infections, dental problems, depressions, are substantially more common in diabetics than non-diabetics [106].

The above statistics have gotten worse since 1995.

Clinical protocol for stem cell transplantation treatment of patients with complications of diabetes mellitus

A proper preparation of the patient for stem cell transplantation is mandatory. A diabetic patient has to be brought into as good a metabolic state as possible by standard therapeutic means, i.e. to carry out stem cell transplantation while the patient is in the state of ketosis, hyperosmolality or prolonged hypoglycaemia is probably minimally effective and should be done only as a last resort. Elimination of ketoacidosis, frequent hypoglycaemia or hyper-osmolality by hospitalization, with intravenous fluids, frequent doses of regular insulin in accordance with glucometer measurements, etc., is mandatory so that the patient's clinical condition will be compensated as well as possible.

Parameters to be followed before and after stem cell xenotrans-plantation, and their frequency:

- ***General***:
    i. level of serum C-peptide once a month x3, then every 3 months

ii. level of HbA$_{1c}$ once a month x3, then every 3 months
iii. level of serum insulin once a month x3, then every 3 months
iv. serum cholesterol, total, LDL, HDL, triglycerides, every 3 months
v. home blood glucose self-monitoring (with diary) several times a day
vi. avoidance of hypoglycaemia, observe if it happens and how often
vii. avoidance of ketoacidosis and hyperosmolality, observe if it happens
viii. decreased requirement of exogenous insulin (with diary)

- ***Immunological***: once a month x3, then every 3 months
    i. total lymphocytes
    ii. T-lymphocytes (CD3$^+$)
    iii. T-helpers (CD4$^+$)
    iv. T-suppressors (CD8$^+$) and CD4/CD8
    v. NK (CD16)
    vi. B-lymphocytes (CD22 and CD19)
    vii. serum IgG, IgA, IgM
    viii. serum complement (CH50)

- ***Special***:
    - *diabetic retinopathy*:
        i. retinal photography: Canon office photographs once a month, 7 standard special photos every 3 months
        ii. visual acuity and visual fields once a month

    - *diabetic nephropathy*:
        i. proteinuria/24 hr urine every 3 months
        ii. microalbuminuria every 3 months
        iii. serum creatinine once a month
        iv. creatinine clearance every 3 months
        v. blood pressure once a month

    - *diabetic polyneuropathy*:
        i. EMG every 3 months
        ii. nerve conduction studies of tibial nerve, sural nerve, median nerve, and ulnar nerve every 3 months
        iii. pain analog scale once a month
        iv. blood pressure lying, sitting, standing once a month

v. orthostatic changes once a month
vi. EKG R-R variation every 3 months

- *diabetic vasculopathy*:
  i. Doppler ultrasound: every month x3, then every 3months
  ii. Doppler probe
  iii. Doppler blood pressure ankle/arm
  iv. Doppler segmental blood pressure
  v. plethysmograph waveform change

- *'brittle' diabetes of children:*
  i. retinal photography every 3 months
  ii. microalbuminuria every 3 months
  iii. serum creatinine once a month

Frequency of office visits: 4 weeks and 48 hours before stem xenotransplantation, 24 hours after and then once a week for the first month after stem xenotransplantation, once a month thereafter.

Other hormone deficiency disorders, where a re-establishment of normal hormonal balance by hormone replacement therapy was not possible, have been successfully treated by stem cell transplantation with increasing frequency.

Adrenal cortex

Two main hormone groups of ***adrenal cortex*** are glucocorticoids and mineralocorticoids, but also androgens, estrogens and progesterons, are produced there. Adrenal cortex is a very important relay point of the whole endocrine system.

All adrenocortical hormones are made from cholesterol. There are eight key enzymes necessary for the production of various adrenocortical hormones, and every one of them may be deficient due to faulty genes. The result is the classical excess of hormone produced in the step just preceding the disruption of biochemical chain reaction, and lack of hormones beyond the point of disruption as *described in chapter45*.

The lack of glucocorticoids leads to an increased release of cortico-trophin-releasing hormone (CRH) of hypothalamus, and thereby of adrenocorticotropic hormone (ACTH) of anterior lobe of pituitary, and that in turn brings about a further increase of concentration of the hormonal precursors just before the disruption of biochemical chain reaction, causing various glucocorticoid, mineralocorticoid androgenic, gestagenic or estrogenic effects in the patient.

The most common of these genetic enzymatic defects is lack of 21β-hydroxylase that leads to the lack of cortisol, increased production of androstendione and testosterone, a cause of *virilisation in females, and adrenogenital syndrome in males, i.e. precocious pseudopuberty.*

Glucocorticoids, mainly cortisol:

- stimulate gluconeogenesis in liver,
- inhibit glucose intake by cells,
- stimulate lipolysis,
- stimulate protein breakdown in tissues,
- stimulate protein production in liver,
- support production of erythrocytes, platelets, and neutrophil granulocytes,
- decrease lymphocyte, monocyte, eosinophil and basophil counts,
- act as immunosuppressants, also by limiting production of antibodies,
- suppress inflammation, and healing by inhibition of connective tissue proliferation,
- lower plasma level of calcium and phosphorus by inhibition of calcitriol.

Mineralocorticoids increase renal retention of Na^+ and water, and stimulate elimination of K^+, Mg^{++}, and H^+, by kidneys, as well as potassium intake.

Adrenocortical hormonal insufficiency can be the result of decreased function of adrenal gland, i.e. Addison's disease, genetic defects, autoimmune inflammation of adrenals, TB, enzymopathies, or of lower level of ACTH, i.e. defect of anterior lobe of pituitary.

The massive therapeutic use of corticosteroids has been one of the big successes of modern medicine but there are many drawbacks to that story as well. The secondary lesions of adrenal glands are more frequent today than primary diseases. The widespread therapeutic use of corticoids in inflammatory conditions, allergies, immune system deficiencies, autoimmune diseases, cancer, skin diseases, etc., brought about an atrophy of adrenal cortex due to competitive inhibition. In other words, the adrenal cortical function is suppressed by exogenous intake of hormones for long periods of time, e.g. for years, often in high doses, and at non-physiological intervals. The functional non-use causes the morpho-logical atrophy of endocrine structures so that eventually adrenal glands can no longer produce sufficient quantities of their hormones. Stem cell transplantation of *diencephalon, entire pituitary, adrenal cortex, liver, spleen, bone marrow*, generally solves this problem.

Growth takes place in three phases:

1. *the 1st phase*, during the first two - three years of life, is *'genetic'*, characterized by a high speed of growth,
2. *the 2nd phase*, from the 4th - 5th to 8th – 12th years of life, is *'pituitary'*, regulated by diencephalon/hypothalamus/pituitary, stimulated by growth hormone system, characterized by a slow and steady growth, with a yearly increase of 4 to 6 cm.
3. hormones of adrenal cortex are responsible for the stimulation of gonads into initiation of the *3rd, i.e. pubertal, phase* of growth, controlled by adrenocortical and sex hormones.

There is an involution of adrenal glands after birth. After the 6th – 8th year of age the adrenal glands and gonads begin to grow rapidly, reaching the culmination between 14 and 18 years of age. Whereas the corticosteroids show a nearly linear rise from birth, the production of gonadotropins, 17-ketosteroids, and sex hormones begins between 6 and 8 years of age only, but then the rise of their levels is parallel with those of corticosteroids.

The growth of the entire body, and bony growth, are controlled by adrenocortical and sex hormones working in synchrony. These two groups of hormones initiate the 3rd phase of growth at the beginning of puberty, and terminate the growth by closure of epiphyses at the end of puberty. The earlier these two groups of hormones act, the earlier the pubertal growth outburst sets in, but is also finished earlier. As a result, the final stature is lower in girls, than in boys, particularly those that start later, as in northern countries. The same applies to some racial groups. To stimulate the 3rd stage of growth and development, stem cell transplants of *adrenal cortex, gonads, and hypothalamus*, are used.

If there is a delay of development in the 2nd phase, then stem cell transplantation of *diencephalon, hypothalamus and anterior lobe of pituitary*, is indicated.

Since the beginning and the end of puberty has moved into earlier years, there is much less time now for the therapy of growth disorders.

Retarded puberty is the result of constitutional factors, malnutrition and other unfavorable environmental conditions, hypogonadism, such as in Turner's syndrome, congenital hypothyreoidism, lack of pituitary gonadotropins in panhypopituitarism, pituitary nanism. Retarded appearance of secondary sex characteristics is due to an insufficiency of adrenal cortex. Stem cell transplantation of *gonads, placenta, adrenal cortex, diencephalon, hypothalamus, pituitary, thyroid, thymus*, is recommended.

Missing puberty is rare and occurs in dystrophia adiposo-genitalis, Prader-Willi syndrome, and various inter-sex conditions.

Gonads

Male infertility is a cause of the infertility of a couple in approximately 50% of instances. The success rate of treatment of male infertility, with azoospermia, oligospermia, or damaged sperm, etc., with modern medical therapies, has been close to zero. With progress of in-vitro-fertilization techniques, male infertility has become a substantially more serious problem than female infertility. It is not surprising that cell transplantation has been tried in such desperate situations [274 - 276].

Enormous advances were made in the diagnosis of male infertility, but not so in therapy. A report of 10 infertile males, two of them with infertile wives, and of another infertile female, treated with cell transplantation of *placenta, gonads and hypothalamus*, with pregnancy in 8 cases, is remarkable, because all these patients had previously been treated for a long time by traditional therapeutic means without success. One of the male patients was found to have an adenoma-like Leydig cell hyperplasia without any seminiferous tubules on testicular biopsy, and no treatment was attempted. In one of the two patients that did not father a child, the problem was his wife, that was found by laparoscopy to have a markedly hypoplastic uterus, and refused any further treatment; in the second, it was a severe damage of seminiferous tubules, possibly of genetic cause, as his brother had azoospermia. Even in such an unfavorable situation, spermiogram improved from a few occasional spermatocytes to 10 million, of which 25% had normal mobility, even though 60% were abnormal, after cell transplantation. This favorable situation lasted 3 months but then spermiogram dropped back to an original state and further cell transplantation did not trigger any response.

Four detailed case histories describe a clinical handling of such patients as individuals and as married couples. Two of the patients were victims of mumps orchitis, one at the age of 20, who following cell transplantation fathered 3 children, and the second at the age of 29. Since the 2nd patient was already a father of 2 children, he served as a temporary control, as his cell transplantation was postponed for 5 months to prove beyond any reasonable doubt that spontaneous regeneration did not take place after orchitis. Two months after cell transplantation his wife became pregnant again. Author advises that two weeks after orchitis no spontaneous regeneration can take place anymore and at that point a patient with mumps orchitis should be treated by cell transplantation without any further delay.

Cell transplantologist must not confuse hormone therapy with cell transplantation. Endocrinologists usually overdose patients, and that is highly inadvisable with cell transplantation. *If the 1st cell transplanttation was not successful, the 2nd must be postponed for 6 – 9 months. Another error is to implant cell transplants of testis only.* It is *mandatory to add hypothalamus and placenta*, and possibly *adrenal cortex and anterior pituitary*, to balance out the regulatory circuits.

One of these male patients, with a biopsy that proved nearly complete atrophy of the seminiferous tubules, was turned away by a university clinic as untreatable, and was impotent as well. After cell transplantation the potency was restored, but sperm count showed only 3 live and 3 dead sperms. The patient was subsequently treated with Mesterolone and chorionic gonadotropin, his sperm count rose to 12.4 million, conception took place, and baby girl was born. Subsequently the patient had azoospermia again. The 2nd cell transplantation was done, and without a success like before, so that another course therapy by Mesterolone and chorionic gonadotropin was planned. In a later follow up-report the author informed that the patient fathered a second child. Author advises that in seemingly hopeless cases before an extensive hormone therapy is begun, all infertile male patients should be treated by cell transplantation in order to stimulate regeneration of testicular epithelium. After cell transplantation it is important to watch for the improvement of sperm motility, as it always precedes the increased sperm count, and pay attention to other ongoing treatments ordered by other physicians, and regularly examine the testicles as they can be palpated easily, and usually in 4 weeks after cell transplantation they become full, tense and tender, i.e. with regenerated seminiferous tubules.

A 30 years' old female with no children after 3 years of marriage had bilateral tubal narrowing and underwent bilateral tuboplasty. Her husband had a low sperm count with 70% immobility. Subsequently, fully synchronized, her ovulation was suppressed for two cycles and her husband received cell transplantation. The conception was prompt and the couple eventually had 3 children.

The sole female patient treated without a husband, 20 years old, had oligomenorhea for 5 years, suffered from erythema nodosum, and 6 years later developed sarcoidosis. For 3 years she took a variety of traditional infertility treatment without success. Cell transplantation of placenta, and ovary, lead to pregnancy, and altogether 3 children.

This success triggered a similar therapeutic program for infertile bulls at the Veterinary Medical School in Munich with comparable results [314].

This is a loose continuation of the previous report. By 1979 the author treated 17 married infertile couples that conceived 29 children. After 1979 only 23 males were treated by cell transplantation of *testis, placenta, hypothalamus, anterior pituitary, adrenal cortex*, three of them fathered a child, 10 did not come for a follow-up and 11 came to one follow-up examination with a spermiogram only: 2 had 15x increased sperm count, one had 8x, one 7x, one 5x, two had 3x, three had 2x, and one had no change in sperm count. One patient had a fructose deficiency, and after two cell transplantations there was an increase of sperm count above normal limit. In 7 patients the sperm mobility significantly improved. It is felt that if the 1st cell transplantation does not give any clinical effect it is probably useless to continue with treatment. If the 2nd cell transplantation is carried out, testis and adrenal cortex only are implanted [315].

Physiology of androgens

Secretion of gonadotropin-releasing hormone from hypothalamus triggers a release of follicle-stimulating hormone (FSH) and luteinizing hormone (LH), while prolactin inhibits it. LH stimulates the secretion of testosterone in Leydig interstitial cells, and that through negative feedback inhibits release of gonadotropin-releasing hormone and luteinizing hormone. FSH supports in Sertoli cells of testis a production of inhibin, which inhibits production of FSH, as well as of androgen binding protein, dihydrotestosterone, and Muller inhibitory factor.

Testosterone is necessary in males for the growth of penis, scrotum and tubuli seminiferi, secretion of prostate, i.e. lowering of ejaculate viscosity, and of tubuli seminiferi, i.e. addition of fructose and prostaglandins, as well as secretion of axillary and inguinal sweat glands, growth of muscles, bones, larynx, pubic, axillary, facial, and chest hair growth, and male pattern baldness. It supports libido and aggressive behavior. It lowers HDL-cholesterol and fertility.

Lack of androgens is due to a lack of gonadotropin-releasing hormone, normally released in pulses, due to disturbances of hypothalamus, i.e. radiation, circulatory dysfunction, genetic defects, inhibition of release of LH and FSH due to pituitary disturbances, i.e. trauma, infarctions, autoimmune diseases, hyperplasias, etc. or due to low production of androgen in testes because of genetic disturbances, or serious systemic diseases.

A 45 year old widower with no children from the first marriage, remarried a 38 years old female and expected pregnancy did not take place. Spermiogram showed lower count and abnormal motility. After the failure of orthodox therapies, including psychological, the patient decided for an alternative treatments, by electroacupuncture and homeopathy. After impotence was admitted, cell transplantation of *testis, mesenchyme, thymus, exocrine pancreas, stomach/intestine, liver*, was carried out. Two months later the patient had a normal erection, 10 months later his wife became pregnant and a baby girl was born [312].

Stem cell transplantation of *testis, hypothalamus, diencephalon, pituitary, adrenal cortex, placenta, prostate, liver, mesenchyme*, is indicated *in all cases of male infertility* even in cases of *azoospermia* if testicular biopsy is normal, or there is a diffuse/focal tubular testicular atrophy but some reproductive epithelium still exists. If there is aspermia on spermiogram, and a total fibrosis by histologic examination, then stem cell transplantation is useless.

We developed a technique, which should be tried in some well selected patients. This protocol requires a full cooperation of an infertility clinic. After a complete diagnostic evaluation, stem cell transplantation is carried out in order to stimulate the 'hypothalamus - pituitary - testes axis', to accomplish an immunomodulation if necessary, and to treat any other existing disease of a patient. After a month or so the patient's ejaculate must be collected every week for 4 weeks, and inspected for normal, mobile, spermatozoa. If any such spermatozoa are found, they have to be concentrated, and frozen. When a sufficient quantity of spermatozoa is accumulated, an artificial insemination is carried out, and repeated as necessary.

As a male is usually not happy with the idea that his child would not be really his, before electing to use a sperm of a donor for *in-vitro-fertilization*, a trial of the above method is worthwhile.

Clinical protocol for stem cell transplantation treatment of male hypogonadism

Parameters to be followed in patients before and after stem cell xenotransplantation, and the frequency:

- **General**: every 3 months, or as clinically necessary
    i. clinical status of pubertal process: symptoms and signs
    ii. measurement of body proportions, body hair and genitalia development
    iii. evaluation of libido and potency
    iv. x-rays of sella turcica
    v. CT scan or MRI of sella turcica and surrounding part of brain
    vi. semen analysis
    vii. buccal smear and/or karyotype if necessary
    viii. testicular biopsy if ever necessary
    ix. test of nocturnal penile tumescence
    x. duplex ultrasonography with intracorporeal injections of vasoactive agents

- **Immunological**: once a month x3, then every 3 months
    i. total lymphocytes
    ii. T-lymphocytes ($CD3^+$)
    iii. T-helpers (CD4)
    iv. T-suppressors ($CD8^+$) and CD4/CD8
    v. NK (CD16)
    vi. B-lymphocytes (CD22 and CD19)
    vii. serum IGG, IGA, IGM
    viii. serum complement (CH50)
    ix. antisperm antibody test

- **Laboratory**: once every 3 months, or as clinically necessary

i. T3, T4, TSH by radioimmunoassay
ii. thyrotropin releasing hormone stimulation test
iii. serum prolactine
iv. serum total and free testosterone and dehydroepiandrosterone sulphate
v. chorionic gonadotropin stimulation test
vi. clomiphene citrate stimulation test
vii. serum FSH and LH levels
viii. gonadotropin-releasing hormone stimulation test
ix. 24-hour urine for free cortisol,17-hydroxycorticosteroids and 17-ketosteroids
x. ACTH stimulation test or Metyrapone test
xi. corticotropin-releasing hormone test
xii. hypo-osmolar swelling test for integrity of spermatocyte plasma membrane
xiii. hemizona assay: sperm binding to oocyte zona pellucida surface receptors
xiv. sperm penetration essay of oocytes

Frequency of office visits: 4 weeks and 48 hours before stem cell xenotransplantation, 24 hours after and then once a week for the first month after stem cell xenotransplantation, once a month thereafter.

Ovarian insufficiency has been treated successfully by cell transplantation for decades, but it has mostly involved patients with a *physiological menopause*. In the last two decades a hormone replacement therapy by estrogen and progesterone became the treatment of choice for a menopause. Today, a growing concern that estrogen causes a variety of side effects, including cancer, brings back the well established fact that cell transplantation is safer than aspirin, and definitely does not cause cancer. In principle, stem cell transplantation of *ovary, placenta, adrenal cortex, hypothalamus, thyroid, epiphysis, entire pituitary including infundibulum, pineal gland*, is recommended.

Premature menopause, where standard hormone replacement therapy has failed, is another group of diseases where stem cell transplantation has been used during the last 10 years with remarkable effectiveness. The number of patients with early menopause treated by stem cell transplantation cannot be compared with those in the usual 'menopause' [277, 278].

The frequency of premature menopause has been increasing with such a speed in the 'civilized' world that there is a talk about a real 'epidemic'. It is apparently due to the stress and pressures of high level jobs, requiring long hours, intense competition, hectic lifestyle, etc., along with the ideal 'thin' body shape, that so many young women in their early thirties stop menstruating, and soon develop classical symptoms of menopause, and of its complications. In not so rare instances it is due to the prolonged use of birth control pills. The high incidence of genital infections among the young people of our modern society plays an unspoken part.

Physiology of female sex hormones

Gonadotropin-releasing hormone of hypothalamus stimulates the release of follicle-stimulating hormone (FSH) and luteotropic hormone (LH) from anterior lobe of pituitary in pulses.

In females FSH supports maturation of follicles and estrogen production in granulosa cells of follicles. Estrogen stimulates at first additional release of gonadotropins up until the full maturation of follicle and creation of corpus luteum, i.e. positive feedback, but from that point on inhibits any further release of gonadotropins, i.e. negative feedback.

LH triggers ovulation and supports the creation of corpus luteum at mid-cycle, and corpus luteum produces progesterons, which inhibits any further release of gonadotropins as well. As a result of inhibition of gonadotropin release the concentration of estrogens and progesterons decreases that eventually leads to menstruation.

Theca cells of corpus luteum also produce androgens.

Estrogens stimulate the development of primary female sexual characteristics, i.e. change of Muller ducts into Fallopian tube, uterus and vagina, as well as of secondary female sex characteristics, i.e. mammary glands, fat distribution, axillary and pubic hair growth (along with androgens), psychic development toward femininity. In uterus they stimulate mucosal proliferation, in uterine cervix and vagina lower the viscosity of cervical mucus and thicken vaginal mucosa, and break down glycogen to lactic acid with help of vaginal microflora. In mammary glands estrogens support development of mammary ducts. They support production of protein, HDL and VLDL, and inhibit levels of LDL, and thereby lower the risk of atherosclerosis. Estrogens increase blood coagulation, retention of salts by kidneys, and bone mineralization.

Progesterons support in uterus the maturation and secretory activity of mucosa and lower the contractility of musculature, and inhibit the motility of Fallopian tubes. In uterine cervix and vagina they increase the viscosity of cervical mucus, narrow cervical canal, inhibit proliferation of vaginal epithelium, in mammary glands support development of alveoli. They increase the basal metabolic rate, body temperature, trigger hyperventilation and lower the sensitivity of peripheral cells to insulin, and decrease the production of cholesterol and plasma concentration of HDL and LDL.

Lack of estrogens and progesterons is often due to lowered release of gonadotropin-releasing hormone (excessive stress, poor nutrition, professional sport, serious systemic diseases, neurotransmitter dysfunction), or of gonadotropins (hemorrhage, infarction, inflammation, trauma of pituitary gland).

With growing ovarian production of androgens, the release of FSH is inhibited, maturation of follicle blocked, and that leads to polycystic ovaries.

Decreased release of gonadotropins is often caused by an *increased concentration of prolactin* due to prolactin producing tumors, lack of inhibition of prolactin secretion, anti-dopaminergic drugs, or by hypothalamic damage: trauma, radiation, degenerative or inflammatory diseases, and defects of biosynthesis.

Decreased production of estrogens and progesterons by ovaries can be due to developmental anomaly of ovaries, damage from radiation or cytostatics, or enzymopathy.

Lack of female sex hormones makes normal menstrual cycle impossible, and the same applies to the excess of female sex hormones, usually a result of use of anti-conception drugs. With lack of estrogen there is no proliferative phase in uterine mucosa, and thereby the progesterons cannot bring it to maturation. In either case the females are infertile. There is amenorrhea, less pronounced secondary sexual characteristics, tendency toward vaginal infections, osteoporosis, and increased risk of atherosclerosis.

Gynecologists have observed that for some reason approximately 50% of patients with early menopause do not respond well to the usual hormone replacement therapy with estrogen and progesterone, for reasons unknown. This was the reason to investigate the treatment of such non-responding patients with cell transplantation.

In the April 1994 issue of the Bulletin of Experimental Biology and Medicine, Volume 117, an official journal of the Russian Academy of Medical Sciences, there are three articles about the results of our controlled study of the treatment of post-castration syndrome, i.e. 'early menopause', by transplantation of human fetal tissues as compared with hormone replacement therapy, and a control group [317 – 320].

Our controlled study, actually a dissertation for 'Doctor of Science' degree at Russian Research Center of Obstetrics Gynecology and Perinatology of Ministry of Health of Russian Federation, included 150 patients from 33 to 43 years of age, that underwent a bilateral total oophorectomy for variety of indications, not including cancer, and were in *early menopause*, and their ovaries were absent as proven by ultrasound. Of this group, 45 patients were treated by human fetal tissue transplantation, 50 patients by a hormone replacement therapy, and 55 patients received a placebo. Cell transplantation of *ovary, adrenal cortex, hypothalamus, placenta, spleen, and liver*, had a 100% success rate.

Figures 1 - 8 show the *serum levels of estradiol, progesterone, follicle-stimulating hormone (FSH), luteinizing hormone (LH), testosterone, prolactine, cortisol, thyroid-stimulating hormone (TSH), all at menopausal levels before stem cell transplantation, that started to return to normal after 4 weeks and remained at low/normal serum levels for 4 – 5 months after the 1st stem cell transplantation.* At that time the level of hormones started to return to menopausal levels again, but *never reached their levels from before stem cell transplantation.*

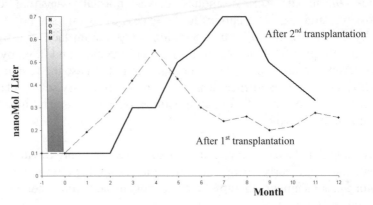

FIGURE 1. Level of estradiol after 1st and 2nd cell transplantation

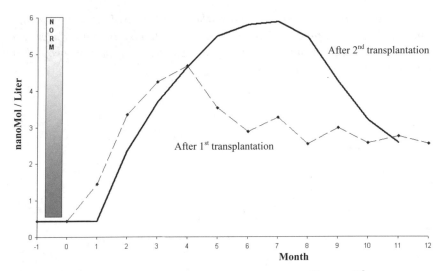

FIGURE 2. Level of progesterone after 1st and 2nd cell transplantation

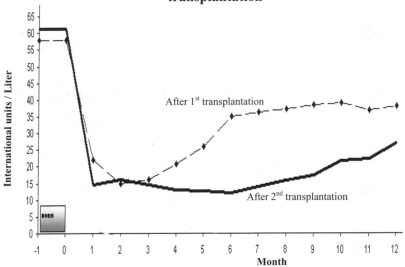

FIGURE 3. Level of FSH after 1st and 2nd cell transplantation

Immediately after the 2nd cell transplantation the level of all hormones goes back to nearly normal and stays there for 6 – 9 months. With each subsequent stem cell transplantations, the duration of clinical effect becomes longer.

Level of prolactine was normal before the 1st cell transplantation and remained so at all times.

The best results were in 4 patients where cell transplant of ovary was implanted endoscopically into an ovarian stump. In two cases an ultrasound examination 6 weeks after cell transplantation proved a temporary presence of follicles.

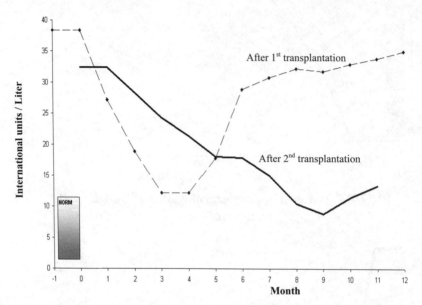

FIGURE 4. Level of LH after 1st and 2nd cell transplantation

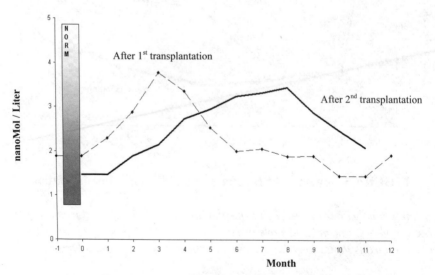

FIGURE 5. Level of testosterone after 1st and 2nd cell transplantation

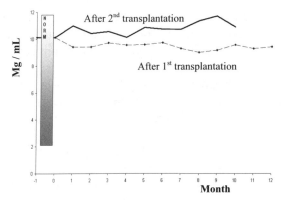

FIGURE 6. Level of prolactine after 1st and 2nd cell transplantation

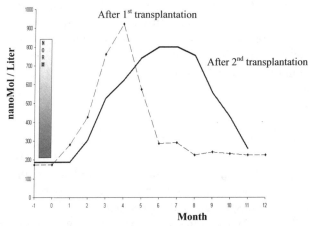

FIGURE 7. Level of cortisol after 1st and 2nd cell transplantation

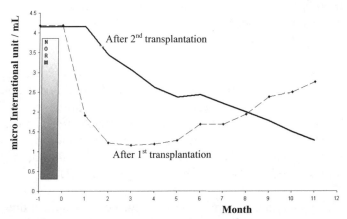

FIGURE 8. Level of TSH after 1st and 2nd cell transplantation

This was a very comprehensive study that included measurements of bone density, evaluation of central nervous system function and autonomous nervous system function, and breast examination [317 - 320].

The *bone density* dropped in control group during 12 months of observation from 90.5% to 87%, while in patients after two cell transplantation treatments, increased from 90.5% to 93%.

In 38 patients of the group treated by cell transplantation, a *functional state of autonomous nervous system was evaluated*. One months after the 1st cell transplantation, patients reported positive changes of general condition, work capacity, mood, sleep, cessation of overreactions to the nuisances of everyday life and excessive concentration on their illness. Reactive anxiety tests dropped from 20 to 9 points. Plethysmographic responses were improved. Responses to cold and mental arithmetics in terms of blood pressure, heart rate, skin galvanic reflex, were improved for the first two months but returned back to the original state in 5 – 6 months along with the return of hormonal indices. The *improvement of autonomous nervous system was attributed to the improved hormonal state after cell transplantation* [318].

In 45 patients of the group treated by cell transplantation, *an EEG study* was carried out before and one month after the 1st cell transplantation, both in the calm state and then during the functional overload of photostimulation, constant light and sound exposure, and hyperventilation. Approximately 2 months after cell transplantation, there was a remarkable improvement of EEG in terms of an adjustment of the relationship between brain cortex and brain stem, a reduction of α-rhythm index, and increased β-activity index. Reactions to light stimuli and the function of brain cortex improved. During the 6th months period after cell transplantation, all improvements disappeared and the pre-transplantations status was restored [319].

Clinical and mammography study of breasts was carried out in 45 patients of the group that received cell transplantation. A drastic drop of estrogen and progesterone and increased gonadotropin levels before the 1st cell transplantation caused involutional process of the breast in all patients regardless of the patient's age. Re-examination 6 – 8 months after cell transplantation showed *an improved skin turgor, but the volume of the glands remained the same on mammography* [320].

Overall, a judicious combination of stem cell transplantation with a hormone replacement therapy can bring patients with premature menopause back to normal.

In animal experiments, Levander proved that implants from tissues obtained from a dead organ could trigger responses and new formations of corresponding tissues in the mesenchyme surrounding the implantation site by a process of induction [323]. It is certain that an explanation of these phenomena is not a continued growth of the implanted cells or cell complexes. Levander observed these *new, induced, organ-specific formations occurred also after the implantation of endometrium, thereby making an important contribution to our knowledge of the pathogenesis of endometriosis.*

In hundreds of experiments with rabbits it could be demonstrated that the subcutaneous injection of various tissues induced only the formation of the tissue that corresponded exactly to the implanted tissue, i.e. local tissue generation is organ-specific. Levander demonstrated pictures of endometrium implantations which always showed new formations of endometrioid tissue [323].

Bernhard verified Lavender's experiments by histological studies to prove that the implants also have a histologically demonstrable organ-specific, organotropic 'distant effects', upon internal organs. He reproduced experiments with endometrium, and proved that the implantation of other organ tissues does not induce the growth of endometrial tissue. He proved this by a process of exclusion, since *implants of liver, spleen, lungs, heart, and placenta, did not produce any new endometrioid tissue formation.*

Organotropic, organ-specific, distant effect on the uterus of the castrated rabbit was seen after castrated rabbits received implantations of rabbit endometrium taken from pregnant rabbits. In all experimental series a regeneration of mucosa with distinct glandular formation was observed in the recipient animal. These effects were not produced by hormonal influence as it was proven that cell transplants did not contain a demonstrable amount of estrogen [323].

In over 70 years' history of stem cell transplantation it has occurred frequently, that it has been used in patients where all known therapies had failed. Among those were patients with intractable **endometriosis**. In our study of 6 such patients treated by cell transplantation of *ovary, adrenal cortex, hypothalamus, placenta, uterus*, at the Russian Research Center of Obstetrics, Gynecology and Perinatology of Russian Academy of Medical Sciences, the success rate was 100% as all patient were pain-free for 6 – 10 months and had normal periods.

Many patients that have undergone hysterectomy for **uterine myomas** because 'the patient was of the age when it makes no difference', learned that their husbands left them because of the lack of uterus, or because they gained too much weight after the operation, etc. Patients with myomas of the uterus, in whom surgery was contraindicated, or who refused it, have been treated by stem cell transplantation of *prostate, ovary, adrenal cortex, hypothalamus*. The size of uterine myomas was decreased by such therapy, and thus hysterectomy could have been avoided or postponed.

In *female infertility*, there are clinical situations, when in-vitro-fertilization had not worked, and repeatedly so, for reasons that cannot be elucidated by even the most sophisticated diagnostic methods. In our experience, stem cell transplantation of *ovary, adrenal cortex, hypothalamus, placenta, liver*, is to be considered in such instances, followed in 4 weeks by another in-vitro-fertilization attempt. Even though the medical reports about such approach are hard to find, this has been a well guarded secret of many gynecologists dealing with infertility long before *in-vitro*-fertilization came to existence.

Our study on treatment of **habitual abortion of adrenal etiology** by porcine stem cell transplantation in 23 patients, with 96% success rate, i.e. 22 out of 23 patients delivered healthy children, proved that routine use of hormones of adrenal cortex, with high risk to the mother and fetus, is not necessary. Habitual abortion due to impaired adrenal function is found in 26.6% of patients with delayed diagnosis, and in 15 – 20% of patients when diagnosis was known before conception or made in early pregnancy. The most common causes of habitual abortion are genetic 21-hydroxylase or 11-hydroxylase deficiencies, and Addison's disease. The usual treatment by gluco- and mineralo-corticoids is fraught with the risk of developmental defects of the fetus, in particular cleft lip and palate, when the treatment had to start in the 1st trimester of pregnancy, or of overall growth retardation, when the treatment had to be carried out throughout the whole pregnancy. The frequency of side effects with the chronic use of glucocorticoids is nearly 50%.

Over the period of 5 years, 23 patients, from 22 to 38 years of age, with a history of one to 9 spontaneous abortions, diagnosis of Addison's disease in 12 patients, or congenital hypocorticism with hyperadrogenism in 11 patients, and a threatened abortion, underwent stem cell transplantation of *porcine adrenal cortex* prepared by tissue culture method at various stages of pregnancy, from 5 to 31 weeks. Implantation was under the aponeurosis of rectus abdominis muscle. A full term delivery of a healthy child of average weight 3,100 gr took place in 22 out of 23 patients. One patient had a spontaneous abortion at 16 weeks. Cortisol level in the late stages of pregnancy was normal. Three detailed case histories are included [316].

Dysfunctional uterine bleeding of unknown cause, when diagnostic steps do not point to a successful treatment, is occasionally an indication for stem cell transplantation of *adrenal cortex, liver, exocrine pancreas, anterior lobe of pituitary, placenta*, usually after surgical or medical D&C has stopped the irregular bleeding [328].

Clinical protocol for stem cell transplantation treatment of premature ovarian failure and female infertility

Parameters to be followed in patients before and after stem cell xenotransplantation, and the frequency:

- **General**: every 3 months or as clinically necessary:
    i. clinical status of hyperandrogenism and galactorrhea, if present
    ii. measure body proportions, body hair, breast and genitalia development
    iii. clinical status of pubertal process: symptoms and signs
    iv. x-rays of sella turcica
    v. CT scan or MRI of sella turcica and surrounding part of brain
    vi. ultrasound of ovaries, serial ultrasound of ovaries, 'folliculogram'
    vii. chromosomal evaluation, if necessary
    viii. progestational challenge test
    ix. basal body temperature
    x. endometrial biopsy during the late luteal phase
    xi. hysterosalpingogram
    xii. hysteroscopy
    xiii. timed cervical mucus examination
    xiv. post-coital test

- **Immunological**: once a month for 3 months, then every 3 months
    i. total lymphocytes

    ii. T-lymphocytes (CD3$^+$)
    iii. T-helpers (CD4$^+$)
    iv. T-suppressors (CD8$^+$)   and CD4/CD8
    v. NK (CD16)
    vi. B-lymphocytes (CD22 and CD19)
    vii. serum IgG, IgA, IgM
    viii. serum complement (CH50)

- **Laboratory**: once every 3 months, or as clinically necessary
    i. CBC, sedimentation rate, serum proteins, A/G ratio, serum Ca, P
    ii. T3, T4, TSH by radioimmunoassay
    iii. thyrotropin releasing hormone stimulation test
    iv. serum estradiol, progesterone, testosterone, dehydroepiandrosterone
    v. serum 17-hydroxyprogesterone
    vi. prolactine level
    vii. serum FSH and LH levels
    viii. gonadotropin-releasing hormone stimulation test
    ix. 24-hour urine for free cortisol, 17-hydroxycorticosteroids and 17-ketosteroids
    x. ACTH stimulation test or Metyrapone test
    xi. corticotropin-releasing hormone test

Frequency of office visits: 4 weeks and 48 hours before stem cell xenotransplantation, 24 hours after and then once a week for the first month after stem cell xenotransplantation, and once a month thereafter.

CASE HISTORY:

A white female, born in 1960, developed endometriosis at the age of 24. None of the treatments could control the disease, and the patient became disabled. At the age of 30, she decided to accept a major surgical procedure: a removal of all pathologic tissues, and that included bilateral total oophorectomy. Postoperatively the patient started a hormone replacement therapy, but regardless of what type of estrogen and progesteron she took, or which program of simulation of the natural cycle of estrogen and progesteron intake her gynaecologists tried, she had persistent severe symptoms and signs of menopause: hot flashes, fatigue, irritability, insomnia, memory loss, lack of concentration, headaches, palpitations, tachycardia, bone pain, atrophic vaginitis, with dyspareunia and lack of libido, and weight gain.

A physical examination on 10/11/94 revealed mild obesity, sallow complexion, atrophic breasts, atrophic vaginitis, and varicose veins. X-rays of sella turcica was within normal limits. Ultrasound of ovaries concurred with the operative report: there was a complete absence of both ovaries. Bone density measurement showed mild osteopenia. Serum estradiol, progesteron, and serum FSH, LH, were at menopausal level. Serum testosterone was normal. Serum cortison was low. Serum prolactine was within normal limits. Serum T4 was low, and serum TSH was higher than normal.

The treatment with Premarin 1.25 mg, and Provera 10 mg for 7 days starting on 17th day of cycle, continued, and on 10/18/94 the patient received stem cell transplantation of ovary, placenta, hypothalamus, liver, adrenal cortex, spleen, and anterior lobe of pituitary.

The post-transplantation course was unremarkable. Within 4 weeks the patient observed a reversal of all symptoms. This favorable clinical course was confirmed by the laboratory testing of hormonal levels.

The serum estradiol increased from very low menopausal levels at one month to 0.2 nanomol/L, at 2 months to 0.35 nanomol/L, at 4 months to 0.6 nanomol/L (which is the lower limit of normal estradiol level), and then dropped to 0.3 nanomol/L, and stayed at this level for the duration of the first year after cell transplantation.

The level of serum progesterone followed the course of estrogen.

The serum FSH decreased from very high menopausal levels at one month to 20 IU/L, at 2 months to 10 IU/L (which is the upper level of normal FSH levels), at 4 months it was at 15 IU/L, at 6 months it increased up to 35 IU/L and remained at this level for the duration of the first year after cell transplantation.

The serum LH decreased from very high menopausal levels at one month to 22 IU/L, at 3 months to 10 IU/L (which is within normal limits), at 4 months was 10 IU/L, at 5 months it increased to 20 IU/L, and one year after cell transplantation it was 25 IU/L.

Serum testosterone increased 3 months after cell transplantation, but generally remained within normal limits for the entire one year.

Serum prolactine remained normal for the entire one year after cell transplantation, without much variation.

Serum cortisol increased from subnormal levels within 4 months to high normal levels and then again decreased to the lower limit of normal 8 months after cell transplantation.

Serum TSH dropped from abnormally high levels within a month to the normal level, and remained normal (with slight variations) for the duration of one year after cell transplantation.

After 12 months, the patient received the 2nd cell transplantation of the same 7 transplants as before. The laboratory testing of the above described hormones revealed the following.

Serum estradiol reached normal level in 3 months, and remained normal for the duration of the follow-up of 12 months after the second cell transplantation.

Serum progesterone reached normal level in 2 months and remained normal for the duration of the follow-up of 12 months after the second cell transplantation.

Serum FSH reached an upper limit of normal after one month and remained at that level until 8 months after the second cell transplantation, but even afterward did not rise over the level of 20 IU/L.

Serum LH decreased to 25 IU/L in 2 months, to 15 IU/L in 5 months, and to the normal level at 9 months after the second cell transplantation, and remained like that for the duration of the 12 months of follow-up.

Serum testosterone remained within limits of normal, although it was slowly moving up to a peak at 8 months after the second cell transplantation.

Serum prolactine remained within normal limits for the entire year after the second cell transplantation.

Serum cortisol reached subnormal levels 12 months after the first cell transplantation, but within 2 months after the second one it was within normal limits again, and it remained so for the duration of the 12 months follow-up.

Serum TSH remained within normal limits after the second cell transplantation.

Overall, the 2nd cell transplantation had a more pronounced effect, and significantly prolonged, as all hormone levels indicated.

Parathyroid glands

Parathyroid insufficiency was the first disease treated by fresh cell therapy/cell transplantation according to the official history, and very successfully, since it saved the life of the dying patient and the patient lived for another 27 years without additional cell transplantation. Despite the fact that cell transplantation of *parathyroid, thyroid, hypothalamus, placenta,* in case of certain genetic disease, *of kidney and adrenal cortex,* has been used extremely rarely, or at the least, there are very few reports. Apparently the thyroid surgeons learned their anatomy, or the parathyroid hormone substitution has worked well in clinical practice, and autoimmune diseases of parathyroid have not become as common as autoimmune diseases of thyroid, i.e. Hashimoto's thyroiditis.

This is a rare case report of a 53 year old female with hypoparathyroidism, after thyroidectomy that suffered for 10 years from inadequate substitution therapy by AT10, vitamin D and calcium. Her condition gradually deteriorated until she became completely disabled. Already the 1st cell transplantation by *parathyroid, thyroid, hypothalamus and placenta*, brought on a marked improvement. Such treatment was repeated every 12 months and the patient remained well [95].

A 33 year old female underwent bilateral thyroidectomy for struma. Immediately after the operation a tetany developed, with marked hypocalcemia and low parathyroid hormone level. Cell transplantation of *parathyroids* brought on extremely fast recovery. Cell transplantation did not have to be repeated [331].

Thyroid glands

Congenital goiter, or athyreosis, with an incidence of 1:4,000 live births, must be diagnosed at birth and treated immediately by thyroid hormones, as severe mental retardation develops quickly, treatable only by stem cell transplantation, but not by hormonal substitution. When in doubt, x-ray determination of bone age confirms the validity of TSH testing. Stem cell transplants of *thyroid, frontal lobe of brain, temporal lobe of brain, thalamus, and hypothalamus*, must be implanted every 3 to 4 months.

Our own study involved two children with congenital hypothyreosis treated by transplantation of human fetal cells at the Endocrinology Research Center of Russian Academy of Medical Sciences in Moscow.

An 18 months old girl was admitted in the state of decompensation, clinically and in terms of laboratory findings, length 76.1 cm, weight 11.3 kg, and extremely high level of TSH. After the 1st cell transplantation of thyroid, hypothalamus, frontal lobe of brain, and with a continuous substitution therapy of 100 mg of L-thyroxin daily, the patient's height increased 5.9 cm within 4 months, and the weight 0.7 kg, the physical development advanced, and 2 months after cell transplantation the patient began to walk without assistance, speak 4 – 5 words, and understand what is spoken to her. Three new teeth appeared. Patient was clinically compensated. After the 2nd cell transplantation, carried out 4 months after the 1st one, the clinical improvement continued.

A 4 1/2 years old boy was admitted with inadequately treated congenital struma and hypothyreosis, and perinatal CNS damage, with marked psychosomatic delay, slight left hemiparesis, strabismus of the left eye, height 94.9 cm, weight 14.9 kg, high TSH, normal T3 and T4. After the cell transplantation of *thyroid, hypothalamus, frontal lobe of brain, brain cortex, medulla alba of brain*, the patient showed remarkable improvement of physical, mental and psychic development.

Although **hypothyroidism** is as common as diabetes mellitus, the statistics of its incidence are not very accurate, because hypothyroidism is rarely the cause of death or seriously disabling complications, and its socio-economic significance is low. Diseases with low function of endocrine glands respond to the hormone replacement therapy not as well as expected today, even in hands of the best endocrinologist. At the same time physicians notice that majority of patients diagnosed with hypothyroidism, Addison disease, etc. developed such endocrine illnesses because of autoimmunity. That explains a lower success rate of a classical hormone replacement therapy in such patients: the relentless progress of an autoimmune damage of hormone producing cells ultimately leaves patient with a very low quantity of functioning endocrine cells, so that even a high dosage of hormones cannot provide the patient with an adequate substitution of missing hormone, but the competitive inhibition, whereby the oral hormone therapy suppresses the function of patient's own same hormone producing cells, plays a part. In such instances it is prudent to consider stem cell transplantation of *thyroid, hypothalamus, anterior lobe of pituitary, thalamus, frontal lobe of brain, medulla alba of brain*.

The goal of stem cell transplantation in the treatment of such autoimmune diseases is mostly immunomodulation, i.e. normalization of immune system function, and thereby suppression of the autoimmune process, and to some degree, a substitution of non-functioning hormone producing cells. It is not a purpose of stem cell therapy to eliminate the need for hormone replacement therapy.

Stem cell transplantation should aim at balancing regulations of the 'axis hypothalamus – pituitary - peripheral endocrine gland, i.e. thyroid in hypothyroidism', disturbed by years of disharmony and demands for over-compensation.

The level of hormones must be measured much more frequently after stem cell transplantation, and the dosage of oral hormones lowered accordingly, but as a rule their intake cannot be discontinued.

If we disregard diabetes mellitus, among hormone deficiency disorders the most common indication for stem cell transplantation in clinical practice is a pronounced hypothyroidism, that is practically always a result of Hashimoto's (autoimmune) thyroiditis. Overall the numbers of patients with hypothyroidism so treated have not been high, and clinical reports are only a few.

Physiology of thyroid hormones

Hormones *thyroxine* (T_4) and *triiodothyronine* (T_3) are produced in the epithelial cells of follicles of thyroid gland. Their synthesis consist of multiple steps, each fraught with possibility of disorder. Iodine from food is mandatory for the synthesis. It is removed from the blood by a Na^+-carrier, taken to the follicular cells, and eventually expelled from the cell into the lumen of follicle by exocytosis.

In the epithelial cells of follicles, *thyreoglobulin*, rich in thyrosin, is created, and secreted into the lumen of follicles. There thyrosyl remnants of globulin are iodinated into diiodinethyrosyl and monoiodinethyrosyl. Two such remnants merge, and attach to thyreoglobulin, which now contains remnants of tetraiodinetyronyl and triiodinetyronyl. This thyreoglobulin colloid in the follicular lumen is the storage form of thyroid hormones. By stimulation of thyroid-stimulating hormone, the thyreoglobulin is taken back into the thyreocytes, and there splits off thyroxin and triiodinethyronine. In the peripheral tissue thyroxine splits off iodine to become more effective triiodinethyronine. Production and release of thyroxine and triiodinethyronine is stimulated by *thyroid-stimulating hormone* (TSH) of anterior lobe of pituitary, and its secretion is regulated by *thyrotropin-releasing hormone* (TRH) from hypothalamus.

Thyroid hormones increase anabolic processes in many tissues, activity of Na^+/K^+-ATP-ase, as well oxygen utilization, and thereby increase the basal metabolic rate and body temperature. They stimulate glycolgenolysis and gluconeogenesis, lipolysis, breakdown of VLDL and LDL, and excretion of bile acids via bile. They stimulate secretion of erythropoietin, sensitize adrenoreceptors and thereby increase the contractility of myocardium and heart rate, stimulate intestinal motility, glomerular filtration rate, and tubular transport, and neuromuscular reaction treshhold. They support intellectual development, and growth of body length, and catabolic process in bones.

The majority of causes of lowered secretion of thyroid hormones lie in the thyroid gland. Disturbance of synthesis and effectiveness of thyroid hormones can happen in any of the several known steps of thyroid hormone synthesis. The most common causes are the inflammations of thyroid gland, and thyroidectomy because of cancer.

Lack of thyroid hormones causes increased levels of TSH, and thereby hyperprolactinemia, that in turn causes disturbance of gonadotropin release and infertility.

Lack of thyroid hormones in fetus and newborn causes irreversible brain damage. *Without thyroid hormones there is no growth of dendrites, axons, and synapses, no glia development, and no myelinization.* Already in utero is the brain development retarded, and if the condition is not recognized at birth, and thyroid hormone substitution started immediately, the ensuing brain damage cannot be repaired later on. There is nanism and deafness as well.

The most common cause of **hyperthyroidism** is LATS (Long Acting Thyroid Stimulator), or TSI (Thyreoid Stimulating Immunoglobulin), that easily bound onto the TSH receptors, as is the case in Graves disease, known also as Basedow disease, as well as thyroid tumors, thyreoditis, increased TSH secretion. *Stem cell transplantation must be used with utmost care, if at all, usually focusing on the autoimmune pathogenesis.*

The exophthalmos, typical of Graves disease, is due to immune reactions against retrobulbar antigens, that are apparently very similar to the TSH receptors. As a result, there is retrobulbar inflammation with edema of extraocular muscles, lymphocytic infiltration, accumulation of acid mucopolysaccharides and of retrobulbar connectiuve tissue.

Clinical protocol for stem cell transplantation treatment of hypoendocrinopathies (for Hashimoto's thyroiditis, Graves disease, Addison's diseases see also the protocol for autoimmune disorders).

Parameters to be followed in patients before and after stem cell xenotransplantation, and the frequency:

- **General**: once a month or as necessary:
    i. growth chart, i.e. height and weight over time
    ii. measurement of body proportions once every 3 months
    iii. observation of symptoms and signs of puberty
    iv. x-rays of sella turcica
    v. CT scan or MRI of sella turcica and surrounding parts of brain
    vi. bone age by hand x-rays
    vii. chromosomal evaluation, if necessary
    viii. clinical status of female or male hypogonadotropism
    ix. clinical status of primary and secondary hypothyroidism
    x. clinical status of primary and secondary hypoadrenalism
    xi. clinical status of primary and secondary hyperthyroidism
    xii. clinical status of hypoparathyroidism

- **Immunological**: once a month for 3 months, then every 3 months
    i. total lymphocytes
    ii. T-lymphocytes (CD3$^+$)
    iii. T-helpers (CD4$^+$)
    iv. T-suppressors (CD8$^+$) and CD4/CD8
    v. NK (CD16)
    vi. B-lymphocytes (CD22 and CD19)
    vii. serum IgG, IgA, IgM
    viii. serum complement

- **Special**: once every 3 months as clinically necessary for the disease (s) under treatment:
    i. T3, T4, TSH by radioimmunoassay
    ii. thyrotropin releasing hormone stimulation test
    iii. growth hormone level

iv. somatomedin C (IGF-1) level
v. insulin tolerance test
vi. 24-hour urine for free cortisol, 17 OH-cortisol and ketogenic steroids
vii. ACTH stimulation test or Metyrapone test
viii. corticotropin releasing hormone stimulation test
ix. prolactine level
x. FSH and LH levels
xi. gonadotropin-releasing hormone stimulation test
xii. simultaneous testing of pituitary secretory reserve, i.e. of insulin, growth hormone, thyrotropin releasing hormone + gonadotropin releasing hormone
xiii. thyroid hormone binding ratio (T3 resin uptake) if necessary
xiv. radioactive iodine uptake if necessary
xv. serum electrolytes: Na, K, Cl
xvi. blood urea nitrogen
xvii. blood glucose
xviii. serum calcium and phosphorus
xix. 24 hour urine for calcium
xx. serum parathyroid hormone level by radioimmunoassay

Frequency of office visits: 4 weeks and 48 hours before stem cell xenotransplantation, 24 hours after and then once a week for the first month after stem cell xenotransplantation, once a month thereafter.

Chapter 50

If ye would go up high, then use your own legs! Do not get yourselves carried aloft; do not seat yourselves on other people's backs and heads!
[Thus Spoke Zarathustra, 1883 – 1981]

No one can draw more out of things, books included, than he already knows. A man has no ears for that to which experience has given him no access. [Ecce Homo, 1888]
[Friedrich Wilhelm Nietzsche, 1844 – 1900]

IMMUNE SYSTEM DISEASES

Immune deficiency disorders, such as AIDS, chronic weakness syndrome, as well as cancer, and *autoimmune diseases*, have been a menace of modern medicine, not only because there is no known cure, but also because the *modern medicine found no effective way to slow down the progress of such illnesses.*

During the last few years, there has been a growing body of peer-reviewed publications reporting on the success of stem cell therapy in the treatment of many cancers, both solid and dispersed. So perhaps the scientific fact that stem cell transplantation is by far the most potent immuno-stimulant known to medicine today, stops being one of the 'best kept secrets'. Immune system testing is still not sufficiently sensitive to assess the degree of benefit from the immuno-stimulating effect of stem cell transplants.

Modern medicine has a very limited armamentarium of therapies for immune deficiencies. With exception of stem cell transplants there are no effective direct immuno-stimulants available for treatment. Stem cell transplantation stimulates immune system spectacularly well, particularly one that is weakened for one reason or another. And that applies to even such deadly diseases of immune system as AIDS, and cancer, in which the immune system is malfunctioning as a result of an illness and a method of treatment used to combat it.

It is also therapeutically effective against autoimmune diseases, apparently functioning as an immuno-modulator in a way that lacks a scientific explanation.

The survival of a live organism without a defense against harmful factors of the outer and inner world, whether living or non-living, is impossible. The defense mechanism that has developed since the inception of life millions of years ago is a complicated and highly organized system which protects the biologic existence of every living being. Contact with, and defense against, the environment are key properties of life. Intake and metabolism of life-sustaining matters are recognized as fundamental biological features, but the defense against damaging and life-threatening matters is on the same level of importance.

As sophisticated as the immune system is, it operates on a very simple basic principle. It distinguishes 'self' from 'non-self' and attacks 'non-self' with the ultimate goal of removing it from the body. Usually this works in our favor, such as when our body is attacked by pathogenic microbes. At other times, it works against us, such as when our life depends on a transplanted organ: heart, liver or kidney, and our immune system attacks it as 'non-self' and causes its rejection. Sometimes the immune system fails to recognize even parts of our own body as 'self' and attacks them as 'non-self', and an autoimmune disease develops.

The immune system consists of four components:

1. *the epithelial surface barrier*, protecting the organism against outside world and the microbial world inside of our bodies, as there are more microbial cells in our body than of our own cells; that is historically, or phylogenetically, the oldest part,
2. *the reticulo-histiocytary system*, spread diffusely throughout our body, that developed next,
3. *thymo-lymphatic system*, consisting of *thymus gland*, and *network of lymphatic vessels* carrying lymph, which is filtered *in lymphatic nodes*, and
4. *spleen*, which filters blood, among other functions, and these last two are phylogenitically the youngest part.

Immune system defends the body against microorganisms, and macromolecules recognized as 'foreign' by *non-specific inborn*, and associated with it *specifically acquired, or adaptive, immunity*. Parts of microorganisms and 'foreign' macromolecules behave as 'antigens', and specifically acquired immune system reacts to them by activation and multiplication of mono-specific T- and B-lymphocytes. Both B- and T-lymphocytes have receptors on their surface for detection of foreign antigens that enable their activities, and production of cytokines, low-molecule soluble polypeptides, and their secretion into the surrounding extracellular space, which participate in elimination of the 'non-self' cells or macromolecules by non-specific mechanisms.

The lymphocytes are the most important cells of our defense system. More than a trillion of them are in the body at once, either circulating in the blood or on guard in the lymph nodes. There are two types of lymphocytes: T-cells and B-cells. Both are formed in bone marrow. B-cells mature in blood, while T-cells must pass through and mature in thymus gland. Thymus instructs the lymphocytes how to recognize 'non-self' and what to do when 'non-self' invades the body.

B-lymphocytes differentiate after stimulation by an antigen into plasma cells, which produce and secrete into body fluids *antibodies*, i.e. immunoglobulins IgA, IgD, IgE, IgG, IgM, that react with antigens that trigger their differentiation, neutralize or opsonize antigen, and activate complement system, i.e. *humoral immunity. They do not enter live cells.* Every B-lymphocyte is programmed to produce one specific antibody. This system has a memory. Once a B-cell produced an antibody against a specific foreign antigen, it remembers it forever. Thus each succeeding wave of the same infection, or the same antigen, is fought off with an increasing efficiency. This is the basis for immunization and explains why we fall victim to several childhood infectious diseases only once. The 'immunological memory' works sometimes in the opposite direction, i.e. in allergic conditions, ranging from hay fever to sudden death due to anaphylactic shock.

T-lymphocytes are the sentries of our body. When the 'non-self' antigen is recognized, they 'sound an alarm' and *direct the cooperation of different cells of immune system*, including histiocytes, macrophages, etc., and various non-cellular components, i.e. complement, cytokines, etc., and *directly attack somatic cells infected by virus*, or those *turned malignant*, and cause a *rejection of tissue transplants*, i.e. *cell immunity.* T-cells are divided into T-helpers, responsible for co-activation of B-lymphocytes and thereby production of antibodies, supporters of function of NK-cells, and T- cytotoxic/suppressors, responsible for uncovering and destruction of virus infected cells.

Any antigen is 'remembered' by T- and B-memory cells. Lymphoid precursor cells without any receptors develop during their 'upbringing period' in thymus for T-cells, and in bone marrow for B-cells, a *repertoire of about 10^8 of various types of lymphocytes, that are mono-specific, i.e. directed against one specific antigen.* Such 'virgin' lymphocytes circulate in the body, between blood, peripheral lymphatic tissue, lymph, and blood again. When such 'virgin' lymphocyte meets 'its' antigen, usually within lymphatic tissues, it multiplies, passes through *clonal selection and proliferation,* and a large number of mono-specific daughter cells is produced. These daughter cells differentiate into required T-cells, or B-cells, which eventually eliminate antigen.

'Virgin' lymphocyte with receptors against own body tissues is eliminated in thymus, i.e. T-cells, or in bone marrow, i.e. B-cells, early enough after recognition of 'its' antigen. Such *'clonal deletion' creates in this way a 'central immunological tolerance'.* This *recognition of difference between foreign antigens and antigens of own body is 'learned' by immune system at the moment of birth.* All substances that come in contact with immune system at that moment are recognized for the rest of life as 'own' and all others that come in contact with immune system later on as 'foreign'. *If this recognition fails, an autoimmune disease develops.*

Immune system cells are characterized by *their own system of membrane antigens,* which appear in cell membrane at certain stage of development, and remain there for a certain period of time, or up until cell death. These membrane antigens are known as *clusters of differentiation (CD).* Some CD's are located on both T- and B-lymphocytes, others are specific for some cells only.

The defense capabilities of immune system have a 'life profile'. After 'immuno-tolerance' of the embryonic and fetal stage of life, when the immune system is not functioning and the entire defense depends on the immune system of pregnant mother and placenta, the immune system gradually 'wakes up', until it reaches the optimal functioning level between 10 and 15 years of age. During puberty the immune system function gets depressed, the exact timing depends on the sex.

Afterward, the immune system works at full capacity for the next 30 to 35 years. *Between 40 and 50 years of age a regression period begins, when the function of immune system decreases relentlessly until a senile 'immuno-paralysis' period is reached when the body becomes defenseless against malignancy and even the most banal infections.*

Non-specific immunity is handled by:

- *dissolved defensive substances*, i.e. lysozym,
- various *complements*,
- *phagocytosis*, carried out mostly by macrophages, developed from monocytes, attracted from blood to tissues where infectious agents are present by chemokines (chemotaxis); here phagocytes trigger via mediator release the inflammatory process, and 'ingest' pathogenic microorganisms and destroy them with lysozym, oxidants, i.e. H_2O_2, and oxygen radicals (O_2-, OH-, $^1O_2$), nitrogen oxide (NO), and 'digest' them by their lysosomal enzymes; phagocytosis is more effective when the surface of antigen is covered by IgM or IgG, or by complement $C3_b$ during the process of 'opsonization',
- pathogenic organisms, 'opsonized', or 'non-opsonized', *trigger* also '*complement cascade*' whereby a membrane attacking complement complex is created which perforates wall of gram-negative bacteria and kills them,
- *non-specific defense against mycobacteria and cancer cells is handled by 'natural killer cells' (NK cells)*, that perforate membrane of target cell and cause its death by cytolysis,
- *macrophages*, developed from monocytes that either traveled to the respective tissue from blood or were fixed in the local tissue, i.e. Kupffer cells in sinuses of liver, lung alveoli, intestinal serosa, sinuses of spleen, lymphnodes, Langerhans cells of skin, synovial A-cells, brain microglia, endothel, etc. that belong to reticulo-endothelial system (RES) or mononuclear-phagocytic system (MFS).

Acquired specific immunity through mono-specific effector T-cells requires that 'modified' antigen is presented to such T-cells by 'professional' antigen presenting cells, i.e. APC's. The 'modification' means that the antigen is built into a molecular capsule of individually specific proteins of MHC class I and II, in humans known also as HLA class I and II. *In lymphatic tissue residing virus-infected dendritic cells serve usually as APC's.* For presentation of antigen by APC a binding between an intracellular adhesive molecule (ICAM) on the surface of APC, and a lymphocyte function associated antigen 1 (LFA-1) on the surface of T-cell, is necessary. When T-cell approaches APC this binding becomes stronger and T-cell is activated by a double signal consisting of:

- *recognition of antigen*, bound to MHC-I or –II, by the T-cell receptor with co-receptor, i.e. CD8 in cytotoxic T-cells, CD4 in T-helpers, and
- *co-stimulatory signal*, i.e. binding of protein B7 (on APC) to protein CD28 of T-cell.

When antigen is bound without a co-stimulatory signal, for example in the liver where there are usually no APC's, T-cell is actually inactivated, i.e. becomes anergic. This is known as 'peripheral immunotolerance'.

Cytotoxic T-cells develop from 'virgin' CD8-T-cells after presentation of antigen associated with MHC-I, during which act MHC-I accepts its antigen mainly from cytosol of APC (antigens are viruses, or cytosol proteins), and for that reason such act is called '*endogenous presentation of antigen*'. Cytotoxic T-cells recognize then by its CD8 associated receptor the respective MHC-I bound antigen on virus-infected cells, cancer cells, or cells of transplanted organs, and kill those cells.

'Virgin' helper CD4-T-cells change after the presentation of antigen (phagocytized bacteria or protein of viral capsules, i.e. 'exogenous antigen presentation') associated with MHC-II into immature effector T-cells (T_{HO}). The T_{HO} cells develop by differentiation into either inflammatory T-helpers (T_{H1}), which activate macrophages, or T-helpers of 2nd type (T_{H2}) necessary for B-cell activation.

Specific humoral immunity is dependent on B-cells.

Disorders of non-specific immunity can be due to:

- *defects of complement system*, i.e. infections by extracellular microorganisms, mainly neisserias,
- *defects of NK cells*, i.e. infections by intracellular organisms, mainly listeria, or herpetic viruses,
- *mannose binding protein*,
- *disturbances of phagocytosis* involving various types of cells, or just functional defects: *leukocyte adhesion defect* (LAD), *syndrome of 'lazy leukocytes'* with slowed down migration, *chronic granulomatous disease* with lack of oxidant production, *Chediak-Higashi syndrome* with disrupted fusion of phagosomes and lysosomes.

Disorders of humoral immunity can be due to defects of maturation, function or activation of B-cells. Without antibodies, the organism is helpless especially against microorganisms causing suppuration, because without opsonization their polysaccharide capsule blocks phagocytosis. Here is a partial list:

- *selective lack of IgG* with insufficient protection of mucosa causes recurrent respiratory and GI infections and predilection to allergies,
- *agammaglobulinemia* where defect of Bruton's tyrosinkinase interferes with maturation of B-cells,
- *syndrome of higher IgM level* characterized by concurrent lowered concentration of IgA and IgG,
- variable defect of immunity with inadequate B-cell stimulation by T-cells.

Defects of cell-mediated immunity occur:

- in thymus aplasia, known as *DiGeorge syndrome*,
- in combination with defects of humoral immunity, covering the whole spectrum of diseases from defects of stem cell differentiation, i.e. *reticular dysgenesis*, through defective HLA production, i.e. *syndrome of naked lymphocytes*, to a very serious combined B- and T-cell insufficiency, i.e. *severe combined immunodeficiency disease*, SCID, caused by a lack of adenosinedeaminase or purinnucleotidephosphorylase.

For direct immunostimulation, stem cell transplantation of *mesenchyme, thymus, spleen, liver, adrenal cortex, mesenterial lymphnode, intestine,* is recommended, with an addition of *lung* when respiratory system defense is at stake, or *skin*, when immune protection of skin is necessary.

AIDS is caused by HIV-1 or HIV-2 viruses. Viruses attack, besides CD8 cells, predominantly CD4 T_H-cells, in which ssRNA is transcribed by virion reverse transcriptase into cDNA, until it is as double chain dsDNA (provirus) placed into the genom of host cell during the latent stage. Between the initial viremia with high level of antigen p24 and production of IgM, and ARC with renewed viremia, without any IgM, many years can pass, during which time proviruses survive in small numbers, such as 10^6, of inactive CD4-cells, mostly in lymphnodes. Activation of CD4 cell, at the beginning of infection and in the late stage, triggers virus expression. Even non-infected CD4 cells die so that in the late stage there is critical lack of CD4 T-cells. Changes of cytokine concentration cause a major elimination of T_{H1} and cytotoxic cells. The organism is now exposed, with growing helplessness, to otherwise unimportant minor infections, i.e. by fungi, and rare cancers, i.e. Kaposi sarcoma, lymphomas.

A case history of AIDS patient treated by cell transplantation is the sole published information about a US clinical trial that began in New York after Prof. Schmid was approached in September 1987 and then visited on November 3, 1987, in the State Pediatric Hospital in Aschaffenburg, where he was a director, by Mr. Ed Kramer and Dr. Kohn, the organizers of the project. Approximately 30 patients were treated, in accordance with the protocol in possession of the author, but the project was stopped because of a lack of funds. The patient described in this publication continued to be treated for free as all expenses were paid for by the German Association for Cell Therapy and German manufacturers [287].

A 39 year old female from Houston, Texas, developed in 1965, at the age of 17, Hodgkin's disease. After 13 surgeries and chemotherapy, since 1971 she was relatively well. In January, 1986 she developed an acute lymphadenitis treated by antibiotics and I&D. In April 1987 a pulmonary aspergillosis was diagnosed, followed by a diagnosis of AIDS Related Complex, with lymphocyte count of 2,200/mm^2, and a weight drop from 144 to 126 lb. On 5/25/87, she received cell transplants of *thymus, mesenchyme, liver, spleen, skin*. One week later her lymphocyte count increased, and after about 8 months, the first monocytes have appeared. The patient was feeling better, and her appetite improved. In October 1987, an implantation of two cell transplants was carried out. WBC had remained normal, lymphocytes rose from 15 to 50%, CD8 cell count rose, CD4 cell count decreased, so that CD4/CD8 ratio improved from 0.60 to 0.88.

Then there was a treatment interruption, and the condition of the patient dramatically worsened. On May 25, 1988 CD4/CD8 ratio was 0.27. After the patient received cell transplantation of *mesenchyme, liver, spleen, thymus, skin, placenta*, in July 1988 the CD4/CD8 ratio went up to 0.40, CD4 T-cells rose from 10% to 24% but also CD8 T-cells from 34% to 63%, the patient was feeling much better and the immune system weakness was diminished [287].

At one of the meetings of the International Society of Cell Therapy, the conclusion of this case history was given. After 2½ years of 'underground' treatment, the immune deficiency appeared again and the patient had to urgently receive another cell transplantation. At that point, US Customs stopped the free shipment of cell therapeutics from Germany twice in a row, and by the time the third shipment arrived the patient was dead.

A 24 year old male homosexual, with a history of mononucleosis 4 years before this report, and gonorrhea and cytomegalovirus infection 2 years later, developed after another two years, a severe herpes zoster. During the examination, hepatosplenomegaly, inguinal, axillary, cervical lymphadenopathy, recurrent bronchial infections, and positive HIV tests, were found. IgG was increased and IgA decreased, CD4/CD8 ratio was 0.34. Cell transplantation with mesenchyme was begun and repeated four times at weeks 2 –4 –8 –16 –24. Splenomegaly subsided; immunoglobulins were within normal limits. Six months after the last treatment the patient was well and working [311].

Therapeutic protocol of the treatment of AIDS requires an avoidance of re-infection, a follow-up every 4 – 6 weeks for immune system function evaluation, and *continuous repetition of cell transplantation whenever the laboratory tests of immune system show that the HIV virus is prevailing again.* Any delays in the cell transplantation treatment are very risky. *When the immune system is at the point of shutdown, the cell transplantation must be done as an emergency*, or there may be no response. *Even patients with ARC-AIDS related complex, with 500 CD4 cells/ml, or those with fully developed AIDS, with 200 CD4 cells/ ml, can reach their normal lifespan, if compliant*, and treated by stem cell transplantation as the therapeutic protocol calls for.

The clinical picture of *immune system deficiencies* is characterized by recurrent, prolonged, often very serious and eventually life-threatening infections, and certain cancers. They are *classified into 5 groups*:

1. **Combined deficit of lymphocytes**

    - *X-linked severe combined immunodeficiency* (SCID) with incidence 1:50,000 to 1:75,000, defect of both T- and B-cells, with low B-cell count and no T-cells, and defect of γ-chain of IL-2 produced by T-cells, causes a severe disorder of both cell and humoral immunity and thereby extreme sensitivity to pathogenic organisms, resulting in candidiasis, chronic otitis media, diarrhea, and sepsis. Treatment is by bone marrow transplant,

- *deficit of adenosinedeaminase*, AR disorder, a purine enzymopathy, leads to accumulation of toxic metabolites damaging T- and B-cells, with pronounced lymphopenia, rachitic rosary on ribs, normal uric acid in urine,
- *deficit of purine nucleosidephosphorylase*, AR disorder, a purine enzymopathy leads to an accumulation of toxic metabolites damaging T- and B-cells, with lowered level of uric acid in urine,
- *defect of class II HLA-antigens, or syndrome of naked lymphocytes*, AR disorder, causes moderate to severe degree of immunodeficiency and thereby serious bacterial infections; there is always a predominance of T-suppressor cells, (while normally the ratio of T-helpers to T-suppressors is 2:1), low level of immunoglobulins, low specific antibody production,
- *reticular dysgenesis*, AR disorder,
- *Omen syndrome*, with immunodeficiency leading to serious infections, and severe erythrodermia, hepatosplenomegaly, lymphadenopathy, continuous diarrhea, persistent leukocytosis with pronounced eosinophilia,
- *immunodeficiency with hyper-IgM syndrome*, XR disorder, causing a failure of interaction of T- and B-cells, responsible for recurrent pyogenic infections, particularly of biliary system, that causes liver damage, with increased levels of IgM, but very low levels of all other immunoglobulins, and persistent neutropenia,
- *DiGeorge syndrome*, AR disorder, with multiple anomalies of structures of 3rd and 4th pharyngeal pouch, i.e. congenital aplasia of thymus, congenital hypothyreosis combined with aplasia of parathyroid glands, heart malformations, particularly conus arteriosus, variable immunodeficiency up to a total absence of T-cells.

2. **Antibody defects**

- *Bruton's X-linked agamaglobulinemia* is the first immunodeficiency discovered, with absent B-cells and plasma cells and thereby decreased levels of all immunoglobulins, normal level of precursors stem cells in bone marrow; at the end of the first 6 months of life repeated bacterial infections, i.e. pneumonia, meningitis, appear, while the sensitivity toward viral infections is not increased, with exception of hepatitis and enteroviroses,
- *deficit of heavy chain of immunoglobulins*, AR disorder, cause IgG deficit, and thereby repeated pyogenic infections,

- *selective IgA deficit* is the most frequent of all immunodeficiency disorders, deficit of IgA is present despite a normal B-cell count, causing recurrent sino-bronchial infections, gastrointestinal diseases, autoimmune diseases, allergies, and malignant diseases.

3. ***Other typical syndromes***:

    - *Wiskott-Aldrich syndrome*, XR disorder,
    - *ataxia-teleangiectasia*, AR disorder, see also in the chapter 'Genetic diseases',
    - *Bloom syndrome*, see also in the chapter 'Genetic diseases',
    - *Hyper-IgE syndrome.*

4. ***Lymphocyte malfunction***:

    - X-linked proliferative syndrome,
    - Chronic granulomatous disease,
    - Leukocyte adhesion deficit,
    - Chediak-Higashi syndrome.

5. ***Complement System Malfunction***

Therapy by bone marrow transplantation from HLA-identical sibling is of great benefit. It has to be carried out before irreversible damage to the organism due to frequent infections takes place. There is much less risk with graft vs. host disease, etc., when stem cell transplantation of *liver, spleen, thymus, mesenchyme, adrenal cortex, intestine*, is used.

CASE HISTORY

The patient worked with the author as an anesthesiologist during the surgical courses that the author used to teach in a major Italian city 3 - 4 times a year from 1989 till 1993. He was an excellent anesthesiologist, very successful in his private practice, vivacious, and a good companion, too. During various social outings he showed great interest in and learned about our work in the field of cell transplantation. In 1992 he 'disappeared' and the writer did not see him again until early 1994, when he desperately sought medical help.

A white male patient, born 1951, developed a flu in early 1992, from which he could not recover. He was continuously fatigued, more so that he ever experienced, and even prolonged sleep did not refresh him. He had muscle pains, constant headaches, and frequent sore throats. Before he could work 12 hours every day, give anesthesia simultaneously in two adjacent operating rooms, now he could not finish a single anesthesia case a day. Gradually, the fatigue became so severe that he became convinced that he is going to die, particularly since no medical professional that he consulted could help him.

He was examined by every professor of internal medicine of reputation in Italy, every imaginable clinical test was carried out, all with negative results, and no one could establish a diagnosis, with the exception of some remarks such as 'that must be some form of depression or psychoneurosis'. In reality everyone who knew this patient well, and the patient himself, were of the opinion that any psychiatric disease is out of question. The sole objective fact that could have contributed to this illness was a 'burn-out' due to long hours of stressful work every day, since his services were in great demand, as he was an excellent anesthesiologist indeed.

The patient took various antidepressants, as advised, but without any effect.

Eventually in 1993, he was referred to a UK physician, who - with his consulting team - made a diagnosis of *chronic fatigue syndrome*, even though all tests were again negative.

The treatment consisted of detoxification: intake of copious amount of distilled water, vegetarian diet, mostly in the form of raw fruits and vegetables, ecologically clean, mega doses of vitamins and minerals, in particular of Niacin, to force salivation.

The patient began to feel better, but his ability to work continued to be minimal. He could do no more than one anesthesia case a day, following which he was completely exhausted. The absence of sexual performance ruined his marriage. His social life was non-existent.

When he met the author again in 1994, he asked if we could help him by cell transplantation.

The patient arrived on April 4, 1994, at Moscow. A complete physical examination was done, which was negative, as always before. Among various laboratory tests that we carried out, a complete blood count, peripheral blood smear, sedimentation rate, total T-cell count, $CD4^+$

count, $CD8^+$ count, serum immunoglobulin electrophoresis, Candida skin test, were all negative. But we finally succeeded where all predecessors failed during the past two years when we found an objective proof of an immune system deficiency: lymphocyte proliferative response test to mitogen, and *in vitro* phagocytosis assays, were both significantly abnormal.

On April 7, 1994, a cell transplantation of adrenal cortex, liver, mesenterial lymphnodes, spleen, thymus, hypothalamus, intestine, mesenchyme, was carried out with an uneventful post-treatment course.

The patient was delighted with the result of cell transplantation. Within 6 weeks he was able to work 8 hours a day without any difficulty, and could do even more, but wisely preferred not to. His social and sexual appetite returned to normal.

Unfortunately he could not find a single laboratory in Italy that could do lymphocyte proliferative response test to mitogens and *in vitro* phagocytosis assay, that would have enhanced our follow-up data, and flatly refused to return to Moscow 'unless he would be in serious trouble again', and that never happened after our treatment.

He waited until we set up a clinical base in Germany, and in March 1999 the patient received cell xenotransplantation of liver, adrenal cortex, thymus, spleen, mesenchyme, mesenterial lymphnodes, testis, of our manufacturing at a clinic in Germany. The post-transplantation course was uneventful.

Today, the patient feels that he is perfectly healthy. But he continues to watch his nutrition and fluid intake.

Thanks to him, to a great degree, that we were able to start to offer cell transplantation in Italy.

The patient underwent his next stem cell transplantation in November 2003, purely as a preventive step.

Clinical protocol for stem cell transplantation treatment of a patient with immune system disorders

A proper preparation of the patient for stem cell transplantation is mandatory. A patient has to be brought into as good a clinical condition as possible by standard therapeutic means, i.e. to carry out stem cell transplantation while the patient is in the condition of insufficiently treated infection, with all the metabolic consequences, is probably minimally effective and should be done only as a last resort. Patient must be detoxified, which means in particular the treatment of the gastrointestinal, respiratory and urinary tract and skin infections and related diseases by antibiotics, etc.

Parameters to be followed in patients before and after stem cell xenotransplantation, and the frequency:

Basic: once a month or as often as clinically necessary:

   i. complete blood count with differential, and platelet count
   ii. peripheral blood smear
   iii. total T-cell count
   iv. serum IgG, IgM, IgA, (and IgE, if necessary)
   v. iso-agglutinin titers: anti-A and/or anti-B to evaluate IgM function
   vi. pre-existing antibody titers after immunization against polio or rubella virus, and against tetanus, diphtheria - to evaluate IgG function
   vii. sedimentation rate
   viii. x-rays of infected organ(s)
   ix. bacterial culture(s) from the infected organ(s)
   x. clinical status of ongoing infectious disease (s) process(es)
   xi. x-rays of chest, also to measure the size of thymus
   xii. delayed hypersensitivity skin tests: Trichophyton, mumps, Candida, fluid tetanus toxoid, to carry out as often as clinically indicated
   xiii. total white blood cell count
   xiv. nitroblue tetrazolium dye reduction test (NBT)
   xv. total serum complement activity (CH50)
   xvi. serum C3 and C4 levels

Special: to be carried out if clinically necessary:

   i. total B-cell count once a month,
   ii. T-subsets counts: T-helpers/inducers (anti-CD4 antibody),T-suppressors/cytotoxic cells (anti-CD8 monoclonal antibody), CD4/CD8 ratio, NK (anti-CD16 monoclonal antibody) once a month,
   iii. antibody response to vaccines: tetanus toxoid, typhoid (for protein

antigen response), pneumococcus, unconjugated H. influenzae (for polysacharide antigen response) as often as needed,
iv. IgG subclass levels as often as needed,
v. lateral x-rays of pharynx: tonsils, adenoids size,
vi. lymphocyte proliferative response test to mitogens, known-to-patient-antigens, irradiated allogeneic white blood cells, (include lymphokines, IFNγ and IL-2 production as clinically required) as often as necessary,
and include the following if clinically necessary as often as needed:
vii. cell movement by Rebuck skin window,
viii. *in vitro* chemotactic essay,
ix. *in vitro* phagocytosis assay (latex particles, bacteria),
x. intracellular microbial killing assay,
xi. complement and inhibitor assays,
xii. classical and alternative complement activity essays.

Frequency of office visits: 4 weeks and 48 hours before stem cell xenotransplantation, 24 hours and then once a week for the first month after stem cell xenotransplantation, and once a month thereafter.

Repeated stem cell transplantation are to be carried as often as clinical course requires maintaining the function of all components of immune system at a normal or near-normal level.

In AIDS, stem cell transplantation should be repeated as often as every 6 weeks depending upon the clinical course of the disease(s).

CASE HISTORY:

In 1991, the author was introduced by a colleague, to a patient, a black male, born in 1942, a top man in the hierarchy of the US Baptist Church, at a political/social function. In May 1993, the author was contacted and asked whether we could treat AIDS, and was sent medical data of the patient.

In early 1992, the patient noticed a gradual development of weakness, malaise, diarrhea, weight loss, and overall wasting, which made it increasingly difficult for him to go through the preaching sermon. In February 1993, a diagnosis of AIDS was established. At the same time, a diagnosis of syphilis was made, and an immediate treatment by depot Penicillin was carried out. As we did not receive an official medical summary from patient's physician, we did not know what type of treatment of AIDS was tried. The patient wished to save his life, but his doctors did not agree that he should seek treatment elsewhere.

The patient arrived Moscow on July 18, 1993, and upon admission to the hospital was found to be in a near moribund state. He was emaciated, dehydrated, and toxic, with a fever of nearly 104 °F, low blood pressure, and tachycardia. He had a right upper lobe pneumonia on the admission chest x-ray. Immediately, an aggressive anti-shock treatment was instituted, including i.v. broad-spectrum antibiotics.

Important laboratory findings on hospital admission: Complete blood count showed minor leukocytosis, with a lymphopenia. Total T-cell count was less than 200/μliter. CD4 count was 0, so that CD4/CD8 ratio was 0 as well. Serum immunoglobulin electrophoresis showed increased IgG, and IgA. Culture and Sensitivity of sputum showed Pneumococcus.

The intensive anti-shock therapy was successful. As the patient arrived at Moscow in a nearly terminal state, which is normally a contraindication for cell transplantation, a deep professional discussion ensued about carrying out the planned treatment.

Eventually, on July 26, 1993, a transplantation of thymus, liver, adrenal cortex, spleen, mesenterial lymphnodes, mesenchyme, and intestine, was carried out. The post-treatment course was uneventful and patient was able to fly back to US on July 30, 1993.

Within 4 weeks of the treatment, the patient began a preaching tour through US baptist churches, openly admitting his past transgressions, that caused his illness, declaring that "God's miracle" in Moscow saved his life, and that he will not sin anymore.

On August 30, 1993, his complete blood count and total lymphocyte count were within normal limits. The patient was clinically in a complete remission.

Our team was at Sansum Medical Research Foundation, Santa Barbara, California, from July 31 until August 6, 1993, to treat 24 US insulin-dependent diabetics with retinopathy and nephropathy, an event widely announced by US media as "Russian rabbit cells treating US diabetics". During this time, we attempted to visit with the patient, but could not get to him even via his private phone number, that he gave the author in Moscow. Finally we spoke to a man who claimed to be his physician.

The author tried to impress upon him that our/his patient needs a very close follow-up, a continuous supportive treatment as per our treatment protocol, and repeated "minor" cell transplantations every 4 - 6 -8 weeks in accordance with the results of laboratory testing of the immune system function.

Despite the best efforts of the patient's friends, who arranged his treatment with our team, we were not able to continue our treatment whether directly or by sending stem cell transplants to the patient to be implanted by his US physicians.

The patient died sometimes in February 1994, allegedly of the lymphoma of the brain.

CASE HISTORY:

In 1980, a two year old boy with Down syndrome was brought from California to the State Pediatric Hospital in Aschaffenburg, Germany, where Prof. Schmid was the director. The complex therapeutic protocol for Down syndrome was begun, which included cell transplantations. The next cell transplantation was carried out in California.

In 1981, the patient was brought to Aschaffenburg again for the 3rd cell transplantation, this time accompanied not only by parents, but also grandparents. The family was pleased with the improvement of symptoms and signs of Down syndrome. After grandson's third cell transplantation was carried out, the grandfather approached Prof. Schmid and asked for an examination, fully aware that he is talking to a pediatrician.

A 55 year old grandfather was a high level manager at film studio. He complained of deepening malaise, lasting for approximately 5 years, which had noticeably lowered his capacity to work and enjoy life on many fronts. During those 5 years, he suffered from frequently recurring attacks of bronchitis and pneumonia, losing many days from work, and his physicians could do nothing about it.

Grandfather received cell transplantation for revitalization (*liver, testes, placenta*), stimulation of immune system (*thymus*), and support of the organs most abused by stress (*hypothalamus, adrenal cortex*).

In 1982, the grandparents brought their grandson back to Prof. Schmid for another cell transplantation treatment. Grandfather was beaming because during the last 12 months he had had neither bronchitis nor pneumonia, and did not lose a single day from work, which made his 'super boss' extremely happy.

The grandfather asked Prof. Schmid if he would be so kind to examine his wife as well.

The 50 year old grandmother, looking older than her age, appeared chronically ill. Her fingers were deformed; the joints of both hands were swollen. She was obviously depressed when she complained about pain, inability to hold a cup of coffee in her hands, or carry many household duties. She barely recovered from one infection when she got the next one. Her circulation was bad, she had low blood pressure, and after being up for two hours she had to lie down again.

Her treatment consisted of nutritional advice, digestive enzymes, and cell transplantation for revitalization (*liver, ovaries, placenta, spleen*), for support of blood circulation and organs abused by stress (*heart muscle, diencephalon, adrenal cortex, medulla*), for immune system stimulation (*thymus, mesenchyme*), and for arthritis (*cartilage*).

In 1983, the grandson and grandparents were back in Aschaffenburg for another treatment. In Prof. Schmid's office, the grandmother was 'playing piano in the air' with her fingers to show off that her arthritis was gone. Her infections did not stop, but were much less frequent, and blood circulation was still somewhat weak.

In 1985, Prof. Schmid received a letter from the grandmother. She was doing relatively well. Her blood circulation was not too bad, but her infections were coming on again, and lasted for along time. She was very disturbed about her positive test for AIDS, in particular, since she could not comprehend how she could have acquired such an illness.

Both she and her husband began to follow therapeutic protocol for AIDS, including frequent cell transplantation to support immune system. Three years later, the immune system was back to normal and the AIDS test became negative.

Chapter 51

Truth has no special time of its own. Its hour is now - always.
Albert Schweitzer, 1875 – 1965 [Out of My Life and Thought, 1949]

AUTOIMMUNE DISEASES

When the immune system continuously produces auto-antibodies against antigens of own body, or activates T-cells that attack self-antigens, it causes damage to the tissues and organs, i.e. autoimmune disease. *Finding of antibody against self-antigens is by itself not a proof of autoimmune disease*, as auto-antibodies are frequently found as a temporary after-effect of tissue destruction.

Organism defends itself against the effect of auto-antibodies by:
- *clonal deletion,*
- *clonal inactivation, or anergy,*
- *immunological ignorance*: AAG-specific cells are sometimes, despite their ability to recognize antigens, not activated.

Apoptosis participates in the peripheral clonal deletion of adult autoreactive T-cells in the peripheral lymphatic system, and elimination of activated T-lymphocytes. In autoimmune diseases there is a resistance of autoreactive T-lymphocytes toward apoptosis, with the *level of resistance being higher in females than males.*

In many autoimmune diseases, mutations of somatic cells, active on various levels of immune system, are considered an important pathogenetic factor.

Possible, or partial, *causes of development of auto-antibodies* are:

1. *Genetic predisposition caused by a certain allele,* i.e. carriers of alleles, HLA-DR-3 and HLA-DR-4 get IIDM 500x more often

than carriers of alleles DR2+DR2,

2. *Hormonal influences*, indicated by sex incidence, particularly during puberty: ratio female/male in systemic lupus erythematosus 10:1, while for ankylosing spondylitis 1:3,

3. *Autoantigens from immunoprivileged areas*, i.e. brain, eye, testis, uterus, that leave those locations, via blood, but not via lymphatic passages, and react with T-cells with release of no auto-antibodies. Auto-antibodies are accompanied by TGFβ (transforming growth factor beta), that causes an activation of T_{H2} cells instead of destructive T_{H1} cells. Despite that autoantigens from such areas trigger autoimmune diseases, i.e. myelin basic protein (MBP) of brain triggers multiple sclerosis, one of the most frequent autoimmune diseases. Similarly, eye injury releases proteins with immune response to them which threaten un-injured normal eye, i.e. sympathetic ophthalmia, and infertility is sometimes caused by spermatozoid antibodies. Contrary to that, embryo, or fetus, with its multiple from father inherited foreign antigens, is immunologically fully tolerated, because placenta makes maternal T-cells anergic.

4. *Infections*, as antibodies against certain microbial antigens, or T-cells, can cross-react with auto-antigens, as it is with antibodies against streptococcus A with autoantigens in heart, causing endocarditis, in joints, causing polyarthritis, and in kidneys, a cause of glomerulonephritis.

Immune mechanisms of autoimmune disease correspond with the allergic reactions of type II through V.

Examples for **allergic reactions type II**, i.e. cytotoxic, are autoimmune hemolytic anemia and Goodpasture's syndrome, where autoantibodies against basal membrane cause destruction of tissues in kidneys and lungs, and IgG is deposited in kidneys along glomerular capillaries that triggers severe inflammatory reaction.

Allergic reactions type III, triggered by production and deposition of immune complexes, or antigen-antibody complexes, take place in systemic lupus erythematosus, serum sickness, exogenous allergic alveolitis, i.e. 'pigeon-breeder's lung' due to antigens in pigeons excreta, or 'farmer's lungs' due to yeast antigens in hay.

Allergic reactions of type IV, or delayed type hypersensitivity, occur in rheumatoid arthritis, multiple sclerosis, IDDM where CD8 T-cells destroy self-β-cells, coeliakia, poison ivy and poison sumac, primary rejection of organ transplant.

Examples for *type V* are auto-antibodies that activate hormonal receptors, as is the case in Graves' disease, or block them, as takes place in myasthenia gravis.

Autoimmune diseases are divided into two groups:

1. diseases where *antigen is organ-specific*, i.e. Hashimoto's thyroiditis, Addison's disease, pernicious anemia, IDDM, etc.,
2. Diseases where *antigen is not organ-specific*, i.e. scleroderma, rheumatoid arthritis, systemic lupus erythematosus, etc.

But there are autoimmune diseases where *antigen is organ-specific but antibodies react also with other antigens*, i.e. idiopathic thrombocytopenic purpura, Sjogren syndrome, idiopathic leukopenias.

For autoimmune diseases stem cell transplantation of *thymus, intestine, adrenal cortex, placenta,* is advised, while specifically for scleroderma, stem cell transplantation of *skin, mesenchyme, placenta, liver, as well as thymus, adrenal cortex, hypothalamus.*

A 72 year old female had rheumatic pains in muscles and joints since puberty. She suffered an acute hepatitis at the age of 35. Nine years earlier, the diagnosis of scleroderma was made: stiffness and swelling of fingers, hand and foot joints, swelling of face, dysphagia, increasing pain in hand joints, and Raynaud-like attacks with change of weather. She had treatment with cortison for 9 years. On April 26, 1984, cell transplantation of *liver, mesenchyme, hypothalamus, anterior pituitary, adrenal cortex, skin,* was carried out. Three months later she stopped taking cortisone, her muscle strength increased, sleep improved, and such improvement continued for 18 months, with no further negative reports [299].

Our experience with treatment of autoimmune diseases by cell transplantation was reported at the 1st Symposium on Human fetal Tissue Transplantation in Moscow, December 4 – 7, 1995, under the title: "Experience of clinical use of transplantation of human embryonic tissues in treatment of rheumatic diseases of children". A heterologous group of patients from the Pediatric Department of the Moscow Medical Academy with different diagnoses, such as scleroderma (2 patients), rheumatoid arthritis (3 patients), dermatomyositis (2 patients), mixed connective tissue disease (1 patient), was treated by cell transplantation of *adrenal cortex, liver, thymus, placenta, hypothalamus, mesenchyme*. This group had one thing in common, i.e. there was no therapy left for them and they were going to be sent back to regional hospitals for palliative care. The patients were from 8 – 14 years of age, 2 males, and 6 females. None of the patients were cured, but all improved so that their label 'incurable' was removed. The formerly called 'collagen diseases', which by definition are still classified as incurable, are successfully treated by stem cell transplantation but the treatment must begin early and not when the patient becomes totally unresponsive to any known treatment.

Clinical protocol for stem cell transplantation treatment of autoimmune diseases

This applies to: Systemic lupus erythematosus (SLE), Rheumatoid arthritis (RA), Scleroderma (PSS), Mixed connective tissue disease (MCTD), Polymyositis (PM), Sjogren syndrome (SS), Polyarteritis nodosa (PN), covered entirely under this protocol; also to: Hashimoto's thyroiditis, Graves disease, NIDDM, some cases of IDDM, idiopathic Addison's disease, failure of other endocrine glands, sometimes combined, covered also under the protocol for 'Hypoendocrinopathies'; as well as to Chronic active hepatitis, Primary biliary cirrhosis, Glomerulonephritis, Goodpasture's syndrome, covered under the respective protocols as well; Myasthenia gravis, unresponsive Bronchial asthma; Pemphigus, Bullous pemphigoid, Vitiligo, Atopic dermatitis; Autoimmune hemolytic anemia, Autoimmune thrombocytopenic purpura, Pernicious anemia.

A proper preparation of the patient for stem cell transplantation is mandatory. A patient has to be brought into as good a clinical condition as possible by standard therapeutic means, while at the same time lowering the dosage of corticosteroids and other immunosuppressants to a necessary minimum, or discontinuing them altogether, and eliminating non-essential drugs.

Parameters to be followed in patients before and after stem cell xenotransplantation, and the frequency:

- **Basic clinical**: once a month:
    i. complete blood count with differential and platelet count,

ii. urinalysis,
  iii. sedimentation rate,
  iv. serum IgG, IgM, IgA once a month x3, then every 3 months,
  v. x-rays of hands or other joints as necessary,
  vi. clinical status of arthritis (RA, SS, SLE, PSS, PM, MCTD),
  vii. status of skin lesions (SLE, PSS, PM, MCTD) and photosensitivity (SLE),
  viii. clinical status of oral ulcers (SLE)
  ix. clinical status of nephritis (SLE, MCTD), tubular acidosis (SS), renal hypertension (PSS, PN),
  x. clinical status of pleurisy, pericarditis (SLE, MCTD),
  xi. clinical status of CREST syndrome (PSS), calcinosis, Raynaud phenomenon (in MCTD too), Esophageal dysfunction, Sclerodactyly, Teleangiectasia,
  xii. clinical status of lung fibrosis (PSS, PM, MCTD),
  xiii. clinical status of arrhytmia (PSS, PM, PN), mitral valve prolapse (MCTD),
  xiv. clinical status of gastrointestinal mucosal atrophy, pancreatitis, biliary disorder (SS, PSS, PN),
  xv. clinical status of proximal muscle weakness (PM, MCTD), flexion, contractures (PSS), mononeuritis multiplex (PN),
  xvi. clinical status of generalized adenopathy (SLE) and fever (PN),
  xvii. Schirmer test for eye dryness, ocular staining (SS),
  xviii. biopsy: skin (PSS), muscle (PM), lesion (PN), labial salivary gland (SS), kidney (SLE), as often as necessary,
  xix. test of salivary flow and salivary scintiscan (SS) every 3 months,
  xx. EMG findings typical of PM every 3 months,
  xxi. angiography (PN) as often as necessary,
  and *once a month x3, then every 3months the following tests*:
    i. total lymphocytes,
    ii. T-lymphocytes (CD3),
    iii. T-helpers (CD4), T-suppressors (CD8) and CD4/CD8 ratio,
    iv. NK (CD16),
    v. B-lymphocytes (CD22 and CD19),
    vi. serum complement (CH50).

- **Special laboratory**: once a month or as often as necessary:
  i. rheumatoid factors (RA, SS, PSS, MCTD),
  ii. latex and bentonite tube dilution tests (RA),
  iii. synovial fluid testing (RA),
  iv. SS-B antibodies (against nuclear antigens) (SS),

v. LE cell preparation (SS, SLE, MCTD),
vi. antinuclear antibody ('ANA') (SLE, PSS, MCTD),
vii. circulating antinuclear antibody to nuclear nucleoprotein antigen (MCTD),
viii. anti-DNA antibodies (SLE, MCTD),
ix. partial thromboplastin time (SLE),
x. anticardiolipin antibodies (SLE),
xi. antibodies to thymic nuclear antigen PM-1, thymic nuclear extract Jo-1(PM),
xii. serum creatin kinase (PM),
xiii. C-reactive protein (SLE).

Frequency of office visits: 4 weeks and 48 hours before stem cell xenotransplantation, 24 hours and then once a week for the first month after stem cell xenotransplantation, and once a month thereafter.

Repeated stem cell transplantation are to be carried as often as clinical course requires maintaining the function of all components of the immune system at a normal or near-normal level.

Chapter 52

Truth is on the march and nothing can stop it.
Emile Zola, 1840 – 1902 [Article in le Figaro, 1897]

Civilization is the progress toward a society of privacy. The savage's whole existence is public, ruled by the laws of his tribe. Civilization is the progress of setting man free from men.
Ayn Rand, 1905 – 1955 [The Fountainhead 1943]

CANCER TREATMENT

Cancer is a disease of the whole organism, physical, mental and spiritual, even if still localized, i.e. without metastases. *The growth of cancer is a regression from the differentiated cell to the non-differentiated state, or from adult to the embryonal stage of development.*

All higher organisms start their lives from one fertilized cell. *As long as there is no connection to the blood, and so there is a lack of oxygen, cells of the developing embryo divide without differentiation.* After nidation of the product of conception in the endometrium at the stage of morula, the oxygen supply starts to develop, and that *triggers the differentiation of up until then uniform embryonic cells into specific tissues and organs.*

Cancer is a regression to the 'pre-nidation stage of division without differentiation'.

Disturbed relationship of Krebs cycle, normally providing 80% of energy supply for the human body, *to* the evolutionary ancient *glycolysis*, normally supplying 20% of energy, is probably the most important cause of the regression of mature differentiated tissue into the immature, undifferentiated, embryonic, tissue of cancer. When the supply of energy via Krebs cycle drops to such a low level that certain part of the normal tissue starts to cover larger than normal part of its energetic needs by glycolysis, that part of tissue switches back into the state of division without differentiation, as it was in the early embryonic stage, and undifferentiated cells easily transform into malignant ones.

Cancerous tissue is an immature, developmentally regressed tissue. Biologically thinking, cancer therapists believe that it is more rational to stimulate this developmentally regressed tissue and give it all support necessary for its maturation and differentiation, because only by differentiation it is possible to re-integrate the cancerous tissue back into the normal organization of the body. Despite some success rate, it appears *illogical to aim the entire therapeutic effort at destruction of the undifferentiated immature cancer cell* with treatment methods that damage healthy tissue, including the immune system, along with the cancer.

Julius Cohnheim, an assistant of Rudolf Virchow, the father of modern pathology, proposed in 1877 an embryonic theory of cancer, whereby cancerous tumor originated from small clusters of embryonic cells which remained unchanged during the development of an organism. In other words, cancer cell is an embryonic cell deprived of an ability to participate in normal embryogenesis, or 'oncogenesis is a blocked ontogenesis'.

Pregnancy is a state of natural parabiosis, i.e. tolerance between two genetically different organisms. Similarities between the functional processes of cancer and the development of embryo have given growing support to this theory, i.e. let's consider what we have learned about oncogenes, growth factors, cell differentiation, etc. Malignant tumors synthesize and release into blood many embryo-specific, and trophoblast-specific, proteins, i.e. α-fetoprotein, carcino-embryonic antigen (CEA), enzymes typical of embryo, many reproductive hormones, i.e. chorionic gonadotropin (HCG), etc.

Organism's immune response to cancer antigens is remarkably similar to its response to an embryo. There are many reports of cross reactions between embryonic and cancer antigens. It is because antigens from fetal tissues, and from malignant tumors, have many common determinants. Onco-fetal antigens are probably evolutionary predecessors of MHC antigens.

So cancer is a 'pathologic embryo', which copies the immune reactions occurring during pregnancy. The biochemical similarities of cancer and embryonic cells have been recognized for many years. Cytoplasm of cancer cells has an embryonic type of organization. Cancer cells copy the key biologic mechanism: ability to reproduce. *Task of treatment of cancer is to create a level of immune reactions characteristic of a spontaneous abortion.*

Malignant properties of cancerous tumors, i.e. invasive growth, unrestricted rapid mitoses, metastases, *are natural functional characteristics of normal trophoblast development.* Embryo, trophoblast and cancer cells, utilize the same mechanisms to avoid immunologic recognition and lysis by effector cells. *Antigens of the developing embryo and trophoblast have exactly the same properties.*

Immunosuppression, as for example after organ transplantation, not only suppresses the rejection, but increases the risk of cancer development. On the other side, pregnancy protects, to a degree, against carcinogenesis. Appearance of cancer in human fetuses or newborns is extremely rare. So cancer can be regarded as a *disease of immunosuppressive reaction in the organism.*

Establishment of normal pregnancy requires not a mother's immunologic tolerance to embryo but an active immunological recognition of paternally inherited proteins in the products of conception. The recognition of MHC and MHC-like paternal antigens during pregnancy stimulates not the cytotoxic effector immunity but the suppressor immunity. So the *recognition of foreign antigens is not accompanied by elimination, but by a maintenance of genetically different cells.* The more active such recognition, the stronger the immunosuppression. Without this, the survival of trophoblast and placenta, or pregnancy-specific immunosuppressive mechanism, is impossible. A deficiency of immunosuppressive mechanism leads to a rejection of the fetus, but the rejection of the cancer as well.

Cancer cells, as well as embryonic cells, frequently do not express class I MHC molecules, and that explains how they escape the immune surveillance.

Lymphocytes of pregnant women react positively to cancer antigens in leukocyte adherence inhibition (LAI) test and similarly the lymphocytes of cancer patients react positively to antigens of embryonic tissues.

Immunosuppression during pregnancy is accomplished through *the joint activity of maternal lymphocytes and humoral products of fetal and placental origin*. Even though *fetal portion of placenta is not genetically identical to the maternal portion*, the placenta is never rejected by the mother. Paternal MHC antigens of fetal portion are not targets for maternal lymphocytes, and rosette cell formation by allogeneic lymphocytes, T-cell response to phytohemagglutinine, or Concavalin A, and other mitogens, are inhibited. Likewise is inhibited the ability of lymphocytes to produce Migration Inhibition Factors (MIF) lymphokines, LAI factors, etc.

Unlike in controlled *in vitro* experiments, lymphocytes with many different functional activities are present in the blood. *In vitro* experiments cannot take into consideration all factors that may affect immunity, and thereby studies of immune regulatory reactions in cancer reveal a lot of contradictory data.

There are *tumor products recognized by the host's immune system that do not cause tumor rejection*. It is related to induction of suppressor T-lymphocytes, decreased level of T-helpers, and autologous serum blocking factors in cancer patients. *Recognition of tumor antigens by the patient's immune system occurs simultaneously with serum suppression of effector mechanisms of cell immunity.*

Cancer is a self-sufficient pathology, capable of neutralizing any number of cytotoxic lymphocytes. Therapeutic effect can be achieved by *inhibition of immunosuppressive properties of embryo-like functions of malignant cells*. In other words, besides an augmentation of the host's immune system, which may weaken to the level of a general anergy in the patients with advanced metastatic cancer, it is necessary to *destroy the 'immunity' of cancer*, not the cancer cells. Destruction of cancer immunity is most important particularly in the early stages of cancer when the immune system functions still well, so that there is no urgent need to support it.

Stimulating the function of T-lymphocytes does not decrease the activity of immunosuppressive products released by the malignant degeneration. This must be remembered in biological treatment of cancer.

Common features of immune reactivity in pregnancy and in cancer are concerned with the presence of characteristic sensitization to embryo antigens and *inhibition of such reaction by serum*. While endogenous immunosuppression serves to protect the embryo in pregnancy, such suppression supports the pathological process in cancer: it distorts the effector immunity. Without eliminating such immunosuppression it is difficult to inhibit the growth of malignant tumor.

Anti-suppression effect can be achieved by a tissue with a high concentration of blocking substances, found for example in chorionic villi that effectively blocks all reactions of cell immunity. *Implantation of trophoblastic cells triggers the production of anti-suppressive antibodies by B-cells of cancer patient*, which neutralize many embryo-like products of cancer cells. Such antibodies form complexes with serum blocking factors, with immunosuppressive agents fixed on circulating lymphocytes and tumor cells. The *complexes of anti-suppressive antibodies and serum blocking substances* are eliminated from the organism probably through liver, (and for that reason a close observation of patients with cancer metastases to the liver is very important after stem cell transplantation). That arms the effector lymphocytes of the patient, while the *neutralization of the suppressor products on the surface of cancer cells* makes them more vulnerable targets for NK cells and cytotoxic lymphocytes.

Implantation of trophoblastic cells causes a direct anti-cancer effect. The greatest *de-blocking effect* is due to antibodies against humoral suppressor products, antibodies against suppressor lymphocytes, and activation of counter-suppressors. By weakening the protective mechanisms of cancer, or tumor immunity, the host's effector immunity realizes its anti-tumor potential with less difficulty.

In 1902 John Beard published in Lancet "Embryological Aspects and Etiology of Carcinoma", his trophoblastic theory of cancer, whereby cancer is a trophoblast tissue that deviated from the proper development by departing from the placenta and dispersing throughout the body. Histological diversity of tumor types can be related to the activation of some genes of somatic nature within cancer cells.

Trophoblast components are inevitable for any malignant tumor. They assure cancer implantation, its trophic support, and invasive growth. Many malignant tumors produce trophoblast-specific hormones, and immunosuppressive substances that defend the cancer against the host immune system.

The initial layer of trophoblast, facing the blastocyst cavity, is cytotrophoblast, a homogenous epithelium with frequent mitoses, relatively poorly differentiated, while the external layer, developing later, is syncytiotrophoblast, with rare mitoses, and a lack of MHC antigen [333].

Principles of biological cancer treatment:

1. Ecological, nutritional and lifestyle modifications, to create an optimal lifestyle, eliminate all noxious elements, etc.

2. Oxygenation, to increase the participation of Krebs cycle in providing for the energy needs up to the normal 80% level, and that includes physical activity and exercise, various forms of oxygen therapy, including hyperbaric oxygen, as well as an improvement of enzyme function of all metabolic pathways, including the respiratory electron transport chain in mitochondria, *by stem cell transplantation*, along with intake of all co-enzymes.

3. Precursor stem cell transplantation that directs de-differentiated cancerous cells back toward natural re-maturation. The effect of stem cell transplantation is tumor-specific and dose-dependent, i.e. primary malignant cell determines the choice of cell type to be used for stem cell transplantation.

4. Stem cell transplantation for direct stimulation of the immune system that fails in its function of immune surveillance, usually as a result of previous orthodox cancer treatments. Stem cell transplants of *thymus, liver, spleen*, are most important for such purpose. Splenocytes of pregnant mother suppress specifically the generation of cytotoxic lymphocytes.

5. Selective stimulation of T-cell activity, such as by transfer factor (see in this book), implantation of autologous or non-autologous dendritic cells or dendritic cell vaccines, passive lymphocyte transfer, etc.

6. Change of antigen structure of cancer cells, by heterogenization *in vitro*, using hyperthermia, deep freezing, etc., and return into the host organism.

7. Lowering the cancer cell count by plasmapheresis: the fewer cancer cells are present in the body of a patient, the greater is the chance of success of stem cell transplantation treatment.

8. Implantation of trophoblastic cells of chorionic villi eliminates blocking factors from the blood of cancer patient.

9. Treatment must be highly individualized.

Stem cell transplantation has to be repeated every 3 to 6 months, as necessary, depending upon the follow-up findings, i.e. therapeutic program is modified to fit the condition of an individual patient.

The biological cancer therapy does not exclude the orthodox treatment of cancer but modifies it:

1. Surgery is limited strictly to the excision of the necrotic center of the tumor. This 'debulking' is quite important at the beginning of cancer treatment to get rid of the 'biologically dead' tissue, that is indeed dead if you would measure its electromagnetic field. The dead tissue is beyond the reach of any treatment. Radical excision with wide margins of healthy tissue must be avoided. It should be noted that old experts of *zellentherapie* believed that cancerous growth of stomach, pancreas, gallbladder and prostate, should never be operated upon.

2. Radiation must be avoided except when 'debulking' is necessary in cases of the advanced dissemination of cancer of hematopoietic and lymphatic systems, when the diagnosis was established too late and the spread of cancerous cells became so massive by then, that the normal cells of those, and other tissues, are 'suffocated' by the cancerous cells. Radiation treatment decreases the effectiveness of stem cell transplantation against cancer, but not as much as chemotherapy.

3. Chemotherapy must be used in lower quantities that do not destroy immune system and other healthy tissue, and do not intoxicate organism. During chemotherapy cancer cells bind molecules of cytotoxic drugs and anti-cancer effect of stem cell transplantation, particularly of trophoblastic cells, is noticeably decreased. After a high dose chemotherapy, stem cell transplantation should be delayed for as long as 3 months, and a minimum of 4 weeks.

4. Stem cell transplantation of *mesenchyme, thymus, spleen, liver, adrenal cortex*, is recommended for immunostimulation, along with *hypothalamus*.

If you give a sufficiently high dose stem cell transplantation of liver and spleen to the patient with any *leukemia*, the typical leukemoid pattern disappears from the blood count and blood smear in 2 – 3 days.

Stem cell transplantation of *mesenchyme, thymus, spleen, liver, mesenterial lymphnodes*, is advised for *Hodgkin's disease*.

In the real world, there are hardly any patients with cancer that received treatment in accordance with above rules. All cancer patients that have ever had stem cell transplantation, have had it after the usual oncologic treatment failed to control their disease and they began to desperately look for something else to save their life. The majority of such patients are still undergoing some form of standard oncologic treatment at the time of their consultation with cell transplantologist.

It is difficult to combine the orthodox cancer therapy with the biological treatment method:

a. Stem cell transplantation must not be used while the patient is taking chemotherapy up until the time the effect of the medications subsides, i.e. ideally 3 months, or when the patient is scheduled to be treated by chemotherapy before the implantation of stem cell transplants, because cytostatica damage implanted stem cell transplants.

b. For the same reason there must be an interval between the implantation of stem cell transplants and beginning of radiation treatment, or between the completion of irradiation and implantation of stem cell transplants, ideally 6 months.

In this situation, it is extremely difficult to create a workable treatment scheme, particularly for patients with advanced cancer, or those with complications of cell destructive therapies.

Due to their direct immunostimulatory effect, the cell transplantation, particularly of *mesenchyme, and thymus*, has been a very useful component of anti-cancer therapy [262].

The case histories of eight patients with advanced cancer, 3 cases of breast cancer, 2 cases of lung cancer, 2 cases of rectal cancer, and one of malignant leiomyoma of tongue, show how to successfully combine cell transplantation with the traditional oncological treatment of surgery, radiation and chemotherapy. Such adjuvant treatment of cancer by cell transplantation apparently prevents the weakening of the immune system caused by chemotherapy and radiotherapy via its immunostimulatory effect. Postoperative adjuvant cell transplantation inhibits the formation of metastases, can reduce their size, or causes them to regress. *Cell transplantation is recommended even in cases of inoperable cancer, as it significantly improves the tolerance of cytostatica* [283].

Lyophilized celltherapeutic preparation of fetal mesenchyme has been used with success as an adjuvant in the treatment of many patients suffering from a variety of cancers that were beyond help of traditional oncology. Case histories of 10 such patients are presented and discussed in this report. Only one patient, who began treatment in moribund condition, at the weight of 35 kg, died of his cancer, at the weight of 52 kg. All other patients lived in remission for the duration of their follow-up [284].

A randomized prospective study was conducted to determine the effect of additional immunostimulation with lyophilized celltherapeutic preparation of fetal mesenchyme, as compared with intensified chemotherapy, in 52 females with recurrent breast cancer treated by radiation and a cocktail of five chemotherapeutic agents. In a group of 24 patients taking implantations of fetal mesenchyme, 9 died, while in a group of 28 patients with intensified chemotherapy, 14 died during a follow-up of 24 months. In another concurrent study, 20 patients with skin and bony metastases were treated by fetal mesenchyme on average 13 times, and the treatment did not cause any significant complications [285].

A 64 year old male became ill 4 years before this report. Four months later an infiltrating adenocarcinoma of minor and major curvature of stomach, pancreas, with metastases of the size of mandarine in both right and left lobe of liver, was resected, leaving many metastases in the liver and mesenterial lymphonodes behind. The patient was given four months to live. The family decided not to inform the patient of his condition and refused any chemotherapy. Biological therapy began 7 weeks after cancer surgery. During the next 24 months the patient received cell transplantation many times: *mesenchyme 18x, thymus 12x, spleen 5x, bone marrow x3, liver twice*, as well as four treatment by Endoxan 250 mg daily for 6 weeks. It took 3 ½ months to see any benefit of such treatment, and during this time the patient's weight dropped from 150 to 110 lb. The patient grew desperate, until one morning he reported that he feels healthy again, the night sweats disappeared, good appetite is back, his big abdomen (due to ascites) is gone, and pain in his spine became bearable. The patient returned back to normal life. CT scan of abdomen was carried out after the last cell transplantation, and there was no evidence of any cancer anywhere, and the same applied to chest x-rays [310].

There are a growing number of reports in peer reviewed journals from the leading oncologic centers, that can be found on MEDLINE, on the success of new therapeutic protocols that encompass conservative cancer surgery, radiation therapy limited to a total of 30 cGy, chemotherapy dosage decreased by 70%, as compared with standard dosages, and stem cell transplantation.

Chapter 53

> Time present and time past
> Are both perhaps present in time future,
> And time future contained in time past.
> *[Four Quartets. Burnt Norton, 1935]*
>
> The only wisdom we can help to acquire
> Is the wisdom of humility: humility is endless.
> *[East Coker, 1940]*
> Thomas Stearns Eliot, 1888 – 1965

HEMATOLOGICAL DISEASES

Hematopoietic tissue, in adulthood in red bone marrow, at fetal stage of development in liver and spleen, contains pluripotent stem cells, which under the influence of hematopoietic growth factors differentiate into erythroid, myeloid and lymphoid precursors. These stem cells replicate themselves, so that their count is maintained the same during the entire life.

While lymphocytes originating from lymphoid precursors require additional 'upbringing' in thymus and bone marrow, and later on are produced not only in bone marrow but also in the spleen and lymphnodes, all other precursor cells proliferate and mature in the bone marrow, and they enter blood from there. These processes are influenced by two renal hormones: *erythropoietin*, necessary for proliferation and maturation of erythrocytes, and *thrombopoietin* for proliferation and maturation of megakaryocytes and thrombocytes.

Mature erythrocytes are without nucleus and cell organelles. Their lifespan is 110 – 120 days, as compared with neutrophil granulocytes which differentiate from precursors in 7 days but their lifespan is only 10 hours.

Stem cell transplantation is of no use to treat disorders of mature erythrocytes. But it can *treat* **disturbances of erythropoiesis**, that normally takes 7 days, with a speed of production of 1.6 million of erythrocytes per second, such as:

1. *insufficient quantity or quality of hematopietic stem cells*, i.e. aplastic anemia, with panmyelopathy, or acute myeloid leukemia,

2. *temporary*, i.e. due to viral infection, *or chronic lack of erythroid precursors* caused by antibodies against erythropoietin, or against membrane proteins of precursor cells,

3. *lack of erythropoietin* due to renal insufficiency,

4. *activation of erythropoiesis suppressing interleukins* by chronic inflammations and tumors,

5. *disorders of cell differentiation* caused by gene defects, lack of folic acid (reserve in liver for 2 – 4 months) or lack of vitamin B12 (reserve in liver for 3 years),

6. failure of hemoglobin synthesis.

Genetic disorders of hemoglobin (Hb) *are the most common single gene disorder.* According to the World Health Organization 5% of world population suffers from various genetic disorders of hemoglobin, and approximately 300,000 severely disabled homozygotes are born every year.

An 80 year old female suffered from recurrent epistaxis, as a result of unsuccessful surgery for nasal septal deviation, and thereby caused persistent anemia, which was diagnosed by bone marrow biopsy as aplastic because the patient's bone marrow could no longer compensate chronic blood loss. In 1982 alone, the patient received 57 blood transfusions. In December 1982, the 1st cell transplantation of *mesenchyme, spleen, liver, bone marrow*, was carried out. In 1983, the patient received 25 blood transfusions, and in November 1983, the 2nd cell transplantation of *mesenchyme, liver, placenta, adrenal cortex, bone marrow*, was done. In 1984, the patient received 17 blood transfusions, and in November 1984, cell transplanttation of *mesenchyme, placenta, liver, bone marrow, osteoblasts*, was carried out. In January 1985, the patient received 4 blood transfusions, but none for the next 13 months, and in February 1986, the blood count was normal. In February 1986, as a result of severe influenza, the aplastic anemia became active again and patient received two units of packed red cells, followed by cell transplantation of *mesenchyme, placenta, liver, bone marrow, osteoblasts*. Since that time the patient has been well [302].

Genetic disorders of hemoglobin are divided into three groups:

1. **Structural hemoglobin variants with qualitative abnormality**, i.e. structural abnormality of polypeptide chains of globin molecules, which amount to about 700.

    Sickle cell anemia (*drepanocytosis*), AR disorder, occurs in Equatorial Africa, and to some degree in Mediterranean region and central India. Substitution of one of 146 aminoacids in the β-chain of Hb A by a point mutation creates Hb S. This new hemoglobin, different in its physical and chemical properties from Hb A, causes deformation of erythrocytes into a sickle or demi-moon shape. Sickling of erythrocytes is observed only in homozygotes, *solely under lower oxygen pressure as found in capillaries and venules*. In homozygotes the severe form of the disease occurs: chronic hemolytic anemia with crises caused by obstruction of blood vessels and painful infarcts in various tissues, such as bones, spleen, lungs. Heterozygotes, i.e. carriers of 'sickle cell trait', AD disorder, are asymptomatic, but have a partially increased resitance to Plasmodium falciparum, because HbS makes replication of this parasites in erythrocytes difficult.

    A 10 year old Turkish boy, diagnosed with sickle cell anemia at the age of 5, was brought to the hospital in Germany at the age of 9 ½ from Turkey in moribund condition, with sepsis, pronounced anemia and no response to any treatment. His height was 132 cm, and weight 18 kg. There was an extreme cachexia, leg ulcers, bilateral basal pneumonia, hepatomegaly, Hb 4.8g%, Hct 27.2, Erythrocytes 1.76 million, anisocytosis, poikilocytosis, and many sickle cells. Stabilization of clinical state by transfusion of whole blood and erythrocyte concentrates was obtained, but sepsis continued unabated. Cell transplantation of *spleen and bone marrow* was carried out and in 3 days fever of over 40 °C finally subsided. The same cell transplants were implanted two more times 4 weeks apart. Skeletal abnormalities were corrected within 6 weeks; patient gained 8 kg, and after 4 months was sent home. There were no sickle cell crises during the next two years [288].

2. ***Quantitative abnormality of hemoglobin***, i.e. where synthesis of structurally normal globin polypeptide chain is decreased or is absent, known as *thalassemias*.

α-thalassemias are usually caused by a major deletion from α-globin gene, which leads to a *blockage of synthesis of α-chain*, which affects production of Hb A, Hb F, and Hb A_2. Patients suffer from microcytic anemia, icterus, splenomegaly with hypersplenism, as well as frequent infections, ulcus cruris, cholelithiasis, and folic acid insufficiency. *α-thalassemia with faulty α-chain leads to death in utero since HbF cannot be produced.*

β-thalassemias are caused by a point mutation in the sole gene for β-globin chain. In homozygotes a serious anemia appears during the 1st – 2nd year of life since faulty β-chain causes a lack of HbA. In untreated children growth retardation, icterus, and hepatosplenomegaly appear, as well as recurrent infections, cholelithiasis, and ulcus cruris. In untreated children, by the age of 10 – 11, there are hepatic, cardiac, and endocrinologic disorders, as well as growth retardation and delay of sexual maturation due to hemochromatosis. Cell transplantation of *spleen, liver, placenta*, is advised, if necessary.

3. ***Genetically caused persistence of fetal Hb***, which is clinically insignificant.

Hemoglobin consists of four subunits and each of them is produced from three components:

    a. protoporphyrin, the lack of which is due to inborn enzymopathies known as porphyrias, or hereditary sideroblastic anemia,
    b. iron: Fe^{2+},
    c. globin.

Properties of Hb depend upon the sequence of aminoacids; 141 in α-chain, 146 in β-chain. Replacement of a single aminoacid by another one leads to sickle cell anemia, where HbS in its deoxygenated form aggregates, which causes a sickle shape of erythrocytes. Such erythrocytes are inflexible and cannot pass through capillaries, and thereby cause an obstruction of small vessels. HbS aggregation takes a few seconds so that obstruction takes place mainly in capillaries with long passage time, i.e. spleen, vasa recta in renal medulla. With systemic slowdown of blood flow, i.e. shock, or with hypoxia, i.e. high altitude, airplane flight, general anesthesia, obstruction can involve other organs, i.e. heart. Blood vessel obstruction causes further drop of pO_2 and thereby additional 'sickling', and a 'vicious circle', or 'crisis', develops.

Hemoglobin can be lost from erythrocytes directly into blood, and this free hemoglobin is destined for degradation. This accounts for about 10% of hemoglobin that is degraded daily. The rest of Hb is broken down when old erythrocytes are removed by the cells of reticulo-endothelial system, i.e. histiocytes, certain splenic cells. Haptoglobin binds Hb in 1:1 ratio, and this complex is quickly taken up by the liver and broken down: in this way iron found in Hb can be preserved.

About 200 billion erythrocytes are broken down per day under normal circumstances, representing the release of about 25 mg of iron, or the volume of 20 mL of erythrocytes.

In principle, stem cell transplantation of *stomach/intestine, intestine, bone marrow, exocrine pancreas, placenta*, is advised for the treatment of aplastic anemias.

Pernicious anemia is due to the lack of intrinsic factor, glycoprotein secreted by stomach mucosa, that binds the vitamin B12, also known as extrinsic factor) from food. The complex of intrinsic factor plus extrinsic factor enters the intestine, and there are receptors in the terminal ileum that recognize the complex so that absorption can take place. Pernicious anemia is caused by the atrophy of gastric mucosa that can be due to autoimmune disease.

Hemolytic anemias: Erythrocytes live 120 days when their flexibility, osmotic and mechanical resistance, redox potential and energy production are normal; if abnormal, their survival is shortened, sometimes to a few days, and they are eliminated prematurely.

Causes of corpuscular hemolytic anemias are:

- **defects of cell membrane** causing hereditary spherocytosis: cytoskeletal defect bring about inability of erythrocytes to assume their normal flexible flat 'target-like' shape, they are

round instead, with lowered osmotic resistance, and thereby prematurely sequestered in spleen,
- ***enzyme defects that disrupt glucose metabolism of cells***, i.e. lack of pyruvatkinase slows down Krebs cycle and OXPHOS with ultimate deficiency of ATP; lack of glucose-6-phosphate-dehydrogenase slows down pentose-phosphate cycle due to which free SH-groups of enzymes and membrane proteins, and phospholipids, are not protected from oxidation, defect of hexokinase leads to the lack of ATP and reduced glutathione,
- ***sickle cell anemia and thalassemias***,
- ***inborn paroxysmal nocturnal hemoglobinuria*** with increased sensitivity of erythrocytes to complement, and resulting perforation of cell membrane.

Causes of extracorpuscular hemolytic anemias:

- ***mechanical damage***, i.e. heart valve or arterial prostheses,
- ***immunological*** *causes*: transfusion reaction, Rh-incompatibility between mother and fetus,
- ***toxic***, i.e. snake venoms.

Erythrocytes are phagocytized and digested in macrophages of bone marrow, liver and spleen, as usually.

Heme synthesis, porphyrias

In addition to utilization in the structure of hemoglobin, *heme is synthetized in nearly all organs* and built *into myoglobin, cytochrome P_{450}, catalase, peroxidase, cytochromes* of the respiratory chain. Lack of heme synthesis means absence of life.

Heme synthesis consists of eight reactions controlled by a heme via negative feedback. The outcome of disorders of heme synthesis depends upon this negative feedback. If lack of heme cannot stimulate sufficiently the activity of δ-ALA-synthase, a *sideroblastic anemia* develops.

Defects of the enzymes of successive 8 reactions via negative feedback cause an enormously increased availability of δ-aminolevulate, and thereby substrates for all subsequent reactions, leading to ***primary porphyrias***, with onset from birth until 20 years of age.

Depending upon their solubility in water or lipids, the intermediary substrates are eliminated via urine, which turns red, or via bile.

Acute intermittent porphyria is due to lowered activity of porfobilinogen-desaminase. There are neurovisceral dysfunctions: tachycardia, nausea, emesis, constipation, and nervous and psychic disorders: pareses, seizures, coma, and hallucinations.

Congenital erythropoietic porphyria is due to excess of uroporphyrinogen I, and from that also of coproporphyrinogen I, both of which do not metabolize further and stain diapers red, and later on also teeth of the patient. There is photosensitivity and hemolytic anemia.

Porphyria cutanea tarda, rather frequent, where due to light absorption ($\lambda=440$ nm) by porphyrins the O_2-radicals are created that damage skin, and non-healing vesicles appear.

Hereditary coproporphyria, with increased levels of δ-ALA and porfobilinogen, causes nervous, psychic and skin symptoms in children.

Protoporphyria is characterized by photosensitivity with burning, itching, skin pain, that follows UV exposure.

Primary hemochromatosis, AR disorder with incidence 1:400, is more common in men, since women lose iron during menstruation. There is a markedly increased absorption of iron in the intestine, serum iron is higher, as well as transferrine iron content. Excessive accumulation of iron in the body, in the parenchymatous cells of liver, pancreas, and other organs, is toxic for cells, with participating creation of oxygen radicals, DNA damage, increased collagen production. If liver fibrosis and cirrhosis develop, the risk of hepatocellular carcinoma grows 200x. Pancreatic fibrosis, caused by siderosis, causes lack of insulin and diabetes mellitus. Accumulation of melanin and hemosiderin in sun exposed skin causes '*bronze diabetes*'. Siderosis causes in myocardium a cardiomyopathy with arrhythmias, and heart failure, with fatal outcome in young patients. Treatment is by phlebotomy once a week for 1 – 2 years. If diagnosed early, stem cell transplantation of *intestine, liver, spleen, placenta, exocrine pancreas, cardiomyoblasts*, is advised.

Disturbances of hemostasis

System of hemostasis protects against bleeding and blood loss. It consists of plasma factors, platelets and vessel wall. *Hemorrhagic diathesis is due to dysfunctions of coagulation or fibrinolytic system, platelets, or vascular wall defects.*

Plasma factors are globular proteins of variable molecular weight. Plasmatic disturbances cause common hematomas and intraarticular bleeding, while damaged platelets and vessel wall are the cause of petechiae.

Hemophilia A, the most frequent genetic disorder of hemocoagulation, is XR disorder with incidence of 1:5,000 to 1:10,000 in newborn boys. Lack of factor VIII, co-factor for the activation of Factor X, vitally important in the hemocoagulation cascade, is the result of faulty genes. Bleeding is most commonly localized in muscles and large joints of lower extremities, which are usually deformed: hemophilic arthropathy.

In Hemophilia A, the risk is 5 – 10 times higher if the maternal grandfather was over 40 years of age at the time of conception: since sons are getting chromosome Y from their fathers, mutation of gene for factor VIII must take place in maternal grandfather's body, and then chromosome X is transmitted via the patient's mother.

Hemophilia B occurs in 1:70,000 of newborn boys, and is due to a lack of Factor IX.

Genetic thromboembolic diseases are the third most common group of acute diseases with lethal outcome, after myocardial infarction and cerebrovascular accident. They must be considered in repeated thromboembolic episodes in younger patients, in several members of the same family, or with involvement of unusual organs or tissues, and inadequate response to anticoagulants.

The process of coagulation is controlled by two groups of inhibitors:

1. System of Protein C:
Activated Protein C resistance due to a mutation in heavy chain FV (Factor V Leiden), present in 3 – 6 % of Europeans, causes thrombofilia predominantly in venous system, and is responsible for approximately 1/3 of all thromboembolic episodes, increased risk of deep venous thrombosis 30 – 140x in homozygotes, as well as of ileofemoral thrombosis, pulmonary embolism, internal carotid artery embolism, etc., particularly where there is a trigger, such as injury, etc.

2. Inhibitors of serine proteases:
There can be either their malfunction or an absence of antithrombin III with a loss of inhibition of coagulation factors IIa, IXa, and Xa in plasma.

Acquired coagulopathies are due to liver damage since most plasmatic factors are produced in the liver, or due to hypersplenism, where blood cells are sequestered.

Hemorrhagic diathesis due to platelet disorder develops when production of platelets is limited, or when their breakdown is increased.

Idiopathic thrombocytopenic purpura, or Werlhof disease, is an acute illness appearing 1 – 3 weeks after virus infection, while a chronic illness is an autoimmune disease. A 62 years old female suffered of this illness for 42 years, and was hospitalized numerous times for skin and mucosal bleeding, menorhagia, splenomegaly. Cell transplantation of *osteoblasts, bone marrow and placenta*, was carried out. Spontaneous bleeding stopped in a few weeks and blood platelet count became normal. Three years later the patient was hospitalized with acute cholecystitis and her physician was surprised to find no evidence of thrombocytopenia. Patient died 12 years later of congestive heart failure, but without any bleeding for the last 15 years of her life [301].

Inborn thrombocytopenic purpura is AD or AR platelet disorder due to:
- *membrane defects*, i.e. Bernard-Soulier syndrome or Glanzmann-Naegeli thrombasthenia,
- *various defects of secretion or storage*.

Acquired thrombocytopenia develops with uremia and with dysproteinemias.

Thrombocytopenic purpura due to blood vessel damage includes:
- various forms of hereditary ***von Willebrand disease***, with vascular endothelial defect and lack of von Willebrand factor, that leads to dysfunction of platelet adhesion and secondarily a lack of Factor VIII, i.e. von Willebrand Factor is a carrier of Factor VIII,
- inborn ***purpura simpex, Osler-Weber-Rendu disease, Schoenlein-Henoch purpura***, or acquired scorbut from lack of vitamin C.

Dissolution of excessive thrombi is carried out by fibrinolytic system. Disturbances are either genetic or acquired.

Disorders of hemostasis have rarely been treated by stem cell transplantation due to the availability of various blood transfusion products. Treatment of genetic thromboembolic diseases by stem cell transplantation should be investigated.

Blood represents 7% of body weight minus fat.

Chapter 54

> Without a shepherd sheep are not a flock.
> *Russian Proverb*

TREATMENT OF RADIATION INJURIES

At the 1st symposium on transplantation of human fetal tissues in Moscow, December 4 – 7, 1995, we presented a report about treatment by cell transplantation of three patients suffering extensive soft tissue injury as a result of carrying containers with radioisotopes on their body for a prolonged period of time, at the Russian Research Center of Biophysics of Russian Academy of Medical Sciences in Moscow. According to all medical knowledge, there was no hope for healing post-irradiation ulcers by any known therapy in all three cases. All three patients healed after cell transplantation.

The same treatment was used for treatment of indolent ulcers after therapeutic radiation at Research Center of Medical Radiology of Russian Academy of Medical Sciences in Obninsk. Every patient responded to cell transplantation by a complete healing.

Systemic therapy of radiation injuries requires stem cell transplantation of *skin, stomach/duodenum, intestine, colon ,mesenchyme, placenta, and thymus, adrenal cortex*, for infection prevention, as well as *hypothalamus, medulla alba of brain, mesencephalon*, in case of CNS involvement.

Chapter 55

All psychical acts without exception, if they are not complicated by elements of emotion ... develop by way of reflex. Hence, all conscious movements resulting from these acts and usually described as voluntary, are reflex movements in the strict sense of the term.

The initial cause of any action lies in external sensory stimulation, because without this thought is inconceivable.
Ivan Mikhailovich Sechenov, 1829 – 1905 [Reflexes of the Brain, 1863]

DISEASES OF CENTRAL NERVOUS SYSTEM

A treatment of advanced **Parkinson's disease** no longer responsive to L-dopa therapy by implantation of human fetal brain cells into the patient's brain, became a landmark in history of stem cell transplantation when a series of such surgical procedures was carried out in Mexico City in 1980's. A term *neurotransplantation* was coined for such treatment.

Treatment of neurological diseases has always been a sad chapter of medicine due to a lack of effective therapy for a great majority of illnesses.

Here Parkinson's disease has been a bright exception because of availability of L-dopa therapy that controls symptoms of the disease quite well for several years. Ultimately, every patient with Parkinson's disease reaches a stage when medications that stimulate production of dopamine by neurons of the basal ganglia of the brain lose effectiveness, whereupon disability becomes severe. Ideally, before that happens, each patient is to receive stem cell transplantation.

But neurotransplantation treatment of Parkinson's disease has not been as successful in clinical practice, with a rate of success 2 - 3 %, as under experimental conditions, with a success rate better than 95%. Such enormous discrepancy between the high success of neurotransplantation in animal experiment and minimal success in clinical practice is unusual. Some of the reasons are known.

The US National Institutes of Health clinical trial completed in 1994, ended in a failure. Scientists believed that the reason was that the neurons in adult human brain and spinal cord could not recover from serious damage, and once absent, could not be replaced. Part of the problem was that researchers were more concerned about fulfilling requirements of double-blind study, including unethical and immoral 'sham surgery', than to help severely disabled patients. Stem cell transplantation, used predominantly for the treatment of untreatable or incurable diseases, is hardly suitable for 'double-blind' clinical studies. And the price tag was very high, in particular when also patients receiving sham surgery had to pay the same amount.

Our BCRO/IIBM team in Moscow devoted an enormous amount of time and energy to find the reasons for the reported failures of neurotrans-plantation in clinical practice worldwide. Under the leadership of S.V. Savel'ev, an excellent comparative embryologist, an extensive experimental research was carried out, and based on that eventually several patients with advanced Parkinson's disease were treated by our method of neurotransplantation.

Based on our analysis the following rules were set:

1. it is mandatory to transplant cells with known and firmly pre-determined properties of establishing synaptic connection with neurons of the host, and human embryonic or fetal brain cells *do not possess such properties by themselves*,
2. transplanted cells must be highly metabolically active, and again human embryonic or fetal brain cells *alone cannot fulfill such requirement*,
3. transplanted cells must be genetically strongly pre-set in the direction of their differentiation, and be independent of environmental influences, and here again human embryonic or fetal cells from the anterior portion of mesencephalon *do not qualify because they are pluripotent*.

Experiments with xeno-neurotransplantation between non-vertebrates and vertebrates, and with xeno- and allo-neurotransplantation between various species of mammals, showed, that *xenotransplants survived in the host brain three times longer than allo-transplant. Xenoneurotransplantation between genetically discordant species was much more successful than between genetically concordant species.*

Primordial brain cells of various genetic mutants of Drosophila melanogaster fulfilled the above three requirements the best, and their neurotransplantation into brain of various vertebrates, including mammals, was unusually successful. Genom of Drosophila had been known in detail for a number of years so that it was not difficult to select the mutants with required properties of the primordial brain cells. The selected mutants survived in the mammalian brain for a minimum of 2 – 3 months, and functioned as a stimulant of human embryonic stem cells, promoting their differentiation and vascularization, as well as *the growth of the host's neuronal processes toward the donor transplant, and vascularization of the adjacent host brain tissue.*

The mixture of human embryonic brain cells from ventral mesencephalon and basal ganglia and of primordial brain cells of the mutants of Drosophila melanogaster in the weight ratio of 50:1 or higher was prepared in the laboratory and then implanted under stereoscopic control into ventrolateral thalamic nuclei of patients.

Three of the several patients who were operated on, two of which had previous cryodestructive stereotactic procedures for Parkinson' disease, are described in the published paper. After 12 months follow-up, there was no recurrence of Parkinsonism. Our overall success was 95% [220].

As described in Chapter 2, another patient of this series died of unrelated cause 8 months later, and a full autopsy of his brain was carried out that proved the full success of described combined xeno-allo-neurotransplantation approach to the treatment of Parkinson's disease [221].

Treatment of diseases of the central nervous system by stem cell transplantation past childhood requires an implantation into the brain and spinal cord, even though not necessarily into the parenchyma of these organs. We advise strongly the *'intrathecal'* implantation, i.e. into the cerebrospinal fluid, vitally important for the function of central nervous system, that vigorously circulates in the preformed spaces around and in the brain and spinal cord, and is completely exchanged every 24 hours.

Our extensive experimental work on xeno-neurotransplantation in Moscow led to a discovery of clinical effectiveness of **'intrathecal' implantation**.

There are two approaches to intrathecal implantation of brain cell transplants in human medicine: via a lumbar puncture or via a 'ventricular tap'. Lumbar puncture implantation is technically simple for any properly trained physician, while ventricular tap is simple for a neurosurgeon.

It is the least traumatic method of neurotransplantation, as there is minimal trauma to the brain tissues of the patient in the course of intraventricular implantation, and no trauma whatsoever when stem cells are implanted via lumbar puncture.

Due to a very narrow connection between a system of four ventricles in the brain parenchyma and a subarachnoid space around the brain and spinal cord via foramina Magendie and Luschkae in the 4th ventricle, an opinionated discussion went on between two of our teams for some time. One group believed that intrathecal implantation via lumbar puncture is dangerous because cell clusters of cell transplants obstructs foramina Magendie and Luschkae and cause obstructive hydrocephalus. The other group believed that it cannot happen. Eventually, the matter was decided in favor of the 2nd group after 3 moribund patients post extensive cerebrovascular accidents were treated with intrathecal implantation of brain cell transplants prepared by our method, and then subjected to a detailed autopsy, and no evidence of obstructive hydrocephalus and a complete patency of foramina Magendie and Luschkae was found [244].

Subsequently, an intrathecal implantation was carried out on many patients suffering from a variety of degenerative neurological diseases, such as amyotrophic lateral sclerosis, multiple sclerosis, Friedreich's ataxia, other spino-cerebellar degenerations, Parkinson's disease, as well as patients in deep coma of various cause, so much so that at our First International symposium in December 1995, in Moscow, several presentations were made about the clinical results, and the total number of patients included in six different reports exceeded 400.

The initial published study of 14 patients, from 29 to 82 years of age, 7 females and 7 males, 4 with cerebrovascular accident, 4 with Parkinson's disease, 2 in coma after clinical death, 1 with toxic encephalopathy, 1 with vascular collapse, 1 with post-traumatic encephalopathy, 1 with Alzheimer's disease, all treated by intrathecal implantation of fetal brain cells via lumbar puncture, describes detailed case histories of 6 patients, and gives overall results. Only one patient had a negative result, i.e. lack of response: a 52 years old female with Alzheimer's disease. All other patients were improved, some spectacularly [244].

The first two patients survived a clinical death and were in deep coma.

A 29 year old female developed anaphylactic shock 30 seconds after I.M. Ampicillin. A resuscitation and intensive care restored spontaneous breathing, and improved cardiac function, but deep coma persisted. On the 16th day, an intrathecal implantation via lumbar puncture of 5 – 6 million of *brain cortex* cells was carried out. Around 18 hours later, the patient opened her eyes, recognized her mother, and began to answer questions in simple words. Left-sided hemiparesis, urinary and fecal incontinence, and dementia persisted. Gradual improvement was observed, and 10 weeks later, a 2nd intrathecal implantation of brain cortex cells was done. Two days later a dramatic improvement was observed by everyone. Athetoid movements of left hand and arm disappeared, spasticity on the left side substantially diminished, and an improvement of speech, reading, writing, comprehension, gait, EEG, was noted.

A 45 year old male was undergoing an uneventful surgery for retinal detachment of the left eye, when a few minutes before the end a sudden bradycardia and blood pressure loss were observed. After the recovery from an operation the patient remained in stupor, and akinesia with rigidity quickly and akinesia developed. On the 22nd day the patient was transferred to a psychiatric ward for rehabilitation of psychic functions. On the 25th day, an intrathecal implantation of *brain cortex and medulla alba of brain cells* was carried out. Two days later a dramatic improvement took place: speech improved, and so did writing, and drawing. Four months later, a 2nd intrathecal implantation was carried out to assure a continuous improvement.

A 36 year old male suffered a massive head injury in a car accident. There was a huge intracranial hematoma and AV malformation. The patient was left with left hemiplegia. Around 6 weeks later, epilepsy developed. A diagnosis of subdural hematoma was made. While the patient was under aggressive medical therapy, 16 months after the accident, an intrathecal implantation of ~ 12 million *fetal cells* of *brain cortex and medulla alba of brain* was carried out. Epilepsy disappeared, EEG slowly returned back to α rhythm, and there was a gradual improvement of neurologic findings.

A 39 year old female was treated for right hemiparkinsonism by L-dopa without any effect, when intrathecal implantation of cells of *basal ganglia* was carried out. At 3-month follow-up a dramatic improvement was noted. There was no tremor in the extremities, the function of right hand was normal, and gait improved. The effect has somewhat diminished subsequently, and 5 months after the first, the 2nd intrathecal implantation was performed. One month later again improvement was noted, tremor disappeared, gait and writing improved.

The other 3 patients with Parkinson's disease were improved as well: tremor, muscle hypertonia, mimicry, and writing, were all improved.

A 65 year old female suffered a cerebrovascular accident. Intrathecal implantation of *brain cortex cells* was carried out immediately. There was a dramatic improvement, so that *rehabilitation could begin 18 hours after intrathecal implantation of fetal brain cells, i.e. the next day after the stroke*. Two days later hemiplegia improved to the level of minor hemiparesis. On the 8th day the patient began to walk with a walker.

A 50 year old male survived an extensive cerebrovascular accident 2.5 years ago, and was left with hemiparesis, aphasia, and Jacksonian epilepsy. The patient received intrathecal implantation of approximately 12 million *brain cortex* cells. Three weeks later he observed an improvement of speech, writing, began to read, and count. Movements of right hand improved noticeably. EEG showed less epileptogenic activity [244].

Apallic syndrome is a persistent vegetative state after the loss of pallium function due to injury, poisoning or anoxia. There is a complete aphasia, apraxia and agnosia, decerebration rigidity, absent corneal reflex, absent papillary reflex, absent deglutition reflex, seizures, trophic disturbances, marasmus, and immune deficiency. CNS functions are reduced below those present at birth. Eyes are open, starring upward and sideways, or vacillating. Optical and acoustic stimuli are not registered. In all 33 patients, between one and 12 years of age, with coma of less than 12 months duration, cell transplantation terminated coma, and the conscious patient recovered with a residual neurological damage. The first step was the removal of all life supports, then implantation of stem cell transplants of *various parts of the brain, and placenta*, and specific metabolic stimulation, followed by peripheral training that took 5 – 6 years before speech and gross motor functions recovered [95].

The existing treatments of all degenerative diseases in contemporary medicine suffer from one common problem: no attempt at regeneration of degenerating cells of diseased organs and tissues is ever made. The sole treatment capable of direct stimulation of regeneration is stem cell transplantation. And that applies primarily to **degenerative diseases of central nervous system**.

In 1996, Diacrin Inc. carried out a clinical trial in which 12 patients with Parkinson's disease and subsequently 12 patients with **Huntington's chorea** underwent unilateral xeno-neurotransplantation of porcine fetal brain cells. The patients with Parkinon's disease received 12 million of *ventral mesencephalic cells*, while those with Huntington's chorea 24 million of cells from *striatum*.

At one year's follow-up, the Parkinson's disease patients had an average of 19% improvement in the Unified Parkinson's Disease Rating Scale 'off' state scores. Some patients had an improvement of as much as 30%. At one year's follow-up of Huntington's chorea patients, there was no change in the functional capacity [245].

In the above study of Parkinson's disease, six patients received an immunosuppression by cyclosporine, and six patients by a monoclonal antibody directed against MHC class I. There were no adverse effects. No transfer of endogenous viruses was detected [246].

One of the patients from the above Parkinson's disease study died of unrelated causes 7 months after the neurotransplantation. Histological analysis of the putamen-caudate nucleus area proved a graft survival: pig dopaminergic neurons, and other pig neurons and glial cells were present and pig axons extended axons from the graft site into the host brain [247].

There are many other neurodegenerative diseases besides Parkinson's disease and Huntington' chorea, and many of them are treatable by stem cell transplantation. Interestingly, there was a temporary success in the past in treatment of Parkinson's disease by cell transplantation without intrathecal implantation. Roeder handled 33 patients with bilateral Parkinson's disease, mostly after previous stereotactic operations on basal ganglia, with deep subcutaneous cell transplantation of substantia nigra, and in 25 patients there was a significant improvement, but only for 2–3 months. The repeated cell transplantation, after 6 months, caused additional improvement, but the next one after another 6 months was without any effect whatsoever. Gianoli treated 18 patients by cell transplantation of *basal ganglia, diencephalon, cerebrum, and placenta*, with greater success. All patients improved for 2–4 months, and several of them that had repeated cell transplantation improved after each treatment. *One patient had 6 cell transplantations during the period of 6 years, and every time with good result, albeit not permanent* [329].

It is advised that *Parkinson's disease* patients receive *intrathecally* stem cell transplants *of basal ganglia and mesencephalon, and subaponerotically cerebellum, frontal lobe of brain, liver, placenta, and adrenal cortex.*

Huntington's chorea patients are to receive *intrathecally stem cell transplants of basal ganglia, diencephalon, and subaponeurotically medulla alba of brain, cerebellum, temporal lobe of brain, liver, placenta, adrenal cortex, intestine, and exocrine pancreas.*

Next to Alzheimer's diseases, the most common disease of the central nervous system in the western countries is a **cerebrovascular accident**. Cell transplantation of *placenta, hypothalamus, liver, spleen, brain cortex, and medulla alba of brain*, 6 months after the stroke was advised, and improvements of dementia, memory loss, intellect, orientation, muscle weakness, and paresthesias, were reported [329].

In 80% of cases where the cause is an obstruction of carotid artery, or its branches, or of vertebrobasilar artery system, the treatment plan was created several years ago but has not been carried out yet. As soon as there is a suspicion of developing stroke and an arterial obstruction confirmed by MRI or CT, a catheterization of carotid or vertebrobasilar arteries must be carried out, a developing thrombus removed, stent placed and immediately intraarterial implantation of stem cell xenotransplants of the respective parts of the brain performed. The sooner such treatment is carried out, the lesser will be the damage to the brain structures from vascular accident, and higher the success rate of stem cell xenotransplantation. The author is not familiar with the reasons for suspension of Diacrin clinical trial of stroke treatment using porcine fetal neural cell transplantation.

In January 2004, we received a SOS E-mail from desperate parents of a 19 year old man who damaged his spinal cord and became quadriplegic from pool diving accident. We offered help, but the authorities in his native land did not give us a permit to treat the patient by stem cell transplantation. Eventually he was treated in Germany 8 months later. The pleas by his parents aroused the consciousness of the country, and patients with old spinal cord injuries flooded the communications lines and eventually some such patients including those with untreatable neurodegenerative diseases came to Germany for treatment. In Table 1 there is a list of the patients with **old spinal cord injuries** treated by stem cell transplants implanted *intrathecally*, usually of *spinal cord and brain stem, or of cauda equina*, in case of lack of urinary bladder or anal sphincter controls, and subaponeurotically of *medulla alba of brain, peripheral myoblasts, mesencephalon, cerebellum, liver, and brain cortex*, but the stem cell transplants used in each individual case varied.

Table 1
Patients with old spinal cord injuries treated by our SCT method

Initials	Age	Sex	Spinal Injury date	SCT date	Diagnosis	Result
E.A.	44	F	18 months ago	11/04	quadriplegia C4/C5	use of hands, can lift silverware, hands more flexible
S.B.	58	M	12 years	1/04	paraplegia	stands on his own
M.F.	37	M	4 years ago	11/04	paraplegia	walking with braces w/ help, drives car with own feet, good leg control
D.K.	19	M	1/04	8/04	quadriplegia	muscle growth, eats w/ help, can open/close hands
H.K.	34	F	2 years	8/04	quadriplegia	good hands movement, eats alone, runs house from wheelchair, controls leg movement, lifts toes
P.M.	46	M	4 years	8/04	Polio age 7 L + paresis, paraplegia	can get up from wheelchair, walks with one brace only, controls both legs
J.O.	29	M	18 Months ago	1/04	paraplegia	can kick a soccer ball
A.P.	23	F	3 years	10/04	paraplegia T6/7	walks in pool, walks with braces & crutches, lifts toes and bends knees, burning in legs
F.R.	30	F	5 years	7/04	quadriplegia	Eats with own hands, walks with brace + electro-stimulator
E.G.	46	F	-	1/05	paraplegia	only 2 months since tx
J.C.	22	M	3 years	8/04	paraplegia	good at first, no follow-up
J.M.	26	M	-	8/04	paraplegia	no follow-up
A.M.	47	M	3 years	5/04	C3 quadriplegia	no change
H.P.	73	M	-	10/04	paraplegia	no change

All patients, with the exception of one, had no bladder and anal sphincter control before stem cell transplantation and there was no improvement after the treatment. One patient catheterized himself before stem cell transplantation and continued to do so after the treatment. One patient happily reported a *return of erection*.

Altogether we treated 14 patients with old spinal cord injuries, and in 9 out of 14 there was a significant improvement, against our expectations. In two patients, there was no change as compared with the condition before stem cell transplantation: one 47 year old male had a C3-C6 level injury, and the other male was 73 year old. In two patients, there was no follow-up, and in one patient less than 2 months transpired since stem cell transplantation at the moment of this writing.

Let's present case histories of *some other neurological patients* treated by our method of stem cell transplantation.

A 46 year old male, from London, UK, a sportsman, developed **encephalitis** 9 years ago, following which he lied in bed motionless. No diagnosis was ever made and no treatment offered. Eventually he was placed in a psychiatric hospital when his wife took him home against medical advice. After a 6 weeks long metabolic preparation to build up his physical stamina, on July 25, 2002, stem cell transplantation of *brain stem, hypothalamus, thymus, lymphnodes, spleen, mesenchyme, adrenal cortex, liver, testis, and stomach/intestine*, was carried out. Within 3 months, the patient was able to move with assistance, and attend an intensive physiotherapy program. During a follow-up examination in October 2003, he was able to walk a short distance without assistance, and capable of self-care in a wheel chair. In June 2004, the patient was walking without any assistance, and gained weight. In October 2004, he became a father of a healthy boy.

A 31 year old male physician from South Africa suffered a fracture of the cervical spine 2 years ago. After his surgery, in the recovery room, a massive embolization of right carotid arteries took place. He was taken back to the operating room and while an attempt was made to remove the emboli, an embolization of the opposite carotids took place. Following that the patient developed a '**locked-in-syndrome**', i.e. a total paralysis of all muscles in his body with the exception of extraocular muscles. His attending physician, a professor of neurology in Pretoria, told the patient's parents (father is a physician) that their son will never swallow, breathe or speak on his own. A very intensive rehabilitation was carried out for 12 months in South Africa. When he arrived at the clinic in

Germany, his breathing was very shallow, and he could not clear any bronchial secretions. His deglutition reflex was absent. He could say a word when someone squeezed the air out of his lungs. All muscles of his body were paralyzed. On November 18, 2004, he received *intrathecally via lumbar puncture* stem cell transplantation of *brain cortex, medulla alba of brain*, and subaponeurotically: *liver, peripheral myoblasts, brain stem, placenta*, and deeply subcutaneously *mesencephalon, frontal lobe of brain, occipital lobe of brain*. Five days after the stem cell transplantation he was able to stand up with assistance, cough up bronchial secretions, speak, swallow, and move his hands. In January 2005, he began a horse riding training, and today he can maintain the balance in the saddle on his own. His speech dramatically improved as well as swallowing and breathing and the same applies to his eyesight in terms of extraocular muscle function, and accommodation.

Four patients with **amyotrophic lateral sclerosis**, 3 males and one female, from 31 to 56 years of age, from 8 months to 30 months since the onset of symptoms, were treated by our method of stem cell transplantation.

A 48 year old male, presented with the first symptoms of amyotrophic lateral sclerosis (ALS) in October 2002. In January 2004, he received stem cell transplantation of *medulla oblongata and brain stem, intrathecally* via lumbar puncture, and subaponeurotically *liver, peripheral myoblasts, exocrine pancreas, stomach/intestine, and hypothalamus*. The disease process was stabilized, and in July 2004, the patient received the 2nd stem cell transplantation of *spinal cord, and rhinencephalon*, intrathecally, and subaponeurotically *peripheral myoblasts, brain stem, adrenal cortex, liver*, and epifascially *medulla alba of brain, hypothalamus*. The progression of the disease stopped from January 2004 on.

A 31 year old male, developed symptoms of ALS in February 2003. On January 15, 2004, he received stem cell transplants of *brain stem, medulla oblongata, intrathecally via lumbar puncture, peripheral myoblasts, liver, exocrine pancreas, stomach/ntestine, and hypothalamus*, subaponeurotically. The deterioration of his condition stopped, the patient still drives a car. The patient reports his progress weekly via E-mail to his attending stem cell transplantologist.

A 56 year old female, developed symptoms of ALS in the Summer of 2003, and the disease was progressing very fast. On March 4, 2004, she received stem cell transplants of *medulla oblongata, brain stem, intrathecally, and peripheral myoblasts, liver, exocrine pancreas, and stomach/intestine* subaponeurotically, and *hypothalamus* epifascially, and her condition was stable for the next 12 months.

A 44 year old male, developed symptoms of ALS in October 2003, and the disease process progressed very fast. He arrived at the clinic in Germany in serious condition: breathing was laborious and shallow, and due to that the patient was unable to speak. The patient was completely helpless. On July 20, 2004, the patient received stem cell transplants of *spinal cord and brain stem intrathecally, peripheral myoblasts, liver, exocrine pancreas, stomach/intestine* subaponeurotically, and *hypotha-lamus and cerebellum* epifascially. The condition of the patient was improved during the next 9 months of follow-up. Breathing is normal at rest; the patient can stand up on his own, move slightly, and walk short distances.

In all four patients the clinical condition stabilized, or slightly improved, and there was no further progression of the disease up until March 2005, and that is about the best that one can expect with ALS if the patient is not treated immediately at the onset of symptoms.

Let's now focus on the *diseases of 'white matter' of the brain* (those marked with * can be found also in Chapter 45).

Neurodegenerative diseases

The ability to accept information from one neuron, and pass it on to another one, requires a *participation of membrane receptors activated by neurotransmitters*. Activity of ion channels is controlled directly or via intracellular transport mechanisms. Acetylcholine opens in respective target cells the non-specific cation channels first, that enable passage of Na^+ and K^+. This leads to depolarization of cell membrane and thereby opening of voltage controlled Na^+- and Ca^{2+}-channels. Ca^{2+} mediates release of neurotransmitters by the target cell. In the long term, cell metabolism and gene expression are modulated in the target cells as well, and thereby production and storage of neurotransmitters.

When axon is interrupted, its distal part dies, i.e. Wallerian axonal degeneration takes place. Axons of CNS neurons do not grow back, and CNS neurons undergo apoptosis. One of the causes is lack of nerve growth factor released by innervated post-synaptic cells that normally keeps pre-synaptic cell alive via axonal transport.

Interruption of retrograde axonal transport with intact axon leads to apoptosis as well.

As compared with CNS neurons, in peripheral axons, the proximal stump can grow back: the necessary proteins are produced in the neuronal cell and transported to the location of injury by axonal transport.

Due to an interruption of axon not only primarily damaged CNS neurons die, but the lack of innervation often leads to the apoptosis of target neurons, i.e. to an *'anterograde transneuronal degeneration'*, and sometimes also apoptosis of neurons innervating the damaged neuron, i.e. to a *'retrograde transneuronal degeneration'*.

Due to *demyelination* of nerve fibers, more electric energy is required for reversal of polarization of internodium, and losses of electric energy are increasing further by loosening of ion channels.

If the electric current produced at internodium 1 is not sufficient to depolarize the next internodium 2, then transmission of the stimulus is interrupted. Lighter lesions of internodia cause slowing down of transmission because it takes more time to reach the threshold at internodium 2. The rate of slow-down can vary in different nerve fibers, and thereby time dispersal of signal ensues.

Eventually, the damaged locus along the demyelinated nerve fiber can spontaneously generate action potentials, with jumping onto the neighboring fibers, or with a retrograde transmission.

Genetic defects of structural proteins of myelin sheath or gap junctions of Schwann cells cause Charcot-Marie-Tooth disease, Dejerin-Sottas syndrome, Pelizaeus-Merzbacher disease, for example.

In etiopathogenesis of neurodegenerative diseases the environmental factors are very important. It is not only the effect of measles, whooping cough, herpetic infections, enterocolitis, or vaccinations, that sometimes trigger neurodegenerative diseases. It is a faulty nutrition as well. It is recognized that due to a poor nutrition in the first 3 years of life, especially deficiency of protein, the brain maturation and intelligence development suffer enormously. But disturbances of the gastrointestinal tract are perhaps even more important. For a long time it was believed that constipation, flatulence, peptic ulcer, mucosal atrophy, and dystrophy, in the face of adequate food intake, are the result of neurodegenerative diseases, but today there is a growing awareness that gastrointestinal disturbances may be a cause of neurodegenerative diseases.

When multiple sclerosis is 5 times more prevalent on Orkney Islands, north of Scotland, than in the Netherlands and 20 times more frequent than in south of France, or when the incidence of intestinal cancer in Iceland is extremely high, or when the prevalence of neurodegenerative diseases in Quebec and Ontario provinces of Canada is the highest in the whole world, it is not due to a racial disposition, as the population in Ontario and Quebec is a mixture of English, Irish, French, Italian, and German immigrants of the past 200 years. The problem is a lack of fresh food, in particular of fresh fruit and vegetables in Orkney Islands as compared with the south of France.

Barbeau in Montreal discovered a deficient fatty acid composition in cholesterol esters of HDL caused by the lack of unsaturated linoleic acid. Overload of defective cholesterol esters causes a deficiency of lipoproteins necessary for myelin production, and other metabolic consequences. Insufficient linoleic acid can cause mitochondrial energy deprivation [248].

The reason for the short discourse on the malfunction of gastrointestinal system and on faulty nutrition is to explain that *stem cell transplantation as treatment of neurodegenerative diseases has to focus on the treatment of gastrointestinal system and metabolism, rather than of central nervous system pathology*. Such changed approach to therapy finally brought on a success in the treatment of such untreatable illnesses.

Stem cell transplants of *small intestine, stomach/duodenum, liver, exocrine pancreas, colon, adrenal cortex, placenta, and peripheral myoblasts*, are recommended, as well as *cerebellum and mesencephalon,* for ataxias, *frontal lobe and basal ganglia*, for coordination malfunctions, *cardiomyoblasts and peripheral myoblasts*, for muscle dystrophies. Stem cell transplants of various parts of CNS are implanted intrathecally [248].

Let's now review neurodegenerative diseases and their treatment by stem cell transplantation.

A. **Leukodystrophies**:

- Metachromatic leukodystrophy*,
- Globoid leukodystrophy, Krabbe disease*,

- Cancellous marrow degeneration, Canavan disease, or van Bogaert and Bertrand disease,
- Sudanophilic leukodystrophies, Pelizeus-Merzbacher disease.

B. **Demyelinization diseases**:

- Diffuse sclerosis, Schilder encephalitis periaxialis,
- Multiple sclerosis,
- Neuromyelitis optica, Devic syndrome.

Myelin is the main component of the 'white matter' of the brain. It consists of lipoprotein layers which surround the axons to insulate the nerve fibers and thereby assure that the impulses are transmitted from the 'grey matter' of the brain to the effector organs without any interference or 'shorting'. This white matter is immature at birth. Even though all neurons are present already at birth, and no new ones are formed during the later stages of development, the brain is the sole organ in the body that is not ready for an independent existence at that time. *Only after the maturation of the secondary structures, i.e. dendrites, axons, synapses, glia, and insulation of nerve fibers by myelin, is the full functioning of brain assured and that takes place in the 4th year of life.*

Since the myelination takes place during the first four years of life, the first defects of medullary sheath maturation become clinically apparent only after that time. When diagnosing myelination defects, it is necessary to distinguish between the *more serious generalized demyelination diseases in early life as a result of inadequate myelination*, and the *more localized manifestation in later life, as an expression of myelin degeneration*. In between, *in the middle decades of life, there are no generalized demyelinations*, although demyelination may be extensive, such as in *Friedreich's ataxia*, which occurs between 10 and 30 years of age, or *multiple sclerosis*, which is prevalent between 20 and 40 years of age, two most common of all degenerative diseases of medulla alba of the brain.

Multiple sclerosis is an autoimmune disease with a typical onset of various neuronal deficits in different parts of CNS at different, variable, unpredictable, time intervals. After inflammation has subsided, a repair of damage takes place and nerves are re-myelinated. It is often a familiar disorder, more common in HLA3 and HLA7 carriers. In multiple sclerosis the main symptoms are disturbances of gait, speech and eyesight, along with manifold neurological symptoms. Periods of progression, an arrest of progression, and even an improvement of clinical status, make an early diagnosis very difficult. Stem cell transplantation of *liver, intestine, exocrine pancreas, adrenal cortex, mesenchyme, placenta,* and *peripheral myoblasts,* are recommended, but **no CNS stem cell transplants are used.**

C. **Cerebro-ocular degenerations**:

- Amaurotic idiocy, infantile form, Tay-Sachs disease*,
  late infantile form, Bielschowsky type amaurotic idiocy*,
  juvenile form, Spielmeyer-Vogt disease*,
- Tapeto-retinal degeneration.

D. **Spino-cerebellar degenerations**:

- Friedreich's ataxia,
- Ataxia-telangiectasia, Louis-Bar syndrome*,
- Abetalipoproteinemia, Acanthosis nigricans, Bassen-Kornzweig syndrome,
- Refsum syndrome*,
- Myoclonus encephalopathy in children, Kinsbourne syndrome.

In *Friedreich's ataxia*, AR disorder with a high penetration, clinical findings are the results of progressive degeneration of *cerebellum and spinal cord*, in particular of spinocerebellar and corticospinal tracts, and dorsal funiculi of spinal cord, i.e. there are gait disturbances, coordination disturbances of arms, speech impairment, hammer fingers, flat feet, scoliosis, and also cardiomyopathy. Stem cell transplantation of *cerebellum, mesencephalon, liver, intestine, stomach/duodenum, placenta, exocrine pancreas, adrenal cortex, peripheral myoblasts, cardiomyoblasts, kidneys, colon*, are recommended.

A 15 year old female wanted to enter a dance school, but she suffered from bilateral pedes valgi and no dancing shoes would fit her. An orthopedic surgery was required, but every surgeon turned her down because she was cachectic, her height and weight were 157 cm and 36.6 kg, respectively. She could not gain weight ever since a severe enteritis that she got in Spain several years ago. Her parents were trying to find a physician who could help her to gain some weight. Finally at one university clinic, a diagnosis of Friedreich's ataxia was made that explained deformity of the patient's feet, and cachexia. Orthopedic surgery was out of question. Cell trans-plantations of *cerebellum, liver, small intestine, peripheral muscle, exocrine pancreas, heart and placenta*, were carried out every 5 months. In two years, the patient gained 4 kg, she could walk more safely, and for a longer periods of time, and was able to go back to a regular school. One year later she was able to participate in her school ski vacation and coping with a 3 hour long uphill walk in deep snow [307].

E. **Cerebro-cutaneous degenerations**:

- Tuberous sclerosis, Bourneville syndrome*,
- Neurofibromatosis, v. Recklinghausen's disease*,
- Angiomatosis retinae et cerebelli, v. Hippel-Lindau disease.

F. **Spino-neuro-muscular degenerations**:

- Neural muscle atrophies: Wolfrath-Kugelberg-Welander,
    Werdning-Hoffman,
    Charcot-Marie-Tooth,
    Dejerine-Sottas,
- Progressive muscle dystrophies: Duchenne,
    Becker muscular dystrophy,
- Myotonia congenita,
- Thomsen myotonia,
- Carnithine myopathy,
- Myasthenia gravis,
- Amyotrophic lateral sclerosis, Motor neuron disease,
- Syringomyelia.

Disorders of motor unit

Motor unit consists of a motoneuron in spinal cord, or in nuclei of cranial nerves, appropriate axon, and all muscle fibers innervated by the same motoneuron. Function can be disrupted by damage to the motoneuron, interruption of nerve conduction, or by a muscle disease.

An α-motoneuron can be attacked by *polio virus*, and partially irreversibly destroyed. In *spinal muscle atrophies*, the groups of neurodegenerative diseases with unknown etiology, these motoneurons are dying. *Amyotrophic lateral sclerosis* develops probably on the basis of genetically induced disorder of axonal transport, which secondarily leads to demise of motoneurons in the spinal cord, as well as supraspinal motoneurons.

Damage or destruction of axons is caused by *autoimmune disease, diabetes mellitus, lead intoxication, alcohol intoxication, genetic defects*, as in Charcot-Marie-Tooth disease.

Peripheral muscles can be damaged by autoimmune disease along with other tissues, i.e. *dermatomyositis*. Additionally, genetic defects cause muscle diseases directly, as *in myotonias, or muscular dystrophies*.

The outcome of lesion of motor unit is a localized paresis of involved musculature regardless whether it is due to lesion of motoneuron, axon, or a muscle proper. With a primary destruction of α-motoneurons, there are typical fasciculations, while with primary destruction of musculature there are fibrillations.

For patients with **Charcot-Marie-Tooth disease,** or **Werdning-Hoffman disease**, stem cell transplantation of *spinal cord, cauda equina, peripheral myoblasts, intestine, and placenta*, is advised.

Amyotrophic lateral sclerosis, is a disease of unknown etiology, although heavy metal poisoning, trauma, especially by electric current, have been implicated, with incidence of 4:100,000 (in Gomoros from Guam 4:1,000), three times more frequent in males, with onset after 40 years of age. Progressive degeneration of pyramidal tract, motor neurons of anterior horn of spinal cord and of cranial nerves, and their axons, with spastic-atrophic muscle pareses, start distally, with muscle fasciculations and spasms. Eventually bulbar paralysis develops with speech and swallowing difficulties, pre-terminally appear sphincter disturbances, vision difficulties, dementia, and death due to paralysis of respiratory muscles. Death ensues after a few years from onset, or after 1 to 2 years from the first symptoms of bulbar paralysis. Stem cell transplantation of *spinal cord, brain stem peripheral myoblasts, liver, stomach/duodenum, exocrine pancreas, adrenal cortex, placenta, and intestine*, is recommended.

Genetic defects of ion channels are a frequent cause of muscle diseases. Normally, depolarization of muscle membrane is triggered after stimulation by voltage dependent Na^+-channels, which control opening of voltage dependent Ca^{2+}-channels. Inflowing Ca^{2+} activates Ca^{2+}-channel in the membrane of sarcoplasmatic reticulum. This leads to release of intracellular Ca^{2+} which mediates muscle contraction.

Repolarization is accomplished by inactivation of Na^+-channels, flow of Cl^- into the muscle cell, and outflow of K^+. Repolarization causes inactivation of Ca^{2+}-channels, so that intracellular concentration of Ca^{2+} is decreased, and muscle relaxes.

Delayed inactivation of Na^+-channels due to a mutation of gene for channel protein can lead to delayed relaxation, increased excitability and spasms, i.e. in **Na^+-channel myotonia**, and *Paramyotonia congenita*. In **Paramyotonia congenita**, AD disorder, the basis is an erroneous opening and closure of voltage controlled Na^+ channel, i.e. at low temperatures the closure of Na^+ channel is too slow, and the opening persists too long. As a result, such patients cannot carry out any muscle activity at low external temperatures.

On the basis of another defect of Na^+-channels, or defective K^+-channels, with high extracellular concentration of K^+, a paralysis takes place, i.e. **Hyperkalemic periodic paralysis**, AD disorder, caused by another mutation of the same gene that causes Paramyotonia congenita.

Genetic defect of voltage dependent Ca^{2+}-channels leads to **Hypokalemic periodic paralysis**.

With defects of Cl^-- channels myotonia develops. Depending upon the severity of molecular defect its inheritance is AD in **Thomsen congenital myotonia and Myotonia Levior**, or AR in **Becker generalized myotonia**, all due to the malfunctions of Cl- channel, caused by different mutations of the same gene.

In some defects of sarcoplasmatic Ca^{2+}-channels of ryanodine type of receptor, an anesthesia gas Halothane can activate this channel independently of the change of potential. Such massively increased use of muscle energy for heat production leads to hyperthermia, i.e. **malignant hyperthermia**. Malignant hyperthermia develops during general anesthesia in 1:15,000 children and 1:50,000 adults. In 50% of cases it is an AD disorder, in 20% AR, and in 30% sporadic condition.

In **Duchenne and Becker muscular dystrophies**, XR disorders, one component of cytoskeleton, dystrophin, is defective. In Duchenne dystrophy, with incidence of 1:3,500 newborn boys, only short and nonfunctioning fragments of dystrophin are produced, and disease is severe and progressive, with lethal outcome in the first 20 years of life. In Becker's dystrophy with incidence of 1:35,000 newborn boys, dystrophin is defective, but to a lesser degree, so that it is still functioning, and the disease begins later in life than Duchenne muscular dystrophy and runs a much less severe clinical course. Stem cell transplantation of *peripheral myoblasts, liver, intestine, spinal cord, exocrine pancreas, placenta*, is recommended.

Our own study, reported at the 1st Symposium on Human Fetal Tissue Transplantation in Moscow, December 4 – 7, 1995, under the title "Preliminary results of treatment of patients with neuro-muscular pathology by implants of human fetal tissues" included the results of treatment of 10 patients with Duchenne and two patients with Becker muscular dystrophies by cell transplantation of *peripheral myoblasts, placenta, and liver*. Diagnosis was established clinically, by EMG, increased serum phosphokinase, and DNA analysis. The response of patients with Duchenne muscular dystrophy was minimal and that applies to repeated cell transplantation as well: some patients were treated three times. On the contrary, both patients with Becker muscular dystrophy increased their muscle strength, and serum creatine phosphokinase was decreased.

Ion channels are specific proteins which can 'open and close', and thereby control movement of ions Na^+, K^+, Ca^{++}, Cl^-, across cell membranes. These ion channels are directed by either

- receptor of the receptor protein complex or
- local changes of transmembraneous voltage.

Clinical entities caused by ion channels abnormalities, called *canalopathies*, are becoming better known and some, those of muscle fibers and peripheral neurons, have a well defined clinical picture already.

Due to the enormous quantity of ion channels in CNS, and their complexity, i.e. they are bound to specific narrow populations of neurons and glia, clinical canalopathies of central neurons are not clearly described to be of use in clinical practice yet. Structural changes of the same ion channel cause different clinical pictures, often even contradictory, or the same clinical picture is due to structural changes of various ion channels.

Defects of ion channels in neurons:

Familial startle disease, known also as familial hyperexplexia, AD disorder, is due to malfunction of glycine type of receptor with Cl^- - channel. Patients respond to an unexpected stimulus by variable movements, such as facial grimacing, unusual arm movements, etc.

Episodic ataxia, AD disorder, is due to a malfunction of voltage controlled K^+- channel. Short attacks of ataxia are caused by unexpected startling stimuli, or by physical exhaustion. Between attacks myokymias are present, usually around the eyes or on hands.

Other *abnormalities of voltage controlled K^+ channel* are benign newborn familial spasms, and various types of prolonged QT interval on EKG.

Among *abnormalities of voltage controlled Na^+ channel* are generalized epilepsy with febrile seizures, and prolonged QT interval on EKG.

Receptor controlled *malfunctions of Ca^{2+}/Na^+ channels* cause various congenital myasthenias, and nocturnal epilepsy of frontal lobe, AD disorder.

Other *abnormalities of voltage controlled Ca^{2+} channel* are progressive cerebellar ataxia, and familial hemiplegic migraine.

Disorders of neuromuscular transmission

Action potential transmitted to the nerve ending by Na^+-channels depolarizes its cell membrane and thereby opens voltage dependent Ca^{2+}-channels. Ca^{2+} flows into nerve ending, and mediates connections of vesicles containing acetylcholine with pre-synaptic membrane so that acetylcholine subsequently pours out of vesicles into the synaptic cleft. Next, acetylcholine binds to the receptors of subsynaptic membrane and thereby opens non-specific cation channels there. Depolarization of membrane in the area of synapse transmits onto surrounding sarcoplasmic membrane, where opening of voltage dependent Na^+-channels triggers action potential, which quickly spreads to the whole membrane of muscle cell. Acetylcholine is broken down by acetylcholinesterase, the split off choline is again taken up by the nerve ending, and used for re-synthesis of acetylcholine.

Myasthenia gravis is the most important disease of neuromuscular synapse. It is a muscle paresis caused by inability to transmit signals from nerve to muscle. The reason is the development of antibodies against acetylcholine receptors of subsynaptic membrane, which suppresses the binding of acetylcholine and speeds up the breakdown of acetylcholine-receptors. This autoimmune disease can be triggered by viruses, and is found in patients with benign thymomas. Repeated simulation of motor nerve leads in patients with myasthenia gravis at first to development of normal muscle summation action potential, but later on with growing tiredness of neuromuscular transmission the amplitude of muscle action potential slowly but steadily diminishes. Stem cell transplantation of *thymus, peripheral myoblasts, spinal cord, liver, intestine, adrenal cortex, and placenta*, is advised.

Myasthenic syndrome of Lambert-Eaton is another autoimmune disease of neuromuscular synapse that occurs in patients with lung cancer of small cell variety.

G. **Degeneration of basal ganglia**:

- Hepatolenticular degeneration, Wilson's disease*,
- Dystonia musculorum deformans, Torsion dystonia,
- Huntington's chorea,
- Pigmentary degeneration of globus pallidus, Hallervorden-Spatz syndrome,
- Parkinson's disease.

For treatment of Parkinson's disease and Huntington chorea by stem cell transplantation see above in this chapter.

Alzheimer's disease is characterized by the following clinical *triad: organic brain disturbances, depression, loss of vitality*, that start between 20 and 30 years of age. Organic brain disturbances are the cause of Alzheimer's disease, while depression is just a symptom of the basic disease, although often a dominant one, and a lack of vitality is the main *clinical* feature of the disease. The dynamic aspects of mental and spiritual processes are the criterion of psychic vitality: the most important are inner drive, mood, sensitivity to stimuli, adaptation ability, stress handling ability, and behavioral contact. Psychopathologic symptoms of a syndrome of brain atrophy can be in general described as lowering of the entire spiritual performance level.

The main goal of therapy is an improvement of the loss of vitality, in line with teachings of Kment of Vienna, Austria, who succeded after decades' long animal experimentation to objectively prove the 'revitalization effect' as the working cytobiological principle. According to Kment revitalization is a preservation of vitality over an extended period of time, or the re-gaining of lost vitality in the later years of life, as objectively proven by statistically significant changes of several parameters of aging, that document an attainment of a younger biological age than the chronological age [256, 257].

Wolf studied 148 female patients of middle age with brain atrophy in the State psychiatric hospital over the period of 20 years. All of them had taken various antidepressants for years without any benefit. The patients were treated by implantation of cell transplants of *frontal lobe of the brain and placenta*, in series of three implantations, given 4 – 6 weeks apart, and repeated after a few months as necessary. After the discharge from the hospital the patients received the same treatment on an outpatient basis as frequently as necessary [249].

There were no complications or death over the period of 20 years, which is another proof of the validity of 'Halsted principle', i.e. when body desperately needs biological therapy, it forgets the laws of immunology. Follow-up consisted of psychological evaluation by the same psychologist, and psychiatric examination. In 40 patients, there were complete psychological and psychometrical evaluation before the patient entered the program and after each treatment, as well as close psychiatric evaluation of all intercurrent issues.

Among those 148 patients, there were 14 patients with advanced brain atrophy, and clinical dementia, 61 to 87 years old, with median age of 74 years, of which 11 were followed for years, one died and two became seriously medically ill. Despite the severity of brain atrophic process, in 6 out of 11 patients, there was an improvement after cell transplantation, and in 4 remarkable improvements [249].

In the previous reports of the same author on the interim results of the cell transplantation treatment of the same patients, one learns that 85% of patients could be discharged from the chronic psychiatric hospital to home care, in 67% the benefit of cell transplantation treatment lasted 18 months, and in 48% as long as 6 years. In the opinion of the psychologist, in 50% of patients the revitalization was so successful that their mental status became normal, and in additional 37% patients, the revitalization reached a lesser degree of success, so that an overall success rate was 87%. Additionally, a consideration must be given to the fact that the brain atrophy is a continuing process, and that an absence of deterioration of patients' condition is to be classified a success as well [250, 251].

The earlier in the course of brain atrophy that cell transplantation is carried out, the better the results will be. However, the improvement is possible also in the advanced stages with dementia, as cell transplantation even in those cases increases the vitality with an overall beneficial effect for the patient, so that it appears that even dementia, i.e. irrepairable loss of intellectual abilities, is improved [252].

A case history covers 30 years of a family history, in which both parents died of dementia at 63 and 66 years of age, two sisters of the mother died of Parkinson's disease, and the patient herself developed Alzheimer's disease in the course of 27 years of observation. Cell transplantation of *mesencephalon, hypothalamus, diencephalon, ovaries and placenta*, were done at that time. Within 8 days, there was speech improvement and disappearance of stuttering. A major diuresis was observed. During the next week the revitalization became apparent with euphoria, 'light and free head', a fluent speech in complete sentences and disappearance of tinnitus. After 3 years, the patient noticed some worsening and 2nd cell transplantation of *thalamus, cerebrum, ovaries and placenta*, was carried out. Within 3 weeks again a major improvement was observed, in particular a normal speech with no stuttering, and that persisted until the time of the report 3 years later [253].

At this time an aggressive treatment of Alzheimer's disease by neurotransplantation is very difficult. Since psychometric diagnosis of dementia is not considered a sufficient proof of diagnosis of Alzheimer's disease, only CT scan or MRI report of brain atrophy is, it is very hard to recommend neurotransplantation to such patients. *By the time CT scan or MRI show brain atrophy, the condition of the patient deteriorates so much, that there is a loss of communination with the closest family and the care of patient becomes an enormous burden on everyone involved,* so that nor the physician, nor the closest family, consider any prolongation of such suffering moral, ethical, and humanitarian. *Neurotransplantation is of value only when carried out at the stage 'when the patient cannot repeatedly find his keys', and shows only subtle symptoms and signs of dementia, that are psychometrically provable* [330].

There is a great dilemma whether to 'treat or not to treat' Alzheimer's disease by neurotransplantation of stem cells. Such indecision can be resolved by using only subaponeurotic implantation of stem cell transplants of *hypothalamus, thalamus, diencephalons, frontal lobe of brain, temporal lobe of brain, cerebellum, brain cortex, medulla alba of brain, and placenta.* Patients, their families, and physicians, are much less concerned about implantation of stem cell transplants under the aponeurosis of rectus abdominis muscle, or deeply subcutaneously, than via lumbar puncture or a Burr hole requiring intraventricular implantation.

In the last few years neuronal stem cells were found in different parts of the adult brain, which implies that regeneration of damaged brain tissue should be possible, and that applies to neurons that carry nerve impulses, as well as to supporting glial cells, without which neurons cannot survive. Since stem cell transplantation is available today to directly regenerate cells, tissues and organs, there is new hope for neurological patients.

An implantation of fetal brain cells, that include stem cells, have been tried during the past 15 years in various countries for treatment of patients with a variety of neurological diseases with no known therapy, such as genetic diseases, injuries, cerebrovascular accidents, etc., or for which treatment had lost its effectiveness in the course of the progression of illness, such as Parkinson's disease, etc., but with very low success rate. *The main reason has been an inadequate viability of implanted human fetal brain cells, used 'fresh' rather than prepared by tissue culture.*

Unless human fetal brain cells are kept in tissue culture up until the last moment before surgery, the viability of implanted cells is always doubtful, and to implant dead brain cells is meaningless.

Ophthalmology

The success of our study at Helmholtz Russian Research Institute of Eye Diseases of Russian Academy of Medical Sciences on treatment of *myopathies of extraocular muscles* by cell transplantation in 8 patients was reported at the 1st Symposium on Transplantation of Human Fetal Tissues in Moscow, December 4 – 7, 1995, under the title: "First experience with treatment of endocrine myopathies by cultures of human fetal myoblasts". At the same research center also a study of treatment of post-radiation eye perforations by cell transplantation was carried out.

A 54 year old male noticed, at the age of 33, a decreased visual acuity. Two years later, in 1971, he underwent operations for *retinal detachment* on both eyes. The following year, a panniculus was removed from the left eye. In 1981, laser coagulation was carried out near the fovea centralis of the right eye. In March 1982, a cataract was removed from the left eye. In 1976, an ophthalmologist advised the patient to have cell transplantation. Between 1976 and 1990 the patient had cell transplantation every year, i.e. 15 times. The retinal disorder stabilized, there was no further decrease of visual acuity. The patient was still working in 1990 in the mail room of a large corporation, although in 1977 was advised to enter the school for the blind [290].

Chapter 56

> I share no man's opinion; I have my own.
> *Ivan Sergeyevich Turgenev, 1818 – 1883 [Fathers and Sons 1862]*

> The civilization under which people are restricted and controlled by a material environment from which they cannot escape, and under which they cannot utilize human thought and intellectual power to change environment and improve conditions, is the civilization of a lazy and non progressive people. It is truly a materialistic civilization.
> *Hu Shih, 1891 – 1962 [La Jeunesse Nouvelle, 1919]*

DISEASES OF LOCOMOTOR APPARATUS

Genetic disorders of structural proteins responsible for connective tissue morphology

Connective tissue contains not only cells, but *mostly intercellular matter*: its quantity, contents, and properties, fit the mechanical requirements of various types of connective tissue. Inter-cellular matter contains two components: *amorphous basic substance* and *fibrillar component*, mostly of protein fibrils. Inter-cellular matter consists of *four main categories of proteins: collagens, elastins, proteoglycans, and glycoproteins*.

Collagen is the most common protein of the body, which grants most of the body tissues, such as skin, tendons, cartilages, bones, tensile strength, organization, and integrity. It is the main constituent of vessel wall, cornea, basal membranes and other tissues and organs. Genetically it is a heterogeneous family, but all molecules have similar structural parameters. Most types of collagen are synthetized by only certain differentiated cells, but *the same type of cell can synthetize multiple types of collagen*.

Berlin nosology of **genetic disorders of connective tissue**, a large group of syndromes, *characteristic by its heterogeneity*:

- Marfan syndrome - AD
- Stickler syndrome - AD
- Ehlers-Danlos syndrome - AD/AR/XR
- Syndrome of familial articular hypermobility - AD/AR
- Larsen or Desbuquois syndromes - AR
- Cutis laxa - AD/AR
- Pseudoxanthoma elasticum - AD/AR
- Epidermolysis bullosa - AD/AR
- Alkaptonuria and Homocystinuria – AR*
- Disturbed media transport: Menkes syndrome* and occipital horn syndrome - XR
- Osteogenesis imperfecta - AD/AR

*See Chapter 45

Marfan syndrome is quite heterogeneous in clinical picture: *skeletal deformities*, especially asymmetrical pectus excavatum or carinatum, dolichostenomelia, arachnodactylia, *joint hypermobility, spinal deformities, and ophthalmologic findings*, such as ectopia lentis, *cardiovascular anomalies*, such as dilatation of ascending aorta, aortic dissecans, mitral valve prolapse, *CNS abnormalities*, such as ectasia of dura mater, dilated cisterna magna, sacral meningocele, learning disabilities, spontaneous pneumothorax, cutaneous striae, hernias, etc. Higher age of father plays a role in neomutations. There is an absence of fibrillin-1, microfibrilar protein component of extracellular matrix of connective tissue. Stem cell transplantation of *mesenchyme, peripheral myoblasts, osteoblasts, cartilage, cardiomyoblasts, liver, and artery,* is advised.

Osteogenesis imperfecta is very heterogeneous in the phenotypic expression: *bone fragility* with frequent spontaneous fractures, *blue scleras, spinal deformities, nanism*, premature deafness, x-ray findings of wide, curved long bones with multiple healing fractures, 'rosary' ribs, etc. There are two forms: advanced, or 'Vrolik type', and mild with retarded manifestations, i.e. Lobstein type. Stem cell transplantation re-stores the healing of spontaneous fractures, in infants for 3 months, in older children for 4 – 6 months. Within 3 weeks after cell transplantation of *cartilage, bone marrow, placenta, mesenchyme, liver, osteoblasts, peripheral myoblasts*, fractures heal, while pain from fractures subsides within a few days. *Cell transplantations must be repeated every 6 months.*

Achondroplasia, or chondrodystrophy, AD disorder, with *nanism, abnormal bony development* of pelvis, hips, femurs, tibias, etc., has been successfully treated by cell transplantation of *cartilage, osteoblasts, bone* *marrow, placenta, liver, mesenchyme, peripheral myoblasts*, repeated every 6 months, for decades. There is usually a growth of 5 - 8 cm per year after cell transplantation, and the final result is about 10 -15 cm increase. Treated children have no hydrocephalus, their back is straighter, and the bizarre deformities are transformed into increasingly regular structures.

Our clinical study at the Endocrinology Research Center of Russian Academy of Medical Sciences involved two female patients, 7 and 15 ½ years old, treated by human fetal cell transplantation.

A 7 year old with pseudoachondroplasia, an extremely rare AD/AR disorder, was admitted with height of 103.4 cm, and weight of 19.0 kg. After the 1st cell transplantation her height increased 2.5 cm and weight 1.0 kg, and after the 2nd cell transplantation carried out 4 months later, her height increased another 3 cm within 4 months.

The 15 ½ year old with hypochondroplasia, with the height of 138.2 cm, and weight of 36.5.kg, slightly higher TSH, minor hypocalcemia, grew after cell transplantation by 5 cm in 4 months.

Ehlers-Danlos syndrome is even more heterogenous in its clinical picture. Cardinal findings are joint hypermobility, skin hyperextensibility, fine velvety surface of skin, which is soft, 'doughy' to touch, fragility of skin and connective tissue with frequent injuries and multiple dystrophic scars.

Arthrogryposis multiplex, or arthro-myo-dysplasia, is characterized by malformed rudiments of joints, tendons, and muscles, causing considerable functional restrictions. Cell transplantation of *cartilage, bone marrow, mesenchyme, placenta, liver osteoblasts, peripheral myoblasts, spinal cord, cauda equina*, repeated at intervals of 5 – 6 months, lead to the restoration of normal anatomy of joints, but not to a perfect posture, gait, and normal speech.

Cell transplantation was tested extensively in **orthopaedic surgery**, and was found to be beneficial in the treatment of aseptic necroses, non-healing fractures, and in chronic osteomyelitis, where cell transplantation of mesenchyme is essential [95]. **Aseptic necroses**, in all their dozens of forms, have been treated successfully by stem cell transplantation of *cartilage, mesenchyme, osteoblasts, and placenta*. For **chronic osteomyelitis** stem cell transplantation of *placenta, mesenchyme, cartilage, and bone marrow*, is advised.

Our own experience in pediatric orthopedic surgery was reported at the 1st symposium on transplantation of human fetal tissues in Moscow on

December 4 – 7, 1995, under the title: "Problem of optimization of regeneration process of bone tissue using fetal tissues in surgical treatment of children and juveniles with inborn anomalies of skeletal system". The presentation described well video-documented treatment of 36 patients with various micromelias treated by an osteotomy of the shortened segment of the limb with fixation of the segments in the Ilizarev apparatus, stretching to the normal length of the limb, and then 2 – 3 days later filling the defect between the ends of the osteotomized humerus or femur by 'bone paste' prepared from human fetal bone tissue. The *bone paste* was injected into a trough made of soft tissues between the osteotomized ends of the bone in the operating room via troacar. X-ray follow-up showed a complete regeneration of the bone in the missing portion within 6 weeks, and ability to use the extremity in every case within 3 months of surgery after proper rehabilitation. In the past this surgical procedure was carried out exactly the same way but without the use of 'bone paste'. There was some degree of regeneration of the bone in the missing portion even without 'bone paste', but it took up to 6 months, and often the new bone tissue was too weak to allow the use of the extremity, i.e. there was some degree of cosmetic correction but not a functional restoration.

Placement of the bone paste into a trough between two ends of osteotomized bone made from soft tissues was found to be a drawback, as the valuable 'bone paste' was misplaced during the blind procedure of application via a troacar. This observation lead us to an idea of *creating live bio-prostheses by combination of already developed and used in surgical practice bio-degradable biopolymers, amorphous or shaped, with live cell transplants*, described *in Chapter 20*. The advantage of such bio-prostheses was a much faster healing, and no need for secondary surgical procedure to remove the fixation prosthesis.

Animal experiments consisted of the use of bio-degradable biopolymer prosthesis called 'straw' soaked in a suspension of bone tissue in physiologic solution to replace a 2.5 cm defect of radius obtained by resection in 20 rabbits. Control group consisted of 5 rabbits. A full regeneration of bone defect occurred in 12 weeks, while in control group, there was no regeneration whatsoever.

Such prostheses have been used for a variety of problems in pediatric orthopedic surgery: correction of coxa vara, Calve-Legg-Perthes disease, epiphysiolysis of femoral head, inborn or acquired hip dislocation, rachitic bone deformities, and correction of pectus excavatum or carinatum.

Extensive clinical experience has been accumulated in the treatment of *osteoarthrosis* and various forms of *chronic arthritis*. Cell transplantation of *mesenchyme, cartilage, osteoblasts, synovial cells, placenta and liver, adrenal cortex, peripheral myoblasts*, is recommended for such indications. The clinical effect depends on the extent of degenerative changes. If the joint is no longer functioning because of loss of cartilage, osteophytes, calcified tendons, or bone alignment deformations, any improvement after cell transplantation can be hardly expected. But even if there is no anatomical regeneration of the worn out cartilage in the joint, the joint function improves and the pain reduces, and such effect lasts up to two years. The benefit of the repeated cell transplantation is the same.

Niehans devoted considerable attention to the treatment of **rheumatoid arthritis** by cell transplantation of *placenta, liver, adrenal cortex, peripheral myoblasts, and in female patients also of hypothalamus and ovary* [18].

A personal experience in the treatment of a variety of 'rheumatic diseases' by cell transplantation, such as rheumatoid arthritis, arthritis due to rheumatic fever, disseminated lupus erythematosus, degenerative osteoarthrosis, in 24 patients, with a success in 22 of them after a minimum of two years' follow-up, is documented in 10 detailed case reports. The article is written for physicians with no prior experience in cell transplantation [291].

A highly qualified orthopaedic surgeon in Vienna, Austria, used cell therapy/cell transplantation in his practice regularly and maintained very detailed records. His *non-surgical indications* for cell transplantation were *arthroses/spondylarthroses, aseptic necroses of bone, non-healing fractures, chronic osteomyelitis, osteoporosis, rheumatoid arthritis, circulation disorders, and adjuvant treatment of bone cancer*. This report includes 10 detailed case histories.

Patients with *arthroses* of knee, hip, proximal and distal interphalangeal joints, were from 17 to 93 years of age, females outnumbered males 5 to 2. Cell transplantation of *placenta, cartilage, synovia and mesenchyme*, were used in every case, while that of *osteoblasts, adrenal cortex, liver, gonads, diencephalon*, when clinically necessary.

Seven patients with mild gonarthrosis were so treated and 6 of them were asymptomatic for 12 months. Of the 39 patients with moderate to severe knee arthrosis, 28 had no improvement, while 6 were asymptomatic for 12 months, and 5 for 6 months. Only 7 patients with severe deforming gonarthrosis were accepted for treatment, and two were asymptomatic for 6 - 12 months.

Three patients with mild to moderate coxarthrosis were treated, and remained asymptomatic for four months. Only one out of 15 moderate and severe coxarthrosis patients was asymptomatic, for 8 months.

Spondylarthrosis treatment results by cell transplantation of *osteo-blasts, bone marrow, mesenchyme, cartilage, synovia, placenta, hypothalamus, peripheral muscle, thymus, liver, adrenal cortex, and gonads*, were not possible to evaluate, because too many factors played a role.

Arthrosis of proximal and distal interphalangeal joints is strictly a postmenopausal disorder. Nine such patients were treated, with a major success: 3 with mild problem became asymptomatic, while 6 with severe pathology were substantially improved.

There is one recommendation for cell transplantation treatment of arthrosis. Treatment must be repeated every year in mild to moderate cases, and every 6 months in severe cases, without waiting for re-appearance of symptoms or worsening.

Cell transplantation of *placenta, cartilage, bone, osteoblasts, mesenchyme, synovia*, was used for treatment of aseptic bone necrosis. There was only one such patient treated, with a complete success.

Senile and postmenopausal osteoporosis was diagnosed in 24 patients, and treated by cell transplantation of *osteoblasts, bone marrow, placenta, hypothalamus, mesenchyme, thymus*: 10 patients remained asymptomatic for 12 months, while 8 were 50% better, and in 6, there was no improvement [292].

The same author reports on his use of cell therapy/cell transplantation in his *surgical orthopedic practice*. His indications for cell transplantation, i.e. *pre-operative and post-operative revitalization in very old patients, amputations for angiopathies or neuropathies of lower extremities*, pre-operative treatment of infections of soft tissues and bones, *pre- and post-operative cell transplantation for poorly developing callus or bone regeneration in the implant surgery*, fusionoperations, etc. are explained also in 10 detailed case histories.

Pre- and post-operative revitalization by cell transplantation of *placenta, hypothalamus, mesenchyme, liver, gonads, adrenal cortex, osteoblasts, thymus, bone marrow*, is essential in the very aged patients who are poor risk for surgical procedures. Post-operative cell transplantation should not be done before 6th – 7th day after surgery, when surgeon is certain of absence of any postoperative infection.

Complications from bone surgeries are usually due to the *poor callus formation or inadequate bone healing*. Cell transplantation of *placenta, osteoblasts, mesenchyme, and bone marrow*, speeds up healing, to make the re-operation possible, but more often is avoided because healing of the damaged bone has already taken place.

Cell transplantation of *placenta, mesenchyme, liver, spleen, hypothalamus, artery, adrenal cortex, and Langerhans islets* in case of diabetes, *permits a very conservative approach to amputations*, whereby a surgeon can amputate at the border between necrosis and living tissue, leaving the wound opened so that it can heal per secundam by granulating and epidermisation. It makes a great difference for the patient's everyday life, if the patient can walk with a special shoe, or a below knee prosthesis [293].

A few case histories

Senile osteoporosis is the most common bone disease, and for 84 year old female patient it meant 8 years of constant pain, and eventual hospitalization. There was marked kyphosis, diminished movement of thoracic and lumbar spine, compression of the body of the 1st lumbar vertebra. Cell transplantation of *placenta, and osteoblasts*, was carried out. Four weeks later, the patient was free of pain on motion, and in another two weeks was able to get out of bed. Three months later the patient walked 4 hours a day. Alkaline phosphatase went up from 83 U/l to 152 U/l. After eleven months, the 2nd cell transplantation of *placenta, hypothalamus, and osteoblasts*, was performed. Two weeks later, the patient could remove her body brace, walk upstairs, and take care of her house. This case proves that it is never too late to treat elderly patients [303].

Chronic osteomyelitis has been one of the established indications for cell therapy. A 40 year old male developed a bilateral chronic osteomyelitis with severe secondary purulent infection, deforming bone healing, and sequestration, following an open fracture of both lower legs

7 years ago. The patient suffered also from lipoproteinemia Type IIA, and hypercholesterolemia. After a continuous hospitalization and multiple procedures on both legs, 2 years after the accident the patient eventually developed an acute osteomyelitis on the right lower leg, non-responsive to any treatment, and 18 months later was advised to have an amputation. Approximately 8 months after the onset of osteomyelitis of right leg, an acute osteomyelitis developed in the left leg as well, again not responding to any treatment.

Eventually, nearly 5 years after the accident, the patient underwent the 1st cell transplantation of *osteoblasts, placenta and mesenchyme*. Seven weeks later, the suppuration stopped, low blood pressure normalized, and cholesterol level became normal. Cell transplantation of *osteoblasts, placenta, and mesenchyme*, was repeated 3 months later, and once more after another 3 months. Six years after an accident, the patient was able to walk on the beach of North Sea for 3 hours without support and swim without any difficulty. Following this encouraging report, the patient had the 4th and the last cell transplantation [306].

A 5 year old female with an aseptic necrosis of the left femoral head was wearing a poorly designed brace for one year, and her condition was not improving. Cell transplantation of *osteoblasts, cartilage, mesenchyme, and placenta*, was given, the brace was removed, and she was walking with crutches. In two weeks after cell transplant-ation, the pain also stopped. In six months her x-rays were showing the healing of femoral head. One month later cell transplantation of *osteoblasts, cartilage, and mesenchyme*, was carried out. In 8 months x-rays showed a complete restoration of the femoral head, and two weeks later the patient was walking without crutches [294].

In the next case report, a medical student described his own case of a *central hip joint dislocation with acetabular fracture* following a motorcycle accident treated by a repositioning, and traction for 3 months. Two years later necrosis of the head of the right femur was diagnosed. The next surgical operation was unsuccessful, and the disability was worse than before the surgery. Due to a defective necrotic femoral head, the patient could not walk at all. The 1st cell transplantation of *placenta, mesenchyme, cartilage and osteoblasts*, was followed by ozonetherapy and magnetic field therapy. Two months later the 2nd cell transplant-ation of *placenta, mesenchyme, cartilage and hypothalamus*, was carried out, and 4 months later followed by the 3rd cell transplantation of *placenta, mesenchyme, cartilage and hypothalamus*. Since that time there was a continuous improvement and x-rays taken 3 years later showed a healing of femoral head, although some flatness, the patient was mobile [304].

A 60 year old female had osteomyelitis of the left femur at the age of 10, which caused a shortening of the left leg by 2 cm, and thereby her foot was in a permanent 'walking on the tiptoes' position, and there was an ankylosis of the left hip joint in adduction-, flexion-, and external rotation, with a pronounced periarthropathy. The severe *coxarthrosis* brought on *the aseptic necrosis* of the femoral head 50 years after the osteomyelitis in childhood, with inability to walk whatsoever. Steroids did not help at all. Cell transplantation was carried out three times, with *intraarticular implantation of cartilage, and systemic implantation of mesenchyme, thymus, liver, placenta, osteoblasts, and adrenal cortex.* The result was excellent; the patient could again work in her food store without crutches that she had to use for years [305].

Clinical protocol for stem cell transplantation treatment of diseases of locomotor apparatus

The patient has to be prepared for stem cell xenotransplantation by elimination of metabolic imbalance, hypoalbuminemia, and chronic infection by hospitalization with intravenous fluids, sufficient doses of antibiotics, pulmonary physiotherapy, proper urinary drainage, etc., so that the patient's clinical condition will be compensated as well as possible.

Parameters to be followed in patients before and after stem cell xenotransplantation, and the frequency:

1. **General**:
    i. complete CBC once a month
    ii. level of serum albumin once a month
    iii. level of serum calcium and phosphorus once a month
    iv. serum chemistry once a month
    v. serum alkaline phosphatase once a month
    vi. x-rays as necessary
    vii. CT scan as necessary
    viii. MRI as necessary
    ix. body weight once a week
    x. bone scan as necessary

xi. 24-h urine calcium as necessary

2. **Immunological**: once a month x3, then every 3 months:

   i. total lymphocytes
   ii. T-lymphocytes (CD3$^+$)
   iii. T-helpers (CD4$^+$)
   iv. T-suppressors (CD8$^+$) and CD4/CD8
   v. NK (CD16)
   vi. B-lymphocytes (CD22 and CD19)
   vii. serum IgG, IgA, IgM
   viii. serum complement (CH50)

3. **Special**: once every 6 months

   i. osteoporosis: - T3, T4, TSH

      - serum protein electrophoresis
      - serum 25-hydroxycholecalciferol and 1,25-dihydro-cholecalciferol

   ii. osteomalacia:

      - serum 25-hydroxycholecalciferol and 1,25-dihydro-cholecalciferol
      - bone biopsy with double tetracycline-labeled histometry

   iii. hyperparathyroidism:

      - circulating immunoreactive parathyroid hormone

   iv. myeloma:

      - serum electrophoresis (monoclonal protein)
      - bone marrow examination
      - urine for Bence Jones protein
      - serum level of monoclonal protein

Frequency of office visits: 4 weeks and 48 hours before stem cell xenotransplantation, 24 hours after, and then once a week for the first month after stem cell transplantation, once a month thereafter.

Chapter 57

> Those who cannot remember the past are condemned to repeat it.
> *George Santayana, 1863 – 1952 [The Life of Reason 1905 – 1906]*

> When you know a thing, to hold that you know it, and when you do not know a thing, to allow that you do not know it – this is knowledge.
> *Confucius, 551 – 497 B.C. [The Confucian Analects]*

DIGESTIVE SYSTEM DISEASES

Living organisms need food to satisfy their needs for substance and energy. Food has to be swallowed, prepared for digestion, digested, absorbed, and remnants eliminated. The extent and depth of pathologic conditions of digestive diseases were not appreciated by medicine for a long time, and that applied to cell transplantation/cell therapy as well. Digestive disorders attracted attention of cell transplantologists only after their role in the pathogenesis of neurodegenerative diseases began to be explored. For this reason, there is not much experience with treatment of diseases of the digestive tube by cell transplantation with the exception of *liver diseases that are discussed in a separate chapter*, and to some degree chronic pancreatitis.

Gastrointestinal tract secretes several peptide hormones, and neurotransmitters, used for regulation and control of digestive tract.

The *surface of digestive tract that amounts to approximately 100 m^2, as compared to the skin surface of less than 2 m^2*, is exposed to food coming from external environment, and is protected against infectious agents. In mouth there are components of saliva, such as mucins, IgA, and lysozym, in stomach HCl and pepsins have bactericidal properties, and then there are Peyer plaques in the intestines, which are a part of immunocompetent lymphatic tissue of digestive tract. Special 'membraneous' M-cells of mucosa enable an access of antigens in the intestinal lumen to Peyer plaques, which then react by release of IgA, i.e. oral immunization. In the intestinal mucosa a 'secretory component' is attached to IgA, that protects IgA against digestive enzymes. Another barrier against infectious agents represents macrophages of intestinal wall and Kupffer cells in sinusoids of liver.

Many chronic diabetics suffering from diabetic complications complain of severe *parodontosis*, not responsive to any stomatological treatment. After cell transplantation they all report dramatic improvement so that there is no need for any further dental treatment. Based on this, a biological treatment of parodontosis was developed with our cooperation with the 1st Stomatological Faculty in Moscow. It entailed the treatment of basic systemic disease(s) of the patient and a local treatment by ultrafiltrates of gum tissues.

Achalasia is due to a lowered count of 'non-cholinergic-non-adrenergic' neurons as well as decreased reactivity of such neurons to acetylcholine released by pre-ganglionic pathways. The result is a markedly increased pressure in lower esophageal sphincter, and delayed relaxation during swallowing act, so that the intra-sphincteric pressure is higher than in the stomach even during the receptive relaxation phase. The swallowed food is accumulated in esophagus, so that intraesophageal pressure keeps on growing and esophagus widens enormously. There are no peristaltic waves.

The reverse condition of esophageal hypomotility occurs in *scleroderma*, an autoimmune disease, with a neuronal defect in the early stages, that causes a disappearance of peristalsis in the lower esophageal segments. Here, the contraction of esophageal sphincter is diminished so that a pathological esophageal reflux develops. For treatment of scleroderma see Chapter 51.

Atrophic gastritis is actually an atrophy of glands in gastric fundus. There are IgG autoantibodies against parts of parietal cells and their products, infiltration by plasma cells and B-cells. The parietal cells atrophy, so that secretion of HCl substantially decreases, i.e. there is achlorhydria. Antibodies block the binding of vitamin B12 to intrinsic factor so that pernicious anemia eventually develops. There is a substantial reactive rise in gastrin release, and G-cells hypertrophy. The high level of gastrin brings on hyperplasia of enterochromaffin-like cells with receptors for gastrin, that are the main producers of histamine in the wall of stomach, and this hyperplasia can become carcinoid. The main risk of atrophic gastritis is an extensive mucosal metaplasia, a precancerous condition.

Peptic ulcer has been treated with cell transplantation of *hypothalamus, placenta, stomach/intestine, and mesenchyme*, for many years with success. As it is a classic hypothalamic syndrome, obviously the cell transplant of *hypothalamus* is of major importance.

Chronic pancreatitis is an inflammatory process destroying exocrine and endocrine tissue, replacing them by fibrous tissue. In 80%, it is due to chronic alcoholism. Tissue lesions are spread irregularly throughout parenchyma with protein drops and stones in major ducts, as well as atrophy and ductal stenosis. There is a decreased secretion of water and HCO_3^- in ducts, so that proteins precipitate in the lumen of ducts and protein drops and deposits are created. Calcium salts deposit into protein drops with creation of stones in small and large ducts. Trypsin is activated in the lumen of ducts and digests pancreatic tissue. Stem cell transplantation of *exocrine pancreas, stomach/duodenum, intestine, and liver*, along with *placenta and adrenal cortex* is advised.

Malabsorption can involve any of three sources of energy: fats, proteins and carbohydrates; as well as vitamins, minerals, and trace elements. Cell transplantation of *exocrine pancreas, stomach/duodenum, small intestine, colon, liver, and placenta*, is highly advisable, although very seldom actually used in clinical practice.

Actual location of absorption varies by availability of specific resorption mechanisms in the respective portions of small intestine. Monosaccharides, i.e. glucose, galactose, are absorbed already at the beginning of duodenum. Disaccharides have to be first split by enzymes of the brush border into monosacharides. Polysaccharides, proteins and fats, have to come into contact with pancreatic juice first, so that their absorption takes place in the middle of jejunum and faster emptying of stomach can move their absorption into the distal jejunum or even into ileum. But some components, i.e. cobalamins or biliary acids, can be absorbed only in terminal ileum.

Causes of malabsorption:

- *stomach surgery* due to a lowered stimulation of hormone secretion, and disturbed synchronization of secretion of pancreatic juices, gallbladder emptying, and choleresis,

- *pancreatic diseases*, such as chronic pancreatitis, mucoviscidosis, due to lack of important enzymes, i.e. lipase, trypsin, chymotrypsin, amylase, etc., and HCO_3^-, necessary for buffering of acid chyme,
- *atrophic gastritis* with achlorhydria, where digestion is slowed down in stomach, and that makes colonization of small intestine by pathogenic bacteria easier. Stasis of intestinal contents due to diverticulosis or 'blind-loop syndrome' facilitates such colonization. Bacteria break the link between cobalamine and intrinsic factors, and thereby cause a lack of cobalamine,
- *lack of disaccharidases in the brush border*: lack of lactase causes lactose intolerance,
- *defects of specific transport systems in mucosa*, e.g. Hartnup disease due to the defective transport system for neutral amino acids, or cystinuria due to the defective transport system for basic amino acids and cystin,
- *global defects of mucosal digestion and absorption* in diffuse mucosal diseases, such as coeliakia, tropical sprue, Crohn's disease, Whipple disease, AIDS, salmonella enteritis, radiation enteritis,
- *defective intracellular digestion of fats*, i.e. production of chylomicrons, the basis of *abetalipoproteinemia*,
- *disturbed blood circulation in intestines*.

Saccharide malabsorption in small intestine leads to further metabolization in colon by bacteria with production of short-chain fatty acids and gases, and flatulence.

Fat malabsorption due to a lack of bile salts or a defect of micelle production, leads to malabsorption of fat-soluble vitamins A, D, E, K, because they reach the absorbing mucosa only in lipophilic environment and that requires the presence of mycelles.

Coeliakia, with incidence 1:100, is handled easily nowadays with the availability of gluten-free food products, but many patients are candidates for the regeneration of intestinal mucosa by stem cell transplantation.

When autoimmune **Crohn's disease** and **ulcerative colitis** stop responding to conservative treatment, cell transplantation should be carried out before proceeding with extensive surgical resection. Stem cell transplantation of *liver, colon, intestine, adrenal cortex, thymus,* *skin, spleen, placenta*, is recommended for ulcerative colitis and Crohn's disease.

Among causes of *constipation* some are possibly treatable by stem cell transplantation:

- *Hirschsprung disease* is a congenital lack of ganglion cells near anus which causes permanent spasm of involved portion of rectum with a lack of receptive relaxation and of recto-anal inhibition reflex: internal anal sphincter does not open when rectum is filled up.
- *Chagas disease* is an infection by Trypanosoma cruci that destroys the nerves of intestinal ganglia and causes dilatation of colon, i.e. megacolon.

Clinical protocol treatment of serious gastrointestinal diseases by stem cell transplantation

This applies to:

1. Malabsorption syndromes (MA),
2. Crohn's Disease, Ulcerative Colitis & variants (CD)

A proper preparation of the patient for stem cell transplantation is mandatory. Patient has to be brought into as good a clinical condition as possible by standard therapeutic means, while at the same time lowering the dosage of corticosteroids and other immunosuppressants to a necessary minimum, (or discontinuing them), and eliminating non-essential drugs.

Parameters to be followed in patients before and after stem cell xenotransplantation, and the frequency:

1. **Basic**: once a month or as often as necessary:
    i. complete blood count
    ii. urinalysis
    iii. sedimentation rate
    iv. serum immunoglobulins
    v. serum albumin
    vi. serum electrolytes
    vii. serum calcium and phosphorus

      viii. serum cholesterol and lipoproteins
      ix. antinuclear antibodies, LE cell prep, Rheumatoid Factor
      x. total lymphocytes
      xi. T-lymphocytes (CD3)
      xii. T-helpers (CD4) and T-suppressors (CD8) and CD4/CD8 ratio
      xiii. NK (CD16)
      xiv. B-lymphocytes (CD22 and CD19)
      xv. serum complement, total (CH50) and C3 and C4
      xvi. serum gamma-Glutamyl transpeptidase

2. **Special**: once every 3 months or as often as necessary:

      i. direct measurement of fecal fat (MA)
      ii. microscopic examination of stool (MA)
      iii. D-xylose absorption test (MA)
      iv. serum ferritin, serum iron levels (MA)
      v. Schiling's test of vitamin B12 absorption (MA)
      vi. Carbon 14-labeled glycocholic acid breath test (MA)
      vii. x-rays: an upper GI + small bowel series (MA, CD)
      viii. small bowel biopsy (MA)
      ix. upper gastrointestinal endoscopy (MA)
      x. lactose tolerance test (MA)
      xi. Chromium 51-labeled albumin test for intestinal protein loss (MA)
      xii. x-rays: barium enema, or double air-contrast barium enema (CD)
      xiii. fiberoptic sigmoidoscopy and total colonoscopy with biopsies (CD)
      xiv. C-reactive protein (CD)

Frequency of office visits: 4 weeks and 48 hours before stem cell xenotransplantation, 24 hours and then once a week for the first month after stem cell xenotransplantation, and once a month thereafter.

Chapter 58

Learn the ABC of science before you try to ascend to its summit.

Learn, compare, collect the facts.
Ivan Petrovich Pavlov, 1849 – 1936 [Bequest to the Academic Youth of Soviet Russia 1936]

LIVER DISEASES

Compensated cirrhosis of the liver and chronic non-aggressive hepatitis have been treated by stem cell transplantation with success for the last four decades. Cirrhosis of the liver and chronic hepatitis were very common in Germany in 1940's, 50's and 60's. This was the result of a severe epidemic of viral hepatitis in Germany during WW2 and thereafter. *Since even today there is no effective therapy for damaged liver, stem cell transplantation continues to be a treatment of choice for serious liver diseases.* Essentially, all patients can be helped *unless their disease is in the stage of acute inflammatory exacerbation or in the stage of decompensated cirrhosis with portal hypertension*, i.e. edema, ascites, bleeding esophageal varices, etc.

Liver cirrhosis is in 50% of cases due to alcohol abuse, particularly due to its metabolite *acetaldehyde*. But cirrhosis can be the end-stage of viral hepatitis, late result of storage diseases, or genetic enzymopathies, or due to blood flow obstruction. Here side-by-side necrosis, inflammation, fibrosis, nodular regeneration and vascular anastomoses development, take place. Hepatocyte damage is from lack of ATP due to disorder of cell energetic metabolism, from increased production of highly reactive oxygen metabolites, i.e. O_2^-, HO_2, H_2O_2, and simultaneous lack of antioxidants, such as glutathione, or a lack of protective enzymes, i.e. glutathionperoxidase, superoxiddismutase, or due to blood flow obstruction.

Damaged hepatocytes release lysosomal enzymes that in turn release cytokines, and cytokines with cellular debris trigger activation of Kupffer cells in liver sinusoids, and attract inflammatory cells. Kupffer cells and inflammatory cells release growth factors and cytokines which:

- change fat collecting Ito cells into myofibroblasts,
- turn incoming monocytes into active macrophages and
- trigger fibroblast proliferation.

Myofibroblasts and fibroblasts increase production of extracellular matrix which fills up Disse space. This fibrosis limits metabolism between blood in sinusoids and hepatocytes.

Increased extracellular matrix can break down and hepatocytes can regenerate. If necrosis took place only in the centers of liver lobules, *'restitutio ad integrum'* is possible. But if necrosis passed beyond the peripheral parenchyma of lobules, fibrotic septa develop and full functional regeneration cannot take place and nodules develop, i.e. cirrhosis, with cholestasis, portal hypertension, and metabolic liver insufficiency.

In 1954, Harbers induced severe liver damage by 24 intraperitoneal injections of carbontetrachloride over 12 weeks and then used bromsulfalein test to determine the extent of liver damage. In controls, the liver disease had a progressive course, and all animals died. After cell transplantation, bromsulfalein test values decreased considerably and animals survived. In 1959, Oetzmann reported on his treatment of rats with an experimental model of liver cirrhosis induced by thioacetamide. Rats treated by cell transplantation showed the highest survival rate of 36.6%, while only 13.3% of those taking only Prohepars survived. In 1958, Rietschel carried out a prophylactic cell transplantation prior to oral feeding via gastric tube of 2.0% solution of allyl alcohol, but that did not work, because one of the cardinal rules for the clinical effectiveness of cell transplants is the presence of damaged organ or tissue in the body of the recipient [321].

After extensive experimental studies, major clinical studies were carried out in Germany by Rietschel [255] and Oetzman [95]. In Oetzman's study, the patients were divided into 3 groups: 1st group was treated by cholin, vitamins and diet, the 2nd group by the same plus prednisone, while the 3rd group was treated with cholin, diet, and cell transplantation of *liver, adrenal cortex, and placenta*. The 3rd group consisted of 210 patients, and the final evaluation was 2 years after cell transplantation. A success rate of 69% was obtained in the 3rd group of patients, for both chronic hepatitis and liver cirrhosis. Clinically, it amounted to a diminished icterus, decreased hepatosplenomegaly, improved appetite and psychic state, normalization of laboratory tests, and even disappearance of palmar erythema and spider nevi. The general physical condition was improved for as long as 6 to 14 months, particularly in patients with chronic hepatitis or with transitional stages of chronic hepatitis leaning toward cirrhosis [321].

A group of 22 patients with chronic liver diseases from a general medical practice that underwent any and all known therapies for chronic liver disease over many years, without any success, was offered a trial of cell transplantation: 7 patients had chronic hepatitis, 5 chronic hepatitis turning into cirrhosis, 3 patients liver cirrhosis, and 7 patients had hepatoses due to chronic alcoholism and drug abuse. Chronic alcoholism was a dominant clinical feature in 40.9% of patients, drug abuse in 22%, diabetes mellitus in 9.1%. The history of ascites was present in 13.6%.

Patients with chronic hepatitis received cell transplantation of *mesenchyme* only, 4 to 6 times a year. Patients with chronic hepatitis turning into cirrhosis received cell transplantation of *liver and mesenchyme*, 4 to 6 times a year. Patients with cirrhosis of liver received cell transplantation of *liver* only, 4 to 6 times a year. Patients with hepatoses received cell transplantation of *liver* only, 4 – 6 times a year, and they were not asked to change their lifestyle, i.e. they could drink or take drugs as before.

The most dramatic changes of SGOT, SGPT and LDH occurred in the group of hepatoses, where SGPT decreased 78%, and SGOT nearly as much, and also LDH improved. Patients with cirrhosis had a decrease of SGOT and SGPT by 38%, and LDH by 63.5%, which is remarkable. Patients with chronic hepatitis had a decrease of SGPT by 29%, SGOT by 26% and LDH by 43%, and those with chronic hepatitis turning into cirrhosis had a decrease of SGPT by 44%, SGOT by 33%, and LDH by 35%. The best results were obtained in patients where the duration of disease was between 1 and 4 years, while after 5 years the success was noticeably lower. In retrospect, the patients with chronic hepatitis should have received cell transplantation of liver as well [322].

German practitioners of cell transplantation recommend that the patients with chronic hepatitis and liver cirrhosis receive cell transplantation of *liver*, but also of *adrenal cortex, spleen, placenta, exocrine portion of pancreas, mesenchyme, stomach/duodenum, intestine, hypothalamus*. Patients with acute hepatitis, chronic hepatitis in active inflammatory stage, decompensated liver cirrhosis with ascites, portal hypertension, esophageal varices, must not be treated by cell transplantation.

A 38 year old male became ill in 1980 with hepatopathy of unknown etiology, as he refused liver biopsy. He was treated by cortisone, etc., but was not feeling well and laboratory tests were abnormal at all times. The patient was advised that there is no treatment for him. The patient sought another opinion and received lyophilized mesenchyme every 6 weeks, altogether 8 times. All laboratory tests improved significantly and patient was feeling well [300].

If chronic alcoholism is the cause of liver cirrhosis, stem cell transplantation would be of no value for a patient that could not stop the addiction. A study of 87 alcoholic patients, one half of them men, with median age of 46 years, treated by a complex protocol of cell transplantation with 12 treatments by autohemotherapy, 1000γ of ozone, psychotherapy, including group therapy, brought on 95 - 100 % success based on a 13 months follow-up after the complex treatment in terms of general condition, overall performance, ability to concentrate, and the relapse frequency were reduced from 85% to 44%. Cell transplantation of *placenta, heart muscle, liver, exocrine pancreas, spleen, thymus, gonads, anterior lobe of pituitary, brain cortex, cerebellum, thalamus, hypothalamus, spinal cord*, was used. Two detailed case histories are included [298].

For patients with **chronic hepatitis**, *it is mandatory to suppress an inflammatory process in the liver first by all other therapeutic means and that is difficult.* Without that, the outcome of SCT cannot be predicted.

The hepatitis C virus (HCV) accounts in the US for 15% of acute viral hepatitis, up to 70% of chronic hepatitis and up to 50% of cirrhosis, end-stage liver disease and liver cancer. Approximately 4 million of US population suffers from chronic hepatitis C, and worldwide that number is 170 million. An estimated 12,000 people dies every year in the US from chronic hepatitis C.

Ultimately 75 – 80% of patients with acute hepatitis C develop chronic hepatitis C, and 80% of them get cirrhosis of liver. Liver failure due to chronic hepatitis C is one of the main indications for liver transplantation in the US Chronic hepatitis is the cause of about one half of all cases of primary liver cancer in the developed world.

Chronic hepatitis C is becoming a major health catastrophy in the world on the same level as AIDS.

One of the reasons is a lack of effective treatment. The currently best therapeutic scheme, a combination of peginterferon α-2 and ribavirin, improves serum ALT levels and HCV RNA disappears in 70% of patients, but in 55% of patients such effect will last for 6 months only. The described therapy is not suitable for children and patients over 60 years of age, and is contraindicated in several frequently occurring medical conditions. There are many side effects, some serious, including worsening of the disease. Besides that this therapy is expensive and hardly affordable in many countries. National Institute of Diabetes and Digestive and Kidney Diseases (NIDDK) recommends that such combination treatment be limited to those patients who have histological evidence of progressive disease, i.e. liver biopsy.

Our own study of children with chronic persistent hepatitis and chronic aggressive hepatitis, was presented at the 1st Symposium of Human Fetal Tissue Transplantation in Moscow, December 4 – 7, 1995, under the title "Experience with the use of human fetal tissues in chronic viral hepatitis and liver cirrhosis in children". In 8 children, from 9 – 12 years of age, with chronic persistent hepatitis, the right lobe of liver decreased in size by 2/3, the left lobe by ½, and spleen by 2/3, 7 days after cell transplantation of *liver, spleen, placenta, stomach/intestine, adrenal cortex, and mesenchyme.* Total bilirubin level dropped 1/3, AST from 41 to 31 U., ALT from 40 to 34 U. Clinical toxicity disappeared in all children, ecchymoses decreased, spider nevi were less pronounced, skin re-gained healthy pink color, and all children were feeling better. Re-testing 4 - 6 months after cell transplantation showed that right lobe of liver was still decreased by 35%, left lobe of liver by 15%, while spleen reached the pre-treatment size. In 2 patients, a Doppler study of portal vein and splenic vein were carried out before and after cell transplantation. The abnormally high parameters for portal vein were further increased after cell transplantation in one patient, but decreased in the 2nd patient. The abnormally high parameters for splenic vein decreased substantially in both patients.

In 8 patients with chronic aggressive hepatitis, from 6 – 12 years of age, the right lobe of liver decreased in size by 45%, left lobe by 30%, and spleen by 60%, 7 days after cell transplantation. Total bilirubin, AST, ALT, were lowered to a similar degree as in chronic persistent hepatitis group. All children were feeling better, the toxicity disappeared, skin became rosy, the ecchymoses were substantially diminished, and so were spider nevi, subicterus present in one child decreased. All children were discharged home after 7 days.

Icterus causing malfunctions: Bilirubin from hemoglobin breakdown enters hepatocytes, and by glucuronyltransferase is transformed into conjugated (direct) bilirubin, more hydrophilic, excreted into biliary tract, and thereby to intestines. There are 3 kinds of disorders:

- pre-hepatic icterus, due to exaggerated bilirubin production, or resorption of large hematomas,
- intrahepatic icterus that develops from the specific defect of bilirubin intake by hepatocytes, i.e. in *Gilbert syndrome* is due to a defect of conjugation, i.e. in *Crigler-Najjar syndrome*, icterus neonatorum, or due to a secretion of bilirubin into biliary pathways, i.e. *Dubin-Johnson syndrome, and Rotor syndrome*,
- post-hepatic icterus, due to blockage of extrahepatic biliary passages.

For treatment of **Crigler-Najjar syndrome** stem cell transplantation of *liver, placenta, basal ganglia, and cerebellum*, is advised.

Portal hypertension: Venous blood from stomach, intestine, pancreas, spleen, gallbladder, is brought via portal vein into liver, where after mixing with oxygenated blood from hepatic artery comes in contact with hepatocytes. Approximately 25% of minute blood volume passes through liver. Resistance in portal vein is small: 4 - 8 mm Hg. With restriction of lumen of portal circulation the pressure in portal vein rises and portal hypertension develops. It can be:

- pre-hepatic: portal vein thrombosis,
- post-hepatic: right heart insufficiency, constrictive pericarditis,
- intrahepatic:
  pre-sinusoidal - chronic hepatitis, primary biliary cirrhosis,
  sinusoidal: acute hepatitis, cirrhosis from chronic alcoholism,
  post-sinusoidal: Budd-Chiari syndrome, i.e. obstruction of large hepatic veins.

Portal hypertension leads to malfunction of all pre-hepatic organs: malabsorption, splenomegaly with anemia and thrombocytopenia, and diversion of blood via porta-caval anastomoses, whereby toxic substances from colon, i.e. NH_3, biogenic amines, short-chain fatty acids, etc., by-pass liver, enter CNS and cause portal encephalopathy.

Intraportal implantation of stem cell transplants is the fastest way to get the clinical response in this therapeutic method, but it must not be done when there is a portal hypertension.

Hepatorenal syndrome: *Liver cirrhosis causes relatively frequently renal ischemia and subsequent oliguric kidney failure*, and such clinical course is known as hepatorenal syndrome. In the liver cirrhosis, there is blood stasis in portal circulation due to fibrosis-caused narrowing of blood vessels. Capillary hydrostatic pressure grows and there is substantial increase of filtration of fluid intraperitoneally, i.e. ascites. As a result of high permeability of liver sinuses for proteins, there is a substantial loss of proteins into extracellular space. Besides that, the damaged liver parenchyma produces less proteins. Hypoproteinemia develops, with increased filtration of plasma water and thereby development of peripheral edemas. In the early stage stem cell transaplantation of *liver, adrenal cortex, spleen, placenta, mesenchyme, stomach/duodenum, intestine, kidneys* should be carried out as there is no other treatment available.

Clinical protocol for treatment of chronic liver disease by stem cell transplantation

This applies to: Chronic Hepatitis, Liver Cirrhosis, Primary Biliary Cirrhosis, and Primary Sclerosing Cholangitis.

A proper preparation of the patient for stem cell transplantation is mandatory. A patient has to be brought into as good a clinical condition as possible by standard therapeutic means, while at the same time lowering the dosage of corticosteroids and other immunosuppressants to a necessary minimum, (or discontinuing them), and eliminating non-essential drugs.

Parameters to be followed in patients before and after stem cell xenotransplantation, and the frequency:

The following parameters will be followed in patients before, and after the stem cell transplantation (SCT), with the following frequency:

General:
       i. level of serum ALT once a month after SCT
      ii. level of anti-HCV once a month after SCT
     iii. CBC, UA, SMA-12 once a month after SCT
     iv. serum HCV RNA once a month after SCT
      v. sedimentation rate once a month after SCT

vi. serum albumin once a month after SCT
vii. prothrombin time
viii. serum alkaline phosphatase
ix. serum transaminases: AST, ALT
x. serum bilirubin
xi. serum cholesterol and lipoproteins

Immunological: once a month after SCT x 2
i. total lymphocytes
ii. T-lymphocytes (CD3+)
iii. T-helpers (CD4+)
iv. T-suppressors (CD8+) and CD4/CD8 ratio
v. NK (CD16)
vi. B-lymphocytes (CD22 and CD19)
vii. serum IgG, IgA, IgM
viii. serum complement

Special:
- CT scan of liver
- liver ultrasound
- liver biopsy
- CT retrograde cholangio-pancreatography

Frequency of office visits: 6 weeks and 48 hours before stem cell transplantation, 24 hours after and then once a week for the first month after the stem cell -transplantation, once a month thereafter.

Chapter 59

> There is no substitute for hard work.
>
> Genius is one percent inspiration and ninety-nine percent perspiration.
> *Thomas Alva Edison, 1847-1931 [Life, 1932]*

METABOLIC DISEASES

Atherosclerosis is the cause of over 50% of deaths in western world. It is slowly progressive disease of arteries, with thickening of intima, fibrotic deposits which gradually narrow the lumen, and simultaneously are the location of bleeding and thrombus development. Atheroma is the most frequent visible sign of atherosclerosis, i.e. subendothelial accumulation of large lipid containing foam cells that later becomes a fibrous plaque. Clinical symptomatology is the result of endothelial dysfunction, coagulation and fibrinolysis. Thrombus, responsible for acute symptoms, is usually triggered by a recent atheroma, without fibrous capsule, that obstructs the arterial lumen only 40% or less.

There are *five risk factors of atherosclerosis that can be influenced*, i.e. hyperlipidemia, smoking, hyperhomocysteinemia, hypertension, diabetes mellitus, and *three that cannot*: older age, male sex, and genetic predisposition. There is some relationship with hyperfibrinogenemia, and gout.

Hyperhomocysteinemia is the sole independent risk factor for early or 'premature' atherosclerosis. Homocystein is a highly reactive amino acid with both direct and indirect toxic effect upon endothel and subsequent thrombogenesis.

According to the hypothesis of a *'response to injury'* in pathogenesis of arteriosclerosis, the first step is an endothelial damage, and a reaction to it that follows in the form of plaques developing on the spots with large mechanical demands, i.e. arterial branching.

Dietary fats, largely triacylglycerides, are hydrolyzed in the intestine by lipases from exocrine pancreas. The breakdown products of triacylglycerides are absorbed by the intestinal mucosal cells, which utilize energy of ATP to reassemble these into triacylglycerides again. Cholesterol from animal fat is absorbed as well, and metabolized into cholesterol ester. Intestinal mucosal cells synthesize certain proteins at the same time, and assemble large lipoprotein particles from these proteins and lipids, called chylomicrons. Chylomicrons are secreted by mucosal cells into blood. Another lipoprotein, VLDL, is assembled from lipids and proteins in the liver and released into blood.

Both VLDL's and chylomicrons function as lipid transporters so that other cells in the body are provided with fuel molecules for metabolism, i.e. muscle cells, or for storage of fat for future needs, i.e. in fatty cells. Lipoproteins cannot unload triacylglycerides into cells directly, they are broken down by lipoprotein lipase, that acts on VLDL and chylomicrons in the blood, into smaller breakdown products, fatty acids. Fatty acids can be taken up by the cells in the vicinity of the breakdown. The VLDL, lipoproteins, decrease dramatically in size by this breakdown, and become smaller lipoproteins, i.e. LDL's. (Note on terminology: the more fat there is in a lipoprotein, the lighter it is. Thus LDL is heavier than VLDL, as it contains a higher percentage of protein and cholesterol and less triacylglycerides than VLDL).

'Bad' cholesterol is associated with LDL, while 'good' cholesterol resides in HDL lipoprotein. HDL is the smallest of lipoproteins, made by the liver, initially rich in protein, with very little cholesterol ester. HDL picks up cholesterol from cells, converts it to cholesterol ester, and carries it to the liver where it can be transferred to LDL or VLDL.

The cause of metabolic disorders is often faulty endocrine regulations, i.e. diabetes mellitus, defects of genes for enzymes, i.e. enzymopathies, or defects of transport proteins, i.e. mucoviscidosis, cystinosis.

Disorders of lipoprotein metabolism

Lipids are transported in blood in the form of globoid molecular complexes, lipoproteins. The *'wrapping'* of the globoid structures is *by hydrophilic lipids, i.e. phospholipids, cholesterol*, and the *'nucleus'* is made of *strongly hydrophobic lipids, i.e. triacylglycerols and cholesterol esters*, that are the transport and storage form of cholesterol. Lipoproteins also contain apolipoproteins.

Lipoproteins are recognized by their size, density, lipid composition, production locus, and their *apolipoproteins, that serve as structural elements of lipoproteins*.

Plasma lipoproteins are macromolecules which enable dissolution of normally water-insoluble cholesterol, triacylglycerol and phospholipids in water, and that takes place in plasma. They also transport such lipids from locations where they enter plasma, by absorption from intestines, or from their production in hepatocytes, to locations where they are catabolized.

By *ultracentrifuge* lipoproteins can be divided into:

- chylomicrones
- VLDL, very low density lipoproteins
- LDL, low density lipoproteins
- HDL, high density lipoproteins.

If only main lipids are taken into consideration, then disturbances of lipid metabolism can be divided into two main groups:

1. *Hyperlipidemias*, i.e. hypercholesterolemias and hypertriacylglycerolemias,
2. *Dyslipidemias*, where *the ratios* of levels of various types of lipoproteins are *abnormal*, i.e. higher level of LDL, lower level of HDL, etc.

Plasma levels of two classes of lipoproteins have a significant relationship to the development of premature atherosclerosis in individuals under 50 years of age: higher concentration of LDL and lower concentration of HDL. In individuals over 60 years of age the prognostic value of high LDL is of not very importance, but lower concentration of HDL is highly significant. The main risk factor for development of atherosclerosis of coronary vessels, *the lowered concentration of HDL-cholesterol in blood serum, is associated with mutation of gene for lipoprotein lipase.*

The second component of lipoproteins are proteins, called *apolipoproteins*, very important for transport and metabolism of lipids:

- *Apolipoprotein A-I* is the main protein component of HDL, that plays a very important role in reversed transport of cholesterol from tissues back to the liver,
- *Apolipoprotein A-II* is the 2nd most important protein of HDL,
- *Apolipoprotein B* is the basic component of LDL: it is 90% of its molecule, and it is the main apolipoprotein of VLDL and chylomicrons,
- *Apolipoprotein C-II* is important for creation of VLDL and HDL,
- *Apolipoprotein E* plays the main role in metabolism of cholesterol and triacylglycerides.

Lipoproteins, especially Lp(a), are the link between atherogenic process and processes of coagulation and fibrinolysis. *At least 17 – 25% of all patients with myocardial infarction have abnormalities of Lp(a), very similar to LDL.*

Lipoproteinlipase (LPL) is a multifunctional enzyme. Besides catalysis of breakdown of triacylglycerides, there are additional structural domains for binding on endothelial cells, chylomicrons, VLDL, proteoglycans, etc., and for that reason the phenotypic expressions of mutation of LPL gene could vary, especially when they are in another domain, i.e. not in the same domain where they were originally created as a result of mutation of LPL gene.

Chylomicrons transport lipids from the intestine via intestinal lymph throughout the body, i.e. skeletal muscles, fatty tissue, where their apolipoproteins activate endothelial lipoproteinlipase that splits off free fatty acids which are then taken up by myocytes and fatty cells. Remnants of chylomicrons are bound in the liver to the receptors, engulfed by endocytosis, and pass on their triacylglycerides, cholesterol and cholesterol esthers. Liver exports imported as well as newly synthetized triacylglycerides and cholesterol in the form of VLDL to the periphery, where lipoproteinlipase, activated by its ApoCII, releases free fatty acids.

HDL picks up extra cholesterol from extrahepatic cells and blood, and carries it, as well as cholesterol esters, to the liver, and steroid hormones producing endocrine glands, i.e. ovaries, testes, adrenal cortex.

Atherogenic lipoprotein phenotype is in 95% of cases caused by genetic metabolic malfunctions, i.e. familial hyperlipoproteinemias and dyslipoproteinemias. A specific patient can be found to have one or more of the following laboratory findings: *hypercholesterolemia, hypertriacyl-glycerolemia, higher level of LDL-cholesterol, apolipoprotein B and lipoprotein(a), or lower level of HDL-cholesterol and apolipoprotein A-I.*

Increased level of lipids in blood applies to cholesterol, triacylglycerides, or both. In a majority of patients with hypercholesterolemia, the real cause is not known, but it often runs in some families, and obesity and improper nutrition play a role.

In *familial hypercholesterolemia*, due to genetic defects of LDL-receptor, a blockage of intake of LDL by the cell takes place, and as a result plasma cholesterol level is higher since birth, and that causes myocardial infarction already in teens. Serum cholesterol rises, because cells do not accept cholesterol-rich LDL, and there is an increased synthesis of cholesterol in extrahepatic tissues. Treatment in heterozygotes is by ion changer Cholestyramin that binds biliary acids in the intestine, and blocks enterohepatic re-circulation, thereby triggering a new production of biliary acids from cholesterol, so that intracellular concentration of cholesterol decreases. In homozygotes only plasmapheresis is of value.

In *combined hyperlipidemia*, another genetic disease, besides cholesterol also levels of triacylglycerides are higher. There is an increased synthesis of VLDL, and thereby also of LDL.

Familial dys-β-lipoproteinemia is characterized by disturbed pick-up of chylomicron remnants in the liver, so that their plasma concentration rises, and thereby a risk of atherosclerosis is very high.

Primary hypertriacylglycerolemia, with an increased synthesis of triacylglycerides in the liver, and low HDL, brings about a higher risk of atherosclerosis, and a predisposition toward pancreatitis.

Hypo-lipo-proteinemias are also pathological. In **Hypo-α-lipoproteinemia**, or Tangier disease, there is a defect of ApoA-lipoproteins, causing low HDL, and thereby high risk of atherosclerosis, ataxia and neuropathy.

In *A-β-lipoproteinemia* there is a lack of LDL in plasma so that chylomicrons cannot be exported from intestinal mucosa, and LDL from the liver, with resulting steatosis of liver. Stem cell transplantation of liver, placenta, stomach/intestine, is advised.

Hyperlipoproteinemia type 1, a rare AR disorder, caused by deficit of Apolipoprotein C-II and of lipoprotein lipase, is characterized by triacylglycerolemia, massive fasting chylomicronemia, and recurrent severe pancreatitis.

Familial hyperchylomicronemia is caused by mutations of LPL gene, and causes very high levels of triacylglycerol, and a risk of severe pancreatitis in early childhood.

Familial hypercholesterolemia, AD disorder, has been found in 5 - 10% of population in the US and UK, causing high levels of LDL cholesterol and premature onset of atherosclerosis. It is the best studied cause of hyperlipidemia. In heterozygotes, with incidence 1:500, the first MI takes place in males before the age of 40, in females before the age of 60, and the level of LDL-cholesterol is twice the norm. In homozygotes, with incidence 1:1,000,000, there is a complete clinical picture with corneal arcus juvenilis, xanthelasma palpebrarum, extensive tuberous xanthomatosis in tendons and skin, extremely high LDL-cholesterol, observed already in childhood.

Familial combined hyperlipoproteinemia is the most frequent genetic metabolic disorder, with incidence of mutant genes 1:300, with high levels of cholesterol and triacylglycerides. Phenotypically, hypercholesterolemia, combined hyperlipidemia, or atherogenic dyslipidemia, are present, along with obesity, hypertension, and insulin-resistance.

Familial dyslipidemia is AD disorder, with higher levels of triacylglycerides, and low levels of HDL-cholesterol, and insulin-resistance.

Familial hypo-α-lipoproteinemia, is characterized by android obesity associated with hypersecretion of lipoproteins containing apolipoprotein B and increased catabolism of apolipoprotein A-I containing lipoproteins.

Familial dys-β-lipoproteinemia, is AD disorder, with high risk of atherosclerosis, where the first clinical finding is peripheral arterial disease appearing at the age of 30, and palmar xanthomas.

Familial excess of lipoprotein (a), AD disorder, leads to premature atherosclerosis, frequently in childhood. Lipoprotein (a) is a risk factor of atherosclerosis with the highest inheritance in population.

There is some confusion about the terminology of various genetic disorders of lipoprotein metabolism. For us the most important fact is that they are frequent, and all of them can be successfully treated by stem cell transplantation.

Family history with presence of risk factors for development of premature atherosclerosis, and presence of any of the just described genetic disorders of lipoproteins and lipoprotein lipase, are important indications for stem cell transplantation of *placenta, heart, liver, artery, gonads, and mesenchyme*. The success rate is high providing that the patient is willing to eliminate the external risk factors.

Gout

Gout is the result of increased concentration of uric acid and urates in plasma. Uric acid is the final product of purine metabolism. Normally, 90% of all metabolites of nucleotides adenine, guanine, hypoxanthine, are re-used after being turned by respective enzymes into AMP, IMP or GMP. Only the remaining 10% is via xanthineoxidase converted into xanthine, and finally uric acid. Uric acid dissolves minimally, particularly in a cold environment, and at low pH, and that is the basis of gout. Since urates dissolve in synovial fluid, but poorly, especially at low temperature, and the most distal parts of the body have lower temperature than the trunk, crystals of urates accumulate frequently in distal joints of the foot. Alcohol ingestion, obesity, some drugs, and presence of lead in the body, contribute to the crystallization process.

Hyperuricemia occurs in 10% of western population, and in 90% of instances it is 'primary gout' with genetic predisposition.

Gout attack develops when a part of microtophi releases some fragments of crystals that act as foreign body, triggering aseptic arthritis. Sudden increase of uric acid level in plasma can cause massive precipitation of urates in collecting tubules of kidneys, which can lead to kidney failure.

Chapter 60

All animals are equal, but some animals are more equal than others.
George Orwell, 103-1950, [Animal Farm, 1945]

He who can does. He who cannot, teaches.
George Bernard Shaw, 1856-1950, [Man and Superman, 1903]

KIDNEY DISEASES

Kidney damage affects blood flow, glomerular function, tubular function, and abnormal urine composition triggers the development of urinary stones. Kidneys play a dominant role in regulation of water, electrolytes, and acid-base balance in the body, and thereby in regulation of blood pressure. Elimination of water and other matter through kidneys is regulated by hormones, i.e. antidiuretic hormone, aldosterone, atrial natriuretic factor, parathormone, calcitriol, calcitonin, cortisol, prostaglandin E2, insulin, estrogens, progesterone, thyroxin, somatostatin.

Twenty-five percent of total blood flow is through kidneys. All water in plasma passes through kidney epithelial cells every 20 minutes, and entire volume of extracellular fluids pass through kidneys every 3 hours.

Kidneys produce hormones: calcitriol, rennin-angiotensin, erythropoietin 40% of insulin breaks down in kidneys, and a significant portion of steroids as well.

Tubular malfunctions

Genetic defect of kidney and intestinal glucose-galactose transport causes ***glucose and galactose malabsorption***. Genetic defect of another glucose transport protein causes ***renal glucosuria***.

With **renal phosphate diabetes** the reabsorption of phosphates decreased, and that leads to bone demineralization (rachitis).

Increased reabsorption of phosphates due to the lack of parathormone or disturbance of its effectiveness, i.e. pseudohypoparathyreosis, leads to **hyperphosphatemia**.

Defect of Na^+-co-transport of neutral aminoacids in kidneys and intestine causes **Hartnup syndrome** with aminoaciduria. Resulting lack of tryptophan leads to the lack of nicotinic acid with damage to CNS and skin.

Defect of aminoacid transport protein for neutral and di-basic aminoacids magnifies losses of ornithin, lysine, arginine, cystin in **cystinuria** with precipitation of cystin in urine into stones.

Reabsorption of basic amino acids is disrupted in **familial protein intolerance**.

Defect of co-transport of cyclic amino acids, i.e. proline, leads to **iminoglycinuria**.

In **acidosis of proximal tubule**, the reabsorption of HCO_3^- cannot be balanced out by transport capacity of distal tubule, and thereby it is excreted in urine even with its normal concentration in plasma.

In **Fanconi syndrome**, several transport systems are malfunctioning, with resulting glycosuria, acidosis of proximal tubule and hypokalemia. We treated a 5 ½ year old boy with otherwise untreatable Debre-De Toni-Fanconi syndrome with cell transplantation of *kidney, liver, cartilage, placenta, and mesenchyme*. Within 5 months, the patient's height increased by 9 cm, weight by 2.1 kg, waddling gate disappeared, the valgus deformity of the left lower leg decreased. The patient did not have a single respiratory infection that he suffered from regularly. Hypocalcemia and hyperphosphatemia disappeared. Hyperphosphaturia decreased. The urinary calcium excretion became practically normal. Hyperaminoaciduria was substantially decreased. Hepatosplenic syndrome was still present but serum transaminases were dramatically lower [282].

In **gout**, the excessive Na^+ and water reabsorption in proximal tubule concentrates uric acid in the lumen, and thereby stimulates its reabsorption with resulting sedimentation of practically insoluble uric acid in joints.

Genetic defect of transport of Cl^-, or K^+ channel, is the cause of ***Bartter syndrome*** with disrupted urine concentration, natriuresis, hypokalemia, and low blood pressure, despite high levels of rennin, angiotensin, aldosterone.

Genetic defect of transport protein causes ***Gittelman syndrome***, a variant of Bartter syndrome.

Hypoaldosteronism leads to Na^+ loss through kidneys, and thereby to lowered volume of extracellular fluid and low blood pressure.

Hyperactivity of Na^+ channels leads to retention of Na^+ and to high blood pressure in ***Liddle syndrome***.

Defect of secretion of H^+ in distal tubule leads to ***acidosis of distal tubule*** with alkaline urine and frequent calciumphosphate stones.

In rare instances of treatment of ***Lowe's oculocerebrorenal syndrome***, stem cell transplantation of *kidney, liver, retina, placenta, exocrine pancreas, and diencephalon*, was used.

Water can reabsorb in the entire nephron, with the exception of an ascending Henle loop, but reabsorption in distal tubule and collecting duct requires ADH. Lack of ADH, or non-responsiveness of nephron to ADH, causes ***diabetes insipidus***, when up to 20 liters of hypotonic urine is excreted. Our experience in treatment of central diabetes insipidus by cell transplantation is *Chapter 45*.

Glomerular defects

Glomeruli are damaged by inflammation, i.e. ***glomerulonephritis***, the cause of which are soluble antigen-antibody complexes which deposit onto glomerular basilar membrane, and by complement activation trigger local inflammation. This damages glomerular capillaries and destroys filtering, i.e. immunocomplex nephritis. As triggers play part many drugs, allergens, pathogenic microorganisms, especially streptococci group A, and IgG, IgM, IgA as antibodies.

Much less frequent is ***Masugi nephritis***, caused by autoantibodies against basilar membrane with proliferation of endothelium, mesangial cells, podocytes, and mesangial matrix.

Glomeruli can be damaged by amyloid deposits in amyloidosis, by high concentration of filtered plasma proteins in plasmacytoma, by high pressure in glomerular capillaries in arterial hypertension, venous thrombosis of renal veins, venous stagnation in right-heart decompensation, hyperfiltration with diabetic nephropathy, as well as by inadequate perfusion in atherosclerosis and arteriolosclerosis.

For treatment of glomerular diseases cell transplantation of *kidney, adrenal cortex, placenta, artery, mesenchyme* are recommended. *Treatment of pyelonephritis by cell transplantation is contraindicated, as it is an inflammatory condition.*

Nephrotic syndrome

Nephrotic syndrome is a triad of proteinuria, hypoproteinemia and peripheral edemas. It is the sole kidney disease that has been treated with cell transplantation, and with success. A 55 year old female with recurrent asthma suddenly developed swelling of both feet and lower legs with dyspnea, nausea, vomiting, loss of appetite, and weakness, so that the patient was confined to bed. The abdominal swelling was increasing, and urinary output was minimal. Cell transplantation of *placenta and kidney*, eliminated most of ascites, restored normal urination, brought back good appetite, within 16 days [18]. Sometimes cell transplants of *liver and adrenal cortex* are added.

Glomerular filter, i.e. fenestrated endothelium, basilar membrane, podocyte slot membrane, has a selective permeability for various components of blood. Molecules larger than pores cannot pass through filter whatsoever while those smaller than pores pass through equally well as water. Electric charge is very important for permeability: positively charged or neutral molecules pass through the filter much better than negatively charged. In glomerulonephritis, the filter integrity can be broken, so that the access to the cavity of Bowman capsule can be gained not only by proteins, but also by erythrocytes. A small transport capacity for proteins cannot 'keep pace' with massive quantity of filtered proteins and proteinuria ensues. This leads to hypoproteinemia.

Lipoproteins cannot be filtered even through damaged filter, and since hypoproteinemia stimulates production of lipoproteins in liver, hyperlipidemia develops with hypercholesterolemia.

Hypoproteinemia causes decrease of blood volume, thirst, ADH secretion, aldosterone secretion. Increased water intake and increase of natrium chloride and water reabsorption brings on edema. Aldosteron causes hypokalemic alkalosis.

Interstitial nephritis is an inflammatory kidney disease where inflammation does not originate from glomeruli. The most common form is bacterial nephritis, or pyelonephritis, with involvement of medulla of kidneys, in which due to marked acidity, hypertonicity and ammonia concentration, all defense mechanisms are weakened. Interstitial nephritis can be caused even without an infection, by deposition of stones of calcium salts or uric acid. Deposits of uric acid in kidney originate from excessive intake of purines in food, but also by excessive endogenous production of uric acid, i.e. after cytostatica for treatment of leukemias. Calcium deposits result from hypercalciuria from increased absorption of calcium in intestine, and excessive calcium mobilization from bones by tumors, or immobilization. Infection by urease-splitting microorganism leads to a breakdown of urea to ammonia in urine. As ammonia binds hydrogen ions, alkaline urine is produced. This helps phosphate sedimentation, stone production causing disruption of urine outflow and thereby support the development of ascending pyelonephritis, i.e. "vicious circle".

In acute kidney failure there is no place for stem cell transplantation and in chronic kidney failure it is too late.

Renal hypertension is a direct cause of arterial hypertension in only 7% of patients, but kidneys play the key role in the causation of arterial hypertension, and its clinical course, even if there is no kidney disease present. Kidney ischemia leads, via stimulation of renin-angiotensin system, to arterial hypertension. Retention of sodium and water causes arterial hypertension even without rennin-angiotensin system.

Every arterial hypertension causes kidney damage. Even primary extra-renal hypertension becomes renal hypertension by development of nephrosclerosis.

Chapter 61

A man is as old as his arteries.
Thomas Sydenham, 1624-1689, [Bulletin of N.Y. Academy at MEDICINE, 1928]

All we know is still infinitely less than all that still remains unknown.
William Harvey, 1578-1657, [De Motu Cordis et Sanguinis, 1628]

CARDIOVASCULAR DISEASES

Conductive system of heart

The heart contains muscle cells which create and conduct electric impulses, as well as those that respond to electric impulse by muscle contraction. In distinction to peripheral muscle, creation of the impulse takes place inside of the organ, i.e. heart has enormous autonomy. Myocardial fibers of atria and ventricles are united into a functional syncytium, i.e. cells are not isolated from each other, on the contrary, they are interconnected through gap junctions. The impulse, created anywhere in ventricles or atria, always leads to a complete contraction of both ventricles and atria in accordance with 'all or nothing law'.

The impulse is normally created in sinoatrial node, and this structure is called cardiac pacemaker. Impulse is spread from it onto both atria toward atrioventricular node, and then passes through His bundle and both its (Towar) branches to Purkinje fibers that transmit impulse to myocardium of the ventricles. There the impulse spreads from endocard to epicard and from apex to the base of the heart.

During action potential Ca^{2+} enters myocardial cell from extracellular space through voltage controlled channels.

Important prerequisites for normal activation of conductive system, but also of working myocardium of atria and ventricles are:

- normal deep and stable resting potential (-80 to –90 mV),
- quick depolarization (dV/dt = 200 – 1000 V/s) at the beginning of action potential,
- sufficiently long duration of action potential.

Any change of impulse creation or conduction that leads to different sequence of electric activation of atria or ventricles, or to disturbance of their mutual interconnection, causes arrhythmia.

In two adult X-linked muscular dystrophy dogs, lacking an expression of dystrophin in both cardiac and skeletal muscles, fetal canine atrial cardiomyocytes, including sinus nodal cells, were injected into the left ventricle. Four weeks later a catheter ablation of AV-node was carried out. Immediately thereafter, a ventricular escape rhythm emerged, that originated from a new pacemaker within the labeled cell transplantation site. This was the first *in vivo* evidence of electrical and mechanical coupling between allogeneic donor cardiomyocytes and host myocardium [209].

Cell transplants of *cardiomyoblasts, hypothalamus, and placenta*, were used for treatment of 10 patients with **intractable arrhythmia** at the Research Center of Cardiology of Russian Academy of Medical Sciences in Novossibirsk. In all 10 patients, cell transplantation reversed the lack of therapeutic response, so that patients were converted to sinus rhythm.

Myocardium

An interesting feature, not seen in voluntary muscle, is that the heart has a number of different receptors located at its sarcolemma that respond to adrenaline (epinephrine), such as α- and β-adrenergic receptors. Adrenaline released into the blood stream increases the heart rate by interaction with β-adrenergic receptors and cardiac output. Myocardium is responsive to adrenaline, noradrenaline, and acetylcholine, while *voluntary skeletal muscle is responsive only to acetylcholine*.

The response of smooth muscle to β-adrenergic stimulation is a muscle relaxation.

Hypertension has incidence of 20% in industrial countries. **Primary hypertension** in the first labile stage can be successfully treated by stem cell transplantation of *placenta, hypothalamus, artery, and liver*. Treatment by anti-hypertensive drugs continues as necessary until the benefit of cell transplantation is known 8 weeks later.

Secondary hypertension is found in 5 - 15% of all hypertensive patients, and is divided into two main types, according to the pathogenesis:

1. ***Renal hypertension***: Every renal ischemia leads to a release of rennin, that separates a peptide angiotensin I from plasma angiotensinogen. By splitting off additional two amino acids from angiotensin I by peptidase, mostly present in lungs, angiotensin II develops, that is a strong vasoconstrictor. It releases aldosterone as well.

2. ***Endocrine hypertension***:
   - ***adrenogenital syndrome***: production of cortisol in adrenal cortex is inhibited, and thereby secretion of ACTH is unblocked, and that leads to a massive production and release of precursors of cortisol and aldosteron in adrenal cortex with mostly mineralocorticoid and androgenic activity,
   - ***primary hyperaldosteronism***, or Conn syndrome: tumor of adrenal cortex produces high quantity of aldosteron without any regulatory limits, with Na^+ retention in kidneys and increase of ECT volume,
   - ***Cushing syndrome***: very high secretion of ACTH by pituitary tumor, or due to neurogenous factors, or autonomous adrenal cortex tumor increases glucocorticoid level in plasma,
   - ***Pheochromocytoma***: tumor of adrenal medulla produces catecholamines with uncontrolled rise of level of adrenaline and noradrenaline and thereby hypertension.

Every chronic hypertension will cause, sooner or later, secondary renal dysfunctions, hypertrophy of vessel wall, and atherosclerosis that makes hypertension permanent despite successful treatment of the primary cause. Kidneys play a leading role in idiopathic hypertension, hypertension in adrenogenital syndrome, and Cushing syndrome.

Hypotension usually goes hand in hand with *autonomous nervous system dysfunction*, and if cell transplantation is necessary, then cell transplants of *hypothalamus, placenta, adrenal medulla, adrenal cortex, cardiomyoblasts*, are advised.

Ischemic heart disease: Characteristic feature is a lowered coronary reserve whereby available oxygen cannot cover the needs. Myocardium gets its energy from free fatty acids, glucose, and lactate. All these substances are used up for production of ATP, and they are all dependant on oxygen.

The main reason is the narrowing of major coronary arteries by atherosclerosis. Cell transplantation of *placenta, heart myoblasts, liver, and artery*, has been used for years for such patients.

For treatment of *unstable angina*, the same cell transplants are advised as for myocardial infarction.

Myocardial infarction: If myocardial ischemia continues for a longer time, then after approximately one hour tissue necrosis will take place, i.e. infarct. In 85% of cases the fault lies with acutely developing thrombus at the point of atherosclerotic coronary stenosis.

During the last three years, many patients with recent extensive myocardial infarction have been treated by stem cell transplantation in various western European countries with remarkably good results.

The purpose is to regenerate as many damaged heart muscle fibers as possible, and thereby decrease the size of myocardial scar, as well as stimulate angiogenesis, i.e. forming new blood vessels from the pre-existing ones.

For patients with massive heart attacks, it is a matter of life or death, or a matter of debilitating disability versus ability to live reasonably well.

Stem cell transplants have to be implanted into heart, either into a re-opened obstructed branch of coronary artery via angiography, or into infarcted heart muscle via heart catheterization.

According to US statistics, 1.1 million people get heart attack every year. There are 4.8 million patients with congestive heart failure, over one half of which dies within 5 years. All patients with extensive myocardial infarction and decompensated congestive heart failure are candidates for stem cell transplantation treatment.

Cardiomyocytes lose their ability to proliferate after birth and so heart muscle fibers cannot regenerate. For that reason, myocardial injury, such as myocardial infarction (MI), heals by replacement of contractile heart muscle fibers with fibrotic tissue scar, which not only cannot participate in pumping of blood, it does not even contribute to passive mechanical function of heart. *Massive loss of cardiomyocytes after MI is a common cause of congestive heart failure.*

Experimental data collected over the years about the ability of implanted myoblastic cells to restore function of damaged cardiomyocytes encouraged cardiologists in Paris, France, and Dusseldorf, Germany, to treat patients with extensive myocardial infarction by cell transplantation. Due to paucity of suitable donors for orthotopic heart transplantation, and severity and risk of such undertaking, success of stem cell transplantation in prevention of massive damage of heart muscle after MI is of enormous significance [279].

Cell transplants used in the above two clinical trials were autologous: skeletal myoblasts in Paris [203], mononuclear bone marrow cells in Duesseldorf [204].

The Duesseldorf group reported clinical data of 10 patients after MI treated with their method of cell transplantation along with their standard therapy, compared with parameters of 10 patients receiving standard therapy only. After 3 months' follow-up, the post-MI scar, measured by left ventriculography, was decreased significantly within the stem cell transplantation group, and was significantly smaller than in standard therapy group. Infarct wall movement velocity increased significantly in the stem cell transplantation group only. Dobutamine stress echocardiography, radionuclide ventriculography, catheterization of the right heart, all showed a significant improvement in stroke volume index, left ventricular end-systolic volume, contractility, and myocardial perfusion of the infarct region [205].

Due to limited availability of human fetal cardiomyocytes, alternative sources of suitable cell transplants for treatment of myocardial infarction, congestive heart failure, dilated cardiomyopathy, and other heart diseases, have been searched for. Here are reports about some laboratory studies. Interestingly, in cardiology experimental data seem to bear a close relationship to clinical data, as compared with neurotransplantation, for example.

A single fiber of skeletal muscle retains skeletal myoblasts beneath basal lamina throughout a lifetime. From these myoblasts skeletal muscle regenerates in case of injury. In two rat models with heart failure, *allogeneic* skeletal myoblasts were injected into four myocardial sites. Within 3 days, the donor single skeletal fibers disappeared, while their myoblasts began to differentiate into multinucleated myotubes. This process took 4 weeks, and caused a significant improvement of cardiac function [206].

Clonal stem cell line WB-F344 from a male adult rat liver was injected as cell xenogeneic transplant into the left ventricle of adult female nude mice. Male WB-F344 cells with the same genotype were identified within the implantation site 6 weeks later. Phenotype of these new 'stem cell derived cells' was that of cardiomyocytes. So adult liver-derived stem cells responded *in vivo* to the tissue environment of adult heart and differentiated into mature cardiomyocytes [207].

Autologous skeletal myoblasts have been favored in clinical practice to-date because of easy availability. In reality, due to lack of connexin43, a gap junction protein, skeletal myoblast transplants should not be as effective as cardiomyocytes to treat MI. Only connexin43 containing cardiomyocyte transplants build intercellular connections with host myocardial fibers, such as gap junctions and desmosomes, and thereby act synchronously with the host heart.

Neonatal cardiomyocytes of 3 day old rats were injected into the border zone of infarct 10 days after injury. Subsequently, 4 to 14 days later, treated hearts were studied by immunohistochemistry. Antibodies against connexin43, desmoplakin, and cadherin, identifying gap junctions, desmosomes, and adherens junctions, respectively, were found between grafted cardiomyocytes, as well as between grafted and host cardiomyocytes. Grafted cardiomyocytes were seen aligning parallel to, and establishing electrical pathways with the host cardiomyocytes [208].

How soon after MI should the cell transplantation be done? Following two studies are not in full agreement, but indicate that CT should be carried out no later than 6 days after MI. When carried out by selective coronary catheterization and infusion of myoblasts, rather than injection into infarcted myocardium, CT can take place at the time of initial balloon angioplasty, stenting or other invasive procedure.

In a rat model of MI, fetal cardiomyocytes were transplanted immediately, 2 weeks and 4 weeks, after myocardial injury. At 8 weeks, studies of heart function, planimetry, and histology were carried out. Inflammatory reaction was greatest during the first week and subsided during the second week after MI. Scar size increased up to 8 weeks after MI. Cardiomyocytes transplanted immediately after MI were absent at 8 weeks and the scar size and heart function were as in untreated group. Cardiomyocyte transplantation should be carried out immediately after the inflammatory reaction is over, but before the scar expansion [210].

Previous studies with bone marrow stromal cells engrafted into *xenogeneic* fetal recipients were repeated: the recipients were fully immunocompetent adults, and *no immunosuppression was used.* Bone marrow stromal cells were taken from C57Bl/6 mice and injected into adult Lewis rats. One week later, the recipients underwent coronary artery ligation and were sacrificed 1 to 12 weeks thereafter. Labeled mice cells were engrafted into bone marrow cavities for the duration of experiment. Circulating mice cells were found only in rats with 1-day old MI. Mice cells were found in the damaged myocardium by immunohistochemistry. This study proved that adult stem cells engraft into a xenogeneic live organism, without immunosuppression, without difficulty. Simultaneously, they can home to injured myocardium, differentiate into cardiomyocytes, and create a stable chimera in the heart [211].

Human mesenchymal xenogeneic stem cells were injected into the left ventricle of CB17 SCID beige adult mice *without immunosuppression.* After 7 days, de novo expression of desmin, beta-myosin heavy chains, alpha actinin, cardiac troponin T, and phospholamban, all typical of cardiomyocytes, could be detected. Human adult xenogeneic mesenchymal stem cells engrafted in the myocardium and differentiated into cardiomyocytes [212].

Embryonic cardiac cells were cultured for 3 days, and then implanted 7 days after extensive MI into myocardium in a rat model, *without immunosuppression.* Engrafment of cell *xenotransplants* was observed 1, 4, and 7 weeks after CT. Differentiation of embryonic cells into cardiomyocytes was proven by antibodies against α-SMA, connexin43, and fast and slow myosin heavy chain. Serial echocardiography revealed that cell transplantation prevented scar thinning, left ventricular dilatation and dysfunction as compared with controls [213].

In five described studies dealing with cell xenotransplantation, no immunosuppression was used, and in 9 of 12 included papers about allogeneic cell transplantation the authors did not utilize immunosuppression either.

Autologous cell transplantation, of skeletal myoblasts, or mononuclear bone marrow stem cells, directly into damaged myocardium, is a reliable treatment for patients with serious myocardial infarction, or heart failure that do not need cell transplantation immediately to save their lives, and are hospitalized in a top hospital, with qualified invasive cardiologists, and excellent tissue culture laboratory.

If this therapeutic method should become important for the health care system worldwide, stem cell xenotransplantation will have to be utilized. *Stem cell xenotransplants can be delivered to any hospital without delay, at all times, and transplanted indirectly into the liver if an interventional cardiologist is not at hand, without immunosuppression.* Subsequently, such patient can be transferred to the high level hospital for the specialist's care.

A report about treatment of 251 chronic cardiac patients with cell transplantation is remarkable, because only one of 251 patients got worse, the rest were improved or unchanged. In 35 patients, 3 - 6 months post-MI the success rate was 51%, in 76 patients with various other types of myocardial damage the success rate was 53%, in 41 patients with 'myodegeneratio cordis' the success rate was 72%, in 9 patients with conduction block of Adams-Stokes type the success rate was 55% [218]. This was before the era of routine heart catheterization and interventional cardiology, and other modern technologies: none of the above patients received cell transplants via injection into damaged myocardium or via balloon catheter in the branch of coronary artery. Fetal cell xenotransplants of *myocardium, placenta, and liver*, were implanted deeply subcutaneously, counting on homing of these fetal progenitor cells into the injured tissue, and their differentiation into cardiomyocytes and vascular cells. The concept of homing was proven in the 1950's in Germany by isotope and intravital dye studies [216, 217, 219, 95], and since 1993 also in other western countries [19 - 21].

In 1993, the author gained his first clinical experience with cell transplantation in cardiology. In a cooperative study of International Institute of Biological Medicine in Moscow and Russian Research Institute of Pediatrics of Russian Academy of Medical Sciences, 7 terminal patients with dilated cardiomyopathy, often with relative insufficiency of 1 - 2 valves, aged 4 to 14 years, were treated by human fetal cell transplantation. Cell transplants of *myocardium, liver, and placenta*, were implanted under the aponeurosis of rectus abdominis muscle above the umbilicus.

One 10 year old female died four days after cell transplantation, and at autopsy it was learned that dilated cardiomyopathy was secondary to anomalous origin of coronary arteries.

One 14 year old female was discharged in improved condition, with liver size decreased by 2.5 cm, lesser crural edema, diminished scleral icterus, and normal auscultation of lungs. She was brought back to ICU 6 weeks later in her home town and died two weeks later.

Another 14 year old male died 9 months later at home.

Remaining patients survived for the duration of the follow-up, and were in good condition: 4 year old female for 14 months, 13 year old male for 17 months, 5 year old female for 15 months, 10 year old male for 17 months. No repeated cell transplantations were carried out.

Only small children in early stages of their illnesses are treated by one cell transplant only. Usually the chronically ill patient requires transplantation of cells of all those organs or tissues which are involved in the pathophysiology of the patient's disease(s). The more exact is the pathophysiological and biochemical diagnosis, the more accurate the choice of cell transplants for treatment will be. Cardiac patients have usually received, besides transplant of *cardiomyoblasts, also cells of liver and placenta, and lungs* in cases of decompensated left heart with pulmonary congestion and hypertension, unless additional malfunctions are discovered which could be corrected by transplants of cells with necessary compensatory functions.

Congestive heart failure: Cardiac insufficiency is a decreased ability of myocardium to carry out its function, mostly applicable to the left ventricle. The most common causes are ischemic heart disease, hypertension, and cardiomyopathies. The body uses compensatory mechanisms to rise the circulating blood volume and blood pressure, mainly the increased tonus of sympathetic nervous system that by the release of additional catecholamines triggers an activation of cardiac β_1-adrenergic receptors, whereby f_S rises, along with tachycardia, and there is a positive inotropic effect as well.

In addition, α_1-adrenergic vasoconstriction limits blood flow through skeletal musculature (tiredness), skin (paleness), and kidneys, since priority is given to the maintenance of blood flow through coronary and cerebral arteries. A decreased flow of blood through kidneys leads to activation of rennin-angiotensin-aldosteron system, rise of filtration fraction and reflexive rise of ADH secretion, and all that is triggered in the atrium of decompensated heart. The final outcome is rising reabsorption of water and salts with peripheral edemas.

Reports by Kleinsorge, Kuhn, Oetzman, and Rietschel, on treatment of over 1,000 of their own patients with *chronic heart failure*, proved the success of cell transplantation of *placenta, heart, and liver*. Besides the general revitalization, placenta stimulates the internal breathing of myocardial cells. Transplants of cardiomyoblasts regenerate contraction ability of damaged heart. Transplanted hepatocytes restore variety of disturbed metabolic functions. Cell transplantation reverses digitalis resistance. Usually 10 - 14 days after cell transplantation, a massive diuresis sets in, lung and liver congestion diminishes, and all parameters of cardiovascular and respiratory functions improve, as well as subjective status of the patient. The success rate in 150 patients of Oetzmann was 73.2%, in 700 patients of Kuhn 67%, in 93 patients of Rietschel 72.1%, and duration of success was 12 - 15 months. Repeated cell transplantation was equally successful [239].

Cardiac decompensation at rest requires implantation of stem cell transplants via heart catheterization.

Peripheral arterial disease

While treating peripheral arterial disease with implantation of cell transplants of placenta, every physician observed how livid and cold feet and lower legs turned warm and pink within 3 – 10 minutes after the implantation. This was due to vasoactive substances in the placenta or hormones; such an immediate effect was only temporary, and was replaced by a permanent positive effect upon peripheral circulation 3 - 4 weeks later.

While developing his surgical method of transplantation of cornea, Prof. Filatov tried to find a way to avoid post-operative clouding of corneal transplants. Once during such an operation he implanted tissue fragments of placenta subcutaneously. After many failures, the corneal clouding finally stopped, and implantation of placental cells became a major topic of Soviet research institutes, and soon spread to the West as 'Filatov treatment'.

The controlled experimental study on the treatment of *arteriosclerotic vascular disease* by cell transplantation of *placenta* showed remarkable improvement in the fresh weight of aortas, significantly lowered calcium content in aortas and kidneys, and positive changes during macro- and micro-scopic examination of the arteries of experimental rabbits. The report also describes studies on clinical application of the same treatment and its success rate in terms of improvement of coronary and peripheral circulation, mental efficiency, degenerative myocardial diseases, and various dyslipoproteinemias [214]. Similar conclusions reached Kleinsorge in rabbits, and Wietek and Taupitz in their study of experimental arteriosclerosis of rats, treated by cell transplantation of placenta.

For years cell transplantation of *placenta* played a major role in the therapy of arteriosclerotic vascular disease, because placenta cells cause generalized vasodilatation, overall circulatory improvement, and increased budding of capillary collaterals.

The level of lipoproteins and cholesterol lowered significantly in all 64 patients with *arteriosclerosis* within 4 – 6 weeks after cell transplantation of placenta. There were no changes in 100 patients that served as controls [280].

Objective and subjective improvements were found in 8 of 15 patients with *advanced peripheral arteriosclerotic vascular disease* after an implantation of cell transplants of *placenta*. Improvements persisted for 8 months, and were recorded ergometrically, oscillometrically and rheographically. In 5 out of 15 patients, cholesterol decreased. Of 3 patients suffering from Raynaud's disease, there was an improvement in two. In another study, the walking distance doubled within 4 - 12 weeks in 8 and tripled in 3 from a total of 21 patients, and 3 patients became completely asymptomatic. Such results persisted for 13 - 16 weeks in 14 out of 21 patients, and for a shorter period in the remaining 7 patients [281]. Similar findings were obtained by Rietschel and Kleinsorge [329].

In a study by Oetzman, 72 patients with *peripheral arterial disease* were treated by cell transplantation of *placenta, liver and gonads*, and 58 patients improved; warming of skin, lowering of cholesterol, and increased walking distances were recorded. In other studies, Kuhn reports 67% success in 700 patients, Rietschel 72.1% success rate in 93 patients, and Oetzman 73.2% success rate in 150 patients. [95]

Scientific explanation of why placenta cells have been the most widely used in cell transplants to-date is limited. Embryonic stem cell research will undoubtedly provide answers because of the close relationship between embryonic stem cells and trophoblastic cells alluded to in other chapters of this book.

Overall, cell transplantation of *placenta, hypothalamus, liver, and spleen*, has been recommended for treatment of peripheral arterial disease caused by arteriosclerosis. Treatment of peripheral arterial disease as a complication of diabetes mellitus is covered under 'Diabetes mellitus'.

Vasculitis

Migraine, or hemicrania, is a well known disease of blood vessel regulation that many famous people suffered from, such as Julius Caesar, von Bismarck, von Beethoven, etc., that has remained incurable. The acute attacks can be treated, but the disease cannot be cured. Cell transplantation has worked wonders in this respect. Cell transplantation of *hypothalamus* is of cardinal importance, as a controlling organ of autonomous nervous system and endocrine system, accompanied by cell transplants of blood circulation regulating *adrenal cortex, liver, kidney, placenta, and pregnant ovaries, i.e. corpus lutem cells, for female patients* since it is a known fact that migraine disappears during pregnancy, and *testis for male patients* [297].

A 57 year old female has suffered from migraines since childhood. In 23 years she had tried so many treatments that she could no longer count them. One son committed suicide, and the second one was a drug addict, in and out of jail. Six years before this report she underwent cell transplantation of *placenta, frontal lobe of brain, temporal lobe of brain, adrenal cortex, and liver*. She has not had any migraines since [308].

Several conditions are triggered by deposition of immune complexes or by cell-mediated immunity, and are treatable by stem cell transplantation *as any other autoimmune disease*:

- *Polyarteritis nodosa*, involving small and medium arteries, the resulting ischemia damages kidneys, heart, and liver.
- *Temporal or arteritis magnocellularis*, involves larger arteries of head, causing headaches or facial pain, claudication of masticatory muscles, sometimes blindness.
- *Thrombangiitis obliterans*, known also as *Burger's disease*, involves medium and small arteries of extremities, and is present mostly in male smokers.
- *Raynaud disease*, painful vascular spasms caused by cold, with anesthesia of fingers or toes, at first white, then cyanotic, and finally red (reactive hyperemia). Stem cell transplantation of *placenta, cardiomyoblasts, and artery*, is advised.

Chapter 62

Nothing great will ever be achieved without great men, and men are great only if they are determined to be so.
Charles de Gaulle, 1980-1970, [Le Fil de l'Épée, 1934]

LUNG DISEASES

The primary function of the lungs is blood oxygenation. Their secondary function is the maintenance of acid-base balance through regulation of CO_2 concentration.

Lung disorders are divided into:

A. **Obstructive** with increased resistance to the air flow in respiratory passages, and thereby limited ventilation of alveoli, which can be global or partial, leading to disruption of distribution of air flow. Bronchial asthma and chronic bronchitis are classical examples.

Bronchial asthma is due to the allergy of inhaled antigens, i.e. pollen, which causes inflammation of bronchial mucosa with subsequent release of histamine and SRS-A, slow reacting substances of anaphylaxis, that bring about contraction of bronchial muscles, mucus secretion, and increased permeability of blood vessels causing edema. Microorganisms in the mucus become antigens as well, and bronchial asthma turns into ***chronic bronchitis***.

Many consider bronchial asthma a contraindication for cell transplantation, but of all lung diseases it has been one most frequently treated by this method. Review of 88 cases, 46 males, 42 females, majority between 60 and 80 years of age, treated by cell transplantation of *lungs, adrenal cortex, thymus, mesenchyme, intestine, placenta, gonads, heart, brain cortex, artery,* but also *liver, diencephalon, mesencephalon, anterior lobe of pituitary, spleen*, over 3 years, each one of them for a classical reason because 'all other treatment methods had failed', showed an absence of any allergic reactions after the treatment, an absence of status asthmaticus and only 3 instances of asthma attack after cell transplantation. A self-evaluation of the results was requested of all 88 patients, and 56 responded: 36 patients reported an improvement of asthma, while 11 reported improved general well-being but no improvement of asthma. All patients that reported an improvement stopped taking cortisol. One patient reported deterioration of his asthmatic condition, and 8 patients did not notice any change.

In the selection of cell transplants for treatment, the author of this report gives credit to P. Janson, who found that cell transplants of *spleen* function as an excellent anti-allergy treatment, causing desensitization, and to P. Niehans, who always treated asthmatics with *hypothalamus, lungs and placenta*, and credited S. Reckeweg with using *spleen, kidneys, adrenal cortex, placenta and hypothalamus*, for his patients. As a precaution, all patients received, 12 hours before treatment, a combination of antihistamin and an injection of cortisone. Based on their experience, the patients with cor pulmonale with dyspnea at rest, and with advanced emphysema, are not to be accepted for treatment by cell transplantation. Seven case histories are included [295].

A 65 year old female suffered from bronchial asthma for over 20 years due to allergies to dust and various kinds of grass. She got worse in the spring and fall when she developed attacks of bronchitis with fever. Five years before this report she developed status asthmaticus for the first time. Laboratory testing proved her allergies as well as immune deficiency. She was treated by γ-globulin as necessary. As her condition was not improving over 21 months, a cell transplantation of *mesenchyme, lungs, adrenal cortex, diencephalon, and thymus*, was carried out. During 3 years of follow-up she has not had a single asthma attack, her immunoglobulins, including IgE, were within normal limits, and other tests indicated no humoral or cellular immune deficiency [309].

Another concept of asthma treatment calls for cell transplantation of *thyroid, thymus, posterior lobe of pituitary, and adrenal medulla*, to which sometimes *liver, parathyroid, anterior lobe of pituitary, and medulla alba of brain*, are added [328].

Cystic fibrosis, or *mucoviscidosis*, is the most frequent lethal AR disorder among Caucasians with incidence 1:2,000. Pathogenesis is due to the deficiency of gene product CFTR, 'Cystic Fibrosis Transmembrane Conductance Regulator', which regulates movement of chloride ions across Cl^- channel. *One type of 850 types of mutations of CFTR gene has been with us for 50,000 years.* There is a malfunction of transport of fluids and electrolytes in exocrine epithelial cells, which causes an increased secretion of sweat in sweat glands with higher concentration of Cl^- than Na^+. There is an increased viscosity of more profuse mucous secretions in small bronchi, because fluids are absorbed rather than secreted, and such protein-rich secretions are the best medium for the bacterial growth, in particular Pseudomonas, that leads to slowly developing chronic pathologic changes of lung, i.e. bronchial obstruction with atelectasis, emphysema, bronchopneumonia, bronchiectases, fibrosis, pneumothorax, and cor pulmonale. That goes hand in hand with insufficiency of exocrine pancreas due to obstruction of pancreatic ducts with viscous secretions that causes chronic pancreatitis, and sometimes liver dysfunction, while in genital tract with blockage of ductus deferens and infertility in men, or lowered fertility in females. In intestines, meconium becomes thickened and gluey and is not eliminated in the usual way, causing meconium ileus in 10% of newborns. Polyps and chronic sinusitis develop in the nose. Stem cell transplantation of *lung, exocrine pancreas, intestine, skin, mesenchyme, and placenta*, are recommended.

Senile lungs with weakened lung retraction force causes obstruction disorder as well. Aging changes mainly the structure of elastic fibers so that their retraction power dwindles, while the proportion of collagen increases. There is a decreased number of alveolar septa, dilatation of alveolar ducts, reduction of capillary network in alveoli, calcification of cartilagineous bronchial skeleton.

B. **Restrictive** with reduction of diffusion area due to loss of functioning lung tissue.

Emphysema is a classical example, where along with reduced diffusion area, there is also a reduced count and increased volume of alveoli. 'Centrilobular emphysema' is brought on by obstructive lung disorders, while in 'panlobular emphysema' there is a loss of interalveolar septa as well.

Primary atrophic, or senile, emphysema has been treated with success by cell transplantation of *placenta, lung, mesenchyme, liver, thymus, hypothalamus, and cardiomyoblasts* if cor pulmonale is present.

In some patients there is an *α₁-antitrypsin deficiency* which normally inhibits the effect of proteases. Such patients suffer from emphysema 15 times more frequently than normal population. This enzyme is produced in the liver, and mutations can disrupt its secretion or function. This enzymopathy leads, in 60% of patients, to disruption of lung tissue and thereby loss of its elasticity. In smokers the α_1-antitrypsin is oxidized and thereby blocked, so that emphysema develops even in genetically healthy individuals. Dominance of elastases leads to breakdown of elastic lung fibers with inflammation.

Limited chest motion, paresis of diaphragm, increased pleural space with pleural effusion, pleural adhesions, or pneumothorax, belong to this group, too.

C. With **impaired perfusion** due to restrictive, obstructive and circulatory disorders, where despite adequate oxygenation and removal of CO_2 from blood in alveoli, there are still decreased concentration of gases in blood, and circulatory overload with serious consequences for the right heart.

D. With **impaired diffusion** due to an increased diffusion distance with **lung edema**, where increased intravascular pressure leads to exsudation of plasma into lung interstitium and eventually into alveoli, or in **pneumonia** where edema and increased production of fibrotic tissue causes thickening of septa between alveoli and blood capillaries, or in **pulmonary fibrosis** where fibrotic tissue pushes capillaries away from alveoli, or in *reduction of diffusion area such as in* **atelectasis** or **pulmonary infarct**.

Lung fibrosis develops after inflammation of connective tissue, i.e. in collagen diseases, or after inhalation of asbestos or silica dust, or sometimes without apparent reason, i.e. Hamman-Rich idiopathic lung fibrosis.

E. Those caused by **malfunction of regulatory neurons in respiratory center**, as well as motoneurons, nerves, neuromuscular synapses and respiratory muscles.

Overall, lung diseases have been treated seldom by cell transplantation in the past for reasons unknown.

Chapter 63

Man is an animal with primary instincts of survival. Consequently, his ingenuity has developed first and his soul afterwards. Thus the progress of science is far ahead of man's ethical behavior.
Charlie Chaplin, 1889-1977, [My Autobiography, 1964]

SKIN DISEASES

Skin is a vitally important organ for defense of our body, and along with gastrointestinal and urinary systems, is important for fluid and electrolyte balance, as well as temperature control of the body. Ten percent of total blood flow is through the skin, mostly for thermoregulation. All internal disorders and external influences can be observed on the skin. Destruction of 30% of the skin surface is dangerous to life, while 70% loss of function is fatal.

The total surface of skin is approximately 2 m^2, and the skin weight is approximately 15% of total body weight. Normal skin cells survive for 30 days. The loss of desquamated cells of stratum corneum amounts to 1.0 g a day.

There are 2 – 4 million sweat glands in the skin which could produce as much as 4 liters of hypotonic fluid every hour. The total number of hair on the body surface is approximately 100,000. One strand of hair survives for 2 ½ years, and eyelid hair 100 to 150 days.

Revitalization by stem cell transplantation makes skin less atrophic, more firm, and more elastic. This applies mostly to the skin of face and hands exposed to the elements most of the time. The skin blood flow is improved, with more rosy color, diminution of wrinkles, dryness and scaling, lid edema, and aging spots. Hair fallout stops, and sometimes new hair growth becomes apparent, occasionally graying of hair improves or disappears. Broken or damaged nails heal. This is a summary of observation made by approximately 4 million patients treated by cell transplantation primarily because of aging disease.

Skin diseases, such as **acne vulgaris, psoriasis, ulcus cruris, and various eczemas**, sarcoid Darrier-Roussy, hereditary keratosis palmaris at plantaris, chronic lichen, **scleroderma**, etc. improve by cell xeno-transplantation [264, 267 - 270]. *Vitiligo* and *frostbite of big toes* were treated by cell transplantation of *placenta and liver,* with success [18].

At the 10th World Congress of Combustology in Paris, France, in June 1994, the author read a paper on **non-surgical treatment of deep (surgical) burns** using human fetal tissues, whereby we proved that patients with burns requiring skin grafting can be treated with nearly 100% success rate by a surface application of a suspension of fetal cells of skin and placenta, faster than with surgery, and with better cosmetic results. In this way skin grafting operations, painful costly, and often repeated many times, could be avoided in the majority of instances [265]. A similar report was read at All-India Congress of Burn Injuries in 1995 at Jaipur.

This idea was born in WW2 during the 9-months long siege of St. Petersburg by the German army, where the number of burned patients reached such proportions that surgeons could not handle the load, and began to use a suspension made from skin of cadavers, frozen in the extremely cold winter, that made burials impossible, to cover the burned surfaces.

The clinical trial took place at the Moscow Burn Center of Sklifasovsky Research Center of Emergency Medicine of Russian Academy of Medical Sciences, where there was an abundance of patients with 3rd degree burns that could not receive skin grafts due to a variety of medical conditions, in particular infections of burned surface not responding to antibiotics, as well as the most experienced burn surgeons.

The published report described the treatment of 20 patients, 17 males and 3 females, from 15 to 53 years of age. *Suspension of fetal skin and placenta* was applied to the burn surface by diluting cells in a physiologic solution, and then dipping the fine gauze in the cell suspension and its application on the burned surface once every 24 hours, preventing dehydration by an external wrapping of cellophane. The treatment of fresh burns began 1 - 3 days after burn injury, and after a very conservative debridement of necrotic skin.

In the 1st degenerative/inflammatory stage, the suspension consisted of 70% of placenta and 30% of skin, as the goal was to take advantage of necrolytic and bactericidal properties of the placenta. In the 2nd inflammatory/reparative stage, the suspension consisted of 50% of placenta and 50% of skin, and finally in the 3rd reparative stage the ratio was 30% of placenta and 70% of skin, as the goal was to use the epidermal growth factors of the skin. Treatment continued until a nearly complete epithelization took place.

The success rate was 100%. The prolonged infections cleared within 24 – 48 hours, and after 24 hours the i.v. antibiotics were discontinued.

Deep burns *healed by a full thickness of exceptionally good quality in 100% of cases.* There were *no atrophic scars and a minimum of hypertrophic scars, so that the cosmetic results were superior to skin grafting* [266].

The main problem was the paucity of preparations of skin and placenta due to the lack of human fetal cadavers, so that only a limited number of patients could be so treated. That was obviously the reason why the method has not been used by anyone else. Due to that, we subsequently developed preparations of rabbit fetal *skin and placenta* for the same purpose, and tested them on patients desiring rejuvenation of skin of the face, neck, and other body parts. In the 1st stage, a controlled chemical burn was created to exfoliate epidermis and the upper layer of dermis, and in the 2nd stage, 48 hours later, a surface application of fetal skin and placenta was carried out varying the ratios of skin and placenta as in the original burn project. The results have been remarkable.

Our study of *alopecia* in children at the Endocrinologic Research Center of Russian Academy of Medical Sciences included 5 children with alopecia areata, one of them with multiple bald areas, one child with subtotal alopecia, and 4 children with total alopecia, 8 to 16 years of age, 2 males, and 8 females. The majority of patients suffered from autonomous nervous system disorder with parasympaticotonic dominance and hypotonia. Blood levels of all hormones were normal in all patients with the exception of a 13 ½ year old female with multiple areas of alopecia areata, mild cataract, and pubertas praecox, where TSH was very low. All patients had a minor hypocalcemia. All patients received human fetal cell transplantation of *adrenal cortex, diencephalon, placenta, liver, and skin*, and the patient with pubertas praecox also received *anterior lobe of pituitary*. All patients with alopecia areata improved within 2 months, while there was no response in patients with total alopecia.

> I am caught like a beast at bay,
> Somewhere are people, freedom, light,
> But all I hear is the baying of the pack,
> There is no way out for me.

Boris Pasternak, 1890 – 1960, [The Nobel Prize, 1959]

BIBLIOGRAPHY

1. Ricordi, C, Lacy, P, Sterbenz, K, Davie J. Low-temperature culture of human islets or *in vivo* treatment with L3T4 antibody produces a marked prolongation of islet human-to-mouse xenograft survival. Proc Natl Acad Sci USA 1987; 84:8080-8084
2. Falqui, L, Finke, E, Carel, J-C, et al. Marked prolongation of human islet xenograft survival (human-to-mouse) by low temperature culture and temporary immunosuppression with human and mouse antilymphocyte sera. Transplantation 1991; 51:1322-1324
3. Goss, J, Finke, E, Flye, W, Lacy, P. Induction of immune unrespon-siveness to concordant islet xenografts by intrahepatic preimmunization and transient immunosuppression. J Clin Invest 1994; 93:1312-1314
4. West, L, Morris, P, Wood K. Fetal liver haematopoietic cells and tolerance to organ allografts. Lancet 1994; 343:148-149
5. Yu, S, Nakafusa, Y, Flye, W. Portal vein administration of donor cells promotes peripheral allospecific hyporesponsiveness and graft tolerance. Surgery 1994; 116:229-235
6. Gaines, B, Colson, Y, Kaufman, C, Ilstad, S. Facilitating cells enable engrafment of purified fetal liver stem cells in allogeneic recipients. Exp Hemat 1996; 24:902-913
7. Goss, J, Flye, W, Lacy, P. Succesful transfer of immune unresponsive-ness to concordant rat islet xenografts. Transplantation 1996; 61:9-13
8. Goss, J, Nakafusa, Y, Finke, E, et al. Induction of tolerance to islet xenografts in a concordant rat-to-mouse model. Diabetes 1994; 43:16-23
9. Aebischer, P, Lacy, P, Gerasimidi-Vazeou, A, Hauptfeld, V. Production of marked prolongation of islet xenograft survival (rat to mouse) by local release of mouse and rat antilymphocyte sera at transplant site. Diabetes 1991; 40:482-485
10. Gehrling, IC, Serreze, DV, Christianson, SW, Leiter, EH. Intrathymic islet cell transplantation reduces beta-cell autoimmunity and prevents diabetes in NOD/Lt mice. Diabetes 1992; 41:1672-1676
11. Morris, C, Simeonovic, C, Ming-Chiu, F, et al. Intragraft expression of cytokine transcripts during pig proislet xenograft rejection and tolerance in mice. J Immunol 1995; 149:2470-2482

12. Satake, M, Korsgren, O, Ridderstad, A, et al. Immunological characteristics of islet cell xenotransplantation in humans and rodents. Immun Rev 1994; 12:191-210
13. Lafferty, KJ, Hao, L. Approaches to the prevention of immune destruction of transplanted pancreatic islets. Transplant Proc 1994; 26:399-400
14. Gage, F. Cell therapy. Nature 1998; 392(supp):18-24
15. Gwinup, G, Elias, AN. Hypothesis: insulin is responsible for the vascular complications of diabetes. Medical Hypotheses 1991; 34:1-6
16. Wahren, J. Does C-peptide have a physiological role? Diabetologia 1994; 37(suppl.2):99-107
17. Sutherland, DRE. Pancreas and islet transplantation: now and then. Transpl Proc 1996; 28:2131-2133
18. Niehans, P. **Introduction to Cellular Therapy**. Pageant Books, Inc, New York, 1960
19. Hendrikx, PJ, Martens, A, Hagenbeek, A, et al. Homing of fluorescently labeled murine hematopoietic stem cells. Exp Hematol 1996; 24:129-140
20. Zanjani, E, Ascensao, J, Tavassoli, M. Liver-derived fetal hematopoietic stem cells selectively and preferentially home to the fetal bone marrow. Blood 1993; 81:399-404
21. Hardy, C. The homing of hematopoietic stem cells to the bone marrow. Am J Med Sci 1995; 309:260-266
22. Sigal, S, Brill, S, Fiorino, A, Reid L. The liver as a stem cell and lineage system. Am J Physiol 1992; 263:139-148
23. Tafra, L, Dafoe, DC, Berezniak, R. Fetal liver and pancreas transplanted as a composite improves islet graft function. Transplant Proc 1991; 23:752-753
24. Dabeva, M, Seong-Gyu H, Vasa SRG, et al. Differentiation of pancreatic progenitor cells into hepatocytes following transplantation into rat liver. Proc Natl Acad Sci USA 1997; 94:7356-7361
25. Dafoe, DC, Xuegong, W, Tafra, L, et al. Studies of composite grafts of fetal pancreas and fetal liver in the streptozotocin-induced diabetic rat In: Vinik AJ (editor). **Pancreatic Islet Cell Regeneration and Growth**. Plenum Press, New York, 1992
26. Adams, G, Xuegong, Wang, Lee, LK, et al. Insulin-like growth factor-I promotes succesful fetal pancreas transplantation in the intramuscular site. Surgery 1994; 116:751-756
27. Eckhoff, D, Sollinger, H, Hullett, D. Selective enhancement of beta-cell activity by preparation of fetal pancreatic proislets and culture with insulin growth factor 1. Transplantation 1991; 51:1161-1165
28. Gittes, G, Galante, P, Hanahan, D, et al. Lineage-specific morphoge-nesis in the developing pancreas: role of mesenchymal factors. Development 1996; 122:439-447
29. Dudek, R, Lawrence, I, Hill, R, Johnson, R. Induction of islet cytodifferentiation by fetal mesenchyme in adult pancreatic ductal epithelium. Diabetes 1991; 40:1041-1048
30. Sykes, M, Yong, Z, Yong-Guang, Y. Tolerance induction for xeno-

transplantation. World J Surg 1997; 21: 932-938
31. Auchicloss, H. The scientific study of xenografting: 1964-1988. In: Cooper, DKC, Kemp, E, Reemtsma, K, White, DJG (Editors). **Xenotransplantation.** Springer-Verlag, Berlin, 1991
32. Paul, LC. Mechanism of humoral xenograft rejection. In: Cooper DKC, Kemp E, Reemtsma, K, White, DJG (Editors). **Xenotransplantation.** Springer-Verlag, Berlin, 1991
33. Bach, FH, Platt, JL, Cooper, DKC. Accomodation - the role of natural antibody and complement in discordant xenograft rejection. In: Cooper, DKC, Kemp, E, Reemtsma, K, White, DJG (Editors). **Xenotransplantation.** Springer-Verlag, Berlin, 1991
34. Moses, RD, Auchincloss, H. Mechanism of cellular xenograft rejection. In: Cooper, DKC, Kemp, E, Reemtsma, K, White, DJG (Editors). **Xenotransplantation.** Springer-Verlag, Berlin,1991
35. Thomas, FT. Isolated pancreas islet xenografting. In: Cooper, DKC, Kemp, E, Reemtsma, K, White, DJG (Editors). **Xenotransplantation**, Springer-Verlag, Berlin, 1991
36. Lanza, RP, Chick, WL. Introduction, Chapter 40. In: Cooper, DKC, Kemp, E, Platt, JL, White, DJG (Editors). **Xenotransplantation**, 2nd ed., Springer-Verlag, Berlin, 1997
37. Thomas, FT. Isolated pancreatic islet xenografting. In: Cooper, DKC, Kemp, E, Platt, JL, White, DJG (Editors) **Xenotransplantation**, 2nd ed., Springer-Verlag, Berlin, 1997
38. Latinne, D, Vitiello, D, Sachs, D, Sykes, M. Tolerance to discordant xenografts. Transplantation 1994;57:238-245
39. Platt, JL. A perspective on xenograft rejection and accommodation. Immunol Rev 1994, No.141:127-149
40. Chen, H-M, Jovanovic-Peterson, L, Desai, T, Peterson, C. Lessons learned from the non-obese diabetic mouse II: amelioration of pancreatic autoimmune isograft rejection during pregnancy. Am J Perinatol 1996; 13:249-254
41. Bartlett, S, Chin, T, Dirden, B, et al. Inclusion of peripancreatic lymph node cells prevents recurrent autoimmune destruction of islet trans-plants: evidence of donor chimerism. Surgery 1995; 118:392-399
42. Sandbichler, P, Erhart, R, Herbst, P, et al. Simultaneous transplantation of hepatocytes mitigates rejection of small bowel allografts in the rat. Transplant Proc 1995; 27:631-632
43. Fuiji, Y, Sugawara, E, Hayashi, K, Sano, S. Neonatal intrathymic splenocyte injection yields prolonged xenograft survival. Acta Med Okayama 1998; 52:83-88
44. Sheffield, CD, Hadley, GA, Dirden, BM, Bartlett, TS. Prolonged cardiac xenograft survival is induced by intrathymic splenocyte injection. J Surg Res 1994; 57:55-59
45. Merino, JF, Nacher, V, Rauell, M, et al. Improved outcome of islet transplantation in insulin-treated diabetic mice: effects on beta-cell mass and function. Diabetologia 1997; 40:1004-1010

46. Beattie, G, Rubin, J, Mally, M, et al. Regulation of proliferation and differentiation of human fetal pancreatic islet cells by extracellular matrix, hepatocyte growth factor, and cell-cell contact. Diabetes 1996; 45:1223-1228
47. Montana, E, Bonner-Weir, S, Weir, G. Beta cell mass and growth after syngeneic islet cell transplantation in normal and Streptozotocine diabetic C57BL/6 mice. J Clin Invest 1993; 91:780-787
48. Vorob'eva, EA. Pokazateli kletochnogo i gumoralnogo immuniteta u bolnych sacharnym diabetom pri transplantacii beta-kletok podzhelu-dochnoi zhelezi. (Parameters of cellular and humoral immunity in diabetic patients treated with transplantation of beta-cells of pancreas.), Summary of dissertation for a degree of a candidate of medical sciences, RITAOMH, Moscow, 1992
49. Smith, DM. Endogenous retrovirus in xenografts. NEJM 1994; 329:142
50. DiGiacomo, R, Hopkins, S. Food animal and poultry retroviruses and human health. Veterin Clin N America 1997; 13:177-190
51. Mare, CJ. Viral diseases. In: Weisbroth, SH, Flatt, RE, Kraus, AL. **Biology of Laboratory Rabbit**. Academic Press, New York, 1974
52. Eastlund, T. Infectious disease transmission through cell, tissue, and organ transplantation: reducing the risk through donor selection. Cell Transplant. 1995; 4:455-477
53. Kalter, SS, Heberling, RL. Xenotransplantation and infectious diseases. Instit Labor Anim Resour J 1995; 37:31-37
54. Fox, JG, Lipman, NS. Infections transmitted by large and small laboratory animals. Inf Dis Clin N Amer 1991; 5:13-163
55. Chapman, L, Folks, T, Salomon, M, et al. Xenotransplantation and xenogeneic infections. N Eng J Med 1996; 333:1498-1501
56. Dylan, D, Gill, R, Schloot, N, Wegmann, D. Epitope specificity, cyto-kine production profile and diabetogenic activity of insulin-specific T cell clones isolated from NOD mice. Eur J Immunol 1995; 25:1056-1062
57. Pittman, K, Henretta, T, McFadden, T, et al. Prevention of primary non-function of xenograft islets. Transplant Proc 1994; 26:1141-1142
58. Kumagai Braesch, M, Groth, C, Korsgren, O, et al. Immune response of diabetic patients against transplanted porcine fetal islet cells. Transplant Proc 1992; 24:679-680
59. Desai, N, Bassiri, H, Kim, J, et al. Islet allograft, islet xenograft, and skin allograft survival in $CD8^+$ T lymphocyte-deficient mice. Transplantation 1993; 55:718-722
60. Buhler, L, Deng, S, Mage, SR, et al. Islets of Langerhans rejection: allo vs xenotransplantation in animals. Transplant Proc 1994; 26:764-765
61. Wolf, L, Coulombe, M, Gill, R. Donor antigen-presenting cell-indepen-dent rejection of islet xenograft. Transplantation 1995; 60:1164-1170
62. Wallgren, AC, Karlsson-Parra, A, Korsgren, O. The main infiltrating cell in xenograft rejection is a $CD4^+$ macrophage and not a T lymphocyte. Transplantation 1995; 60:594-601
63. Thomas, FT, Pittman, K, Thomas, JM. Induction of functional xenograft tolerance of pig islets in the autoimmune NOD mouse. Transplant Proc

1995; 27:3323-3325
64. Mandel, TE, Kovarik, J, Koulmanda, M. A comparison of organ cultured fetal pancreas allo-, iso-, and xenografts (pig) in non-immunosuppresses non-obese diabetic mice. Am J Pathol 1995; 147:834-843
65. Kondratiev, YY, Sadovnikova, NV, Petrova, GN, et al. Islet cell transplantation in type 1 diabetes mellitus: evaluation of humoral immune response. Exp Clin Endocrin. 1989; 93:147-150
66. Morozov, YI, Kirdei, EG, Kim, AY. Vlianie ksenotransplantatsii ostrovkovykh kletok podzheludochnoi zhelezi na immunny status bolnyckh sacharnym diabetom. (Effect of xenotransplantation of islet cells of pancreas on the immune status of diabetic patients). Klinicheskaia Medicina, Moscow, 1995; 73:32-34
67. Lodish H, Baltimore D, Berk A, et al. **Molecular Cell Biology**. 3rd ed., Scientific American Books, New York, 1995
68. Zubkova, ST, Danilova, AI, Kovpan NA. Sostoianie sosudov glaznogo dna i nizhnykh konechnostei u bolnykh sacharnym diabetom posle trans-plantatsii kultury ostrovkovych kletok podzheludochnoi zhelezi. (Condition of vessels of retina and of lower extremities in diabetic patients after transplantation of cultures of islet cells of pancreas). Summary, In: Proceedings of 4th Congress of Ukrainian Endocrino-logists, Kiev, Ukraine, 1987, 153
69. Boiko, NI, Pavlovsky, MP, Stefaniuk, AM, Lebedovich, AI. Immuno-logocheskiye aspekty transplantatsii endokrinnoi tkani podzheludochnoi zhelezi. (Immunological aspects of transplantation of the endocrine tissues of pancreas). Summary, In: Proceedings of 3rd Congress of Endocrinology, Tashkent, Turkestan, 1989, 159
70. Leinieks, AA, Rozental, PL, Ligere, RY, et al. Korrelacia t'azhesti neiropatii i gastrinemii u bolnykh sacharnym diabetom posle transplantatsii kultur ostrovkovych kletok podzheludochnoi zhelezi. (Correlation of severity of neuropathy and gastrin level in diabetic patients after transplantation of cultured islet cells of pancreas). Summary, In: Proceedings of 3rd All-USSR. Congress of Endocrinology, Tashkent Turkestan, 1989, 257
71. Evseiev, Yu N. Sravnitelnaja ocenka intramuskularnoi i intraportalnoi transplantatsii kultur ostrovkovykh kletok podzheludochnoi zhelezi u bolnych sacharnym diabetom I tipa. (Comparative evaluation of intramuscular and intraportal transplantation of cultured islet cells of pancreas in patients with type 1 diabetes mellitus). Dissertation for the degree of "Candidate of Medical Sciences", RITAOMH, Moscow, 1993
72. Skaletsky, NN. Ksenotransplantatsia kultur ostrovkovykh kletok podzheludochnoi zhelezi plodov cheloveka krysam s eksperimentalnym sacharnym diabetom. (Xenotransplantation of cultured human fetal islets of pancreas to the rats with experimental diabetes mellitus). Summary of dissertation for the degree of "Candidate of Medical Sciences", RITAOMH, Moscow, 1987
73. Ignatenko, SN. Transplantologicheskiye metodi lecheni'a sacharnogo diabeta. (Transplantologic methods of treatment of diabetes mellitus). Dissertation for the degree "Doctor of Medical Sciences", RITAOMH,

Moscow, 1990
74. Leinieks, AA. Otsenka effektivnosti transplantatsii kulturi ostrovkovykh kletok podzheludochnoi zhelezi u bolnykh sacharnym diabetom. (Evaluation of effectiveness of transplantation of cultured islet cells of pancreas in diabetic patients). Dissertation, "Candidate of Medical Sciences", Latvian Republic's Center of Transplantology, Riga, 1989
75. Podshivalin, AV. Otsenka effektivnosti transplantatsii ostrovkovykh kletok podzheludochnoi zhelezi u bolnykh sacharnym diabetom radionuklidnymi metodami. (Evaluation of the effectiveness of transplantation of islet cells of pancreas in diabetic patients with radioisotope methods). Dissertation for the degree "Candidate of Medical Sciences", RITAOMH, Moscow, 1994
76. Ministry of Health of USSR. O rezultatach klinicheskoi aprobatsii transplantatsii ostrovkovykh kletok podzheludochnoi zhelezi bolnym sacharnym diabetom i podgotovke metodicheskykh ukazanii s cel'u shirokogo vnedrenia metoda v praktiku. (About results of clinical approbation of transplantation of islet cells of pancreas to diabetic patients, and preparation of instructions about the method, with the goal of widespread use of the method in the clinical practice). Moscow, December 13, 1983
77. Ministry of Health and Health Care Industry of Russian Federation Order: O sovershenstvovanii okazania meditsinskoi pomoshchi bolnym sacharnym diabetom (Order: On accomplishment of handling of medical care to diabetic patients). Moscow, November 2, 1994
78. Ministry of Health of USSR. Metodi poluchenia kultur ostrovkovykh kletok iz podzheludochnoi zhelezi trupov plodov cheloveka i nekotorykh mlekopitaiuschikh zhivotnykh. Metodicheskiye rekomendatsii. (Methods for obtaining cultures of pancreas from fetal cadavers of humans and of some mammals. Recommendations on method). Moscow, 1995
79. Skaletsky, NN, Zagrebina, OV, Kirsanova, LA, et al. Rabbit pancreas as a source of islet cell cultures for transplantation. Summary, In: Abstracts of the 4th International Symposium "Transplantation of Endocrine Pancreas", Belgrade, Yugoslavia, 1990
80. Suskova, VS, Shalnev, BI, Vorobeva, EA, et al. The indexes of the cell and humoral immunity of the insulin dependent diabetics in the earlier period after xenotransplantation of the rabbit pancreatic islet cell cultures. Summary, In: Abstracts of the 4th International Symposium "Transplantation of Endocrine Pancreas", Belgrade, Yugoslavia, 1990
81. Ignatenko, SN, Skaletsky, NN, Bulatova, OS. Preliminary results. Transplantation of rabbit pancreatic islet cells. Summary, In: Abstracts of the 4th International Symposium "Transplantation of Endocrine Pancreas", Belgrade, Yugoslavia, 1990
82. Ablamunits, VG, Baranova, FS, Ignatenko, SN, et al. Recipient's own C-peptide in type 1 diabetic patients after rabbit islet cell transplantation. Summary, In: Abstracts of 3rd International Symposium "Transplan-tation of Endocrine Pancreas", Vrnjacka Banja, Yugoslavia, 1989
83. Skaletsky, NN, Kirsanova, LA, Zagrebina, OV, et al. Poluchenie kultur

ostrovkovykh kletok iz podzheludochnoi zhelezi krolika dlia transplantatsii. (Obtaining of cultures of islet cells of rabbit pancreas for transplantation). Summary, from Proceedings of All-USSR Symposium on Organ Transplantation, Lvov, Ukraine, 1990, 238-239

84. Abdul, M, Danilova, AI, Zubkova, ST, Sidorenko, LN. Vlianie xenotransplantatsii tkanevykh kultur ostrovkovykh kletok podzheludochnoi zhelezi na techenie diabeticheskoi angiopatii. (Effect of xenotransplantation of tissue cultures of islet cells of pancreas on the course of diabetic angiopathy). Summary, from Proceedings of All-USSR. Symposium on Organ Transplantation, Lvov, 1990, 89-91

85. Kirsanova, LA, Zagrebina, OV, Leonova, LN, Ermolenko, AE. Podzheludochnaya zheleza krolika kak vozmozhny istochnik ostrovkovykh kletok dlia peresadki. (Pancreas of rabbit as possible source of islet cells for transplantation)., Summary, In: Proceedings of Symposium "Transplantologic Methods of Treatment of Diabetes Mellitus", Riga, Latvia, 1988, 24-25

86. Kravchenko, VI. Sravnitelnaya otsenka effektivnosti allo- i ksenotransplantatsii insulinovykh ostrovkov u krolikov c eksperimentalnym diabetom. (Comparative evaluation of effectiveness of allo- and xeno-transplantation of insulin islets in rabbits with experimental diabetes). Summary, In: Proceedings of Symposium "Transplantologic Methods of Treatment of Diabetes Mellitus", Riga, 1988, 29-30

87. Balakirev, EM, Kuznetsova, LA, Bliumkin, VN. Razrabotka problemy klinicheskoi svobodnoi transplantatsii ostrovkovykh kletok bolnym sacharnym diabetom v Sovetskom Soiuze i za rubezhom. (Elaboration on the problem of clinical free transplantation of islet cells to diabetic patients in USSR and abroad). Summary, In: Proceedings of Symposium "Transplantologic Methods of Treatment of Diabetes Mellitus", Riga, 1988, 50-52

88. Danilova, AI. Osobennosti techenia diabeticheskykh retinopatii u bolnych sacharnym diabetom pod vlianiem allo- i ksenotransplantatsii ostrovkovykh kultur podzheludochnoi zhelezi. (Peculiarities of the course of diabetic retinopathies in diabetic patients after allo- and xenotransplantation of cultured pancreatic islets). Summary, In: Proceedings of Symposium "Transplantologic Methods of Treatment of Diabetes Mellitus", Riga, 1988, 65-67.

89. Zubkova, ST, Naumenko, VG, Lis'anskaya, SM. Sostoianie gemodynamicheskykh pokazatelei u bolnych sacharnym diabetom s angiopatiami nizhnych konechnostiei posle transplantatsii kultury ostrovkovykh kletok podzheludochnoi zhelezi. (Status of haemodynamic parameters in diabetic patients with angiopathies of lower extremities after transplantation of cultures of pancreatic islets). Summary, In: Proceedings of Symposium "Transplantologic Methods of Treatment of Diabetes Mellitus", Riga, 1988, 69-70

90. Efimov, AS, Tronko, ND, Komissarenko, IV, et al. Vlianie allo- i ksenotransplantatsii ostrovkovykh kletok podzheludochnoi zhelezi na

techenie insulinzavisimogo sacharnogo diabeta i diabeticheskykh angiopatii. (Effect of allo- and xeno-transplantation of pancreatic islet cells on the course of insulin-dependent diabetes mellitus and diabetic angiopathies). Summary, In: Proceedings of Symposium "Transplan-tologic Methods of Treatment of Diabetes Mellitus", Riga, 1988, 71-72

91. Kazarian GA, Basmadjian ME, Ovanesian PA, et al. Vlianie transplantatsii kultur ostrovkovykh kletok podzheludochnoi zhelezi na techenie angiopatii u bolnykh sacharnym diabetom. (Effect of transplantation of cultured pancreatic islet cells on the course of angiopathies in diabetic patients). Summary, In: Proceedings of Symposium "Transplantologic Methods of Treatment of Diabetes Mellitus", Riga, 1988, 74-75

92. Kondratiev, Ya Yu, Sadovnikova, NV, Fedotov, VP, et al. Antitela k poverchnosti ostrovkovykh kletok podzheludochnoi zhelezi pri transplantatsii kultur ostrovkovykh kletok bolnym sacharnym diabetom tipa 1. (Antibodies to the surface of pancreatic islet cells with transplantation of cultured islet cells to patients with type 1 diabetes mellitus). Summary, In: Proceedings of Symposium "Transplantologic Methods of Treatment of Diabetes Mellitus", Riga, 1988, 78-79

93. Leinieks, AA, Shtifts, AK, Vasipa, CB, et al. **Izmenenie immunoglobulinov u bolnykh sacharnym diabetom do i posle transplantatsii kultur ostrovkovych kletok podzheludochnoi zhelezi**. (Changes of immuno-globulins in diabetic patients before and after transplantation of cultured pancreatic islet cells) Summary, In: Proceedings of Symposium 'Transplantologic Methods of Treatment of Diabetes Mellitus', Riga, 1988, 79-80

94. Skaletsky NN, Kirsanova LA, Bliumkin VN. Poluchenie kultur ostrovkovykh kletok iz podzheludochnoi zhelezi i ich transplantatsia. (Obtaining of cultures of pancreatic islet cells and their transplantation). In: Problemy transplantologii i iskusstvennych organov. (Problems of transplantology and artificial organs), Anniversary Collection of Papers, RITAOMH, Moscow, 1994, 71-80

95. Schmid, F. **Celltherapy, a New Dimension of Medicine**, Ott Publishing, Thun, Switzerland, 1983

96. Sadykova, RE, Skaletsky, NN, Dreval, AV, et al. Vlianie ksenotransplantatsii kultur ostrovkovykh kletok na techenie alloksanogo diabeta u krys nachodivshichsia na diete s raznym soderzhaniem belka. (Effect of xenotransplantation of cultured islet cells on the course of Alloxan diabetes in rats kept on diets with variable protein content). Problemi endokrinologii, Moscow 1994; 4: 45-47

97. Shumakov, VI, Skaletsky, NN. Transplantatsia ostrovkovykh i drugikh endokrinnykh kletok. (Transplantation of islet and other endocrine cells). In: Shumakov VI, (Editor). **Transplantologiya – rukovodstvo**. (Transplantology – manual), Medicina (Moscow) and Reproniks Ltd. (Tula), 1995, 317-331

98. Shumakov, VI, Skaletsky, NN, Evseev, Yu N, et al. Intraportal transplantation of islet xenografts in diabetes mellitus patients. Biomaterial-

Living System Interactions, Moscow, 1993; 1:175-181
99. Shishko, PI, Dreval, AV, Babicheva, MG, et al. Islet cell transplantation in induction and prolongation of insulin-dependent diabetes remission. Transplant Proc 1992; 24:3040
100. Dreval, AV, Shishko, NN, Skaletsky, NN, et al. Parameters of the immune status in patients with newly diagnosed type 1 diabetes mellitus after islet cell transplantation. Transplant Proc 1992; 24:3041-3042
101. Shumakov, VI, Ignatenko, SN, Bliumkin, VN, et al. Effect of clinical transplantation of fetal islet cell cultures on late diabetic complications. Diabetes 1989, Suppl 1; 38:314
102. Mumladze, RB, Moshetova, LK, Chudnykh, SM, et al. Lechenie sacharnogo diabeta v chirurgicheskoi klinike. (Treatment of diabetes mellitus in surgical clinic). Annali chirurgii, Moscow 1996; 1:35-39
103. Skaletsky, NN, Shalnev, BI, Bliumkin, VN, Kirsanova, LA. Xenotransplantation of human and animal fetal pancreas in diabetic rats. Diabetes 1989, Suppl 1; 38:317
104. Bundesgesundheitsamt: Gutachten zur therapeutischen Anwendung injizierbar Frischzellenpraparatonen beim Menschen. (German Federal Health Office: Report on therapeutic use of injectable fresh cell preparations in man of 3/16/94) and Stellungnahme vom 20.12.1994 des Bundesverbandes Deutscher Arzte fur Frishzellen-Therapie zum Gutachten des Bundesgesundheitsamtes vom 16.3.1994. (Statement of Association of German Physicians for Fresh Cell Therapy of 12/20/94 to the Report of German Federal Health Office on the Therapeutic Use of Injectable Fresh Cell Preparations in Man of 3/16/94)
105. National Diabetes Data Group. **Diabetes in America**, 2nd ed., National Institutes of Health, National Institute of Diabetes and Digestive and Kidney Diseases, NIH Publication No. 95-1468, 1995
106. Diabetes Statistics, NIDDK, world wide website: http://www.niddk.nih.gov/health/diabetes/pubs/dmstats.htm#comp
107. Kidney Disease of Diabetes, NIDDK, world wide website: http:/diabetes.niddk.nih.gov/dm/pubs/statistics/index.htm
108. Stites, D, Terr, A, Parslow, T. **Basic and Clinical Immunology**. 8th ed, Appleton & Lange, 1994
109. Shumakov, VI, Bliumkin, VN, Skaletsky, NN, et al. Transplantatsia ostrovkovykh kletok podzheludochnoi zhelezi. (Transplantation of pancreatic islet cells), Kanon publishing, Moscow, 1995
110. Cunningham, FG, MacDonald, PC, Leveno, KJ, et al. **Williams Obstetrics**. 19th ed, Appleton and Lange, 1993
111. Bio-Cellular Research Organization LLC website: www.stem-cell-transplantation.com
112. Memo to Mr. Snyder, General Counsel, US-FDA, of 4/28/97, by BCRO
113. Los Angeles Times article by T H Maugh: Transplants of Cells Aided Diabetics, of 4/12/95
114. Molnar, EM. Report on medical research project in transplantation of human fetal tissues in Russia. Medorganica 1993; 17: 57-61

115. Jovanovic-Peterson, L, et al. of Sansum group, Molnar, EM, et al. of BCRO group. An international collaborative study of human fetal islet tissue transplantation in insulin-dependent diabetic patients. (The Russia - United States Collaborative Transplant Study Group), manus-cript, read at the International Symposium on Cell Transplantation Treatment of IDDM, Santa Barbara, Calif, October 1994
116. Lernmark, A, Freedman, ZR, Hofmann, C, et al. Islet-cell-surface antibodies in juvenile diabetes mellitus. N Eng J Med 197; 299:375-380
117. Kondrat'ev, Ya Yu, Sadovnikova, NV, Liozner, AL, Fedotov, VP. Autoantitela k poverchnosti ostrovkovykh kletok podzheludochnoi zhelezi: immunofermentnoie opredelen'e c ispolzovan'em kletok-myshenei krys. (Antibodies to the surface of pancreatic islet cells: immunoenzymatic determination using rat target cells), Problemi endokrinologii, 1986; 32:39-43
118. Hopf, U, Meyer zum Buschenfelde, KH, Freudenberg, J. Liver-specific antigens of different species. Clin Exp Immunol 1974; 16:117-124
119. Baekkeskov, S, Nielsen, JH, Marner, B, et al. Autoantibodies in newly diagnosed diabetic children immunoprecipitate human pancreatic islet cell proteins. Nature 1982; 298:167-169
120. Robertson, RP, Sutherland, DE. Pancreas transplantation as therapy for diabetes mellitus. Annu Rev Med 1992; 43:396-415
121. Barker, CF, Naji, A. Perspectives in pancreatic and islet transplant-tation. N Eng J Med 1992; 323:271-273
122. Morris, PJ, Gray, DW, Sutton, R. Pancreatic islet transplantation. Brit Med Bull 1989; 45:224-241
123. Moskaleski, S. Isolation and culture of the islet of pancreas of the guinea pig. Gen Comp Endocrin 1965; 5:342-353
124. Hellerstrom, S, Swenne, I, Andersson, A. **Islet cell replication and diabetes**. Plenum Press, New York, 1988
125. Voss, F, Brewin, A, Dawidson, J, et al. Transplantation of proliferated human pre-islet cell into diabetic patients with renal transplants. Transplant Proc 1989; 21:2751-2756
126. Thomson, NM, Hancock, WM, Lafferty, KJ, et al. Organ culture reduced Ia-positive cells present within the human fetal pancreas. Transplant Proc 1983; 15:1373-1376
127. Lafferty, KJ, Prowse, S, Simeonovic, CJ, Warren, HS. Immunobiology of tissue transplantation: A return to the passenger leucocyte concept. Annu Rev Immunol 1983; 1:143-147
128. Hegre, OD, Ketchum, RJ, Popiela, H, et al. Allotransplantation of culture-isolated neonatal rat islet tissue. Absence of MHC class II positive anigen-presenting cells in non-immunogenic islets. Diabetes 1989; 38:146-151
129. Harrison, DE, Christie, MR, Gray, DWR. Properties of isolated human islets of Langerhans: insulin secretion, glucose oxidation and protein phosphorylation. Diabetologia 1985; 28:99-103
130. Warnock, GL, Dabbs, KD, Evans, MG, et al. Critical mass of islets that function after implantation in a large mammalian. Horm Metab Res, Suppl

1990; 25:156-161
131. Cossel, L, Wohlrab, F, Blech, W, Hahn, HJ. Morphological findings in the liver of diabetic rats after intraportal transplantation of neonatal isologous pancreatic islets. Wirchows Arch 1990; 59:65-77
132. Federlin, KF, Bretzel, RG. The effects of islets transplantation on complications in experimental diabetes of the rat. World J Surg 1984; 8:169-178
133. Cuthbertson, RA, Hopper, JL, Mandel, TE. Difference in effect of cultured fetal pancreas transplants on retinal and renal capillary basement membrane thickness in diabetic mice. Transplantation 1989; 48:218-223
134. Laky, SP, Anderson, J, Chamberlain, J, et al. Bovine serum albumin density gradient isolation of rat pancreatic islets. Transplantation 1987; 43:805-809
135. Najarian, JS, Sutherland, DE, Matas, AJ. Human islet transplantation: a preliminary report. Transplant Proc 1977; 9:233-236
136. Socci, C, Davalli, AM, Maffi, P, et al. Allotransplantation of fresh and cryopreserved islets in type 1 diabetes in patients: two years experience. Transplant Proc 1993; 25:989-991
137. Farney, AC, Najarian, JS, Nakhleh, R, et al. Long-term function of islet autotransplants. Transplant Proc 1992; 24:969-971
138. Miller, JO, Wright, NM, Lester, SE, et al. Spontaneous and stimulated growth hormone release in adolescent with type 1 diabetes mellitus: effects of metabolic control. J Clin Endocrin Met 1992; 75:1087-1091
139. Sacca, L, Sherwin, R, Hendler, R, Felig, P. Influence of continuous physiologic hyperinsulinemia on glucose kinetics and counterregula-tory hormones in normal and diabetic humans. J Clin Invest. 1979; 64:949-957
140. Unger, RH, Orci, L. The essential role of glucagone in the pathogenesis of diabetes mellitus. Lancet 1975; 2:14-16
141. Powell, HC. Pathology of diabetic neuropathy: new observations, new hypothesis. Lab Invest 1983; 49:115-119
142. Pyzdrowski, KL, Kendall, PM, Halter, JB, et al. Preserved insulin secretion and insulin independence in recipients of islet autographs. N Eng J Med 1992; 323:220-226
143. Block, S. Frishzellentherapie - eine Erfahrungswissenschaft. (Fresh cell therapy - an empirical science). Biologische Medizin 1986; 15:116-122
144. Panchenko, EI, Sukhikh, GT, Molnar, EM. A comparative study of the institutionalized children with Down syndrome. Medorganica 1993; 17:124-125
145. Panchenko, EI, Burkova, MI, Molnar, EM. An experiment with the transplantation of human fetal tissues in children with Down syndrome. Bull Exp Biol Med 1994; 117:374-376
146. Malaitsev, VV, Molnar, EM, Sukhikh, GT, Bogdanova, IM. Transplantation of human fetal tissues as a promising method in the treatment of diabetes mellitus. Bull Exp Biol Med 1994; 117:351-357
147. Skaletski, NN, Fateeva, NL, Molnar, EM. Transplantation of cultured fetal pancreatic islet cells in the treatment of insulin-dependent diabetes

mellitus. Bull Exp Biol Med 1994; 117:357-365
148. Gilbert, SF. **Developmental Biology**. 4th ed, Sinauer Associates, Sunderland, MA, 1994
149. Steiner, DF. On the role of the proinsulin C-peptide. Diabetes 1978, Suppl 1; 27:145-148
150. Auchinloss, H, Sachs, DH. Xenogenic transplantation. Annu Rev Immunol 1998; 16:433-470
151. Williams, PL, Warwick, R, Dyson, M, Bannister, LH (Editors). **Gray's Anatomy**. 37th ed., Churchill-Livingstone, Edinburgh, 1989
152. Rouviere, H, Delmas, A. **Anatomie Humaine**. 13th ed, Vol 2: Trunk, Masson Publishing, Paris, 1992
153. Romanes, GJ (Editor). **Cunningham's Textbook of Anatomy**. 11th ed, Oxford University Press, London, 1972
154. Hollinshead, WH, Rosse, C. **Textbook of Anatomy**. 4th ed, Harper Row, Cambridge, 1985
155. West, JB (Editor). **Best and Taylor's Physiological Basis of Medical Practice**, 11th ed, Williams Wilkins, Baltimore, 1985
156. Hall, VF (Editor). **Handbook of Physiology**, Vol.2 (Neurophysio-logy), Am Physiol Soc, Washington, D.C., 1971
157. Niehans P. **Introduction to Cell Therapy**, 4th ed., Editions Clinique La Prairie, Clarens, 1978
158. **Literaturverzeichnis der Zelltherapie**. (Literature Index of Cell Therapy), Internationale Forschungsgessellschaft fur Zelltherapie (publisher: International Research Association for Cell Therapy), Stand vom Dezember 1974 (situation as of December 1974)
159. Reynolds, BA, Weiss, S. Generation of neurons and astrocytes from isolated cells of the adult mammalian central nervous system. Science 1992; 255:1707-1710
160. Netter, FH. **Atlas of Anatomy**, 2nd ed, Novartis, E Hanover (NJ), 1996, plates 238, 239, 288, 293
161. Netter, FH. **Nervous System**. CIBA Collection of Medical Illustrations, vol 1: Nervous System, Suppl on the Hypothalamus.
162. Berne, RM, Levy, MN. **Principles of Physiology**, 2nd ed, Mosby, St. Louis, 1996
163. McGee, J O'D, Isaacson, PG, Wright, NA. Oxford **Textbook of Pathology**, Vol.2b: Pathology of Systems, Oxford University Press, Oxford, 1992
164. Rubin, E, Farber, JL. **Pathology**, 2nd ed, JB Lippincott Co, Philadelphia, 1994
165. Janeway, CA, Travers, P. **Immunobiology**, 2nd ed, Churchill Livingstone, 1996
166. Roitt, I, Brostoff, J, Male, D. **Immunology**, 5th ed, Mosby, London, 1998
167. Charlton, HM. **Hypothalamic transplantation**, CIBA Foundation Symposium No. 166, 1992, 268-286.
168. Rahier, J, Goebbels, RM, Henquin, JC. Cellular composition of the human diabetic pancreas. Diabetologia 1983; 24:366-371

169. Lacy, PE, Davie, JM, Finke, EH. Transplantation of insulin-producing tissue. Am J Med 1981; 70:89-594
170. Lafferty, KJ, Hao, L. Fetal pancreas transplantation for treatment of IDDM patients. Diabetes Care 1993; 16:383-386
171. Lacy, PE, Kostianovsky, M. Method for the isolation of intact islets of Langerhans from the rat pancreas. Diabetes 1967; 16:35-39
172. Koesters, W, Seelig, HP, Strauch, M. Reversibility of functional and morphological glomerular lesions by islet transplantation in long-term diabetic rats. Diabetologia 1977; 13:409
173. Mauer, SM, Steffes, MW, Sutherland, DER, et al. Studies of the rate of regression of the glomerular lesions in diabetic rats treated with pancreatic islet transplantation. Diabetes 1975; 24:280-286
174. Lacy, PE, Davie, JM, Finke, EH. Effect of culture on islet rejection. Diabetes 1980; 29:93-97
175. Altman, JJ, Cugnenc, PH, Tessier, C, et al. Epiploic flap: a new site for islet implantation in man. Horm Metab Res, Suppl 1990; 25:136-137
176. Steiner, DF. Pro-insulin and the biosynthesis of insulin. N Eng J Med. 1969; 280:1106-1113
177. Ricordi, C, Socci, AM, Davalli, C, et al. Swine islet isolation and transplantation. Horm Metab Res 1990, Suppl; 25:26-30
178. Calafiore, R, Calcinaro, F, Basta, M, et al. The massive separation of adult porcine islets of Langerhans. Horm Metab Res 1990, Suppl; 25: 30-31
179. Papayannopoulou, T, Craddock, C. Homing and trafficking of hemopoietic progenitor cells. Acta Hemat 1997; 97:97-104
180. Springer, TA. Traffic signals for lymphocyte recirculation and leukocyte emigration: the multistep paradigm. Cell 1994; 76:301-314
181. Ricordi, C, Starzl, TE. Cellular transplants. Trans Proc 1991; 23:73-76
182. Gotoh, M, Porter, J, Kanai, T, et al. Multiple donor allotransplantation. Transplantation 1988; 45:1008-1012
183. Shumakov, VI, Bljumkin, VN, Ignatenko, SN, et al. The principal results of pancreatic islet cell culture transplantation in Diabetes Mellitus patients. Trans Proc 1987; 19:2372
184. Schmid, F. Personal communications, 1983 – 1996
185. Goldstein, H. Siccacell therapy in children. Arch Pediatr 1956; 73: 234-249
186. Goldstein, H. Siccacell therapy for retarded children. Gen Practice 1961
187. Griffel, A. The latest development in dry cell therapy (Siccacell). Arch Pediatr 1957; 74:325-342
188. Smith, LF. Species variation in the amino acid sequence of insulin. A J Med 1966; 40.662-666
189. Weiss, P, Andres, G. Embryonic transplantation by the vascular route. Science 1950; 111:456
190. Weiss, P, Taylor, AC. Reconstitution of complete organs from single-cell suspensions of chick embryos in advanced stages of differentiation. Proc Nat Acad Scien 1960; 46:1177-1185
191. Biocell Corp: Internal pre-clinical testing of organ cultures, 1997.

192. International Institute of Biological Medicine (IIBM)'s R&D cooperation agreements with top Russian research institutes, and areas of cooperation, 1992-1996.
193. **The Merck Veterinary Manual**, 8th ed, Merck & Co, Whitehouse Station, NJ, 1998
194. Popesko, P, Rajtova, V, Horak, J. **Atlas of topografickej anatomie laboratornych zvierat**. (Atlas of topographic anatomy of laboratory animals), Volume 1 and 2, Priroda Publishing, Bratislava, 1990
195. Krieg, NR, Holt, JG (Editors). **Bergey's Manual of Systematic Bacteriology**, Williams & Wilkins, Baltimore/London, 1984
196. Jurcik, R, Lencuchova, A, Salaj, J, et al. Empfanglichkeit von Feldhasen fur die infectiose hamorrhagische Erkrankung der Kaninchen under experimentellen Bedingungen. (Susceptibility of hares to the infectious Haemorrhagic Disease of Rabbits under experimental conditions), Z Jagdwiss, Verlag Paul Parey, Hamburg/Berlin 1992; 38:34-41
197. Goldstein, H. Treatment of mongolism and non-mongoloid mental retardation in children. Arch Ped 1954; 71:77-81
198. Destunis, G. The treatment of mental defficiency and of encephalo-pathies in childhood by means of fresh tissue and Siccacell. Arch Ped 1957; 74:285-290
199. Briusov, PG. personal communication, 1996
200. Murphy, FA, Fauquet, CM, Bishop, DHL, et al. **Virus Taxonomy**, (Sixth Report of the International Committee on Taxonomy of Viruses), Springer Verlag, Vienna - New York, 1995
201. Fauquet, CM, Pringle, CR. Abbreviations for vertebrate virus species names. Arch Virology 1999; 144:1865-1880
202. Murphy, AF, Gibbs, EPJ, Horzinek, MC, Studdert, MJ. **Veterinary Virology**, Academic Press, San Diego, New York, London, etc., 1999
203. Menasche, P, Hagege, A, Scorsin, M, et al. Autologous skeletal myoblast transplantation for cardiac insufficiency. First clinical case. Arch Mal Coeur Vaiss 2001; 94:180-182
204. Strauer, BE, Brehm, M, Zeus, T, et al. Intracoronary, human autologous stem cell transplantation for myocardial regeneration following myocardial infarction. Dtsch Med Wochenschr 2001;126: 932-938
205. Strauer, BE, Brehm, M, Zeus, T, et al. Repair of infarcted myocardium by autologous intracoronary mononuclear bone marrow cell transplant-tation. Circulation 2002; 106:1913-1916
206. Suzuki, K, Murtuza, B, Heslop, L, et al. Single fibers of skeletal muscle as a novel graft for cell transplantation to the heart. J Thorac Cardiovasc Surg 2002; 123:984-992
207. Malouf, NN, Coleman, WB, Grisham, JW, et al. Adult-derived stem cells from the liver become myocytes in the heart *in vivo*. Am J Pathol 2001; 158:1929-1935
208. Matsushita, T, Oyamada, M, Kurata, H, et al. Formation of cell junctions between grafted and host cardiomyocytes at the border zone of rat myocardial infarction. Circulation 1999; 19 (Suppl II): 262-268

209. Ruhparwar, A, Tebbeenjohans, J, Niehaus M, et al. Transplanted fetal cardiomyocytes as cardiac pacemaker. Eur J Cardiothorac Surg 2002; 21:853-857
210. Li, RK, Mickle, DA, Weisel, RD, et al. Optimal time for cardio-myocyte transplantation to maximize myocardial function after left ventricular injury. Ann Thorac Surg 2001; 72:1957-1963
211. Saito, T, Kuang, JQ, Bittira, B, et al. Xenotransplant cardiac chimera: immunotolerance of adult stem cells. Ann Thorac Surg 2002; 74:19-24
212. Toma, C, Pittenger, MF, Cahill, KS, et al. Human mesenchymal stem cells differentiate to a cardiomyocyte phenotype in the adult murine heart. Circulation 2002; 105:93-98
213. Etzion, S, Battler, A, Barbash, IM, et al. Influence of embryonic cardiomyocyte transplantation on the progression of heart failure in a rat model of extensive myocardial infarction. J Mol Cell Cardiol 2001; 33:1321-1330
214. Dornbusch, S. The effect of placenta on experimental cholesterin-sclerosis. In:Schmid, F, Stein, J, **Cell-research and Cellular therapy**, Ott Publishers. Thun, Switzerland, 1967
215. Cunningham, FG, MacDonald, PC, Leveno, KJ, Gant,NF, Gilstrap, LC, **Williams Obstetrics**, 19th ed, Appleton&Lange, 1993
216. Schmid, F, Stein, J. **Cell-research and Cellular therapy**, Ott Publishers, Thun, Switzerland, 1967
217. Schmid, F, Stein, J. **Zellforschung und Zelltherapie**, Verlag H. Huber, Bern, Stuttgart, 1963
218. Oetzmann, HJ, Cell therapy for diseases of organs. In: Schmid, F, Stein, J. **Cell-research and Cellular therapie**, Ott Publishers. Thun, Switzerland, 1967
219. Schmid, F. **Zelltherapie-Grundlagen-Klinik-Praxis**, Ott-Verlag, Thun, Switzerland, 1981
220. Savel'ev, SV, Lebedev, VV, Vojtyna, SV, Korochkin, LI, Molnar, EM. Transplantation of Fetal and xenogeneic nervous tissue in parkinson's disease. Bull Exp Biol Med 1994; 117:370-373
221. Savel'ev, SV, Lebedev, VV, Evgeniev, MR, Korochkin, LI. Chimeric Brain: Theoretical and Clinical Aspects. Int J Dev Biol 1997; 41:801-808
222. Benikova, EA, Turchin, IC. Transplantatsia kultur beta-kletok v lechenii insulinzavisimogo sakharnogo diabeta u detei. (Transplantantation of cultures of β-cells as a treatment of diabetes mellitus in children.). Problemy endokrin. 1991; 4:17-19
223. Lawrence, HS. The cellular transfer of cutaneous hypersensitivity to tuberculin in man. Proc Soc Exp Biol Med 1949; 71:516-521
224. Lawrence, HS. The transfer in humans of delayed skin sensitivity to streptococcal M-substance and to tuberculin with disrupted leukocytes. J Clin Invest 1955 ; 34:219-225
225. Wilson, GB, Paddock, GV, Fudenberg, HH. Bovine 'transfer factor': an oligoribonucleopeptide which initiates antigen-specific lymphocyte responsiveness. Thymus 1982; 4:335-350

226. Wilson, GB, Newell, RT, Burdash, NM. Immunochemical and physical-chemical evidence for the presence of thymosin α-peptide in dialyzable leukocyte extracts. In: Kirkpatrick, CJ, Lawrence, HS, and Burger, DR. Fourth International Transfer Factor Workshop in Denver, Acad Press Inc, New York, 1983.
227. Fudenberg, HH. Transfer Factor: 'Past, Present, and Future'. In: Mayer V, Borvak J (Editors). Proceedings of Fifth International Symposium in Transfer Factor, Bratislava, Slovakia, 1987.
228. Fudenberg, HH, Wilson, GB, Keller, RH, et al. Clinical applications of the leukocyte migration inhibition assay - new method for determining transfer factor potency and for predicting clinical response. In: Kirkpatrick, CJ, Burger, DR, Lawrence, HS (Editors). **Immunobiology of Transfer Factor**. Acad Press, 1983
229. Kirkpatrick, CJ, Rozzo, SS, Mascali, JJ. Murine transfer factor III. Specific interactions between transfer factor and antigen. J Immunol 1985; 135:4035-4039
230. Schmid F. Mitochondriale Enzephalo-Myopathien, (Mitochondrial Encephalo-Myopathies), Biol Med, 1994, 23:38-44
231. Schmid F. Lysosomen, (Lysosomes). Cyt Rev 1987; 11:23-30
232. Keuser, I. Krankheitebilder des Zentralnervensystems, (Atlas of diseases of central nervous system). Cyt Rev 1987; 11:165-171
233. Margraf, O. Minder- und Zwergwuchs, (Microsomia and dwarfism). Cyt Rev 1979; 3:122-123.
234. Schmid, RG. Stoffwechselstorungen. (Disorders of Metabolism). Cyt Rev 1979; 3:151-154
235. Schmid, F. **Das Mongolismus-Syndrom**, (Mongolism syndrome).Hansen u Hansen Verlag, Munsterdorf, 1976
236. Schmid, F. Beeinflussung der mongoloiden Dysencephalie durch Injections-Implantationen fetaler heteloger Gehirngewebe. (Influence upon mongoloid dysencephaly by injections/implantation of heterologous brain tissue). Fortschr Med 1972; 90:1181-1197
237. Schmid, F. Down syndrome: Situations-Analyse, (Down syndrome: Analysis of situation). Cyt Rev 1981; 4:184-197
238. Schmid, F. Down syndrome. Eine bio-soziale Situations-Analyse. (Down syndrome Bio-social analysis), Kinderarzt 1985; 16:526- 536
239. Schmid, F, Braun, P, et al. The personality of Down Child. Cyt Rev 1983; 7:106-114
240. Schmid, F, Pedrero, FA. Down-Syndrom. Revista Cytobiol. 1981; 4:2-17
241. Grebennikova, NV, Burkova, MI, Fisenko, AP, Molnar, EM. Vli'an'ie transplantatsii fetalnykh tkanei cheloveka na razvit'ie vysshikh psykhicheskich funtsii u detei s bolezn'iu Dauna. (Influence of transplanttation of human fetal tissues on the development of higher psychic functions in down syndrome children). lin Vestnik 1995; 3:44-45
242. **The Merck Manual of Geriatrics**, 2nd edition, Merck Research Laboratories, Whitehouse Station, NJ, 1995
243. Wolf, N. Katamnesen nach cytobiologischer Revitalisierung. (Katam-neses

after cytobiological revitalization). Cyt Rev 1987; 11: 80-83
244. Mironov, HV, Shmyr'ev, VI, Bugaev, VS, Molnar, EM. Endoliumba-lnyi metod neirotransplantatsii fetalnykh kletok golovnogo mozga cheloveka v nevrologii. (Endolumbar method of neurotransplantation of human fetal brain cells in neurology). Klin vestnik 1995; 3:84-87
245. Fink, JS, Schumacher, JM, Ellias, SL, et al. Porcine xenografts in Parkinson's disease and Huntington's disease patients: preliminary results. Cell Transplant 2000; 9:273-278.
246. Schumacher, JM, Ellias, SA, Palmer, EP, et al. Transplantation of embryonic porcine mesencephalic tissue in patients with PD. Neurology 2000; 54:1042-1050
247. Deacon, T, Schumacher, J, Dinsmore, J, et al. Histological evidence of fetal pig neural survival after transplantation into a patient with Parkinson's disease. Nat Med 1997; 3:350-353
248. Schmid, F. Die degenerativen Krankheiten der weissen Gehirnsub-stanz. (The degenerative diseases of the white matter of brain). Cyt Rev 1982; 6:189-197
249. Wolf, N. Klinische Behandlungsergebnise bei Patienten mit Alzheimerscher Krankheit mit zwei berichten zum Krankheitsverlauf. (Clinical experience in handling patients with Alzheimer disease and two case reports). Medorganica 1996; 18:25-27
250. Wolf, N. Revitalisierung bei psychischen Storungen des mittleren und hoheren Lebensalters durch Zelltherapie. (Revitalization of psychic disturbances of middle and higher age by cell therapy). Erfahr Heilkunde 1981; 30:26-32
251. Wolf, N. Die hirnatrophischen Prozesse des mittleren und reifen Alebensalters als Indikation for eine Zelltherapie. (Brain atrophic processes of middle and ripe age as indication for cell therapy). Rev Cytobiol 1984; 8:202-205
252. Wolf, N. Behandlungsergebnisse der Zelltherapie bei Patienten mit fortgeschrittenen cerebralen Abbau-erscheinungen. (Results of cell therapy treatment of patients with manifestation of advancing cerebral deterioration). Cyt Rev. 1980; 4:128-132
253. Camerer, W. Genetish bedingte progrediente Demenz bei Verdacht auf Morbus Alzheimer. (Genetically conditioned progressive dementia with a suspicion of Alzheimer disease). Cyt Rev 1987; 11:89-90
254. Ries, W. Methodische probleme bei der Ermittlung des Biologischen Alters. (Methodical problems of determination of biological age). Innere Medizin 1996; 4:109-106
255. Rietschel, IIG. **Problematik und Klinik der Zelltherapie**, (Problems and clinical practice of cell therapy) Urban und Schwarzenberg, Munich-Berlin, 1957
256. Kment, A. Altern und Geriatrica aus der Sicht der experimentalen gerontology. (Aging and geriatrics from the viewpoint of experimental gerontology). Akt Gerontol 1978; 8:241-252
257. Kment, A, Hofecker, G, Niedermueller, H, Skalicky, M. Neue ergebnisse

aus der Revitalisierungforschung. (New results from revitalization research). Cyt Rev 1979; 3:4-48
258. Gianoli, AC. Revitalization. Cyt Rev 1980; 4:12-17
259. Hofecker, G, Kment, A, Skalicky, M, Niedermueller, H. Messungen des biologischen Alters. (Measurements of biological age). Rev Cyt 1979; 3:49-53
260. Schmid, F. Lebensbehinderungen. (Life handicapped). Cyt Rev 1978; 2:3-22
261. Stuhlinger, H. Beobachtungen uber die Latenzzeit zwischen Zellimplantation und Wirkungseintritt. (Observations on the latency period between implantation of cells and the beginning of offect). Cyt Rev 1979; 3:157-161
262. Schnitzer, A. Wirkungsmechanismen bei der Zelltherapie. (Mechanisms of effectiveness of cell therapy). Cyt rev 1978; 2:33-38
263. Buscha, J, Sontag, M, Frank, T, Hager, ED. Antikorperuntersuchungen nach Zelltherapie. (Antibody testing after cell therapy). Cyt Rev 1987; 11:84-88
264. Neubert, H. Die Haut - ein wichtiges Erfolgsorgan der Frischzellentherapie. (Skin- an important organ of success with fresh cell therapy). Read at German Cell therapy Days, Hamburg, May 11-13, 1984.
265. Smirnov, V, Shakhlamov, M, Molnar, EM, et al. Non-surgical treatment of deep (surgical) burns using human fetal tissues, Read at 10th World Congress of Combustology, Paris, June 12-17, 1994.
266. Smirnov, V, Shakhlamov, M, Molnar, EM, et al. Non-surgical treatment of deep burns using human fetal tissues. Bull Exp Biol Med 1994; 117:376-379
267. Ackermann, G. Systematisierte Elastorhexis-Sarcoid Darier-Roussy, Behandlungversuch mit Humanplazenta. (Systemic Elastorhexis-Sarcoid Darrier-Rousy, Therapeutic attempt with human placenta). Dermat Wschr Leipzig 1956; 134:946-949
268. Hasselmann, H. Zum Problem einer Therapie der Keratosis palmaris at plamtaris hereditaria. (To the problem of treatment of Herditary kera-tosis palmaris at plantaris). Hippocrates, Stuttgart 1959; 30:184-187
269. Janson, P. Behandlung des Lichen Chron simplex. (Treatment of chronic lichen simplex). Arztl Praxis, Munich 1955, VII/51
270. Janson, P. Therapie der Sclerodermie. (Therapy of sclerodermia). Med Klin 1956; 51:2152-5
271. Doderlein, G. Die Indikation zur Implantation von Kalbs- oder Schweine-Hypophysen. (Indication for implantation of calf- or pig-pituitary glands). Munch Med Wschr. 1953; 95:969-975
272. Ehni, L, Duve, G. Zur Beurteiling und Therapie hypophysar-diencephaler Regulationstotungen in Entwicklungsalter. (Assessment and treatment of disorders of pituitary-diencephalic regulation in developmental period). Medizinische, Stuttgart 1957; 38:1381-1384
273. Janson, P. Zur therapie der Dystrophia adiposogenitalis, des Klimakterium virile und des Eunuchoidismus. (Therapy of dystrophia adiposogenitalis, male menopause, and eunuchoidism). Arztl.Praxis, Munchen 1955, VII/23

274. Camerer, W. Behandlung der Infertilitat des Mannes. (Treatment of male infertility). Therapie-Woche 1956; 7:13-18
275. Nikolowski, W. Behandlung mannlicher Potenzstorungen. (Treatment of male impotence). Therapie-Woche 1956, 7:604 - 608
276. Janson, P. Probleme des mannlichen Klimakteriums und der sexualitat des alternden Mannes. (Problem of male menopause and of sexuality of aging man). Hippocrates, Stuttgart 1952; 23:539-546
277. Holmer, AJM. Implantation von embryonalen Eierstocksgewebe in Fallen vo gonadaler Agenesie. (Implantation of embryonic ovarian tissue in cases of agenesis of ovary). Geburtsh.u.Frauenhk. 1958;18: 621-626
278. Vorster, R. Zur Siccacell-Behandlung von Amenorhoe und Sterilitat. (About Siccacell treatment of amenorrhea and sterility). Hippocrates, Stuttgart 1958; 29:565-570
279. Molnar, EM. Stem cells and myocardial regeneration. In: Kipshidze, NN, Serruys, PW (Editors). **Handbook of Cardiovascular Cell Transplantation**, Martin Dunitz, London UK, 2004
280. Kuhn, W, Knuchel, F. Zur Wirkung von Placenta-Trockengewebe auf arteriosclerotische Veranderungen. (About the effect of dehydrated placenta tissue on arteriosclerotic changes). Med Klin 1954; 48:1363-1366
281. Stepantschitz, G, Schreiner, B. Erfahrungen mit der Siccacell-Therapie bei Gefasserkrankungen. (Experience with dehydrated celltherapeu-tica in vascular diseases). Therap Umschau 1956; 10
282. Panchenko, EL, Naumova, VI, Shelija, NS, Molnar, EM. Debre-De Toni-Fanconi-Syndrome: Treatment of childhood kidney disease by the transplantation of human fetal tissues. Med Organ 1994; 18:16-18
283. Muller, A. Biologische Zusatztherapie in der Krebsbehandlung. (Biological adjuvant therapy in handling of cancer). Cyt Rev 1985; 9:32-36
284. Hagmaier, W, Hoepke, H, Landsberger, A, Renner, H. Erfolgreiche Behandlung Krebskranker durch Immuntherapie mit fetalem Mesenchym-Lyophilisat. (Succesful treatment of cancer patients by immunotherapy with lyophilisate of fetal mesenchym). Cyt Rev 1979; 3:10-14
285. Renner, H, Bendel, R, Bendel, V, et al. Erfahrungen mit Resistocell als Zusatztherapie beim metastasierenden Mamma-Carcinom. (Expe-rience with resistocell as adjuvant treatment of metastasizing breat cancer). Cyt Rev 1980; 4:109 -115
286. Schneider, H. Die Uberlebenszeit lebenswichtiger Organe. (Survival time of vital organs). Cyt Rev 1978; 2:19
287. Schmid, F. AIDS-Ist die therepeutische Resignation berechtigt? (AIDS – is the therapeutic resignation justified?). Cyt Rev 1988; 12:117-120
288. Schmid, F. Sichclzell-Anamie. (Sicke cell anemia). Cyt Rev 1988; 12:52-56
289. Blaney, GR. Paralysis of muscles of deglutition. Cyt Rev 1988; 12:86
290. Block, S. Ein optimaler Behandlungserfolg durch Freschzellentherapie bei schwersten Sehstorungen. (Optimal result of treatment of the most severe eye disorder by fresh cell therapy). Biol Med 1990; 19:244-247
291. Ortiz, FR. Citoterapia en las enfermedadez reumaticas. (Cell transplantation in rheumatic diseases). Cyt rev 1981; 5:30-37

292. Schenk, S. Zelltherapie in der konservativen Orthopadie. (Cell therapy in non-surgical orthopaedics). Erfahr.-heilkunde 1985, 34:30-37
293. Schenk, S. Zelltherapie in der operativen Orthopadie. (Cell therapy in surgical orthopaedics). Erfahr.-heilkunde 1985; 34: 38-50
294. Blaney, GR. Calve-Legg-Perthes disease. Cyt Rev 1988; 12:87
295. Buscha, J. Zelltherapie bei Asthma bronchiale? (Cell therapy for bronchial asthma?). Cyt Rev 1979; 3:174-179
296. Weber, T, Weber, D. Zelltherapie bei Anorexia nervosa - ein Behandlugsplan. (Cell therapy in anorexia nervosa - a therapeutic program). Cyt Rev 1984; 8:153-157
297. Babilotte, J. Die Migrane - Indikation fur eine Zeltherapie. (Migraine – indication for cell therapy). Cyt Rev 1979; 3:117-121
298. Brammer, H. Neue Wege in der Behandlung von Alkoholkranken. (New way of treatment of alcoholics). Cyt Rev 1981; 5:73-75
299. Camerer, W. Fortgeschrittene Sclerodermie. (Advanced scleroder-ma). Cyt Rev 1987; 11:34
300. Dufek, V. Zelltherapie bei chronisch aggressiver Hepatitis. (Cell therapy for chronic aggressive hepatitis). Cyt Rev 1987; 11:33-34
301. Camerer, W. Morbus Werlhof. (Idiopathic thrombocytopenic purpura). Cyt Rev 1987; 11:27
302. Kollersbeck, E. Erfolgreicher Einsatz der Cytotherapie bei hamatologischen Erkrankungen. (Succesful use of cytotherapy in hematological diseases). Cyt Rev 1987; 11:26-27
303. Schenk, S. Senile Osteoporose. (Senile osteoporosis). Cyt Rev 1987; 11:22-24
304. Schneider, U. Anwendung der Zytotherapie bei Huftkopfnekrose. (Application of cytotherapy in necrosis of the head of femur). Cyt Rev 1987; 11:21-22
305. Marzheuser, F. Femurkopfnekrose links bei Coxarthrose nach Osteomyelitis. (Necrosis of the head of the left femur in coxarthrosis after osteomyelitis). Cyt Rev 1987; 11:20
306. Eickschen, H. Chronish persistierende Osteomyelitis. (Chronic persistent osteomyelitis). Cyt Rev 1987; 11:18-20
307. Schmid, F. Friedreich'sche Ataxie. (Friedreich's ataxia). Cyt Rev 1987; 11:15-16
308. Muller, A. Migrane. (Migraine). Cyt Rev 1987; 11: 14
309. Muller, A. Asthma bronchiale. (Bronchial asthma). Cyt Rev 1987; 11:13-14
310. Dorr, HW. Multipel metastasierendes Magenkarzinom. (Cancer of stomach with multiple metastases). Cyt Rev 1987; 11:8
311. Berger, J. Therapie mit dem Immunomodulator Resistocell bei AIDS-Patienten. (Treatment of AIDS patient with immunomodulatoir Resistocell). Cyt Rev 1987; 11:5-6
312. Weber, T, Weber, D. Potenz- und Fertilitatstorungen. (Disorders of potency and fertility). Cyt Rev 1987; 11:4
313. Follmer, W. Zelltherapie im Klimakterium - Vorlaufige Mitteilung. (Cell therapy in menopause - a preliminary communication). Cyt Rev 1986;

10:204-207
314. Camerer, W. Infertilitat - Diagnostik und Therapie. (Infertility - diagnosis and treatment). Cyt Rev 1978; 2:12-17
315. Camerer, W. Behandlung mannlicher Fertilitatsstorungen mit Siccacell-Praparaten. (Treatment of male infertility with Siccacell preparations). Medorganica 1987; 18:84-86
316. Egorov, YI, Marshalko, VI, Orlov, VI, Molnar, EM. Experimental treatment of habitual abortion of adrenal etiology by transplantation of tissue culture of newborn pig adrenals. Bull Exp Biol Med 1994; 117:389-39
317. Alikhanova, ZM. Treatment of patients with postcastration syndrome by transplantation of human fetal tissues. Dissertation for the degree of "Doctor of Medical Sciences", Russian Research Center for Obstetrics, Gynecology, Perinatology, (Kulakov VI), and International Institute of Biological Medicine, (Molnar EM), Moscow, 1995
318. Kulakov, VI, Alikhanova, ZM, Il'ina, EM, Molnar, EM. The state of autonomic regulation with postcastration syndrome after transplantation of human fetal tissues. Bull Exp Biol Med 1994; 117:379-382
319. Kulakov, VI, Alikhanova, ZM, Tkachenko, NM, Molnar, EM. Effect of transplantation of human fetal tissue on central nervous system function in patients with the post-castration syndrome. Bull Exp Biol Med 1994; 117:383-386
320. Kulakov, VI, Alikhanova, ZM, Burdina, LM, Molnar, EM. Status of the breasts in patienst with the postcastration syndrome treated by transplantation of human fetal tissue. Bull Exp Biol Med 1994; 117: 387-389
321. Neumann, K. The influence of tissue injections on experimental liver damage. In: Schmid, F, Stein, J. **Cell-research and Cellular therapy**, Ott Publishers, Thun, Switzerland, 1967.
322. Dufek, V. Wirksamkeit lyophilisierter fetaler Zell-praparate in der Therapie chronischer Lebererkrankungen. (Effectiveness of lyophilized cell preparations in the treatment of chronic liver disease). Cyt Rev 1987; 11:63-67
323. Bernhard, P, Krampitz, W. The organ specific cellular effect of implanted rabbit endometrium upon the uterus of castrated rabbits. In: Schmid, F, Stein, J. **Cell-research and Cellular therapy**, Ott Publishers, Thun, Switzerland, 1967
324. Neumann, KH. Induction of growth in organs by the implantation of homologous tissues. In: Schmid, F, Stein, J. **Cell-research and Cellular therapy**, Ott Publishers, Thun, Switzerland, 1967.
325. Weiss, P, Taylor, AC. Reconstitution of complete organs from single-cell suspensions of chick embryos in advanced stages of differentiation. Proc Nat Acad Sciences USA 1960; 46:1177-1185
326. Stein, J. Objective demonstration of the organ-specific effectiveness of cellular preparations. In: Schmid, F, Stein, J. **Cell-research and Cellular therapy**, Ott Publishers, Thun, Switzerland, 1967
327. Stein, J. Specific effect of implanted endocrine tissues. In: Schmid F, Stein J. **Cell-research and Cellular therapy**, Ott Publishers, Thun, Switzerland,

1967
328. Trudy Nauchno-issledovatelskogo Instituta Obmena Veschestv I Endokrinnykh Rasstroistv NKZ RSFSR, Vypusk 1, **Teori'a i praktika lizatoterapii po metodu IN Kazakova**, Gosudarstvennoe Medicinsko'e Izadtelstvo, Moskva, Leningrad, 1934. (Papers of Research and Scientific Institute of Metabolism and Endocrine Disorders of National Comissariat of Health, Edition 1, Theory and Practice of Lysatetherapy by method of IN Kazakow. State Medical Publishing, Moscow, Leningrad, 1934)
329. Stein, J. Die Zelltherapie in der inneren Medizin. (Cell therapy in internal medicine). Heilkunst 1974; 87:11/1-7
330. Korsakova, NK, Dybovskaia, NP, Roschina, IF, Gavrilova, SI. Uchebno-metodicheskoe posob'e po neiropsykhologicheskoi diagnostike dementsii alcgeimerovskogo tipa [bolezn Alcgeimera i senilnaia dementsia] (Teaching Manual of Method of Neuropsychological Diagnosis of dementias of Alzheimer's type [Alzheimer's disease and senile dementia]) Research Center of Psychic Health of Russian Academy of Medical Sciences, Moscow 1992
331. Muller, A. Postoperative parathyreoprive Tetanie. Cyt Rev 1987; 11:3-4
332. Paracelsus, PA. Chirurgia Magna. Basel, 1579 [Peter Perna]. (from amazon.com is available, the translation by HE Sigerist of 1941: Four Treatises of Theophrastus von Hohenheim Called Paracelsus)
333. Govallo, VI. **Immunology of Pregnancy and Cancer**, Nova Science Publishers, New York, 1993

ABBREVIATIONS

AAALAC	American Association for Accreditation of Laboratory Animal Care
AAG	(or aAg) Allogenic Antigen or Alloantigen
ACE	Angiotensin Converting Enzyme
ACTH	Adrenocorticotropic Hormone
AD	Autosomal Dominant
ADH	Anti-Diuretic Hormone
ADP	Adenosine diphosphate
AIDS	Acquired Immunodeficiency Syndrome
ALS	Amyotrophic Lateral Sclerosis
ALT	Alanine Aminotransferase (formerly SGPT)
AMP	Adenosine Monophosphate
APC	Antigen-Presenting Cell
APHIS	Animal and Plant Health Inspection Service
AR	Autosomal Recessive
ARC	AIDS Related Complex
AST	Aspartate Aminotransferase (formerly SGOT)
AT	Allo-Transplantation
ATP	Adenosine Triphosphate
BaEV	Baboon Endogenous Retrovirus
BCRO	Bio-Cellular Research Organization
BIO	Biotechnology Industry Organization
BSL	Biosafety Level
BUN	Blood Urea Nitrogen
CBC	Complete Blood Count
CBS	Cystathionine-β-Synthase
CD	Crohn's Disease
CDC	Centers for Disease Control and Prevention
CEA	Carcino-Embryonic Antigen
CFR	Code of Federal Regulations
CFTR	Cystic Fibrosis Transmembrane Conductance Regulator
CIS	Commonwealth of Independent States
CJD	Creutzfeldt-Jakob Disease
CLIA	Clinical Laboratory Improvements Act
CMV	Cytomegalovirus
CNS	Central Nervous System
CRH	Corticotropin Releasing Hormone
CSF	Cerebrospinal Fluid
CT	Coaxial Tomography
CVA	Cerebro-vascular Accident
DCCT	Diabetes Control and Complication Trial
DHHS	Department of Health and Human Services (USA)

DLE	Dialysable Leukocyte Extract
DM	Diabetes Mellitus
DNA	Deoxyribonucleic Acid
DOPA	Levo-dopa, metabolic precursor of dopamine
DRS	Diabetes Retinopathy Study
EC	European Commission
ECT	ECT Growth Factor and ECT antibody
EDTA	Ethylene-diamine-tetra-acetate
EEG	Electroencephalogram
EKG	Electrocardiogram
EMG	Electromyogram
ERB-B	Erythroblastic leukemia viral oncogene homolog
ESRD	End-Stage Renal Disease
FADH	Flavin Adenine Dinucleotide H^+
FCT	Fresh Cell Therapy
FDA	Food and Drug Administration (USA)
FSH	Follicle-Stimulating Hormone
GABA	Gamma-amino-butyric Acid
GALT	Gut-Associated Lymphoid Tissue
GCP	Good Clinical Practice
GH	Growth Hormone
GHRF	Growth Hormone Releasing Factor
GHRH	Growth Hormone Releasing Hormone
GMP	Good Manufacturing Practice; also Guanosine-mono-phosphate
GRH	Gonadotropin-Releasing Hormone
HCG	Chorionic Gonadotropin
HCV	Hepatitis C Virus
HDL	High Density Lipoprotein
HIV	Human Immunodeficiency Virus
HLA	Human Leukocyte Antigens
HPV	Human Papilloma Virus
HTLV	Human T-Cell Lymphotropic Virus
IACUC	Institutional Animal Care and Use Committee
IBC	Institutional Biosafety Committee
ICAM	Intracellular Adhesive Molecule
IDDM	Insulin Dependent Diabetes Mellitus
IFN	Interferon
IGF	Insulin Growth Factor
IIBM	International Institute of Biological Medicine
IMP	Inosine-mono-phosphate
IND	Investigational New Drug
IRB	Institutional Review Board
LAD	Leukocyte Adhesion Defect
LADA	Latent Autoimmune Diabetes Mellitus of Adults
LAI	Leukocyte Adherence Inhibition

LATS	Long Acting Thyroid Stimulator
LcD	Leukocyte Dialysate
LDH	Lactic Dehydrogenase
LDL	Low Density Lipoproteins
LEAD	Lower Extremity Arterial Disease
LH	Luteinizing Hormone
LPL	Lipoproteinlipase
MA	Malabsorption Syndromes
MALT	Mucosa-Associated Lymphoid Tissue
MBP	Myelin Basic Protein
MCTD	Mixed Connective Tissue Disease
MFS	Mononuclear-Phagocytic System
MHC	Major Histocompatibility Complex
MI	Myocardial Infarction
MIF	Migration Inhibition Factors
MODY	Maturity-Onset Diabetes of the Young
MPS	Mucopolysacharidoses
MRI	Magnetic Resonance Imaging
NAD	Nicotinamide Adenine Dinucleotide
NADH	Nicotinamide Adenine Dinucleotide H^+
NADPH	Nicotinamide Adenine Dinucleotide Phosphate H^+
NHIS	National Health Interview Survey
NHP	Nonhuman Primates
NIDDK	National Institute of Diabetes and Digestive and Kidney Diseases
NIDDM	Non-Insulin Dependent Diabetes Mellitus
NIH	National Institutes of Health
NO	Nitric Oxide
OBA	Office of Biotechnology Activities
OECD	Organization for Economic Cooperation and Development
ORDA	Office of Recombinant DNA Activities
OXPHOS	Oxidative Phosphorylation
PBMC	Peripheral Blood Mononuclear Cells
PHS	Public Health Service (USA)
PKU	Phenylketonuria
PM	Polymyositis
PN	Polyarteritis Nodosa
PP	Pharyngeal Pouch
PSS	Scleroderma
RA	Rheumatoid arthritis
RAS	Ras Protein or ras Gene
RDDP	RNA-Directed DNA Polymerase
RER	Rough Endoplasmic Reticulum
RES	Reticulo-Endothelial System
RIH	Release Inhibiting Hormones
RITAOMH	Research Institute of Transplantology and Artificial Organs of the Ministry of Health (USSR)

RNA	Ribonucleic Acid
SACX	Secretary's Advisory Committee on Xenotransplantation (USA)
SBE	Spongiform Bovine Encephalitis
SCID	Severe Combined Immunodeficiency Disease
SCT	Stem Cell Transplantation
SCXT	Stem Cell Xeno-Transplantation
SFV	Simian Foamy Virus
SGOT	Same as AST
SGPT	Same as ALT
SIS	Sis Oncogene
SLE	Systemic Lupus Erythematosus
SMA	Laboratory Chemistry Screen
SPF	Specific Pathogen Free
SRS-A	Slow-reacting substance of anaphylaxis
SS	Sjogren Syndrome
TFN	Tumor Necrosis Factor
TGF	Transforming Growth Factor
TORCH	Toxoplasmosis, Rubella, Cytomegalovirus Herpes
TRH	Thyrotropin-Releasing Hormone
TSEs	Transmissible Spongiform Encephalopathies
TSH	Thyroid Stimulating Hormone
TSI	Thyreoid Stimulating Immunoglobulin
USDA	US Department of Agriculture
UV	Ultra Violet
VLDL	Very Low Density Lipoproteins
VS	Veterinary Services
WAGR	Wilms Tumor with Aniridia, Genital anomalies and Mental Retardation
WESDR	Wisconsin Epidemiologic Study of Diabetic Retinopathy
WHO	World Health Organization
XR	X-linked Recessive
XT	Xeno-Transplantation

Index

Aarskog syndrome 345
Abetalipoproteinemia 524
Acanthosis nigricans 524
Accessory portal system 270
A-cells 467
Acetylcholine 300
Acetyl-CoA 150, 151, 152
Achalasia 546
Achondroplasia 178, 341, 536
Acne vulgaris 590
Acquired specific immunity 467
Acute hepatitis 556
Acute intermittent porphyria 503
Acute leukemia 203, 278
Autosomal dominant (AD) disorder 201, 204
Addison's disease 307, 344, 436, 484
Adenocarcinoma 202
Adrenal cortex 144, 281, 182, 297, 435
Adrenaline 300, 416
Adrenocortical hormones 435, 436
Adrenocorticotropic hormone 300, 436
Adrenogenital syndrome 348, 575
Adrenoleukodystrophy 358, 359
Adult rheumatoid arthritis 278
Adult stem cells 138
Agammaglobulinemia 278, 344
Aging disease 177, 307, 387, 391, 394, 396
AIDS 134, 277, 305, 469, 470, 471, 478, 548
Albinism 349
Alkaptonuria 343, 349, 536
Allergic reaction 335, 482
Allo-transplant 6, 187, 198
Allo-transplant recipients 196
Allo-transplant rejection 188
Allo-transplantation 7- 10, 13, 16, 23, 192
Alopecia 591, 592
Alopetia areata 278
Alport syndrome 349
Alzheimer's disease 10, 134, 278, 512, 516, 530, 532, 533
Amaurotic idiocy 524
Aminoaciduria 361

Amyotrophic lateral sclerosis 278, 519, 525, 526
Androgens 440, 441, 444
Anemia 355
Anencephaly 379
Anergic 190, 191
Anergy 189, 190
Angelman syndrome 159, 372
Angiokeratoma corporis diffusum 354
Angiomatosis retinae et cerebelli 525
Angiopathies 540
Animal organ extracts 24
Animal procurement sources 88
Animal sources 76, 87, 225
Anorexia neurosa 407
Anterograde transneuronal degeneration 521
Anti-aging treatment 391
Antidiuretic hormone 408
Antigenic overload 223
Antigenic tumor cells 278
Antigenicity 122, 188
Antigens 134, 162
Apallic syndrome in children 308, 514
Apert syndrome 178
Aplastic anemia 498
Aponeurosis 270, 316
Aponeurosis of rectus abdominis muscle 271
Apoptosis 127, 133, 166, 189, 200, 481, 521
Archiving of records 245
Arhinencephaly 379
Arrhythmias 361
Arteriolosclerosis 570
Arteritis magnocellularis 584
Arthrogryposis multiplex 537
Arthropathy 349
Arthroses 539
Artificial organ 209, 213
Aseptic necroses 537, 539
Aspartylglucosaminouria 354
Astrocytoma 204
Ataxia 159, 177, 201, 343, 356, 359, 373, 380, 524

Atelectasis	588
Atherosclerosis	287, 351, 559, 561, 563, 564, 570
Athetosis	380
Athyreosis	381
Atopic dermatitis	278
Atrophic gastritis	546, 548
Atrophic state	144
Atypical retinitis	361
Autism	278
Auto-antibodies	194, 481
Auto-antigens	193, 482
Auto-transplantation	9, 192
Autoimmune disease	134, 187, 211, 307, 457, 481, 526
Autonomic neuropathy	260, 294
Autosomal chromosomes	364
Autosomal dominant	340
Autosomal recessive (AR) disorder	159, 201, 202, 342, 346
A-β-lipoproteinemia	563

B cell 184, 185, 191, 292, 412, 413, 414, 465, 466, 468, 469, 471, 472, 491, 546

B lymphocytes	184
Bartter syndrome	569
Bassen-Kornzweig syndrome	524
Becker muscular dystrophy	525
Beckwith-Wiedeman syndrome	204
Behcet syndrome	278
Bielschowsky type amaurotic idiocy	524
Biliary cirrhosis	556, 557
Bio-Cellular Research Organization	27, 28
Bio-compatible artificial materials	210
Biological age	388
Biological cancer treatment	492
Bio-prostheses	209
Birth damage	379
Bleeding disorders	346
Blindness	356, 357
Bloom syndrome	201, 347, 473
B-lymphocytes	184, 185, 465
B-memory cells	465
Bone anomalies	204
Bone cancer	539
Bone deformities	354
Bone marrow	137, 140, 171, 184, 303, 471
Bourneville syndrome	525
Bourneville-Pringle disease	341
Brain atrophy	395, 531
Brain damage	308, 380
Breast cancer	202, 203
Brittle Diabetes of children	306, 418, 426
Bronchial asthma	277, 585
Bronchiectases	346
Budd-Chiari syndrome	556
Bulimia	407
Bullous pemphigoid	278
Burger's disease	584
Burkitt lymphoma	203, 278

C cells	301
Cachexia	200, 355
Café-au-lait spots	204
Calve-Legg-Perthes disease	538
Canavan disease	523
Cancer	136, 199, 487, 491, 463
Cancer cells	177, 200, 201, 203, 278, 279, 467, 491
Cancer of urinary vesicle	202
Cancerogenesis	202
Carcino-embryonic antigen	488
Cardiac insufficiency	581
Cardiomegaly	354
Cardiomyocytes	574
Cardiomyopathies	361, 581
Carnithine myopathy	525
Carpal tunnel syndrome	260
Cartilage cells	171
Cataract	358
Catecholamines	300
Causes of extracorpuscular hemolytic anemias	502
Cell allotransplantation	28
Cell allotransplants	186
Cell immunity	490
Cell lines	137
Cell therapy	25, 26, 117, 119,
Cell transplant	213
Cell transplantation	5, 129, 340, 367
Cell xenotransplant	4, 33, 119, 186, 197, 206, 124
Cell xenotransplantation	10, 28, 118, 182, 189, 196
Cell xenotransplantation surveillance	328
Cell-mediated immunity	276, 278

Index 621

Cellular cytotoxicity	186	Cirrhosis of liver	551
Cellular immunity	426, 431	Cleft lip	379
Centrilobular emphysema	587	Closed colony	77, 122, 123, 219, 221, 231
Centroacinar stem cells	303	Coccidiomycosis	277
Ceramidosis	354	Cockayne syndrome	177, 347, 548
Cerebellar ataxia	380	Color blindness red/green	344
Cerebellar syndrome	361	Coma	308
Cerebral palsy	377, 378, 379, 383	Comatose patients	308
Cerebro-cutaneous degenerations	525	Combination of stem cell xenotransplants	333
Cerebrohepatorenal syndrome	359	Combinations of cell transplants	333
Cerebro-ocular degenerations	524	Combined deficit of lymphocytes	471
Cerebro-spinal ataxia	380	Combined hyperlipidemia	563
Chagas disease	549	Complement System Malfunction	473
Charcot-Marie-Tooth disease	521, 525, 526	Complications of DM	285, 410
Chediak-Higashi syndrome	468, 473	Concordant	185
Cherry-red-spot-myoclonus syndrome	354	Concordant species	228
Children's gout	351	Congenital adrenogenital syndrome	343
Chondrodysplasia punctata	359	Congenital disease	339
Chorda-mesoderm	169	Congenital erythropoietic porphyria	503
Chorea	380	Congenital goiter	457
Choreoathetosis	346, 351, 380	Congenital hypothyreosis	343
Choriomammotropin	416	Congenital methemoglobinopathy	159
Chorionic adrenocorticotropin	295	Congestive heart failure	576, 581
Chorionic gonadotropin	162, 295	Constrictive pericarditis	556
Chorionic somatomammotropin	162	Contiguous gene syndromes	340
Chorionic thyrotropin	295	Contraindications	305, 308
Chorionic villi	303	Cor pulmonale	355
Chorioretinopathy	358	Cornelia-de-Lange syndrome	341
Chromosomal aberration	201, 203, 363	Coronary stenosis	576
Chromosomal disease	308, 372, 379	Corpuscular hemolytic anemias	501
Chromosomal disorders	382	Corticoids	144
Chromosomal inborn diseases	308	Corticosteroid hormones	162
Chromosomal Instability Syndrome	201	Corticosteroids	300
Chronic alcoholism	554	Corticotropin-releasing hormone	296, 298, 300
Chronic arthritis	539		
Chronic bronchitis	585	Cortisol	285, 288, 297, 298, 416, 446, 456
Chronic cystitis in children	278	Cortisone	281
Chronic fatigue syndrome	277, 474	Co-transplantation	334
Chronic granulomatous disease	473	Co-transplants	288
Chronic hepatitis	278, 551, 553, 554, 556, 557	Craniofacial dysmorphism	358
		Cri du chat syndrome	371, 383
Chronic hypertension	575	Crigler-Najjar syndrome	556
Chronic leg ulcer	263	Criteria of success after cell transplantation	419
Chronic leukemia	201, 203	Criterion of rejection	419
Chronic lichen	590	Critical islet mass	146
Chronic obstructive pulmonary disease	277	Critical mass of the transplanted endocrine tissue of islets	145
Chronic osteomyelitis	537, 539		
Chronic pancreatitis	547, 548	Crohn's disease	278, 548, 549
Chronic pyelonephritis	278		

Cryptococcosis	277
Cryptosporidiosis	277
Cushing syndrome	575, 401
Cutaneous leishmaniasis	277
Cutis laxa	536
Cystic fibrosis	343, 586
Cystinosis	343, 349
Cystinuria	343
Cytomegalovirus infection	277
Cytosol	156
Cytotoxic cells	470
Cytotoxic lymphocytes	492
Cytotrophoblast	162, 295, 492

D cells 301, 412, 413

Deafness	356
Decerebration state	357
Decidual cells	303
Dedifferentiation	200
Deep burns	4
Defects of cell-mediated immunity	469
Defects of ion channels in neurons	529
Degeneration of basal ganglia	530
Degenerative diseases of central nervous system	514
Dejerin-Sottas syndrome	521
Dementia	360
Demyelinization diseases	523
Dendrites	166, 168
Dendritic cells	182, 185, 192
Dentinogenesis imperfecta	341
Denys-Drash syndrome	204
Dermatomycosis	197, 526
Desbuquois syndrome	536
Devic syndrome	523
Devitalization	388, 389
Diabetes	257, 258, 260
Diabetes insipidus	344, 408, 569
Diabetes mellitus	140, 144, 147, 255, 256, 285, 287, 290, 306, 331, 409, 410, 412, 413, 416, 428, 432, 526, 559
Diabetes mellitus in pregnancy	418
Diabetes mellitus type 1	414
Diabetes mellitus type 2	415
Diabetic complications	273, 274, 332, 411
Diabetic fetal distress syndrome	428
Diabetic fetopathy	306
Diabetic lower extremity arterial disease	259, 263, 418, 432, 433
Diabetic microangiopathy	285, 286
Diabetic nephropathy	261, 263, 418, 420, 432, 433, 260
Diabetic polyneuropathy	261, 264, 265, 294, 418, 432, 433
Diabetic retinopathy	258, 262, 418, 428, 429, 432
Dialysable leukocyte extract	276, 279
Diencephalon	165
Differential growth	166
Diffuse sclerosis	523
DiGeorge syndrome	472
Dilated cardiomyopathy	580
Direct stimulation by cell transplantation	141, 332
Direct stimulation of regeneration	3, 4
Discoid lupus erythematosus	278
Discordant cell xenotransplantation	119
Discordant species	228
Diseases of white matter of the brain	520
Disorders of humoral immunity	469
Disorders of motor unit	525
Disorders of neuromuscular transmission	529
Disturbances of erythropoiesis	497
Disturbed media transport	536
Disturbed neurosecretory regulations	144
DNA	132, 157, 158, 165, 177, 178, 200, 201, 202, 227, 278, 345, 359, 360
Dolichocephalia	352
Dominant oncogenes	201
Dominant otosclerosis	341
Dopamine	300
Down syndrome	177, 201, 365, 366, 367, 369, 375, 376, 381, 383
Drosophila	11, 12
Drosophila melanogaster	511
Dubin-Johnson syndrome	343, 556
Duchenne and Becker muscular dystrophies	528
Dwarfism	405
Dysfunctional uterine bleeding	453
Dyslexia	380
Dyslipidemias	561
Dysmorphic syndromes	379
Dystonia musculorum deformans	530

E

Early menopause	445
Ectoderm	8, 163, 171

Index 623

Ectodermal	174
Edwards syndrome	369
Ehlers-Danlos syndrome	536, 537
Electromagnetic fields	137
Electron transport cascade	150
Embryo	8
Embryogenesis	173
Embryonic cells	5, 6, 136
Embryonic development	162
Embryonic epiblast	161
Embryonic stem cell transplantation	11
Embryonic stem cells	5, 7, 13, 135
Embryonic theory of cancer	488
Embryo-producing cells	5, 295
Emphysema	587
Encephalitis	117, 518
Endocardium	171
Endochondral ossification	170
Endocrine gland	143, 144, 401, 404
Endocrine hypertension	575
Endocrine myopathies	534
Endocrine nanism	405
Endocrine system	404
Endoderm	163
Endogenous antigens	184
Endogenous retroviruses	195
Endogenous viruses	195, 196
Endometriosis	451
Endothelial cells	139, 192, 302, 303
Endothelial venules	139
Endothelium	139, 200, 286
End-stage renal disease	257
Enzymatic events	149
Enzyme reactions	150
Enzymes	149, 150
Enzymopathies	347, 348, 349, 352, 379, 436, 551
Ependyma	166
Ependymal cells	166
Epiblast	161
Epidermolysis bullosa	536
Epilepsy	278
Epimyocardium	171
Epiphyseal plates	170, 171
Epithelial cells	131
Epithelial progenitor cells	289
Epizootiologic data	220
Epizootiology	232
Epstein-Barr virus	202
Erythroid precursors	498
Erythropoietin	498
Esophageal hypomotility	546
Estradiol	296, 455, 456
Estriol	296
Estrogen	144, 171, 296, 444
Eukaryotes	161
Eukaryotic cells	13, 157, 175, 205
Exogenous insulin	274, 332, 414
Exophthalmos	460
Extracellular matrix	132, 140
F cells	412, 413
Fabry's disease	344, 354, 357
Familial adenomatous polyposis of colon	204
Familial dysautonomy	343
Familial dyslipidemia	564
Familial dys-β-lipoproteinemia	563, 564
Familial excess of lipoprotein	564
Familial hereditary retinoblastoma	203
Familial hypercholesterolemia	563, 564
Familial hyperchylomicronemia	564
Familial hyperuricemia	345
Familial hypo-α-lipoproteinemia	564
Familial melanoma	201
Familial protein intolerance	568
Familiar combined hyperlipidemia	341
Familiar hypercholesterolemia	341
Fanconi pancytopenia	201
Fanconi syndrome	346, 354, 356, 361, 568
Feeder cells	12
Feeder layer of cells	137
Feeder mouse cells	135
Female infertility	452
Fertilization	6, 452
Fetal adrenal gland	162
Fetal allo-transplantation	30
Fetal islet cells	145, 186
Fetal liver cells	289
Fetal tissue transplantation	5
Fibrosarcomas	202
Floppy infant syndrome	379
Foam hydrogel	212
Follicle-stimulating hormone	440, 444, 446
Follicular cells	301
Fresh cell therapy	26, 117, 120
Friedreich's ataxia	512, 523, 524
Fucosidosis	354

G6PD deficit 344
Galactose metabolism 350
Galactosemia 343, 350
Gangliosidoses 344, 357
Gangrene 264, 286
Gardner syndrome 201
Gargoylism 352
Gastrin 293
Gastrulation 133
Gastrulation movements 161
Gaucher cells 355
Gaucher disease 343, 354, 355, 356
Gene disorder 339
Gene mutations 158
Genetic abnormalities 122
Genetic and chromosomal diseases 255
Genetic code 157
Genetic defects 526, 527
Genetic diseases 307, 333
Genetic disorders 498, 535
Genetic encoding 14
Genetic events 200
Genetic inborn diseases 308
Genetic mutants 11
Genetic mutations 158
Genetic thromboembolic diseases 504
Genital hypoplasia 159
Genome 157
Germ cells 177
Germ layer 173
Germinal layer 166
Germinal neuroepithelium 165
Gestation diabetes mellitus 417
Gilbert syndrome 556
Gittelman syndrome 569
Glial cell 166- 168, 301, 304, 381
Gliomas 202
Globoid leukodystrophy 354, 522
Glomerular diseases 570
Glomerulonephritis 569
Glomerulosclerosis 286
Glucagon 285, 290, 294, 416
Glucocorticoids 297, 298
Gluconeogenesis 152, 154, 156
Glycogen 152, 155, 416
Glycogenoses 347, 350
Glycoproteinsialidosis 354
G_{MI} gangliosidoses 354, 357, 357
Gonadotropin 144, 296, 300, 440, 441

Goodpasture's syndrome 482
Gout 565
Graves disease 460
Gray matter of the brain 166
Growth hormone 171, 296, 299, 405
Growth hormone releasing factor 406
Growth retardation 355, 361
Guillain-Barre syndrome 278
Gut-associated lymphoid tissue (GALT) 291

Habitual abortion of adrenal etiology 452
Haematopoietic stem cell transplantation 6
Haematopoietic stem cells 303
Hallervorden-Spatz syndrome 530
Halsted principle 140, 142, 146
Hamman-Rich idiopathic lung fibrosis 588
Handicapped individuals 378
Hartnup disease 548
Hartnup syndrome 343, 568
Hashimoto's thyroiditis 307, 457, 459, 483, 484
Heart attack 261
Heart myocytes 132
Hematopietic stem cells 137, 140, 171, 177, 191, 268
Hemicrania 584
Hemofilia A and B 344
Hemoglobin 500, 501
Hemolytic anemias 501
Hemophilia A and B 504
Hemopoietic cells 140
Hemorrhagic diathesis 355, 503
Hemostasis 503, 506
Hepatitis 202, 551, 554
Hepatocellular carcinoma 202
Hepatolenticular degeneration 530
Hepatomegaly 355, 358, 359
Hepatorenal syndrome 557
Hepatosplenic syndrome 568
Hepatosplenomegaly 352, 355, 357, 358
Hereditary bullous epidermolysis 278
Hereditary coproporphyria 503
Hereditary fructose intolerance 350
Hereditary hypophosphatemic vitamin-D resistant rachitis 345
Hereditary spherocytosis 341, 501
Herpes simplex 277
Herpes virus 198

Herpes zoster	277	Hypotonic cerebral palsy	381
Hirschsprung disease	549	Hypotonic disorders	381
Histoplasmosis	277	Hypoxia	286
Hodgkin's disease	278, 494	Hypo-α-lipoproteinemia	563
Homing	128, 129, 139-142, 174, 331, 378		
Homocystinuria	351, 536		
Homologous organs	142	Iatrogenic diseases	281
Hormonal therapy	143	Idiopathic thrombocytopenic purpura	505
Hormone deficiency disorders	435	Iminoglycinuria	568
Hormone replacement therapy	307, 445	Immune deficiency	382, 383, 463
Human embryonic stem cell transplantation	9	Immune reaction	6, 8, 118, 120, 122, 145, 334
Human fetal brain cells	11, 12	Immune response	139, 140, 162, 332, 333
Human fetal tissue transplantation	23	Immune system	145, 212, 276, 278, 463, 471, 491
Human leukocyte antigens (HLA)	183		
Human retroviruses	228	Immune tolerance	329
Humoral immunity	190, 426, 431, 465	Immunity	490
Hunter's syndrome	344, 352, 353	Immunocompetent	134
Huntington's chorea	515, 516, 530	Immunocompetent cells	134
Hydraencephaly	379	Immunodeficiency	277, 472
Hyperaminoaciduria	568	Immunogen	189, 276
Hypercholesterolemia	561, 563, 570	Immunogenicity	124, 137, 139, 187, 221
Hyperfibrinogenemia	559	Immunologic reactions	335
Hyperglycemia	145, 146, 285, 286, 287, 349, 412	Immunologic stimuli	191
		Immunological problems	206
Hyperhidrosis	354	Immunological reactions	228, 429
Hyperhomocysteinemia	351, 559	Immunological tolerance	121
Hyper-IgE syndrome	473	Immunologically privileged regions	144
Hyperimmunoglobulinemia	278	Immunomodulator	275
Hyperkalemic periodic paralysis	527	Immuno-paralysis	466
Hyperlipidemia	559, 561	Immunoprivileged areas	482
Hyperlipoproteinemia type 1	564	Immunoprivileged sites	145
Hyperoxaluria	349, 359	Immunoprotective	270
Hyperphosphatemia	568	Immunoreactions	193
Hyperprolinemia	349	Immunostimulation	495
Hypertension	286, 287, 559, 574	Immunosuppressants	6, 8, 228, 330
Hyperthyroidism	460	Immunosuppression	7, 8, 26, 27, 119, 122, 124, 128, 129, 137, 182, 196, 197, 212, 223, 313, 330, 333, 335, 489, 491, 579
Hypertriacyl-glycerolemias	561		
Hypertrophic scar	591		
Hyperuricemia	565	Immunosuppressive	490, 491
Hypoaldosteronism	569	Immunosuppressive reaction	489
Hypo-endocrinopathies	143, 306, 461	Immuno-tolerance	134
Hypofunction of the immune system	307	Impaired diffusion	588
Hypokalemic periodic paralysis	527	Impaired perfusion	588
Hypophosphatemia	345	Implantable artificial organs and tissues	209
Hypotension	575		
Hypothalamic pituitary system	285	Implantation Scheme	314, 315, 316, 317
Hypothalamic syndrome	547	Implantation sites	269, 270
Hypothalamus	299	Impotence	264
Hypothyroidism	366, 458, 459	Inborn errors of metabolism	347, 379

Inborn paroxysmal nocturnal hemoglobinuria	502	Langerhans islands	193, 284, 285, 290, 301, 303, 332, 411- 417, 418, 541
Inborn thrombocytopenic purpura	505	Laron nanism	406
Incontinentio pigmenti	345	Larsen syndrome	536
Indications of SCT	305	Latent autoimmune DM of adults	415
Individual xenotransplant recipient health records	327	Laurence-Moon-Biedl syndrome	343
		Lead intoxication	526
Infection control	77, 104	Learning disorders	380
Infertility	281, 307, 428	Leber hereditary optic nerve neuropathy	361
Informed consent	69, 84, 327		
Institutional xenotransplantation record	327	Leigh disease	361
Insufficient peripheral arterial circulation	263	Leprosy	277
		Leptospirosis	197
Insulin	146, 259, 290, 293, 306, 332, 409, 410, 417	Lesch-Nyhan syndrome	344, 351
		Lethal anencephaly	165
Insulinitis	140	Leukemias	202
Insulin-like growth factor	171, 288	Leukodystrophies	522
Insulin-resistant lipoatrophic diabetes	417	Leydig cells	302
Intercellular matrix	132, 535	Liddle syndrome	569
Inter-species barrier	277	Lifespan	177, 388
Interstitial nephritis	571	Li-Fraumeni syndrome	203
Interstitial pneumonia	277	Lipidoses	288, 347, 354
Intracoronary implantation	307	Lipoproteinlipase	562
Intractable arrhythmia	574	Live human placental tissue implantation	5
Intraventricular bleeding	308		
Ischemic heart disease	575	Liver cancer	554
Islet cell	193, 198, 206, 301, 414, 422, 430	Liver cirrhosis	358, 551, 553, 554, 557,
		Liver diseases	551, 554
Islet xenotransplants	187	Liver fibrosis	288
		Liver hematopoietic cells	191
Juvenile diabetes mellitus	414	Leukemoid reactions	201
Juvenile rheumatoid arthritis	278	Locked-in-syndrome	518
		Louis-Bar syndrome	346, 524
Kaposi sarcoma	202	Lowe's oculocerebrorenal syndrome	344, 569
Kearns-Sayre syndrome	178, 361	Lower extremity arterial disease	255
Kidney failure	359	Lower extremity vascular disease	256
Kimmelstiel-Wilson syndrome	286	Lung cancer	202
Kinsbourne syndrome	524	Lung edema	588
Klinefelter syndrome	178, 371	Lung fibrosis	588
Krabbe disease	354, 356, 522	Lupus vulgaris	278
Krebs cycle	151, 152, 153, 154, 156, 200, 487, 502	Luteinizing hormone	295, 440, 444, 446
		Lymphoid cell	291, 302, 303
Kupffer cells	187, 302, 467, 552	Lymphoid organ	139, 140
Kyphoscoliosis	353, 361	Lymphoid tissue	140
		Lymphokines	277
Labeling	249	Lymphomas	202
Lambert-Eaton syndrome	530	Lysosomal enzymopathies	352
		Lysosomal storage diseases	352

Index

Macrocephaly 357
Macroglossia 357
Macrophages 140, 171, 192
Macular degeneration 357
Mad Cow Disease 220, 221, 228
Major histocompatibility complex 182
Malabsorption 547, 549
Male hypogonadism 307
Male infertility 438, 441
Male pattern baldness 169
Malignant hyperthermia 527
Malignant melanoma 278
Mannosidosis 354
Manufacturing 220
Manufacturing process 248
Maple syrup disease 343, 349
Marfan syndrome 178, 341, 536
Maroteux-Lamy syndrome 353
Masugi nephritis 569
Melanoma 202
Menkes disease 344, 345
Menkes syndrome 536
Menopause 395
Mental retardation 204, 308, 351, 355- 359, 360, 370, 380, 384
Mesenchymal cells 170, 173, 174
Mesenchymal tissue 170
Mesenchyme 169, 172
Mesoderm 8, 162, 169, 170, 173
Metabolic pathways 152
Metabolic regulation 154
Metachromatic leukodystrophy 354, 356, 522
Metastases 199, 200
Metastatic cancer of lungs 278
Microalbuminuria 257, 262
Microangiopathic changes 332
Microangiopathy 286
Microcephaly 379
Micromelias 538
Migraine 584
Missing puberty 438
Mitochondria 133
Mitochondrial diseases 361
Mitochondrial DNA 157
Mitochondrial encephalomyelopathy 361
Mitochondrial genetic diseases 359, 362
Mitochondrial myopathy 361
Mitochondrial theory of aging 178

Mitosis 131, 135, 165, 199, 200
Mongolism 365, 366
Monitoring of closed colonies 238
Monoclonal origin 279
Mononucleosis 277
Monosomy X 370
Morquio syndrome 353
Motor disturbances 378
Motor neuron disease 525
Mucolipidosis 354
Mucosa-associated lymphoid Tissue (MALT) 284, 291
Multiple exostoses 201
Multiple sclerosis 134, 278, 523
Muscle dystrophy Duchenne 344
Muscular dystrophies 526
Muscular dystrophy Becker 344
Mutation 157, 200
Myasthenia gravis 525, 530
Myasthenic syndrome 530
Mycosis fungoides 277
Myelination 523
Myelitis 134
Myeloblastic crisis 203
Myeloid leukemia 201, 203
Myocardial infarction 286, 307, 576
Myocardial ischemia 576
Myoclonic epilepsy 361
Myoclonus 360
Myoclonus encephalopathy 524
Myogenesis 170
Myopathies of extraocular muscles 533
Myositis ossificans 178
Myotonia congenita 525
Myotonia Levior 527
Myotonias 526
Myotonic dystrophy 178

Nanism 536
Nanismus 405
Nasopharyngeal cancer 202
Natural killer cells 278, 467
Neimann-Pick disease 354
Nephrolithiasis 359
Nephropathy 255, 256, 257, 286, 306, 412
Nephrotic syndrome 570
Neural crest cells 168, 169
Neural muscle atrophies 525
Neural tube cells 166

Neural tube	164, 165, 169
Neuroblastoma	202, 278
Neurodegenerative diseases	520
Neuroepithelial cells	164
Neurofibroma	204
Neurofibromatosis	201, 204, 341, 525
Neurofibrosarcoma	204
Neuromyelitis optica	523
Neuronal ceroidlipofuscinoses	355
Neuropathy	260, 540
Neurotransmitters	300, 520
Neurotransplantation	11, 12, 509, 510, 532
Niemann-Pick disease	357
NK cells	292, 465, 467
Non-healing fractures	307, 539
Non-Hodgkin lymphomas	203
Non-spherocytic hemolytic anemia due to G6PD deficit	344
Non-surgical treatment of deep burns	590
Noonan syndrome	341, 370
Norepinehrine	300

Obesity	408
Occipital horn syndrome	536
Ochronosis	349
Ocular albinism, types I and II	345
Ocular herpes	277
Omen syndrome	472
Oncogene viruses	202
Oncogenes	200, 202, 203
Optic nerve atrophy	361
Optic nerve dysplasia	358
Organ specific antibodies	329
Organ transplantation	6
Organ xenotransplant	186, 206
Organ xenotransplantation	185
Organogenesis	136, 163
Organospecificity	14, 16, 24, 129, 140-143, 161, 163, 174, 193, 205, 206, 331
Organotropic	451
Organotropic effect of cell transplants	141
Organ-specific	142, 451, 483
Orniti-ntranscarbamylase deficiency	345
Osler-Weber-Rendu disease	505
Osteoarthrosis	539
Osteogenesis	170, 536
Osteogenic sarcoma	278
Osteomyelitis	307
Osteoporosis	351, 539

Osteosarcoma	202, 204
Osteosynhesis	212
Ovarian failure	307
Ovarian insufficiency	443
Oxidative phosphorylation (OXPHOS)	150, 153, 359, 360

Pancreatic islets	14, 186
Pancreatic stem cells	302
Pancreatic β-cells	145
Panmyelophthisis	346
Papillomatosis of larynx	278
Paramyotonia congenita	527
Parathyroid insufficiency	457
Parkinson's disease	11, 12, 134, 509, 511, 512, 515, 530
Parodontosis	546
Partial monosomy	372
Patau syndrome	369
Pathophysiologic diagnosis	267, 268
Pearson syndrome	362
Pelizaeus-Merzbacher disease	521, 523
Pemphigus vegetans	278
Peptic ulcer	547
Peripancreatic block	289, 300, 302, 418
Peripheral arterial disease	286, 306, 582
Peripheral myocytes	132
Periventricular malacia	377
Pernicious anemia	501
Peroxisomal enzymopathies	358
Perthes disease	355
Phacomatoses	201
Phenylketonuria	343, 348
Pheochromocytoma	575
Physiological menopause	443
Phytanic acid storage disease	359
Pigmentary degeneration of globus pallidus	530
Pituitary nanism	406
Placenta	294
Platelet disorder	505
Pluripotential embryonic cells	7
Pneumonia	355, 588
Polyarteritis	584
Polyarthritis	143
Polyneuropathy	255, 260, 286, 306, 412
Polyposes syndromes	201
Polyposis coli familiaris	201
Polyposis of colon	341

Index   629

Porenecephaly	379	Purpura simpex	505
Porphyria cutanea tarda	503		
Porphyrias	502		
Portal hypertension	551, 556	**Q**uality control of stem cell transplantation manufacturing	247
Post-menopausal women	144		
Post-natal damage	379		
Post-natal diagnosis	339		
Post-SCT infection	335	**R**abson-Mendelhall syndrome	417
Posttraumatic aphasia patients	11	Radiation enteritis	548
Prader-Willi syndrome	159, 438	Radiation injuries	507
Precursor cells	135, 167, 171, 305, 498	Radiation	493, 495
Precursor (or progenitor) stem cells	7	Raynaud disease	584
Pregnancy	488, 489	Recklinghausen disease	341
Pregnant diabetic	428	Recurrent aphthous stomatitis	278
Premature atherosclerosis	561	Recurrent otitis media	278
Premature menopause	443	Red spots on retinal macula	357
Prenatal damage	379	Refsum disease	359
Prenatal diagnosis	339	Rejuvenation	179, 388
Preparation of stem cell transplants	137	Rejuvenation therapies	391
Pre-xenotransplantation screening	93	Renal diabetes insipidus	408
Primary amenorrhea	143	Renal glucosuria	567
Primary cell culture	137	Renal hypertension	571, 575
Primary hemochromatosis	503	Renal insufficiency	498
Primary hyperaldosteronism	575	Renal phosphate diabetes	568
Primary hypertension	574	Reproduction	131
Primary hypertriacylglycerolemia	563	Respiratory infections, frequent	354
Primary porphyrias	502	Retarded puberty	438
Primary tissue culture	121, 137, 138	Retinal detachment	534
Principle of homology	14	Retinoblastoma	201, 202
Principle of organospecificity	14	Retinopathy	255, 256, 258, 306, 412
Procurement of stem cell transplants	121, 241	Retrobulbar implantation	428, 429
		Retrovirus infections	198
Progeria	177	Retroviruses	226, 279
Progesterone	296, 445, 455, 456	Revitalization effect	531
Progressive vaccinia	277	Revitalization	179, 388, 541
Proliferation	138	Revitalization therapies	391
Proliferative retinopathy	262, 263	Reye syndrome	360
Proportional nanism	406	Rheumatoid arthritis	539
Proteinuria	257, 261	Right heart insufficiency	556
Proteolytic activity	162	Riley-Day syndrome	343
Proteolytic enzyme	137, 150, 162, 199	RNA	278
Protooncogenes	202	RNA-genome	202
Protoporphyria	503	RNA-oncogene viruses	202
Pseudoachondroplasia	537	RNA-viruses	202, 227
Pseudo-Hurler syndrome	357	Rotor syndrome	556
Pseudoxanthoma elasticum	536	Russell-Silver syndrome	343
Psoriasis	278, 590		
Psychiatric disorders	351	**S**almonellosis	197
Pulmonary fibrosis	588	Sandhoff syndrome	358
Pulmonary infarct	588		

Sanfillipo syndrome	353
Sarcoid Darrier-Roussy	590
Sarcomas	202
Scheie syndrome	353
Schilder encephalitis periaxialis	523
Schoenlein-Henoch purpura	505
SCID	469, 471
Scleroderma	546, 590
Sclerosing Cholangitis	557
Secondary amenorrhea	281
Secondary hypertension	575
Seip syndrome	177
Seizures	351, 357, 360, 378, 381
Senile lungs	587
Serotonine	300
Sertoli's cells	300
Severe combined immunodeficiency	469, 471
Sex chromosomal disorders	383
Sex chromosome aberrations	370
Sex-chromosome mosaicism	364
Sheehan syndrome	407
Sickle cell anemia	342, 499, 502
Sideroblastic anemia	502
Single gene abnormalities	340
Single gene disorders	201, 351
Sipple syndrome	201
Sites of implantation	335
Site of implantation of stem cell transplants	144
Sjogren syndrome	484
Skeletal dysplasia	352
Skin abnormalities	352
Sly syndrome	353
Somatomedins	299
Somatostatin	293
Somatotropin	285, 405
Spastic hemiplegia	379
Sphingomyelinase	357
Spielmeyer-Vogt disease	524
Spina bifida	165, 379
Spinal cord injuries	516
Spinal muscle atrophies	526
Spino-cerebellar degenerations	524
Spino-neuro-muscular degenerations	525
Splenomegaly	355
Spondylarthroses	539
Spondylarthrosis treatment	540
Stem cell allo-transplants	7
Stem cell of human origin	7

Stem cell transplantation	3, 5, 9, 15, 23, 27, 127, 128, 132, 144
Stem cell transplants	165, 307
Stem cell xenotransplantation	13, 120, 182, 192, 327
Stickler syndrome	536
Stroke	261
Sturge-Weber syndrome	341
Subacute sclerosing panencephalitis	278
Subacute toxicity of SCT	124
Subaponeurotic implantation	315, 316, 335
Subaponeurotic sites	335
Subaponeurotic space	272
Subponeurotic sites	335
Sudanophilic leukodystrophies	523
Sudden infant death syndrome	360
Surveillance of xenotransplant recipient	325
Surveillance plans	84
Surveillance program for infectious agents	231
Syncytiotrophoblast	162, 295, 296, 492
Syndaktylia	134
Syndrome of Fanconi anemia	346
Syndrome of lazy leukocytes	468
Syndrome of naked lymphocytes	472
Syndrome of testicular feminization	345
Syndromes of defective DNA	345
Syndromes of spontaneous chromosomal instability	345
Syringomyelia	525

T cell
    189, 291, 188, 140, 182, 184, 188,
    276, 278, 279, 292, 405, 466-469, 471,
    481, 482, 490

T cell reactivity	188
T cell tolerance	191
T lymphocytes	140, 188
Tapeto-retinal degeneration	524
Tay-Sachs disease	342, 358, 524
T-cell activity	492
T-cell defficiency	277
T-cell leukemia	202
Testosterone	171, 436, 441, 443, 446, 448, 449, 454, 455, 456
Thalassemias	500, 502
Thomsen congenital myotonia	527

Thomsen myotonia	525	Unified Parkinson's Disease Rating Scale	515
Three germ layers	163		
Thrombangiitis obliterans	584	Universal stem cells	295
Thrombocytopenia	355	Unstable angina	576
Thrombocytopenic purpura	505	Usual aging	391
Thromboembolism	287	Uterine myomas	452
Thyroid gland insufficiency	143	Uveitis	278
Thyroid stimulating hormone	293, 446		
Thyrotropin-releasing hormone	296		
Timing of stem cell transplantation	147	**V**. Hippel-Lindau disease	525
Tissue allo-transplants	188	v. Recklinghausen's disease	525
Tissue immunogenicity	188	Vagal and sacral neural crest	169
Tissue transplantation	5	van Bogaert and Bertrand disease	523
Tissue xenotransplants	206	Varicosities of veins	271
Torsion dystonia	530	Various eczemas	590
Toxicological studies	124	Vasculitis	584
Transfer factor	278, 279	Venous thrombosis	351
Transfer of xenoses	129	Virgin lymphocyte	466
Transmissible spongiform encephalopathies	79	Vitality	179, 180, 388, 396
		Vitamin-D resistant rachitis	345
Transmission of infection	6	Vitiligo	590
Transmission of xenogeneic infections	327	Von Hippel-Lindau syndrome	201
Treatment procedure	313	von Recklinghausen disease	204
Trisomy 13	369	von Willebrand disease	505
Trisomy 18	369	von Willebrand Factor	505
Trisomy 21	365, 366		
Trisomy X	371		
Trophic disturbances	380	**W**aldens-trom's macroglobulinemia	278
Trophoblasts	5, 162, 296, 489, 492	Wallerian axonal degeneration	520
Trophoblastic cell Implantation	13	Warts	278
Trophoblastic cells	5, 12, 13, 162	Werdning-Hoffman	525, 526
Transfer factor	276	Werner's disease	177
Tuberculosis of bone	277	Whipple disease	548
Sarcoidosis	277	White matter of the brain	166, 520
Tuberculosis of lungs	277	Willi Prader syndrome	372
Tuberous sclerosis	201, 341, 525	Wilms tumor	204
Tumor growth	200	Wilson's disease	342, 343, 530
Tumor immunity	491	Wiscott-Aldrich syndrome	277, 473
Tumor suppressive genes	202	Wolf syndrome	372
Turner syndrome	178, 370	Wolfrath-Kugelberg-Welander	525
Two hits hypothesis	203	Wolman disease	355, 358
Type 1 diabetes mellitus	409, 416		
Type 2 diabetes mellitus	409		
		Xenogeneic class II MHC protein/antigen	189
Ulcerative colitis	548, 549	Xenogeneic infections	313, 325, 326
Ulcus cruris	590	Xenogeneic infectious agents	79
Umbilical cord blood stem cell transplantation	9	Xeno-neurotransplantation	510
		Xeno-organ	185

Xenoses 117, 195, 196, 197
Xenotransplantation 5, 7, 9, 10, 14, 67, 185, 186, 192, 195, 197
Xenotransplants 187, 188
Xeno-tropic 195
Xeno-zoonoses 195, 325
Xeroderma pigmentosum 201, 343, 346
X-linked dominant 345
X-linked mental retardations 344
X-linked proliferative syndrome 473
X-linked recessive 344
XR disorder 344, 472

Y-linked genetic disorders 345

Zellentherapie 10, 25, 26, 181, 359
Zellweger syndrome 359
Zollinger-Ellison syndrome 201
Zoonoses 79, 80, 196, 221

α_1-antitrypsin deficiency 588
α-cell 293, 301, 412, 413
α-motoneuron 526
α-thalassemias 500

β-cell 134, 140, 145, 146, 291, 274, 332, 409, 413, 414, 415, 417, 428
β-oxidation pathway 153, 154
β-thalassemias 500